Seminars in Forensic Psychiatry

College Seminars Series

For details of available and forthcoming books in the College Seminars Series please visit: www.cambridge.org/series/college-seminars-series.

Seminars in Forensic Psychiatry

Second Edition

Edited by
Mary Davoren
Trinity College Dublin
Harry Kennedy
Trinity College Dublin

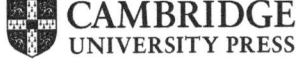

CAMBRIDGE
UNIVERSITY PRESS

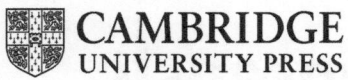

CAMBRIDGE
UNIVERSITY PRESS

Shaftesbury Road, Cambridge CB2 8EA, United Kingdom

One Liberty Plaza, 20th Floor, New York, NY 10006, USA

477 Williamstown Road, Port Melbourne, VIC 3207, Australia

314–321, 3rd Floor, Plot 3, Splendor Forum, Jasola District Centre,
New Delhi – 110025, India

103 Penang Road, #05–06/07, Visioncrest Commercial, Singapore 238467

Cambridge University Press is part of Cambridge University Press & Assessment,
a department of the University of Cambridge.

We share the University's mission to contribute to society through the pursuit of
education, learning and research at the highest international levels of excellence.

www.cambridge.org
Information on this title: www.cambridge.org/9781911623816

DOI: 10.1017/9781911623809

First published 1995
Second edition 2024

A catalogue record for this publication is available from the British Library

A Cataloging-in-Publication data record for this book is available from the Library of Congress

ISBN 978-1-911-62381-6 Paperback

....

Every effort has been made in preparing this book to provide accurate and up-to-date information that
is in accord with accepted standards and practice at the time of publication. Although case histories are
drawn from actual cases, every effort has been made to disguise the identities of the individuals involved.
Nevertheless, the authors, editors, and publishers can make no warranties that the information
contained herein is totally free from error, not least because clinical standards are constantly changing
through research and regulation. The authors, editors, and publishers therefore disclaim all liability for
direct or consequential damages resulting from the use of material contained in this book. Readers are
strongly advised to pay careful attention to information provided by the manufacturer of any drugs or
equipment that they plan to use.

Contents

Contributors

Gwen Adshead
Consultant Forensic Psychiatrist and
Psychotherapist, Personality Disorder
Directorate, Paddock Building, Broadmoor
Hospital, Crowthorne, England, UK and
West London NHS Trust, London,
England, UK.

Saima Ali
Senior Registrar in Forensic Psychiatry,
West London NHS Trust, London,
England, UK.

Ai-Li W. Arias
Assistant Clinical Professor of Psychiatry,
Department of Psychiatry, University of
California–Irvine and University of
California–Riverside, USA.

Harm Boer
Consultant Forensic Psychiatrist and
Clinical Lead, Learning Disabilities and
Autism West Midlands Partnership
Alliance, Kings Norton, England, UK.

Penelope Brown
Clinical Research Fellow, Institute of
Psychiatry, Psychology and Neuroscience,
King's College London, London, England,
UK; South London and Maudsley NHS
Foundation Trust, London, England, UK;
West London Mental Health Trust,
London, England, UK.

James Cavney
Deputy Clinical Director, Auckland
Regional Forensic Psychiatry Services,
Auckland, Aotearoa, New Zealand.

Jeremy W. Coid
Professor of Epidemiology in Psychiatry,
West China Brain Research Centre, West
China Hospital, Sichuan University,
Chengdu, Sichuan, China; Visiting
Professor to Institute of Psychiatry,
Psychology and Neuroscience, King's
College London, London, England, UK;
Emeritus Professor of Forensic Psychiatry,
Queen Mary University of London,
London, England, UK.

**Ian Cumming, Consultant Forensic
Psychiatrist**
HMP Belmarsh and South London and
Maudsley NHS Foundation Trust, London,
England, UK.

Michael A. Cummings
Clinical Professor of Psychiatry and
Associate Clinical Professor of Psychiatry,
Department of Psychiatry, University of
California–Irvine and University of
California–Riverside, USA.

**Mary Davoren, Consultant Forensic
Psychiatrist**
Central Mental Hospital, Dublin, Ireland;
Clinical Senior Lecturer in Forensic
Psychiatry, Trinity College Dublin, Ireland;
Visiting Professor of Forensic Psychiatry,
University of Bari 'Aldo Moro', Bari, Italy.

Enys Delmage
Consultant in Adolescent Forensic
Psychiatry, Inpatient Forensic Child and
Adolescent Mental Health Services,
Porirua, New Zealand.

Frank Farnham
Consultant Forensic Psychiatrist, North
London Forensic Service, Barnet, Enfield
and Haringey Mental Health Trust, London,
England, UK; Honorary Associate Professor
of Security and Crime Science, University
College London, London, England, UK.

Paul Gill
Department of Security and Crime Science, University College London, London, England, UK.

Heidi Hales
Consultant in Adolescent Forensic Psychiatry, Llandudno Child and Adolescent Mental Health Services, Betsi Cadwaladr University Health Board, Bangor, Wales, UK.

Harry Kennedy
Professor of Forensic Psychiatry, Trinity College Dublin, Ireland; Honorary Skou Professor of Forensic Psychiatry, Aarhus University, Aarhus, Denmark; Visiting Professor of Forensic Psychiatry, University of Bari 'Aldo Moro', Bari, Italy.

Richard Latham
South London and Maudsley NHS Foundation Trust, London, England, UK.

John Marshall
Head of Psychological Services and Consultant Clinical and Forensic Psychologist, The State Hospital, Carstairs, Scotland, UK.

Brian McKenna
Professor of Forensic Mental Health, Auckland University of Technology, Auckland, New Zealand; Associate Clinical Director for Improvement, Auckland Regional Forensic Psychiatry Services, Auckland, Aotearoa, New Zealand; Adjunct Professor, Centre for Forensic Behavioural Science, Swinburne University of Technology, Victoria, Australia.

Damian J. Mohan
Associate Professor of Forensic Psychiatry Trinity College Dublin and Consultant Forensic Psychiatrist, National Forensic Mental Health Service, Dublin, Ireland.

Raj Mohan
Consultant Forensic Psychiatrist, South London and Maudsley NHS Foundation Trust, London, England, UK.

Paul E. Mullen
Emeritus Professor of Forensic Psychiatry, Monash University, Melbourne, Victoria, Australia; Visiting Professor to the Institute of Psychiatry, Psychology and Neuroscience, King's College London, London, England, UK.

Kevin Murray
Honorary Consultant Forensic Psychiatrist, Broadmoor Hospital, Crowthorne, England, UK; West London NHS Trust, London, England, UK; Member, Parole Board, London, England, UK.

Sajida Nabi
Consultant Forensic Psychiatrist and Associate Clinical Director, Broadmoor Hospital, Crowthorne, England, UK; Lead for the National High Secure Consultants Forum, London, England, UK.

Krishna Pillai
Clinical Director and Consultant Forensic Psychiatrist, The Mason Clinic, Auckland, New Zealand.

George J. Proctor
Associate Clinical Professor of Psychiatry, Department of Psychiatry, Loma Linda University, Loma Linda, USA.

Shubulade Smith
Consultant Psychiatrist, South London and Maudsley NHS Foundation Trust, London, England, UK; Visiting Senior Lecturer, Institute of Psychiatry, Psychology, Neuroscience, King's College London, London, England, UK.

Stephen M. Stahl
Professor of Psychiatry, Department of Psychiatry, University of California–San Diego, USA; Professor of Psychiatry, Department of Psychiatry, University of Cambridge, Cambridge, England, UK.

Carolyn Stanley
Consultant Forensic Psychiatrist and
Clinical Director, North London Forensic
Services, Barnet, Enfield and Haringey
Mental Health NHS Trust, London,
England, UK.

Danny H. Sullivan
Executive Director of Clinical Services,
Forensicare, Victoria, Australia; Honorary
Senior Fellow, University of Melbourne
(Department of Psychiatry and Justice
Health Unit, Melbourne School of
Population and Global Health), Melbourne,
Australia; Adjunct Research Fellow, Centre
for Forensic Behavioural Sciences,
Swinburne University, Melbourne,
Australia.

Pamela J. Taylor
Professor of Forensic Psychiatry, Cardiff
University, Wales, UK.

Alexis Theodorou
Specialist Trainee in Forensic Psychiatry
and Medical Psychotherapy, West London
NHS Trust, London, England, UK.

Lindsay Thomson
Professor of Forensic Psychiatry,
University of Edinburgh, Edinburgh,
Scotland, UK; Medical Director of the State
Hospitals Board for Scotland and the

Forensic Mental Health Managed Care
Network, Scotland, UK.

Peter Turner
Safety Without Compromise Expert
Group – Retired Violence Reduction Nurse
Specialist and Lead for Professional
Management of Violence and Aggression
Team, Broadmoor Hospital, Crowthorne,
England, UK.

Vivienne de Vogel
Professor, Forensic Mental Health Care at
the Faculty of Psychology and
Neuroscience, Maastricht University,
Maastricht, the Netherlands; Professor at
the University of Applied Sciences Utrecht,
Centre for Social Innovation, Utrecht, the
Netherlands; Researcher De Forensische
Zorgspecialisten, Utrecht, the Netherlands.

Katherine Warburton
Statewide Medical Director, California
Department of State Hospitals, Sacramento,
USA; Associate Clinical Professor,
University of California–Davis, USA.

Treena Wilkie
Forensic Psychiatrist; Chief, Forensic
Service, Complex Care and Recovery
Program, Centre for Addiction and Mental
Health; and Associate Professor, University
of Toronto, Toronto, Canada.

Foreword

It is a pleasure to welcome this second edition of *Seminars in Forensic Psychiatry* in the College Seminars Series. We have no doubt readers will find it has been well worth the wait. The book is more than a simple update. Rather, it has successfully sought to include discussion of those developments that continue to shape the evolving practice of forensic psychiatry.

In the last 25 years forensic psychiatry has been required to adjust to a variety of changes and challenges. In particular, we have seen increased public and political concern with the safe management of offender patients in the community; rising rates of mental illness, particularly in prisons that are frequently overcrowded; disquiet about the standards of care in some in-patient settings; a much-expanded role for independent and third-sector service providers; increased accountability to, and a more intrusive role for, statutory agencies; and increasing expectations of service provision from the police, courts, prisons and from our psychiatric colleagues in general adult, adolescent, older-age and intellectual disability services. Some of these are contentious issues but readers will find that this book does not side-step them.

Clinical practice in forensic psychiatry must be underpinned by a sound theoretical and evidence-based approach. Advances that have been made in the reliability of risk assessment, in the vexed issue of the relationship between mental illness and violence, and difficult contemporary issues regarding culture, terrorism and medical negligence are fully examined. The book is intended for practitioners and so, along with discussion of relevant law and its application, the reader will find valuable advice and guidance on professional practice issues such as consultant responsibility and leadership.

Harry Kennedy, Mary Davoren and their contributors have put together a highly informative book. We hope it will become the go-to book for a new generation of trainees and consultants in forensic psychiatry, for other professionals involved in the care and treatment of offender patients and for those practitioners who wish to keep abreast of what is a rapidly changing clinical specialty.

Derek Chiswick
Rosemarie Cope
Editors of the First Edition

Introduction

Mary Davoren and Harry Kennedy

It is a privilege to edit a textbook in the subject to which we devote our professional lives. We were both influenced by Derek Chiswick and Rosemary Cope's text that set out a list of essential topics. Part of the reward for the work of renewing this textbook has been to nudge new topics into the canon of forensic psychiatry.

Forensic psychiatry is the interface between psychiatry and the law. It is a complex and challenging discipline encompassing clinical care and treatment for a highly vulnerable patient group with some of the most complex presentations in psychiatry, legal knowledge and ability, as well as leadership and academic expertise. The forensic psychiatrist must be the experts' expert, a shrewd clinician with serious attention to detail. It is not for the faint-hearted. We hope this book will inspire the brightest and the best to undertake training in this discipline.

Forensic psychiatry is often thought of only in terms of violence risk, and clearly the assessment and management of violence is key to this discipline. 'Risk' is the name of a popular board game in which war and diplomacy are pitched against each other by rolling the dice. Clinical ability in the area of risk assessment is often seen as the defining skill and characteristic of the very best forensic psychiatrists, though actually the best forensic psychiatrists must excel in multiple areas. Forensic psychiatry can also be understood as an uneven distribution of risk in which professional expertise and practice generate means of either regulated redistribution of risk or unregulated accumulation. The risk of violence arising from mental illness, substance misuse and delinquency can only be partly quantified and even more imperfectly regulated. Unregulated, relapses and interactions in these three domains lead to disorder, damage and occasionally death. The risk accumulates non-randomly among the vulnerable – those with mental illnesses, substance misuse issues and personality disorders. The victims are also seldom random: parents, spouses and friends, others with the same vulnerabilities, and sometimes professionals. Most patients in forensic hospital settings are both victims and perpetrators of violence – when the consultant forensic psychiatrist can see only the victim or only the perpetrator, they are unlikely to succeed. A nuanced understanding of both sides is required for excellence in this complex area.

Forensic psychiatry services provide care and treatment to mentally disordered offenders for whom violence linked to mental disorder is also an unmet treatment need. The purpose of these services is to reduce both the probability of violence and the serious-ness of violence if it occurs. This is accomplished first through a process of redistribution of risk – placing the high-risk patient in the most therapeutically safe and secure setting, while those who are at a lesser risk, or a less serious risk, can be placed in or moved to medium or lower levels of therapeutic security. Restrictive practices such as seclusion, restraint and forced medication may be medically necessary to prevent imminent violence while treatments, both pharmacological and psychological, are implemented and take gradual effect. Reducing and eliminating the cycle of violence and providing a safe space for therapeutic engagement and the challenge inherent in good therapy are vital.

There are competing models for how such risks should be managed or regulated. A libertarian approach would hold the mentally disordered to be strictly liable for their acts and would use compulsion under almost no circumstances. Like any unregulated economy, great inequalities in the distribution of risk follow, with prisons becoming the main centres for coping with severe mental illnesses, comorbidities and disadvantages. A bygone era of moral regulation confined the mentally disordered away from civil society in asylums and 'colonies'. A more recent era of risk consciousness and risk aversion also confines but more selectively and with greater attention to selective triage, risk stratification and legally regulated recovery pathways. Modern specialist forensic psychiatry services should provide culturally sensitive services, women's services and specialist services for uniquely vulnerable groups such as children and adolescents and those with intellectual disability.

This second edition of *Seminars in Forensic Psychiatry* aims to find clinical relevance across services and across jurisdictions insofar as this is possible, since we believe that this will reflect the needs of a forensic psychiatry readership. We are confident that this will also benefit forensic psychiatry patients.

Chapters commence with two approaches to the psychiatry of violence in mental disorder (Chapters 1 and 2). Next (Chapter 3) is a chapter on the history of how modern forensic psychiatry services have evolved in Britain, through inquiries and reports that shaped policy. A chapter on psychiatry in prisons follows (Chapter 4). A review of legal issues (Chapter 5) may represent a watershed between psychiatry in the courts and legislation as a gateway or pathway into treatment. A later chapter also addresses questions of medical negligence (Chapter 16). Chapters then deal with structured professional judgement and risk as ways of understanding expertise in forensic psychiatry (Chapter 6); models of care in forensic psychiatry (Chapter 7); the pharmacology of aggression and violence (Chapter 8); the clinical management of in-patient violence (Chapter 9); and community forensic psychiatry (Chapter 10). There are then four chapters covering special subjects such as personality disorder, stalking, sex offenders and terrorism (Chapters 11, 12, 13 and 14, respectively), followed by chapters on psychotherapies and psychological treatments (Chapter 15); forensic child and adolescent psychiatry (Chapter 17); forensic psychiatry and women (Chapter 18); intellectual disability (Chapter 19); cultural psychiatry (Chapter 20); ethnic inequality (Chapter 21); and academic forensic psychiatry (Chapter 22). The book concludes with some no-nonsense guides (Chapter 23) that we hope will be useful prompts and supports as readers set out on their forensic careers.

Forensic psychiatry is much more than medico-legal psychiatry. Dr Katherine Warburton says we must be advocates and educators, as well as treatment providers. An essential aspect of being a consultant forensic psychiatrist is working to attract the very best psychiatry trainees into our discipline; this is what is required to reach the top of this challenging field, and it is what our patients, with their very high levels of vulnerability and complexity, deserve.

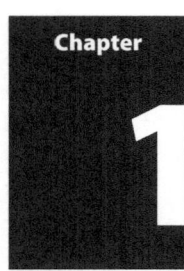

Violence and Mental Disorder
The Evidence

Jeremy W. Coid

The assessment of violent behaviour and its association with mental disorder is at the core of clinical practice in forensic psychiatry. It is the main clinical skill that a forensic psychiatrist needs to develop. This chapter will concentrate on the evidence for the association between psychotic illness and violence. Most persons referred for assessment of violence to a forensic psychiatrist in the UK present with psychotic illness, mainly schizophrenia, and to a lesser extent personality disorders and sexual deviation. However, this does not reflect violence in the UK general population but a system of referral and gatekeeping of patients and clients assessed in what is a relatively small tertiary care service. Although forensic psychiatrists should be experts in the assessment of violence among people with mental disorder, it is essential to develop expertise with those who have no evidence of mental disorder. Paradoxically, these cases are often the most challenging to understand and evaluate.

Training in UK forensic psychiatry is based primarily on an 'apprenticeship' model and does not require passing additional examinations after becoming a specialist in psychiatry. This means that it is essential to obtain further specialist training in assessment techniques and to have some understanding of criminology. It is also important to have as much experience as possible of the different healthcare and prison facilities for violent individuals and at different levels of security. For many psychiatrists, Broadmoor, Ashworth and Rampton high-secure hospitals represent the most severe level of risk for violence, but in fact there are a group of individuals contained in special prison units who represent an ongoing level of risk for violence that cannot be contained within a high-secure hospital, some with severe mental illness.

Assessment of violence will sometimes require courage and the ability to monitor one's personal safety based on observation, experience and training. It also requires an ability to remain objective and detached from the personal feelings that can interfere with giving a sound and helpful opinion. With experience, one's own personal response to a potentially violent individual can be highly important in an assessment. What is it that makes one uncomfortable around or even afraid of the patient? Why is it that the patient appears to have a good relationship with one member of the clinical team but no-one else? This means learning to be aware of and overcoming the strongly negative feelings held by most persons when encountering violence and violent individuals. It helps if a forensic psychiatrist has a natural interest in violence. If not, it will be necessary to develop one.

This chapter is intended for trainees in forensic psychiatry but may be of help to more experienced practitioners because it is based on personal clinical experience, as well as involvement in research into violence. The aims are, first, to help trainees refine forensic assessments of offender patients so they can give advice to courts in determining an offender's legal responsibility for a criminal act. Second, the chapter aims to help increase understanding of the motivation for violent offending and the pathways to violence. This is not only necessary for giving expert evidence in courts but is also essential in choosing the treatment that should be offered to a patient and the level of security required in which to deliver treatment, and in some cases it may be relevant to the likelihood of a successful response to the treatment. Third, the chapter shows that associations between criminal behaviour and mental disorder may be highly important in the assessment of risk for future reoffending, although this chapter does not deal with risk assessment as currently operationalised in many North American and European forensic services. Finally, and most importantly, the chapter emphasises that a good forensic assessment should concentrate on the future management and prevention of further violence.

Evaluating Research, Risk Assessment and Considering Causation

This chapter covers a wide-ranging area of research and clinical observation and should be considered as an overview. When considering research, it is important to evaluate the current literature on mental disorder and violence, what it means for the practice of forensic psychiatry and why some is highly limited and even unhelpful. The chapter also aims to give some indication of future directions for research into violence for forensic psychiatrists.

This chapter will not consider risk assessment for violence, which is covered in Chapter 6 and by means of specific training. However, the assessment of violence for planning a treatment intervention or giving evidence to court should not be confused with an assessment of future risk for violence. For example, many current research limitations derive from an overemphasis on research methods used to develop instruments which aim to predict violence. Some disciplines have even come to confuse assessment of violence with assessment of risk. There is no reason not to carry out both forms of assessment. From the perspective of the assessment of violence, a numerical score of future risk can be helpful in a limited sense by categorising individuals based on their previous behaviour and demography. However, these predictions stand a good chance of being wrong in the narrow sense of estimating future likelihood of violence.

There is no current high-grade research evidence which demonstrates that a structured clinical risk assessment instrument or an actuarial risk instrument can prevent an act of violence following discharge from hospital or release from prison. The only randomised controlled trial to date which tested a structured professional judgement instrument against management as usual failed to show a significant reduction in violence following hospital discharge [1]. There are two randomised controlled trials which demonstrate a significantly reduced count of violent acts among patients in hospital who were assessed for short-term risk by nurses [2, 3]. However, closer examination reveals these risk assessments were tied to the requirement by clinical teams in the intervention arm of these studies to select, then carry out, active interventions based on a score of risk.

These findings indicate that it was very likely that the clinical preventative intervention was the active and effective component resulting in reduction of violence and not the risk assessment. Clinical experience with violent patients soon reveals a range of different chance events and circumstances that can interfere with one's predictions of future behaviour. The most important clinical use of risk assessments should therefore be to determine the necessary treatment and management options to prevent future violence rather than categorising patients according to risk scores, or speculative notions of future risk based on a training session in structured clinical judgement. No risk instrument can consider all possibilities and the increasing proliferation of these instruments for different forms of violence emphasises these clinical limitations. No new statistical development or advance in machine learning can substitute for professional experience. However, they can help as an important aide-memoire and ensure that key areas are not forgotten in an assessment.

Multiple limitations of violence research are shown when attaching too much importance at the individual level to results from surveys and, most importantly, to case register studies – no matter how large the sample size and despite claims the sample represents the entire population of a country. It is important to question whether the published research has any bearing on forensic clinical practice. The forensic psychiatrist should have multiple sources of information before conducting an assessment, and experience soon shows that most epidemiological studies are remarkably short of the key variables that determine violence. These studies are important in suggesting avenues for future research and creating new hypotheses. However, interpretations such as violence being substantially determined by genetic factors, while a possibility, cannot be relied upon in studies that use data that was never intended for the purpose of genetic study and that depend entirely on sparse data on siblings and criminal records to determine genetic association.

Forensic psychiatrists should have a healthy scepticism of studies where the statistics are so dense and complex that they are incomprehensible to the average clinician. There have been a series of studies of violence using the Scandinavian case registers where patients – sometimes all patients in a country captured by the register with a psychiatric diagnosis who have had contact with hospital and out-patient/community services – are linked with police records. Apart from the fact that neither register was designed for the study of either complex criminal acts or mental illness and that both are merely administrative registers to record the performance of services, criminal records are a poor indication of violence in a population and convictions and arrest records represent the last stage along the criminal pathway in which mentally ill persons are disadvantaged at each stage. Most Western countries now rely on self-report surveys of victims of crime to get a picture of crime trends and do not rely on official police statistics alone. But more importantly, the presence of a categorical diagnosis in a register does not mean that symptoms of mental illness or intoxication from drugs or alcohol were actually present at the time the violence occurred.

This key data is simply not available in the Scandinavian case registers. Closer examination shows that this is an unsubstantiated assumption on which to base conclusions such as that depression causes violence, drugs and alcohol cause violence among persons with schizophrenia (but not their schizophrenic illness), a substantial proportion of all violence in a population is genetically determined and so on. If the data does not include the social circumstances and other potential social determinants of violence and whether symptoms of mental illness were present at the material time, together with observational effects of those symptoms on the violence, it cannot be determined whether any of these factors had any impact or whether unknown confounders not included in the register were the key drivers.

Epidemiology of Violence

Violence, according to the World Health Organization [4], is 'the intentional use of physical force or power, threatened or actual, against oneself, another person, or against a group or community that either results in or has a high likelihood of resulting in injury, death, psychological harm, maldevelopment, or deprivation'. Although violence is a criminal behaviour, before it is formally deemed a crime the violence must have been observed and reported to the police, the individual must be arrested, a decision must be made to prosecute, and the offender must appear at trial in court before a final conviction. The verdict may be 'not guilty'. It is therefore important to remember that the overwhelming proportion of violence in all countries is not reported to or detected by any official agency. Criminologists refer to the 'dark figure' of crime: that which is not reported in official criminal statistics, which only represent the 'tip of the iceberg' of actual crime in a population. This means that when evaluating epidemiological research evidence, it is essential to be fully aware of the limitations of the measures of violence in the research study.

Psychiatric studies of violence are bedevilled by poor measures of violence. If a study relies entirely on criminal convictions, this means the majority of violent events in the population have been missed and cannot be included in the study. It is estimated that 95% or more of all violent events will not be reported to the police. Although it is argued that if more serious crimes such as homicide are studied, then more violence will be included, it still has to be remembered that even in Western countries with resources to conduct careful investigations, a proportion of offenders will never be arrested or convicted. In countries with exceptionally high homicide rates, such as in Central and South America, nearly half of offenders may never be arrested. Most importantly, persons with mental illness are more likely to be detected, arrested and convicted than other offenders. Furthermore, for those who are violent in hospital, the violence may not be reported to the police unless serious injuries occur. In the UK, however, this is changing as staff become less able to respond to and less willing to accept violence from patients, particularly in community-based services.

Homicide and Mental Disorder

It is important to place violence in the UK in an international context. The most extensive information for comparison purposes is recorded for homicide. Rates vary greatly between world regions [5]. Homicide is considered the best comparator for international purposes because it is seen as the most serious violent offence and more time, effort and financial expenditure is invested in its investigation. However, not all deaths are accurately identified as homicides or the perpetrators identified. Overall, less than 1% of all global deaths are due to homicide, but in some countries this is as high as 10% and a leading cause of death. Rates are highest in Central and South America and South Africa and lowest in certain East Asian countries and western Europe (see Figure 1.1).

Figure 1.2 shows the number of deaths internationally by cause for all ages. Homicides are not the leading cause of death. However, if the histogram includes younger persons aged 15–49 years, it rises to the ninth most common cause. If the data is applied to Venezuela in 2017, homicide was the third, in Honduras the fifth and in Guatemala the sixth most common cause of death. Looking at younger adults aged 15–49 years in Latin American countries, homicide is the highest-rated cause of death.

Homicide rates appear to have fallen in all regions over the last quarter century. But because the global homicide rate is calculated as a proportion of the population, it has declined only because the global population has risen. The overall number of people killed worldwide in homicides actually increased from 1990 to 2017. During this same period, homicides due to criminal activity caused as many deaths as armed conflicts and terrorism combined. Women and girls account for a far smaller share of victims of homicide in general than men. The majority of all homicides involve young men, both as perpetrators

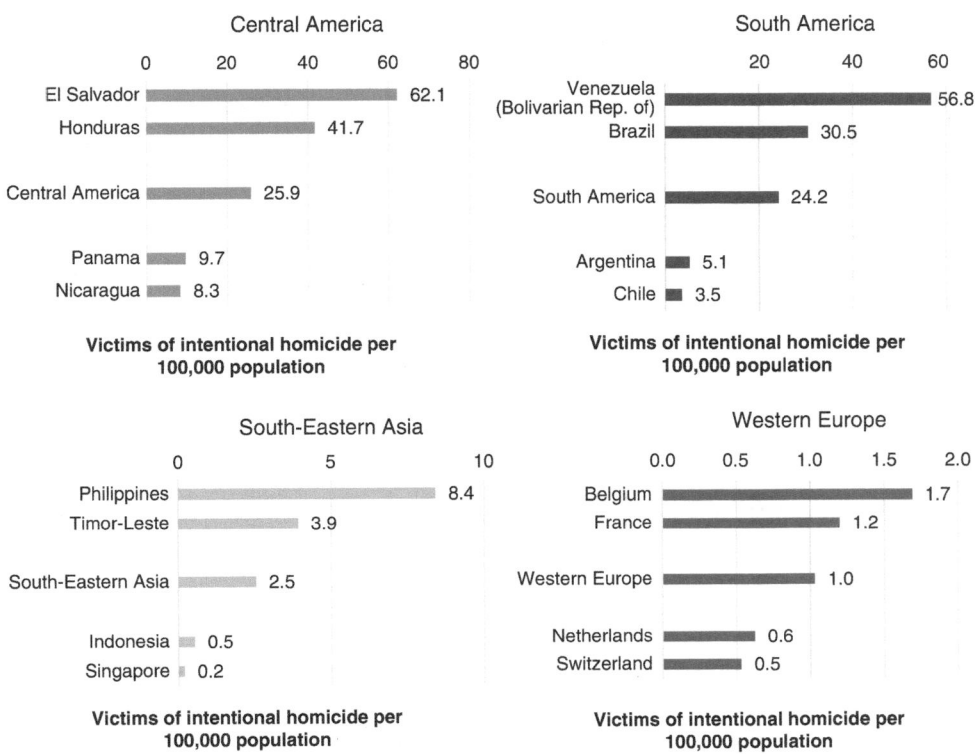

Figure 1.1 Countries with the highest and lowest homicide rates in selected subregions, 2017. United Nations Office on Drugs and Crime homicide statistics. From *Global Study on Homicide* by the United Nations Office on Drugs and Crime. © (2019) United Nations. Reprinted with permission of the United Nations.

and victims. However, women bear by far the greatest burden of family-related and intimate partner homicide as victims.

Rises and falls in homicide rates in most countries are largely explained by changes in rates among young adult males with no mental illness. Pinker has argued that there has been a dramatic fall in homicide since the Middle Ages, measured largely in Europe and more recently North America, and that humans are becoming less violent and more altruistic [6]. However, not all academics agree in that violence changes in its form and fluctuates over time. For forensic psychiatrists, a key issue is whether violence has fluctuated over time among the severely mentally ill. However, there is little evidence to indicate change over time using homicide statistics, which may be the best data available but are dependent on processing through the criminal justice system; also, different jurisdictions differ in how they deal with mentally disordered offenders. If this data can be relied upon in England and Wales, homicide rates for the mentally ill appear to have remained the same, while those for other offenders have changed over time [7].

To understand violence in a single country, it is necessary to observe fluctuations in rates rather than relying on cross-sectional surveys and case register studies, which take measures over short time periods – although these often represent the only detailed data available. Changes in exposure to risk factors affecting this subgroup of the population include the

Causes of death, World, 2019

The estimated annual number of deaths from each cause. Estimates come with wide uncertainties, especially for countries with poor vital registration[1].

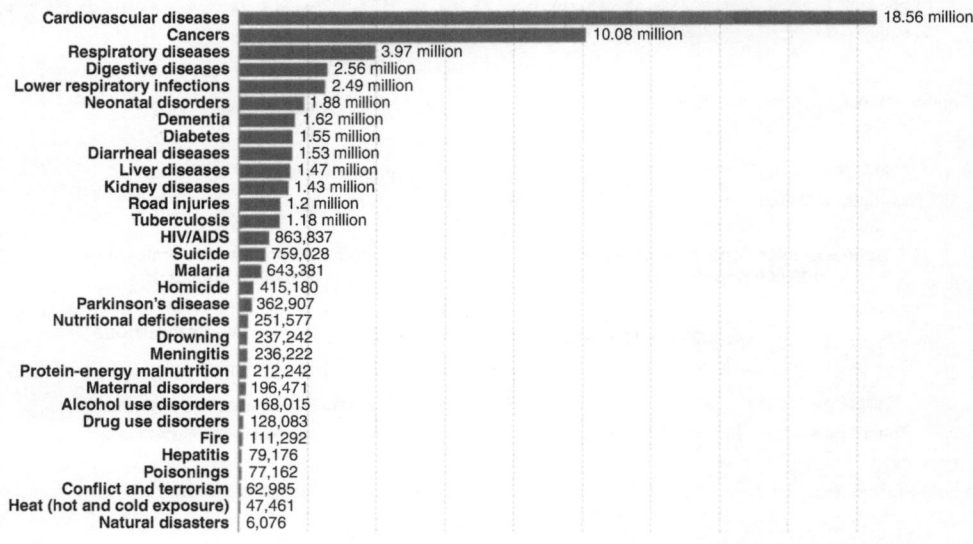

1.**Civil and Vital Registration System:** A Civil and Vital Registration System (CVRS) is an administrative system in a country that manages information on births, marriages, deaths and divorces. It generates and stores 'vital records' and legal documents such as birth certificates and death certificates. You can read more about how deaths are registered around the world in our article: How are causes of death registered around the world?

Figure 1.2 Causes of death. Source: Institute for Health Metrics and Evaluation, *Global Burden of Diseases* (2019) (https://ourworldindata.org/causes-of-death, https://ourworldindata.org/grapher/share-of-deaths-from-major-caus es?time=1990).

availability of firearms, gang involvement, changing involvement in criminal activity (particularly drug trafficking and sales) and the consumption of alcohol. The impact of these social and environmental factors means that the public health problem of violence has to be considered. Forensic psychiatrists should be aware of local, population-based factors in their catchment-area populations and when giving opinions on cases in other jurisdictions. Changes in homicide rates involving women rarely make an impact on fluctuations or changes in national homicide rates. For example, the homicide rate for Scotland became the highest in western Europe by the 1990s, but then fluctuated. Further rises and subsequent falls in homicide rates in Scotland between 2000 and 2014 were entirely accounted for by men. Meanwhile, women showed a small, progressive *decline* over the same period.

There is also no current evidence that *changing* rates of homicides are explained by persons with mental illness. Although it may make complete sense to a forensic psychiatrist that the closure of the mental hospitals and shift of patients into the community should have led to an increase of recorded violence by mentally ill persons, this has not been convincingly established and study findings remain controversial. In 1939, English mathematician, geneticist and psychiatrist Lionel Penrose hypothesised that the numbers of psychiatric hospital beds and sizes of prison populations were inversely related. The hypothesis fell out of favour in the 1980s, by which time bed closures had become a more accepted aspect of ongoing changes in psychiatric provision in most of Europe and North America. The hypothesis was revived by the work of Mundt and colleagues more recently in South America, showing that the prison populations in 17 Latin American countries had substantially increased and that they had increased more where more psychiatric beds were removed [8]. These findings held up when introducing per-capita income and income inequality as co-variates. However, it remains unclear and controversial whether serious violence by persons with severe mental illness has increased as a result of bed closures.

An earlier study in England and Wales [9] observed the overall rise in homicide rates in England and Wales but demonstrated that court adjudications, resulting in successful diminished responsibility and insanity defences, had remained remarkably stable over a 30-year period, during which the overall rises had occurred. Subsequently, it was claimed there had been a rise and then a fall in homicides attributed to mental disorder over a 50-year period, the fall coinciding with a fall in the overall homicide rate [10]. However, these observations were dependent on small numbers of cases each year and, most importantly, processing through the criminal justice system to identify the mental disorder. The change was more likely due to a change in the willingness of psychiatrists giving evidence in courts to recommend defendants for a defence of diminished responsibility and offer a hospital bed, particularly for those with personality disorder, rather than a true rise and fall in homicides involving mental disorder. It is worth reflecting that in Western countries, particularly in Europe, where there are few homicides, a larger proportion (but not rate) with mental disorder will make it appear that there is a large problem of violence by the mentally ill. In countries with very high rates of homicide, homicides by the mentally ill may appear to be negligible. Paradoxically, stigmas involving the mentally ill are often similar in both locations.

A key unresolved question is whether rates of homicide by mentally ill persons are the same or differ between different countries. An early study showed that they were apparently very similar, but this was based on countries with low overall homicide rates [7]. A later study criticised this argument and suggested that if countries with higher overall rates were included, then the rate among the mentally ill would correspond to the overall rate [11]. This would imply that in countries with high overall rates, with specific risk factors influencing these high rates such as firearm availability, persons with mental illness would be proportionately influenced by these same risk factors – in the same way that persons without illness are affected. In a country such as the USA, with ready availability of firearms, rates should therefore be higher for persons with severe mental illness than in the UK. However, this possibility ultimately remains unresolved due to a lack of data from countries with high homicide rates. Countries with the highest homicide rates tend to have low clear-up rates or do not routinely screen for mental disorder. In countries with multiple unsolved murders, drug cartels and readily available firearms, mental illness is simply not considered a likely or relevant factor in the overwhelming majority of cases. This is an important consideration in countries with low homicide rates. If media attention and public opinion does not keep these issues in perspective, concern can arise that homicide by the mentally ill is a major problem when it is in fact exceptionally uncommon. It is therefore essential not to confuse percentages of the total number of homicides with age-standardised population rates.

A key epidemiological finding with regard to psychotic illness and homicide is that, for schizophrenia, it is the prodrome and during a first episode of psychosis (often the period of greatest symptomatic disturbance over the lifespan) that is most strongly associated with homicide – a relatively short timespan over the entire life course. In a meta-analysis, approximately 30% of homicides in a range of countries were found to have occurred prior to ever receiving treatment. The risk during this period was 12 times that during the rest of the lifespan following a diagnosis of schizophrenia [11]. As the first episode of psychosis is relatively short compared to the total duration of the illness, the risk of homicide during a first episode is therefore considerably greater than the annual risk among individuals with treated psychosis. This confirms that a first episode is a medical emergency and suggests that reducing the duration of untreated psychosis might save lives. However, because many individuals committing homicide during a first episode will not be known to mental health services, this may be difficult to achieve. Furthermore, the illness may only be identified as a result of the homicidal behaviour.

In a national nested case–control study of previously admitted male patients diagnosed with schizophrenia in England and Wales, those who were convicted of homicide were statistically more likely to be non-adherent to their treatment plan; had lost contact with services prior to the offence; had a history of violent criminality, comorbid personality disorder or drug use disorder; had been admitted to hospital multiple times; and belonged to a black and minority ethnic group. Homicide perpetrators were less likely to have had recent routine contact with services and to have been recently discharged from hospital [12]. It was subsequently argued that these findings showed that much of the risk of serious violence in schizophrenia is related to comorbidity with alcohol or drug misuse, corresponding to previous research, with similar conclusions to the national Scandinavian case registers study and a related meta-analysis [13, 14]. However, none of these studies had information on whether psychotic offenders were actually intoxicated or had even taken any drugs or alcohol at the time of the violence to confirm this assumption and rates for schizophrenia in England and Wales were not standardised to be able to tell if there had really been a trend over time. They did, however, show that 90% of homicide offenders with schizophrenia had psychotic symptoms at the time of the killing, meaning that intoxicated or not, psychotic symptoms may have driven the homicide in a proportion of cases. Substances may have interacted with the acute psychotic process at the time, but no data was available to confirm this.

This is an important study with important epidemiological findings, but methodological limitations make it difficult to interpret the implications of substance misuse for homicide by persons with schizophrenia. The uncertainties of these study findings directly impact on clinical forensic practice because it is the role of a forensic psychiatrist to be absolutely sure when giving an opinion to the court whether psychotic symptoms were a causal factor at the material time of the homicide, and to give a precise opinion on the role of substance misuse. Such opinions cannot rely on a comorbid diagnosis of substance misuse at some undefined time in the past. Furthermore, when giving opinions on treatment and management, ensuring compliance with treatment and follow-up is highly important in preventing future violence in persons treated for schizophrenia. Patients who abuse substances are more likely to be non-compliant with medication and follow-up and thereby are at greater risk of relapse.

Non-lethal Violence

Homicide is an unusual violent crime with particular characteristics. The overall level of violence in a population can be obtained from non-lethal violent crimes which are recorded by the police, but many countries also record self-reported violence using surveys carried out at regular time intervals. These can give a different picture. For example, an earlier study of crime rates in the USA and England and Wales covering 1981–96, comparing New York and London, showed a considerably higher homicide rate in New York, whereas common assault and robbery were somewhat higher in London [15]. A fuller picture can be obtained if these statistics are further supplemented with hospital episodes, where violence victims are registered at hospitals. However, definitions of violent offences vary between countries due to legal differences and statistical recording methods. Useful comparisons may be adversely affected by these differences. Violent crime in England and Wales is measured using two different sources: the British Crime Survey (BCS) and police-recorded crime. Police-recorded crime is a good measure of trends in well-reported crime and also of less common but more serious crimes. However, the BCS provides the most reliable measure of victimisation and national trends over time and is not affected by whether the public report crime or by changes in the way the police record crime. It is essential to be aware of the context of these trends over time when carrying out an assessment, as well as when evaluating research. From the epidemiological perspective, it can then be questioned whether psychiatric morbidity has any impact on these trends. Apart from changes in patterns of drug and alcohol misuse, there is little evidence that it does.

Crime in England and Wales, including violent crime, increased between 1981 and 1995, after which it fell sharply but then stabilised, according to the BCS, with a fall in violent crime of 41%, or half a million fewer victims, after 1995. This was accounted for by large falls in both domestic and 'acquaintance' violence, whereas stranger violence remained stable. Those most at risk of violence are young men aged 16–24 years and unemployed people. The risk of violence varies according to lifestyle characteristics, reflecting differences in social interaction. For example, people who visit pubs and bars are more at risk of violence than those who do not. Figures for 2000 onwards showed a progressive fall in violence using police-reported incidents, the BCS and hospital-treated injuries [16]. However, during the period after 1995, a steady rate of violence was observed in certain UK inner-city areas, particularly London. These observations are important because they show that violence in a population can both rise and fall over time and clinicians should be aware of whether they are in one of these time periods. There is no convincing evidence that severe mental illness has an impact on rises or falls in violence, but this must be considered in the context of studies not yet carried out to test this possibility and where many studies are conducted in countries with good data, social stability and consequent low rates of violence.

Violence is a highly social activity and patterns of self-reported violence in England and Wales during the COVID-19 pandemic were influenced by government instructions to limit social contact. Although there was no change in the total number of violent incidents, the total number of victims of violent crime decreased by 28% in the year ending March 2021 compared to the year ending 2019. The number of homicides fell by 16%. A fall in violent crime was driven by decreases in violence where the offender was a stranger, corresponding to a fall in violence in public spaces. However, when considering the effects of COVID-19 on violence, it is important to also consider the international perspective. Violent crime in the USA had also shown a progressive fall over a similar time period, as shown in Figure 1.2. However, for the year 2020, homicide showed the sharpest increase in certain states and among poorer persons and minorities for many years.

An alternative source of information regarding the prevalence of violence is self-reported violence obtained from national surveys. The national survey of psychiatric morbidity among adults living in households in the UK in 2000 was the first in the UK to include questions on violent behaviour and to compare violent behaviour with psychiatric morbidity in a representative sample of the population [17–20]. Figure 1.3 demonstrates the prevalence of self-reported violence among adults in the UK aged 16–74 years over the previous five years, in a survey in 2000 and 2007. This shows findings repeatedly found in international studies, indicating violence decreases with age and is less prevalent among women. Figure 1.4 compares reported victims of violence, according to the sex of the respondent. It confirms that the primary public health problem among the British household population is violence from men towards strangers or other persons known to them. These patterns are partly reflected in the national homicide statistics, as described earlier. Violence outside of the home and involving strangers can be thought of as just one among a series of hedonistic and negative social behaviours (including hazardous drinking, drug misuse, sexual risk-taking and non-violent antisocial behaviour) exhibited by a subgroup of young men [21].

However, Figure 1.4 also shows another unexpected and controversial finding. Using self-report data, women report more violence towards an intimate partner than men and more violence towards a child than men [22]. These observations contrast with victim reports which suggest that intimate partner violence (IPV) is experienced more by women. However, most studies show that reporting injury is more likely when the victim of IPV is a woman. Considering these findings, the primary public health problem of most countries is not IPV but male-on-male violence among young men. Furthermore, self-report data from UK national surveys indicates that a minority of men who are violent to their partners are only violent to their partners, and that men who perpetrate IPV tend to be generally violent with more than one type of victim [22]. This epidemiological finding has major implications for treatment interventions and prevention of IPV, suggesting that focussing on IPV alone will be ineffective for the majority of these men.

Violence by Women

Men are more violent than women. Sex differences in aggression are thought to be explained by greater male physical strength and testosterone, as well as socialisation in childhood to be more aggressive. A key issue is whether psychiatric morbidity has an impact on violence by women relative to men. Population studies show that men are more likely to abuse alcohol and be dependent on drugs and alcohol, and to have antisocial personality disorder (ASPD), conditions associated with violence in general population studies. Women are more likely than men to receive 'no psychiatric diagnosis' or a diagnosis of affective or anxiety disorder; the latter is associated with somewhat higher risk but at a level lower than other diagnostic categories. One study [22] found that although ASPD was more common in men at the population level, when it occurred in women it posed a greater risk of violence than in men, although this might be because it was more likely to be comorbid with anxiety and affective disorders, including borderline personality disorder, than in men. However, the 'threshold of risk' (gender paradox or group resistance) hypothesis argues that females who develop antisocial behaviour have a higher threshold of risk than males and that violent females are more severely afflicted with mental disorder than males. The female threshold is presumed to be raised by the gender-role socialisation against aggression of women at the level of culture. The push over this threshold is presumed to come from psychobiological or developmental factors at the level of the individual. If more severe aetiology is found for women, then the inference is made that a higher threshold for women therefore exists. A population study found that women who were violent experienced more severe anxiety, affective disorder and personality disorders than men who were violent [22].

Public Health Implications of Psychiatric Morbidity and Non-lethal Violence

Using the British National Household survey, psychiatric diagnoses that had relatively high prevalence in the population, such as affective/anxiety disorder and personality disorder, accounted for a large proportion of all violent incidents. Hazardous drinking, which involves intermittent bouts of heavy drinking, was associated with half of all incidents. In contrast, people who screened positive for psychotic illness constituted a very small percentage overall of people with psychiatric morbidity and accounted for a very small percentage of all violent incidents. However, people with alcohol dependence, drug dependence and ASPD, while having a relatively low prevalence in the population, did account for a relatively high proportion of all incidents [20].

One approach to measuring the impact of a disease at the population level is to calculate the population attributable risk (PAR), which is the incidence of a disease in a population associated with (or attributable to) exposure to the risk factor and is used by epidemiologists to consider which preventative interventions should be used, particularly whether these should be targeted towards individuals or at the population level. This is often expressed as a percentage. Using Swedish case register data, Fazel and colleagues [14] estimated that 1 in 20 persons with schizophrenia and associated psychoses diagnosed by clinicians and included in a national case register were convicted of violent crimes in Sweden. Looked at differently, this means that if the risk exposure of severe psychosis could be eliminated in Sweden, there might be 5% fewer violent convictions in Sweden. However, reliance on criminal records data means that the overall impact of psychotic illness on violence may be greatly overestimated. Using self-reported violent behaviour but using a screen for psychosis (a less robust diagnostic measure), the PAR for violence was only 0.7% in a representative population sample of England, Scotland and Wales [20]. Furthermore, persons who screened positive for psychosis only accounted for 2% of all self-reported violent events over a five-year time period in this population. This difference may have been partly due to the diagnostic measures used. However, it was more likely due to an underestimation of the overall level of violence using criminal records and where persons with severe mental illness are more likely to be convicted.

In contrast, hazardous drinking (a pattern of intermittent bouts of excess drinking) was found among 27% of the British population with a PAR of 47%, and with over 50% of all violent events over the past five years self-reported by this population. Drug misuse was found among 10% of the population (most frequently cannabis) and showed a PAR of 37%, with drug users accounting for 42% of all violent events. Overall, these findings do not suggest that targeted interventions for people with major psychosis would have a large impact on the overall level of violence. A reduction by 5% might include a large number of violent incidents across an entire country. But this needs to be considered in the context of a country such as Sweden with a relatively low rate of serious violence and in the context of the measure of violence used in the case register study – violent convictions in a criminal court. If the aim were to reduce a larger amount of violence using a population approach, then limiting access to alcohol and reducing alcohol consumption among hazardous and harmful drinkers is likely to have the largest impact nationally, particularly among young men. The figures also suggest that reducing drug consumption may have a major impact. However, when using PAR measures to estimate the impact of interventions, it is important to consider their main limitations. A PAR assumes that the condition being eliminated from the population has a direct *causative* effect on the violent behaviour. This cannot be assumed for factors such as drug misuse, where associations are highly complex and can include reverse causation.

Overall, the largest public health impact on serious and repetitive violence was exerted by hazardous drinking. The relationship between drinking and violence was strong among young people and those who conducted a high percentage of their drinking in bars. These findings indicate that public health population approaches involving risk reduction programmes to encourage healthy drinking and control of outlets, particularly those associated with drunken disorder, many within the 'night-time economy', are the most appropriate preventative interventions.

The position with regard to ASPD differed from that of alcohol. Despite a relatively low prevalence in the population, individuals with ASPD make a substantial contribution to violence and serious violence. Eliminating exposure to this disorder would have reduced the proportion of individuals who reported injuries to other persons by almost a quarter. This indicates a subgroup suitable for targeted (or secondary and tertiary) prevention strategies. This group were more likely to injure victims and their violence was repetitive. They assaulted multiple different victims and in different locations. However, targeting this group poses logistical and moral problems. They represent approximately 2% of the population in different Western populations. This is a substantial number of individuals, far beyond the scope of mental health and criminal justice services for interventions such as selective incapacitation [23]. There is also no intervention that is currently known to be successful with this subgroup. Furthermore, if reliance were placed on the diagnosis of ASPD to identify these individuals, despite a high prevalence of violence among this subgroup, half were not found to have been violent in the past five years despite living an otherwise highly antisocial lifestyle [17–20].

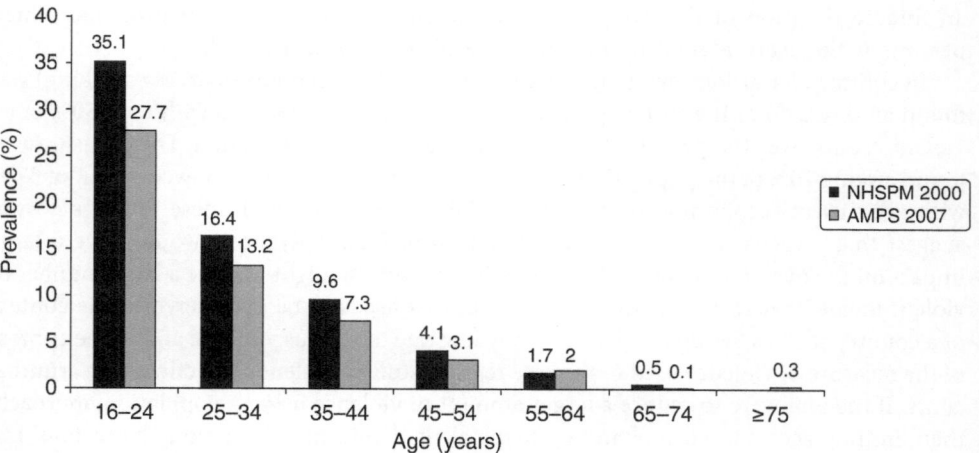

Figure 1.3 Prevalence of any violence in the past five years in the UK by age group and survey. From Coid JW, Ullrich S, Kallis C et al. Improving risk management for violence in mental health services: a multimethods approach. *Programme Grants for Applied Research* 2016; 4(16).

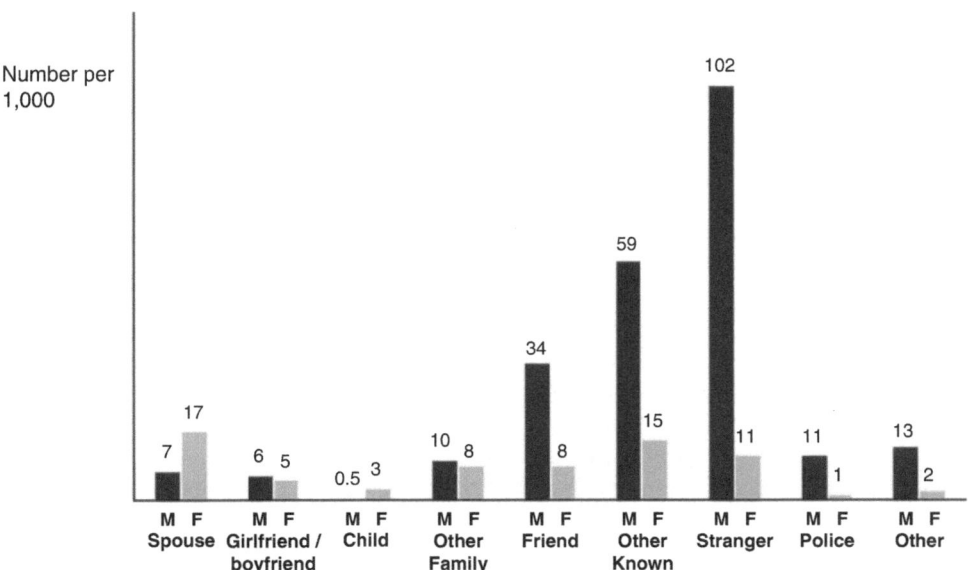

Figure 1.4 Number of subjects (per 1,000 persons) reporting violence towards victims by sex. From Coid, State-of-Science Review: SR-B11, *Epidemiological Linkages between Mental Ill-Health and Violence: Risk Factors and Wider Consequences*, 2008. Open Government Licence.

Psychosocial Risk Factors and Mental Illness

It is correct to say that certain social characteristics of an individual are often more strongly associated with future involvement in violence than the presence of mental illness [25]. However, this argument was based on simple statistical associations in a literature review. This review is sometimes used to incorrectly claim that it is psychosocial risk factors and not the mental illness that causes violence among the mentally ill. It is indeed correct that there are strong interactions between different psychiatric conditions and the psychosocial circumstances of people with mental illness. A good forensic assessment will disentangle these components. Unfortunately, few research studies investigate these interactions. This has also led to simplistic claims that it is rare that the presence of a mental illness will provide a causative explanation for an act of violence [26, 27]. Careful examination of this research shows it was based on an earlier misunderstanding of the associations between risk factors in statistical models used to create predictive models for future risk for violence. Mental disorder appeared to come out worse in the models in terms of its relative predictive power when the usual measure of a mental disorder was a diagnostic label which paid no attention to whether symptoms of the disorder were present or absent at the time of the violence. In most of these studies, the diagnosis had been made well in advance of the violence. These risk prediction models are seriously flawed, as described earlier, and did not consider the possibility that mental disorder could be causal, as in the case of when symptoms are present at the time and drive the violent behaviour.

More recently, it has become more important in research to consider whether symptoms of mental disorder were actually present at the time of the violence to be directly relevant to the violence, and this is a key requirement in a forensic assessment. Forensic psychiatrists should not engage in an 'either/or' debate as to whether it was the mental disorder or the psychosocial circumstances that caused the violence. Both are likely to be important. Unless symptoms of mental illness can be ruled out as being present at the material time, a more sophisticated analysis involves understanding how psychosocial factors influenced mental disorder, and vice versa, along the pathway to violence. Nevertheless, it is rare to find that psychosocial factors had no impact on mental illness to result in violence. Mental disorder, particularly severe conditions like schizophrenia, tends to be found among persons of lower social class and living in areas of higher socioeconomic deprivation. Persons with severe mental illness tend to drift down the social scale, with difficulty managing finances, debt, housing instability and increased likelihood of homelessness. They often live in social environments where there is increased risk of being preyed upon by others, resulting in violent altercations and where the violent incident may not have had a direct association with their symptoms, apart from the symptoms making them more likely to be identified as a target of violence by others. At the same time, they are often socially withdrawn and come into contact with fewer persons, mainly carers, who may be at risk from them during episodes of psychosis. A forensic assessment of an individual should not be influenced by overarching statements based on the theoretical position of a discipline striving for dominance in the field of violence studies and stick to the facts of the case at hand.

Causation

At the heart of a good assessment is an understanding of the cause or causes of the violence by the forensic psychiatrist to be able to prepare a report and give useful advice to colleagues in second opinions. Courts expect psychiatrists to be able to explain the violent offence and assume that psychiatry has something special to offer that other disciplines do not. Courts will rigorously test expert evidence if they say the defendant has a defence at law for their behaviour due to a mental illness. Colleagues will expect a forensic psychiatrist to be able to explain why a patient under their care does not respond to their interventions, why they continue to be violent and what to do about it. They will want to know whether the patient is in the correct level of security for the protection of staff and other patients.

In clinical practice, there will seldom be a single cause for violence. It is important to be able to assemble the multiple factors leading directly to violence, together with the factors that did not cause the violence but made it more likely to occur when it did and where it did. It is helpful to consider a pathway to violence. Although focussing on psychiatric morbidity, it is important to remember that situational factors are of considerable and often prime importance, sometimes involving unique and unexpected occurrences in an individual's social environment. There is also usually more than one motive for violence that can be identified and it is important to be clear about whether violence is driven by symptoms of mental disorder, whether there are elements of intoxication with disinhibition, whether there is mood disturbance such as irritability and anger, whether the violence was provoked by the behaviour of others or triggered by certain key factors, and whether there was evidence of planning beforehand. Experienced forensic psychiatrists typically put together a causal chain, or pathway, as a mechanism to understand violence, considering the above and multiple other factors they identify during a good-quality assessment. In assessing previous violent behaviour, the psychiatrist is examining a process of what are usually multiple causes in the past and effects which lie in the future in terms of time and space (or place). In the case of assessment of disturbed and violent inpatients, these causal factors may be directly observable during the examination of the patient and in the patient's physical environment, such as the hospital ward, together with the social interactions between the patient and other patients, friends, and relatives and staff. Problems arise, however, when attempts are made to extend the assessment to future behaviour if no causal associations can be established as a target for intervention.

Many statistical predictors of future violent behaviour such as young age, number of previous convictions and so on, typically used in a risk assessment which uses actuarial scores to determine future risk based on statistical models, are not amenable to clinical intervention. Using a statistical 'predictive' model of future behaviour, these have stronger statistical power because past behaviour is a reasonably recurring statistical predictor of future behaviour – but with considerable limitations in the real world. More importantly, few are causal factors for violence and, paradoxically, causal factors are often poor predictors in statistical models. If the intention is to effectively intervene and prevent violence, then it will be necessary to identify the factors which are causal, even if the causal factor does not appear to currently be in operation. The art of assessment is to understand the causal chain and determine whether it is likely to re-occur and to understand if and when there should be an intervention. If the individual has multiple previous violent convictions, this gives some strong indication statistically of future risk but little indication of causation.

However, if each of these offences were against victims who had been incorporated into delusions of persecution, typically occurring when the patient ceased to take medication and the symptoms re-occurred, this would give some indication of the cause or causes of the violence and a possible solution to future prevention. But the latter would then involve assessment of whether the individual responded to treatment for delusions, whether they were likely to cooperate with treatment again in the future and how this might be assured, and multiple other factors based on extensive clinical experience that cannot be packaged into a course on risk assessment by trainers who are not clinically experienced and licensed to administer certain treatment options such as medication. Having said this, clinical assessment of violence can and sometimes should include a structured assessment of future risks. However, this is peripheral to the main task of understanding why an individual has been violent and most importantly what has caused the violence. Despite an earlier, negative commentary on the standard method of medical history-taking when assessing potentially violent persons for an assessment of future risk [4], forensic psychiatrists should ignore this and continue to use the standard approaches they have been taught during their medical training, and ignore spurious criticisms from other disciplines of the 'medical model'.

Research into violence and mental disorder remains short on studies that attempt to establish causation. Using a predictive approach in what are usually pseudo-longitudinal designs, research studies have typically used 'lagged' statistical models. For example, a factor occurring in the past six months is used to predict violence occurring in the subsequent six months (or over a longer period). In a temporal proximity or causal model, both the predictor and outcome are measured in the same time window (e.g. the same six months, or more ideally during shorter time periods). The former, lagged or 'predictive' model is used in all studies which attempt to create new risk assessment instruments and also to validate these instruments. However, this model cannot evaluate causation for violence because the factor found associated with and sometimes incorrectly thought to have caused the violence may not have actually been present at the time the violence occurred. A good example is the Swedish case register studies which concluded that violence in schizophrenia was due substantially to substance misuse [5, 6]. However, having drawn this conclusion, closer examination shows that it is impossible to conclude, firstly, that symptoms of schizophrenia were present at the time of a violent offence and, secondly, that persons diagnosed with schizophrenia had taken drugs or alcohol at the material time the violence occurred.

Symptoms of psychosis fluctuate, sometimes on a day-to-day basis, and it is necessary for a forensic psychiatrist to have a considerable degree of certainty that they were present at the time of the violence when giving evidence in court, otherwise their evidence will be discredited. The best example of the confusion that can occur in research is shown in the re-analysis of the MacArthur study data [7] where it had originally been asserted that delusions did not either cause or predict violence [8]. Most experienced forensic psychiatrists will find such assertions counter-intuitive and not based on their clinical experience. Patients with schizophrenia frequently explain their violence on the basis of their delusional beliefs. Depositions and sometimes witness statements will reveal assertions by a patient that violence was due to a delusional belief. In this context, re-analysis of the same MacArthur data using a causal model, aiming to demonstrate causality, revealed that the predictive model had missed the fact that the delusions were strongly associated with violence, but that only certain delusions caused violence, and that angry affect due to the delusions had to be present for violence to occur. Because the delusions had fluctuated in severity over a one-year follow-up period, unless the measures were taken at frequent intervals over this time period and a statistical method was used to test whether symptoms and violence coincided during a narrowed timespan, the statistical association between the two would be totally missed. Interestingly, the re-analysis found that it was entirely correct that if an observation of delusions was made at the time of discharge from hospital and then tested to see if they statistically predicted violence over the follow-up, delusions could not accurately predict violence occurring at either 6 or 12 months later using a lagged model. Delusions did indeed not *predict* future violence among released psychiatric patients. However, using a causal model, delusions were found to have *caused* violence.

These criticisms of existing research are important for clinical assessment. For example, violence among persons with schizophrenia can occur at times when no symptoms are present and when the patient is intoxicated. It is unlikely a defence can be established in court if no symptoms were present, and courts are not sympathetic to excuses of intoxication for violence. Intoxication and repeated episodes of substance misuse can precipitate symptoms of psychosis in predisposed individuals, but it will be necessary to give supporting evidence that it was the symptoms that caused the violence and not the intoxication. When giving evidence, that may be hard to achieve. Correspondingly, it would be poor clinical practice to conclude that because an individual had a history of substance abuse in the past, violence during an acute psychotic episode when there was no evidence of substance misuse was primarily due to the latter. Because establishing associations between violence and psychosis is so important, the present mental state at interview should never be relied on alone when forming an opinion. It is important to seek all sources of information prior to and following the violent act from case records and from witnesses, or their statements, and to get the client's account of the symptoms' progress over time and how they think they influenced the violence, then come to their own opinion. The most relevant information in the case of a serious offence may be the police interrogation because it is close in time to the offence and the individual is under pressure to give an explanation. It is particularly helpful to have training in using standardised research instruments, which include a comprehensive series of questions to elicit psychotic symptoms such as the World

Health Organization's Schedules for Clinical Assessment in Neuropsychiatry (SCAN), but also to know how to elicit lifetime diagnoses using instruments such as the World Health Organization's Composite International Diagnostic Interview (CIDI). During assessment, it will be necessary to focus on whether they were experiencing these symptoms at the time of the offence and elicit whether symptoms motivated or 'drove' the behaviour.

Research into Causal Effects of Psychotic Symptoms on Violence

A clinical diagnosis is a construct created for research and clinical purposes and is unhelpful and can be misleading when applied to the study of violence, apart from grouping patients into broad categories. Surprisingly, there has been only limited study of the associations between violence and psychotic symptoms, even though clinicians need to establish that symptoms were present at the material time of the violence and explain how they cause violence. Sadly, at the time of writing this chapter, there has been only limited progress in this area, probably because these studies are difficult to conduct and require more complex statistical analyses and study methods that can be difficult to set up. They also require face-to-face interviews with patients and cannot rely on existing datasets such as cross-sectional surveys and case registers. However, cross-sectional surveys can be a starting point to establish the direction of future study and whether symptoms apply differently to categorical diagnoses at the population level. For example, a meta-analysis of seven UK general population surveys measured psychotic symptoms of hypomania, thought insertion, paranoid ideation, strange experiences and hallucinations. It also created a categorical diagnosis of 'psychosis', using a cut-off to compare with other studies [28]. Using the categorical construct, psychosis was not found to be associated with violence after controlling for confounding from demography and comorbid conditions such as ASPD, substance dependence and anxiety disorder. This is similar to findings from case register studies. Depressive disorder also showed no association after adjustments. However, one symptom, paranoid ideation, showed strong independent associations with more serious violence where a perpetrator or victim had been injured, repetitive violence, violence involving the police and where victims were more likely to be strangers. The other four symptoms showed no associations after adjustment including adjustment for other symptoms.

These findings appear supportive of the notion that paranoid ideation could cause violence but a cross-sectional survey cannot establish causation. The five symptoms are surprisingly common in the general population and do not necessarily mean a person reporting them is psychotic. What about in the case of established clinical psychotic illness? To study this, a first episode study of psychosis in East London, UK was used which measured psychosis using face-to-face, structured clinical interviews administered by psychiatrists and with questions to establish whether violence had occurred in the year before the interview [29]. Most patients were psychotic at the time of the interview and many were in a psychiatric hospital in the first or second week of admission. They were also administered questionnaires to establish whether they were impulsive, had state or trait anger, and had psychopathic traits, and to test their reactions to a wide range of delusional beliefs and other symptoms established from the structured interview. Importantly, any patients who did not have psychotic symptoms at the time of the violence were excluded from the analyses. The study found a strong, independent relationship between delusions and violence in the year prior to first contact. This effect was greater for more serious violence. The association was not confounded by other psychotic symptoms, psychopathy or trait anger. The structured clinical interview included 32 possible delusions but only 6 were associated with angry affect: being spied upon, familiar people impersonated, persecution, conspiracy, threat/control override and misidentification. Most importantly, mediation analysis established that violence was dependent on whether the delusion made the patient angry.

The East London study findings were replicated in a re-analysis of the US MacArthur dataset, a prospective longitudinal study of violence among patients discharged from hospital and interviewed face-to-face at baseline before discharge and on five subsequent occasions in the community [30]. Nine of 15 delusions showed strong associations with violence, following adjustments, and included being spied upon, being followed, being plotted against, being able to hear others' thoughts, being under the control of a person/force, thought insertion, strange forces working on them and having special gifts/powers. As with the East London study, being spied upon, being under external control and thought insertion were mediated by angry affect due to the delusions, suggesting a different, indirect pathway to serious violence. There was a direct pathway between certain symptoms and violence, but in these cases the violence was less serious.

A further UK study of patients discharged from medium-secure services to the community measured symptoms and violence at baseline (pre-discharge) and at 6 and 12 months in the community [31]. The aim was to look at shifts in symptoms over time. The study found that an overall shift in positive symptoms was associated with violence. The larger the symptom shift, the more likely that violence would occur. Negative symptoms appeared to shift in the same direction as positive, corresponding to an overall increase in severity of illness. However, closer examination indicated that negative symptoms exerted protective effects. But there was no clinically observable effect because the protective effect of increasing negative symptoms was overwhelmed by the positive symptoms and, most importantly, the shift to increasing anger which accompanied the positive symptoms, particularly delusions. There was a relationship between stable paranoid delusions and violence but also between intensifying delusions accompanied by intensifying anger. Shifts and instability in the psychotic process were themselves causally associated with violence.

A final study in this series, which aimed to investigate causal links between symptoms and violence, included a prospective longitudinal study of prisoners released from prison and followed up in the community at a mean of 39 weeks later [32]. A subgroup had been diagnosed as suffering from schizophrenia, delusional disorder or drug-induced psychosis by researchers (but not necessarily the healthcare staff of the prison who were unaware of certain cases) prior to release. First examination of the data showed that prisoners diagnosed with schizophrenia did not have higher rates of violent behaviour than those with no mental disorder, including criminal reoffending once they returned to the community. However, when the data was re-examined to identify those who had *not* received any treatment for psychosis in prison, this subgroup were highly likely to become violent again. Untreated schizophrenia was associated with the emergence of persecutory delusions at follow-up, which were in turn associated with violence. Mediation analyses confirmed the effects of the persecutory delusions on the violence.

Using a causal approach in data analysis and concentration on symptoms rather than studying whether violence is associated with a diagnostic category resulted in new findings to guide future research. This approach corresponds to clinical experience and a forensic clinical assessment of psychosis and violence. Persecutory delusions appear to be the key symptoms, but these need to be accompanied by angry affect and/or anger for violence to occur. Although delusions were of prime importance, it is likely that other symptoms played a part. Although anxiety symptoms did not exert effects in the models in these studies, clinical experience shows that anxiety does have an effect in some cases, contributing to violence. The other aspect indicated by this work was that the intensity of the psychotic illness was of considerable importance, and also when symptoms were shifting or fluctuating, a key feature of an acute and severe episode of psychosis. It is also clear that prevention of relapse leading to further violence is dependent on maintaining anti-psychotic treatment and mental stability, and that the key preventative strategy is to avoid the re-occurrence of delusions associated with violence. The importance of associated anger with the delusions questions whether targeting anger as an associated affect should be the primary strategy for treatment intervention in future.

Violence Pathways

Forensic assessments of violence typically include two types of pathway analysis: firstly, an understanding of the life-course development of the individual from childhood to the violent incident or incidents under investigation, typically in adult life, together with examination of corresponding factors that may have had an impact and are known from research and experience to be strongly associated with future violence; and secondly, a painstaking forensic examination of the key components of the violent acts leading to a referral for a professional opinion. For example, this might be the prosecution case against the defendant in depositions and statements, or a series of worrying assaults on other patients and nurses by a patient detained in hospital, based on reading documented accounts, asking nurses for their account and interviewing the patient for their account and explanation. In clinical practice, opinions are usually presented in written form, with the recent pathway to the presenting events coming first and the lifetime understanding of the antecedents to the violence coming later in the report to establish links. It is usually necessary to set a starting timepoint and clarify the context of the assessment, such as who made the referral and why, the information available and the nature of the examination conducted to form an opinion. The life-course analysis is then used to support the opinion based on the recent violence and how this corresponds to or in some cases diverges from it.

Vignette 1

A man has a history of life-long antisocial behaviour and repetitive involvement in violence, starting with childhood maltreatment in his family of origin and being taken into care, then childhood conduct disorder and persistent criminality in early adulthood, before developing schizophrenia in his mid-20s, subsequent refusal to cooperate with aftercare between episodes, frequent relapses, and a criminal history suggesting acquisitive offences such as theft and burglary together with assaults, where it is not always possible to be sure whether these are driven by the underlying antisocial personality or psychosis. However, it is apparent that some offences have been followed by hospital admission in an acute state of psychosis requiring treatment. Witness statements indicate that for some violent offences in public places, the individual has been acutely psychotic, but also intoxicated with both drugs and alcohol at the same time. He is currently charged with a serious wounding of another man in a bar with a beer glass where he got into an altercation due to his bizarre and provocative behaviour towards the victim. Other drinkers have given witness statements describing him as talking to himself, shouting at them and making threats of violence for no apparent reason.

Vignette 2

In a contrasting case, a man in his early 30s is charged with the attempted murder of his next-door neighbours. He has no previous convictions and had ceased working at a bank and become socially isolated over a one-year period. He had developed schizophrenia following the death of his mother 18 months earlier and has lived alone in the family home, unemployed but caring for himself, with no previous criminal convictions or contact with mental health services. He had recently made a complaint to the police regarding the behaviour of his neighbour which was found to have no basis in fact and no action had been taken. He had bought knives and an axe and had made a determined homicidal attack on his neighbour when the latter returned in the evening from work. He described an elaborate delusional system of persecution by his neighbour and his family, including the belief they had built a machine on behalf of the government, which was now causing damage to his internal body organs in a medical experiment. Police found detailed writings suggesting plans for the offence, but with multiple biblical references and scientifically unrelated research findings regarding experimentation on animals.

Using an actuarial measure of future risk, the first case will score higher on an actuarial measure of risk of future violence, leading to an expectation of prioritisation by services responsible for him. It can be argued that he has shown a lifetime of high risk of violence towards others. There is considerable scope for rejection of the first man from mental health services on the grounds he has ASPD and polysubstance abuse, and because experts are arguing over whether he was psychotic at the time of the latest episode of violence. However, experience demonstrates that many cases of schizophrenia with similar features can show considerable improvement with sustained pharmacological treatment over time, starting in a secure hospital setting, and continued medication, together with regular court-ordered follow-up in the community. In contrast, the second case shows a high risk of extreme violence towards others of a homicidal nature. Relapse of the illness in future and re-appearance of similar delusional beliefs (which cannot be accurately predicted) would render him a clear and immediate danger to persons in the local proximity. Both patients require long-term surveillance and monitoring for the safety of others. But for each, the risk assessment using a pathway model and future process of risk management are very different.

A Theoretical Model of Risk Pathway to Violence

A model that can be incorporated into clinical practice is based on empirical research and clinical experience [33]. It is based on a longitudinal approach that aims to capture the evolution of risk over time, typically from when an offender is released from custody or a patient is released from hospital. This type of assessment might at first appear more useful for the first of the two examples given in the vignettes, both for the assessment of the latest criminal charge of violence and for the purpose of managing the risk of future violence, although it is equally applicable to the second. A typical actuarial risk assessment instrument using a score based on previous behaviours would suggest the first case is considerably more dangerous than the second, but this would be incorrect.

The clinical risk assessment using this model would proceed through each of the of the five stages shown in Figure 1.5. This would be based on previous behaviour and a full assessment of the individual's previous history, including current circumstances and reason for the assessment, detailed assessment of previous and more recent violent and criminal behaviour, family history, and developmental history from childhood to the present day.

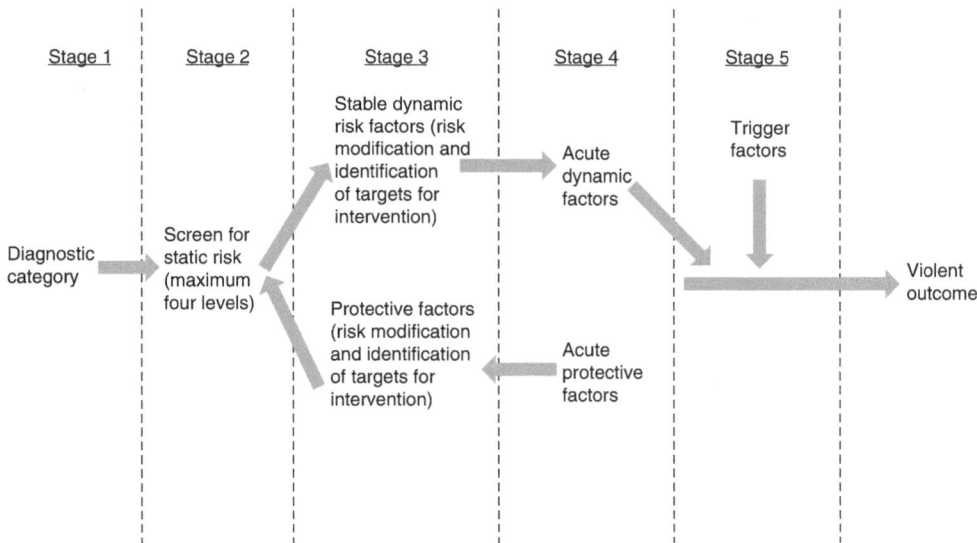

Figure 1.5 Theoretical model of risk pathway to violence. From Coid JW, Ullrich S, Kallis C et al. Improving risk management for violence in mental health services: a multimethods approach. *Programme Grants for Applied Research* 2016; 4(16).

Although Figure 1.5 shows that the first stage of the assessment is to make a diagnosis, most clinicians would correctly point out that this is usually completed towards the end of a clinical assessment. However, research has shown that pathways to violence and other offending are different according to different diagnoses in clinical forensic practice [34]. The model therefore differs from psychological assessments which do not always recognise the considerable differences in pathways determined by diagnosis and include diagnosis as one among multiple risk factors. (It is not recommended that forensic psychiatrists adhere to this simplistic approach. Clinical experience will soon reveal that different psychiatric conditions have very different pathways to violence.)

The model is similar to a risk assessment in that it includes a series of stages in which risk factors could potentially be measured quantitatively using risk assessment instruments and was used in a research study to test the accuracy of these measures. However, that was not its primary intention, which was the formulation of a risk management plan or alternatively a retrospective analysis of an offence pathway according to the impact of exacerbating and protective factors over time. It would include assessment of current and previous mental state to obtain a formal diagnosis, and would include personality disorder and substance misuse, for example as in the first vignette, as well as schizophrenia. These further diagnoses would add to the complexity of the model. The figure also forms the basis of a risk formulation which follows from the full clinical assessment. If the patient is already known to services or if the forensic psychiatrist is approaching a case with a considerable body of knowledge and information available, this model may be particularly helpful.

Stage 1: Figure 1.5 begins with establishment of a psychiatric diagnosis at the outset together with (Stage 2) the level of static risk for future violence, based on actuarial measures. We have already referred to the considerable problems of the actuarial approach using static measures but believe they have some limited value as long as they are combined with an in-depth analysis of dynamic risk factors. A clinician may want to know a score for risk based on previous offending and this may be helpful in a more in-depth profiling of qualitative as well as quantitative aspects of previous offending. But it should not be the basis for major decisions such as release from hospital or prison. It is also of some help in indicating when an in-depth clinical assessment is required. It will be of little or no use in formulating a treatment plan. For the two case vignettes, it is the second which may concern many forensic psychiatrists most of all because of the risk of future homicidal violence towards others. However, when combined with dynamic factors, a static or actuarial measure of risk can provide a more clinically helpful assessment, which can then be used to formulate factors for risk management that will be targeted in a future intervention.

Stage 3 requires an assessment of ongoing dynamic risk factors. These are changeable and should be targets for future intervention if the aim is risk management or if they are identified as having an impact on the violent events in an assessment for court. An interaction can occur between dynamic risk and protective factors whereby the protective factors reduce risk or whereby risk is seen to increase when the protective factors are no longer present. Examples include alcoholism, mood disorder, moving into the vicinity of a group or class of previous victims, reducing the level of supervision by professionals and social support, refusal to take medication, and attitudes which condone violence or other hate crimes. There is debate over the extent to which dynamic risk factors can truly be considered causal factors for violence but can be considered as contributing to the violence to varying degrees and by different means. These have also been referred to as 'criminogenic needs' by psychologists with the theoretical question of whether the offence would have occurred if the 'need', or what had been lacking, had been redressed. Few of these factors are directly related to a violent act in terms of constituting an immediate, demonstrable cause. But they are nevertheless major contributing factors which make the violence more likely to occur.

In Stage 4, the individual may encounter acute dynamic risk factors that have a direct influence on subsequent behaviour; for example, acute intoxication, being involved at the time in a group or gang, sudden removal of social support, or sudden loss of a close relationship. These have a more immediate bearing in time on the violent outcome than ongoing or chronic risk factors. Descriptions of the effect of these factors by the patient or witness statements indicating change in behaviour or emotional presentation are important in formulating an assessment of causal effects on violence. For example, intoxication with alcohol could not be considered to have a direct, causal effect on violence. However, when combined with other factors such as provocation by the victim, intoxication may greatly increase the likelihood of a violent response through factors such as cognitive impairment, disinhibition and so on.

At Stage 5, certain trigger factors which have an immediate and causal effect on the violent outcome may be encountered. These are very common in reactive, impulsive acts. Alternatively, the violence may have been planned for some time, although a sudden triggering factor can sometimes occur in cases where planning may have been present and determine the time and place when the violence occurred. Trigger factors are factors which, like the trigger on a gun, cause something to happen and can be an event or situation that *causes* something to start – in this case, a violent retaliation. The key definition which distinguishes a trigger from a dynamic risk factor is the timing of the event in terms of its occurrence before the violence and the direct relationship between the trigger and the violent act. There should be a very short period before the occurrence of a triggering factor and the violent act, where anything more than 1 hour is likely to be considered as occurring after a 'cooling-off' period in a court and would strongly suggest planning. Research with recidivists indicates that the majority are highly impulsive and do not consider or plan their next behaviour any more than 15 minutes before the criminal act [35].

A study proposed that trigger factors exist that could be considered 'super-acute' risk factors that have an immediate, moment-to-moment impact in precipitating a violent incident [36]. These are best referred to as 'situational variables' and conceptualised as external environmental effects that have an immediate effect on the appraisal of a situation. They correspond to reactive aggression in response to frustration or threat and are unlikely to be present in most cases of instrumental aggression, where there is more likely to be forethought or planning before the aggressive act. In this study of violent prisoners, external triggers were found to be random events that could not be predicted by either static or dynamic risk factors but were linked to specific psychological characteristics of the violent offender, for example features of their personality disorder. The personality features rendered the individual more likely to respond violently to the trigger, but the causal factor was the trigger itself.

There should not be any confusion between triggers and the dynamic risk factors which are incorrectly defined as 'triggers' in a Scandinavian case register study [37]. These included exposure to violence, parental bereavement, self-harm, traumatic brain injury, unintentional injuries and substance intoxication in the week before the violent act rather than on the day of the act, which excludes them as trigger factors. Immediate retaliation to an assault or becoming involved to help a friend being assaulted may be triggers if occurring very close to the violence, but it is unclear how self-harm and death of a parent can trigger violence if it occurred up to a week before. These did not appear to be credible or sufficient 'triggers' in themselves to result in violence. Forensic psychiatrists will not fare well when giving evidence in court if they attempt to mitigate previous violent behaviour as a 'causal' factor for violence and even less so for a bout of intoxication. These findings would be best described as dynamic factors that increased risk for a subsequent violent act rather than a 'trigger'.

Violence: Impulsive/Reactive and Targeted/Predatory Dichotomy

The model in Figure 1.5 does not take into account specific qualities of the violent action being assessed. Aggression is complex and heterogeneous, which often explains the limitations of both epidemiological studies which have minimal data to differentiate between different types and biological studies which combine more than one type. There are different typologies and a single individual can show different types at different times. However, a longstanding system for codifying aggression is the impulsive/reactive and targeted/predatory (the latter including instrumental aggression) dichotomy, with differing pathways. The two cases of schizophrenia described in the vignettes will fit into differing categories using this dichotomy. With experience, however, trainees will find that violent acts will sometimes fit into both categories. Nevertheless, being aware of this dichotomy is useful; firstly, because it is thought there may be different underlying neurobiology which explains these pathways [38]; secondly, a full understanding of the different components of each give a more nuanced picture of the patient's diagnosis and the links to their behaviour and will help formulate a treatment plan; and thirdly, because it has been used for the development of threat assessments for future harm reduction.

The Pathway to Violence

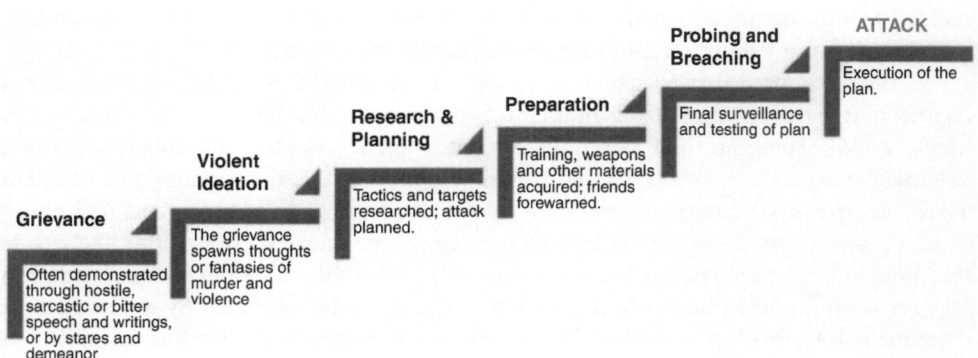

Figure 1.6 The pathway to violence, reproduced with permission from TorchStone Global. Source: U.S. Department of Homeland Security. Copyright TorchStone Global (2020). www.torchstoneglobal.com.

Impulsive/reactive aggression is driven by internal emotion, it tends to be reactive, the violence is likely to be immediate, it is likely to be triggered by an external event which occurs only a short time before the violent act (typically minutes or seconds), and it is carried out against perceived threats where the goal is threat reduction, primarily defensive, aiming for rapid displacement of the violence with the reaction being time-limited.

In contrast, targeted/predatory aggression is less reactive and emotional, it is planned and purposeful, it is thought out in advance (often with a decision made well before the violent act), it has a specific target, it is carried out to achieve a goal or goals, it is cognitive and attack orientated, and it is not time-limited. Targeted violence is rarely impulsive or random and most individuals think through and plan out the violence so that it is much easier to discern and follow a 'pathway' to the violent act. Figure 1.6 shows a US Homeland Security Pathway stepwise model which applies to the targeted/predatory pathway and was developed from experience with mass killings in the USA with the aim of disrupting or getting potential offenders off the pathway to violence [39, 40]. Features of this model can be considered within forensic assessments and apply equally to psychotic offenders as to those with no mental disorder. Most steps of the model apply to the second case of schizophrenia described in the vignettes.

There can be multiple reasons for an individual embarking on the pathway; for example, a grievance due to problems needing to be solved, drawing attention to a cause, personal pain and anguish, an unresolved or unresolvable grievance, paranoid delusions, no longer wanting to live, and so on. In studies carried out after mass killings, most perpetrators were actively suicidal or at a point of desperation prior to their attacks. Figure 1.6 shows how the grievance progresses from violent ideation to research and planning followed by subsequent preparation, including access to weapons and other equipment needed for the attack. The preparation stage is often short before the person engages in violence. In terms of prevention, the first question is whether it is possible to identify that a person is on a pathway to violence. Secondly, and if so, how far down the pathway are they in terms of idea, plan, preparation or implementation? Thirdly, why are they on the pathway and resorting to violence? And fourthly, is it possible to divert them to a better path?

Retrospective observations show a change in identification behaviour, such as joining right-wing or other terrorist organisations, but also what enforcement agencies refer to as 'emotional leakage', with many actually stating that they will do it or posting threats in some form online in over 60% cases. Less than 20% directly threaten victims in mass killings, but in many cases of violence in psychosis the victim may have been threatened or even been a victim of violence on a previous occasion, particularly relatives. Probing and breaching includes 'try-outs' of the eventual violent act, sometimes with visits to the planned location. Try-outs are also a particular component of serious sex offences when there is a sadistic motive [41] and where this may be the only overt indicator of the future behaviour, which is otherwise concealed within an undisclosed sadistic fantasy. There may also be examples of 'short-term' behaviour such as closing bank accounts or ominous texts of farewell to close persons. There are occasional last-resort warnings, but the perpetrator may no longer expect this to have any effect. The timing of an attack may be brought forward when it is thought that the victim may no longer be in the location or soon inaccessible. In psychotic patients, increasing symptoms such as hostility and anger, threat perception, grandiosity and dysphoria may be seen in cases where there has been treatment non-adherence.

Criminal Records – Criminal Careers

A criminal career has a beginning (onset), an end (desistence) and a career length in between (duration) [42]. Criminal records are essential for a forensic assessment of violence and may reveal multiple pathways. It is important to go through a criminal record with the offender during an assessment, particularly when alternative sources of information are unavailable. Typically, convictions represent only a fraction of the offences committed by an offender and better research in the field includes self-report data, so it is important to ask the patient about other violent events over the lifespan. Individual offenders tend to commit offences at a fairly constant frequency during their criminal careers. However, those first convicted at a young age have more prolonged careers. Furthermore, when looking at an entire population, a minority account for the majority of all offences. Violent offenders tend not to be specialist offenders in most studies, although these will sometimes be encountered in clinical forensic practice where it is important to understand similarities between individual incidents. Sex offenders tend to be most specialised and fraud offenders most persistent. Most offenders will commit a single offence and not be reconvicted. However, some will be persistent and a subgroup will be chronic offenders.

Chronic offenders are more likely to have histories of maltreatment in childhood and come from families where a member also has a criminal history. Debut offence is important and those who commit a robbery are more likely to go on to commit serious offences such as violence and become chronic offenders. Late-onset offenders after the age of 18 years tend to have been more anxious in childhood with fewer social contacts and with a proportion showing evidence of social decline leading to criminality from alcohol dependence and after developing severe mental illness. Previous studies of these groups in childhood and adolescence showed that childhood-onset delinquents had inadequate parenting, neurocognitive problems, under-controlled temperament, severe hyperactivity, psychopathic personality traits and violent behaviour. Adolescent-onset delinquents were not distinguished by these features.

A New Zealand cohort followed to age 26 years showed that the childhood-onset delinquents were the most elevated on psychopathic personality traits, mental health problems, substance dependence, numbers of children, financial problems, work problems, and drug-related and violent crime, including violence against women and children [43]. The adolescent-onset delinquents at 26 years were less extreme but elevated on impulsive personality traits, mental health problems, substance dependence, financial problems and property offences. A third group of men who had been aggressive as children but not very delinquent as adolescents emerged as low-level chronic offenders who were anxious, depressed and socially isolated, and had financial and work problems. These findings support the theory of life-course-persistent and adolescence-limited antisocial behaviour among offenders, but also extend it to include other groups.

The first vignette earlier is clearly a case of an early-onset offender and delinquency preceded the development of schizophrenia. Because there are important additional components to early-onset cases which will impact on other psychopathology and behaviour, including behaviour in security while undergoing treatment and after return to the community, it is recommended that when carrying out a forensic assessment this should routinely include assessment for the presence or absence of ASPD using the US *Diagnostic and Statistical Manual*. This requires three or more criteria to be present before the age of 15 years and three or more after the age of 15 years (see criteria in box). It is generally the case that the earlier the onset, the more severe and persistent the condition. Forensic psychiatrists should not be confused by criterion D which specifies that ASPD should not occur in the context of schizophrenia or conduct disorder. In forensic practice many patients will have comorbid ASPD with a psychotic illness – although it will be necessary to disentangle whether the criminal behaviour being assessed was due to the psychosis or ASPD, which is not always straightforward.

Antisocial Personality Disorder *DSM*-5 301.7 (F60.2)

A. Disregard for and violation of others' rights since age 15, as indicated by one of the seven sub features:

1. Failure to obey laws and norms by engaging in behavior which results in criminal arrest, or would warrant criminal arrest
2. Lying, deception, and manipulation, for profit or self-amusement
3. Impulsive behavior
4. Irritability and aggression, manifested as frequently assaults others, or engages in fighting
5. Blatantly disregards safety of self and others
6. A pattern of irresponsibility
7. Lack of remorse for actions (American Psychiatric Association, 2013)

The other diagnostic criteria are:

B. The person is at least age 18
C. Conduct disorder was present by history before age 15
D. The antisocial behavior does not occur in the context of schizophrenia or bipolar disorder (American Psychiatric Association, 2013)

Conduct Disorder 312.8x (F91.x)

1. A repetitive and persistent pattern of behavior in which the basic rights of others or major age-appropriate societal norms or rules are violated, as manifested by the presence of at least three of the following 15 criteria in the past 12 months from any of the categories below, with at least one criterion present in the past 6 months:

Aggression to People and Animals

1. Often bullies, threatens, or intimidates others.
2. Often initiates physical fights.
3. Has used a weapon that can cause serious physical harm to others (e.g., a bat, brick, broken bottle, knife, gun).
4. Has been physically cruel to people.
5. Has been physically cruel to animals.
6. Has stolen while confronting a victim (e.g., mugging, purse snatching, extortion, armed robbery).
7. Has forced someone into sexual activity.

Destruction of Property

8. Has deliberately engaged in fire setting with the intention of causing serious damage.
9. Has deliberately destroyed others' property (other than by fire setting).

Deceitfulness or Theft

10. Has broken into someone else's house, building, or car.
11. Often lies to obtain goods or favours or to avoid obligations (i.e., 'cons' others).
12. Has stolen items of nontrivial value without confronting a victim (e.g., shoplifting, but without breaking and entering; forgery).

Serious Violations of Rules

13. Often stays out at night despite parental prohibitions, beginning before age 13 years.
14. Has run away from home overnight at least twice while living in the parental or parental surrogate home, or once without returning for a lengthy period.
15. Is often truant from school, beginning before age 13 years.

2. The disturbance in behaviour causes clinically significant impairment in social, academic, or occupational functioning.
3. If the individual is age 18 years or older, criteria are not met for antisocial personality disorder.

Specify whether:

312.81 (F91.1) Childhood-onset type: Individuals show at least one symptom characteristic of conduct disorder prior to age 10 years.

312.82 (F91.2) Adolescent-onset type: Individuals show no symptom characteristic of conduct disorder prior to age 10 years.

312.89 (F91.9) Unspecified onset: Criteria for a diagnosis of conduct disorder are met, but there is not enough information available to determine whether the onset of the first symptom was before or after age 10 years.

Moffitt proposed that delinquency conceals two distinct categories of individuals, each with a unique natural history and aetiology: a small group engages in antisocial behaviour at every life stage, whereas a larger group is antisocial only during adolescence. According to the theory of life-course-persistent antisocial behaviour, children's neuropsychological problems interact cumulatively with their criminogenic environments across development, culminating in a pathological personality. According to the theory of adolescence-limited antisocial behaviour, a contemporary maturity gap encourages teens to mimic antisocial behaviour in ways that are normative and adjustive, although this group will mature out of the behaviour by adulthood [44].

The appearance of a series of violent offences occurring in later life is unusual and should prompt investigation of the onset of psychiatric morbidity as a causal factor. Heavy use of alcohol is the most common factor associated with late onset, but this group is also associated with more forms of ill-health and hospitalisations [45]. However, it can be seen that the second vignette earlier fits this category. Experience will reveal that a proportion of patients with psychotic illness begin to show recorded criminal offences for the first time following development of a psychotic illness, sometimes with re-admissions to hospital following arrests by the police, and coinciding with re-appearance of symptoms due to failure to take medication and accept follow-up in the community. Hodgins proposed that among violent offenders with schizophrenia, there are three distinct types defined by the age of onset of antisocial and violent behaviour [46]. The early starters display a pattern of antisocial behaviour that emerges in childhood or early adolescence, well before illness onset, which remains stable across the lifespan. The largest group of violent offenders with schizophrenia show no antisocial behaviour prior to the onset of the illness and then repeatedly engage in aggressive behaviour towards others. A small group of individuals who display a chronic course of schizophrenia show no aggressive behaviour for one or two decades after illness onset and then engage in serious violence towards, often killing, those who care for them. This typology, while not fitting all cases encountered in forensic practice, does correspond to many a trainee will encounter in the future.

Drug and Alcohol Misuse

The associations between alcohol and drug misuse and violence are probably the most complex on which to give an opinion in forensic assessments. This chapter has explained why current research into the relationship between psychosis and substance misuse has been unhelpful and misleading. It has also suggested a new approach to the study of symptoms of psychosis and violence. However, in the latter, there has been no investigation of the effects of substances on symptoms leading to violence and this will be important in future research. It is therefore important to look at previous research findings and see to what extent these can guide a forensic assessment. Forensic psychiatrists will frequently be required to decide whether substances were relevant to violent behaviour and should be well acquainted with criminal law in relation to intoxication.

White [47] describes three basic explanatory models for the relationship between alcohol/drug use and violence: (a) substance use causes violence; (b) violence leads to substance use: (c) it is spurious, or coincidental, being explained by a set of common causes. These need to be considered when evaluating epidemiological research findings, but also when considering individual cases in a forensic assessment.

Causal Relationships

There is more than one causal model. The first is due to psychopharmacological properties of intoxication which can include disinhibition, cognitive-perceptual distortions, attention deficits, bad judgement and neurochemical changes. In addition, chronic intoxication may result in withdrawal, sleep deprivation, impairment of neuropsychological functioning or exacerbation of personality disorders, including borderline personality disorder leading to violence.

The second model is economic motivation to obtain income to buy drugs, typically robbery. The third systemic model argues that a system of drug distribution and use is inherently connected with violence. This includes violence for territory where drug sales take place, particularly involving street gangs, enforcing rules, punishments for non-payment of debts, arguments during transactions, robberies from drug dealers or buyers, and where dissatisfied parties cannot go to the police or courts to resolve disagreements. A key public health consideration is that drug markets can create community disorganisation, which in turn affects the behaviour of others in the community and increases violence among many other persons.

A final model is that drug and alcohol misuse are part of a causal pathway leading to violence which is mediated by symptoms of mental disorder. For example, persons with schizophrenia who abuse drugs such as stimulants, hallucinogens and cannabis can relapse into an acute psychotic episode or their symptoms may be exacerbated, leading to violent behaviour. Similarly, patients who chronically abuse drugs and alcohol may fail to take medication, leading to relapse. However, it is the symptoms of psychosis that have a direct causal effect on the violence and not the drugs or alcohol, and where the latter may not be directly and immediately relevant at the time of the violence. However, if both symptoms which had a causal relationship with violence are present at the same time as intoxication, it can be difficult to disentangle the effects of each separately. In most cases, it may be possible to differentiate the symptoms as having a causal effect and the substances as further disinhibiting behaviour driven by symptoms or exacerbating the symptoms. However, it is important to be aware of the law regarding intoxication. Voluntary intoxication leading to exacerbation of symptoms which in turn leads to violence may not convince a court that there is a defence against conviction, despite clear evidence of symptoms, for example *R v Quick* in a defence of insanity.

Forensic psychiatrists will occasionally be asked to give an opinion as to whether an individual showed an abnormal violent reaction to a prescribed drug when there have been similar adverse drug reports. These cases are best argued in court together with an expert in psychopharmacology. It is important to be aware that the relationship may not be causal and that evidence may be produced to attribute a motive and to challenge evidence in court, requiring a careful assessment of the circumstances and the individual's history. However, factors indicative of an adverse reaction include cases when there appear to be more reports than would be expected for a particular drug considering the number of prescriptions in the populations (proportional reporting ratio), unusual demographics (older and female), early onset of psychiatric symptoms (usually within a few days), a senseless act of aggression/violence directed at anyone who happened to be nearby, and resolution of the symptoms upon discontinuation of the drug.

Violence Leads to Substance Misuse

Individuals who are aggressive are more likely to become involved in situations and subcultures in which drug and alcohol use are encouraged. This can include a professional criminal lifestyle. Aggressive individuals are also more likely to use drugs to self-medicate, for example cannabis to make violence less likely and to calm themselves. However, it can also be used to give individuals an excuse or courage to act aggressively.

Spurious Relationship

Substance use and violence are related coincidentally because they share common causes, for example genetic or temperamental traits and ASPD, and consequently there is no causal relationship. White [47] describes the 'routine activities' perspective where violence occurs most often when and where people are drinking, particularly in certain bars where social controls are weakened. Similarly, it can occur in subcultures where violence and heavy drinking are considered proof of masculinity, which would spuriously inflate the relationship and where situational factors increase violence risk.

A spurious relationship needs to be considered in certain epidemiological studies of violence which assert that conditions such as schizophrenia do not cause violence and that the association is due to substance misuse. This is a common conclusion using case registers and some surveys where drug misuse is recorded in case files or a comorbid diagnostic category of drug misuse disorder is recorded as well as a diagnosis of schizophrenia. In some studies, statistical adjustments are then made for the substance misuse disorder and the odds of association with schizophrenia are then attenuated, leading to the conclusion that the association was confounded. However, unless it can be established when the drugs had been used and whether this coincided with the violence, and also whether symptoms had been present at the material time, these conclusions cannot be drawn. Taking the case of the first vignette earlier with a comorbid diagnosis of ASPD, it is likely that many violent events, probably the majority over the patient's life course, had occurred at times when the patient was *not* psychotic. However, that does not necessarily mean that psychotic symptoms had never had a direct causal effect on the patient's violence. Because of downwards social drift and because schizophrenia is more common among the poor, persons with schizophrenia often reside in communities with high levels of crime and drug misuse, where violence is more common, and as a result of their illness they also misuse drugs which are more freely available to them in these areas.

References

1. Trochette NAC, van den Brink RHS, Beintema H et al. Risk assessment and shared care planning in out-patient forensic psychiatry: cluster-randomised controlled trial. *British Journal of Psychiatry* 2013; 202 (5): 365–71.

2. Abderhalden C, Needham I, Dassen T et al. Structured risk assessment and violence in acute psychiatric wards: randomised controlled trial. *British Journal of Psychiatry* 2008; 193: 44–50.

3. van de Sande HLI, Nijman EO, Noorthoorn AI et al. Aggression and seclusion on acute psychiatric wards: effect of short-term risk assessment. *British Journal of Psychiatry* 2011; 199: 473–8.

4. Krug E, Dahlberg L, Mercy J, Zwi A, Lozano R. *World Report on Violence and Health*. Geneva, World Health Organization, 2002.

5. United Nations Office on Drugs and Crime. *Global Study on Homicide*. 2019 edition. www.unodc.org/unodc/en/data-and-analysis/global-study-on-homicide-2019.html.

6. Pinker S. *The Better Angels of Our Nature: Why Violence Has Declined*. New York, Viking, 2011.

7. Coid J. The epidemiology of abnormal homicide and murder followed by suicide. *Psychological Medicine* 1983; 13: 855–60.

8. Siebenforcher M, Fritz FD, Irarrazaval M et al. Psychiatric beds and prison populations in 17 Latin American countries between 1991 and 2017: rates, trends and an inverse relationship between the two indicators. *Psychological Medicine* 2022; 52 (5): 936–45.

9. Taylor PJ, Gunn J. Homicides by people with mental illness: myth and reality. *British Journal of Psychiatry* 1999; 174: 9–14.

10. Large M, Smith G, Swinson N, Shaw J, Neilssen O. Homicide due to mental disorder in England and Wales over 50 years. *British Journal of Psychiatry* 2008; 193 (2): 130–3.

11. Nielssen O, Large M. Rates of homicide during the first episode of psychosis and after treatment: a systematic review and meta-analysis. *Schizophrenia Bulletin* 2010; 36 (4): 702–12.

12. Baird A, Webb RT, Hunt IM, Appleby L, Shaw J. Homicide by men diagnosed with schizophrenia: national case–control study. *BJPsych Open* 2020; 6 (6): e143.

13. Fazel S, Gulati G, Linsull L, Geddes JR, Grann M. Schizophrenia and violence: systematic review and meta-analysis. *PLOS Medicine* 2009; 6 (8): e1000120.

14. Fazel S, Langstrom N, Hjern A, Grann M, Lichtenstein P. Schizophrenia, substance abuse, and violent crime. *Journal of the American Medical Association* 2009; 301 (19): 2016–23.

15. Langan PA, Farrington DP. *Criminal Justice in the United States and in England and Wales 1981-96.* Washington, DC, Bureau of Statistics, Office of Justice Programs, US Department of Justice, 1998.

16. Sivarajasingam V, Page N, Green G, Moore S, Shepherd J. *Violence in England and Wales by 2018: An Accident and Emergency Perspective.* Cardiff, Cardiff University, Crime and Security Research Institute, 2019.

17. Singleton N, Bumpsted R, O'Brien M, Lee A, Meltzer H. *Psychiatric Morbidity among Adults Living in Households, 2000.* The report of the survey carried out by the Social Survey Division of the Office for National Statistics on behalf of the Department of Health, the Scottish Office, and the National Assembly for Wales. London, The Stationery Office, 2001.

18. Coid J. State of Science Review: SR-B11. *Epidemiological Linkages between Mental Ill-Health and Violence: Risk Factors and Wider Consequences.* London, Government Office for Science. UK Government's Foresight Project, Mental Capital and Wellbeing, 2009.

19. Coid J, Yang M, Roberts A et al. Violence and psychiatric morbidity in the national household population of Britain: public health implications. *British Journal of Psychiatry* 2006; 189: 12–19.

20. Coid J, Yang M, Roberts A et al. Violence and psychiatric morbidity in a national household population: a report from the British National Household Survey. *American Journal of Epidemiology* 2006; 164: 1199–208.

21. Shepherd J, Farrington DP. The impact of antisocial lifestyle on health. *British Medical Journal* 2003; 326 (7394): 834–5.

22. Yang M, Coid J. Gender differences in psychiatric morbidity and violent behaviour among a household population in Great Britain. *Social Psychiatry and Psychiatric Epidemiology* 2007; 42: 599–605.

23. Davoren M, Kallis C, Gonzalez RA, Freestone M, Coid JW. Anxiety disorders and intimate partner violence: can the association be explained by coexisting conditions or borderline personality traits? *Journal of Forensic Psychiatry and Psychology* 2017; 28 (5): 639–58.

24. Haapanen RA. *Selective Incapacitation and the Serious Offender: A Longitudinal Study of Criminal Career Patterns.* New York, Springer-Verlag, 1990.

25. Bonta J, Law M, Hanson K. The prediction of criminal and violent recidivism among mentally disordered offenders: a

meta-analysis. *Psychological Bulletin* 1998; 123: 133–42.

26. Monahan J, Steadman HJ. Extending violence reduction principles to justice-involved persons with mental illness. In Dvoskin JA, Skeem JL, Novaco RW, Douglas KS (eds) *Using Social Science to Reduce Violent Offending*. New York, Oxford University Press, 2012.

27. Skeem JC, Kennealy P, Monahan J, Peterson JK, Appelbaum PA. Psychosis uncommonly and inconsistently precedes violence among high risk individuals. *Clinical Psychological Science* 2015; 4 (1): 4–49.

28. Coid JW, Ullrich S, Bebbington P, Fazel S, Keers R. Paranoid ideation and violence: meta-analysis of individual subject data of 7 population surveys. *Schizophrenia Bulletin* 2016; 42 (4): 907–15.

29. Coid JW, Ullrich S, Kallis C et al. The relationship between delusions and violence: findings from the East London first episode psychosis study. *Journal of the American Medical Association Psychiatry* 2013; 70: 465–71.

30. Ullrich S, Keers R, Coid JW. Delusions, anger, and serious violence: new findings from the MacArthur violence risk assessment study. *Schizophrenia Bulletin* 2013; 40: 1174–81.

31. Coid JW, Kallis C, Doyle M, Shaw J, Ullrich S. Shifts in positive and negative psychotic symptoms and anger: effects on violence. *Psychological Medicine* 2018; 48: 14.

32. Keers R, Ullrich S, DeStavola BL, Coid JW. Association of violence with emergence of persecutory delusions in untreated schizophrenia. *American Journal of Psychiatry* 2014; 171: 332–9.

33. Coid JW, Ullrich S, Kallis C et al. Improving risk management for violence in mental health services: a multi-methods approach. *NHS National Institute for Health Research* 2016; 4 (16).

34. Coid JW, Yang M, Ullrich S et al. Psychiatric diagnosis and differential risks of offending following discharge.

International Journal of Law and Psychiatry 2015; 38: 68–74.

35. Zamble E, Quinsey VL. *The Criminal Revidivism Process*. Cambridge, Cambridge University Press, 1997.

36. Freestone MC, Ullrich S, Coid JW. External trigger factors for violent offending: findings from the UK Prisoner Cohort Study. *Criminal Justice and Behavior* 2017; 44 (11): 1389–1412.

37. Sariaslan A, Lichentstein P, Larsson H, Fazel S. Triggers for violent criminality in patients with psychiatric disorders. *JAMA Psychiatry* 2016; 73 (8): 796–803.

38. Rosell DR, Siever LY. The neurobiology of aggression and violence. *CNS Spectrums* 2015; 20: 254–79.

39. Calhoun FS, Weston S. *Contemporary Threat Management*. San Diego, CA, Specialised Training Services, 2003.

40. *Disrupting the Path to Violence*. Trainer manual. Nebraska Emergency Management Agency, Two Rivers Public Health Department, University of Nebraska Public Policy Center, 1 January 2019. cve.unl.edu.

41. MacCulloch MJ, Snowden PR, Wood PJ, Mills HE. Sadistic fantasy, sadistic behaviour and offending. *British Journal of Psychiatry* 1983; 143: 20–9.

42. Farrington DP. Criminal career research in the United Kingdom. *British Journal of Criminology* 1992; 32 (4): 521–36.

43. Moffitt TE, Caspi A, Harrington H, Milne BJ. Males on the life-course-persistent and adolescent-limited antisocial pathways: follow-up at age 26 years. *Developmental Psychopathology* 2002; 14 (1): 179–207.

44. Moffitt TE. Adolescence-limited and life-course-persistent antisocial behaviour: a developmental taxonomy. *Psychological Reviews* 1993; 100 (4): 674–701.

45. Skinner GM, Farrington DP, Shepherd JP. Offender trajectories, health, and hospital admissions: relationships and risk factors in the longitudinal Cambridge Study in Delinquent Development. *Journal of the*

Royal Society of Medicine 2020; 113 (3): 110–18.

46. Hodgins S. Violent behaviour among people with schizophrenia: a framework for an investigation of causes, and effective treatment, and prevention. *Philosophical Transactions of the Royal Society of London.* *Series B, Biological Sciences* 2008; 363 (1503): 2505–18.

47. White HR. Alcohol, illicit drugs, and violence. In DM Stoff, J Breiling, JM Maser (eds) *Handbook of Antisocial Behaviour.* New York, John Wiley, 1997, pp. 511–23.

Violence and Mental Disorder
Clinical Considerations

Harry Kennedy

Introduction

Violence is common. Children play at it, team sports permit it and computer games simulate it. Archaeological studies suggest that violence was one of the most common causes of death up to relatively recent times. One scholar claims that in modern times violence has never been so rare [1]. However rare, immoral or socially dysfunctional violence may be, none of these imply that violence is necessarily pathological in origin or evidence of psychopathology. Violence is, however, a public health issue. All psychiatrists will need to be able to assess and treat problems related to violence occurring in the mentally ill and mentally disordered. Forensic psychiatrists offer treatment for the small amount of serious violence in society that is due to mental disorder.

Violence may be defined as the intentional use of physical force, either threatened or actual, against persons that either results in or has a high likelihood of resulting in injury, psychological harm or death. This definition identifies four means by which violence may be inflicted: physical, sexual and psychological attack, and (illegal) deprivation of liberty. A dangerous offender is a person who has been convicted of a very serious sexual or very serious violent crime against persons and who presents a high likelihood of reoffending with further very serious sexual or very serious violent crimes against persons [2].

Violence is strongly influenced by social factors such as population density, material deprivation and lack of social cohesion. In this there is a similarity between violence to others and suicide, as well as violence to self [3]. Population surveys suggest that interpersonal violence is very common. Surveys in the USA and the UK yield a recent six-month prevalence of 2% for adults, with the majority of this perpetrated by men, the majority being within the home and within family or intimate relationships, mainly against women and girls, but also against elders, children, the mentally ill and healthcare workers, including mental health professionals.

The psychiatry and psychology of violence are related but must be distinguished. A psychological explanation for violence is not evidence of abnormality of mind. Nor does explanation always excuse. Explanations in psychology and psychiatry are not the same as explanations in physics and engineering. A causal explanation should always be sought but is seldom found.

Meaningful explanations are satisfying, more so when in the form of a narrative that tends to ameliorate responsibility, justify morally or forgive guilt. But such explanations are often unrelated to causation. There is some evidence that in the months before onset of a relapse of schizophrenia there may be more life events, at least when elicited retrospectively. But retrospective recall is biased and not all life events are independent of the patient and their developing illness [4]. The statistical approach adopted in early studies of life events, difficulties and vulnerabilities in depression was quickly found to be flawed in the way the statistical model was designed. Where an effect can arise from several causes, the best that can be done is to offer a weak inference; to say 'in some cases of A, some instances of B may follow' [5, 6]. Predisposing vulnerabilities and sensitisers, trigger events and provocations may make meaningful sense but may not be as independent and causal as they appear. For example, life events appear to run in families so that 'independent' life events may still be non-independent from a nature–nurture perspective [7]. This is not to deny that all violence is a contextual and interpersonal event; what matters is the extent to which a violent person influences or shapes their own context and generates or at least shapes their interactions.

A causal factor should be antecedent, proximate and explanatory. A good explanation should be parsimonious, compatible with known facts and processes, hard to vary, falsifiable and a better explanation than other possible explanations. It may have 'reach', explaining other phenomena too. The relationship between a violent act and antecedent circumstances can to some extent be divided into remote causes or predispositions, proximate causes and immediate precipitants [8]. Epidemiological studies of case register material tend to emphasise stable and long-term risks or exposures, dispositions and traits such as antisocial personality and aggressive traits, low empathy, and pro-violent attitudes, while underestimating the effects of short-term but proximate causes such as mental state, intoxication and affect. Psychiatric explanations often make unwarranted assumptions about which is cause and which is effect. Self-reported explanations concerning early or antecedent experiences are often examples of striving after meaning rather than causal. Subjective recollection may itself be regarded as a mediating factor [9].

Violence is not a unitary concept. Violence may be minimally harmful or it may be fatal; planned (deliberative) or impulsive; instrumental (a means to an end) or direct; rational or (expressive) emotional; offensive or defensive; moral or amoral. While some of these characterisations may seem naturally related, they can all be independent of each other. The causes and associations of each type of violence will be different while also overlapping in ways that may reflect common underlying causes or confounding by common social associations.

Epidemiology and Evidence for a Link between Mental Illness and Violence

Although the criminal courts have recognised that mental illness is relevant to crimes of violence in some cases, and may represent mitigation or complete excuse, mental illness was not scientifically linked to violence when early scientific studies tested the clinical and legal consensus [10]. There was a general acceptance that there was no valid link between crime (broadly defined) and mental illness (broadly defined). For fatal or near fatal attacks over a 10-year period in former West Germany, 3% (5% of fatal attacks) were by the mentally abnormal (schizophrenia 53%, affective psychosis 7%, intellectual disability 13%, other organic disorders 22%, epilepsy 5%), comparable to the population prevalence of these disorders (approximately 3–5%). But the risk of violence was 10 times higher for people with schizophrenia than affective or intellectual disability. People with schizophrenia were 100 times more dangerous to themselves than to others, but people with affective disorders were 1,000 to 10,000 times more dangerous to themselves, and people with intellectual disability about equal. Overall, 23% of mentally abnormal violent offenders also attempted suicide (47% of women) at the time or soon after the offence. Violent schizophrenics were older than other violent offenders, had been ill for several years, had dropped out of treatment and offended mostly against first-degree relatives [10–12].

The next development in research recognised that prison samples were biased by discrimination against the mentally ill, while domestic violence by others often went unreported or the perpetrator was not arrested, tried or convicted. Even community clinical samples were biased by those who were in need of assistance due to involvement with the criminal justice system. Some evidence emerged, however, that those with severe mental illnesses such as schizophrenia were over-represented among homicides [13–15]. For men on remand in London, 11% of homicides, 9% of non-fatal assaults and 21% of criminal damage was committed by men with schizophrenia versus a population prevalence in Greater London of 0.1–0.4% [13]. This apparent link between schizophrenia and homicide could not be explained by the closure of asylums [16–18]. First episodes were more strongly linked to violence [19] and homicides, along with lack of treatment [20, 21].

The Epidemiological Catchment Area study in the USA [22, 23] provided an epidemiologically unbiased population sample to examine the prevalence of mental disorders. It demonstrated that all of the common severe mental disorders (schizophrenia, bipolar disorder, delusional disorder, depressive psychosis) were associated with excess rates of interpersonal violence when compared to community controls; violence was also associated with misuse of (not just dependence on) all intoxicants including alcohol, cannabis, stimulants, sedatives and hallucinogens. Severe mental illness appeared also to predispose to substance misuse problems and an interactive effect could be shown between mental illness, substance misuse and violence [22]. This held true even taking into account the effect of urban drift or urban incidence of mental illness and crime at an ecological level [24].

Subsequent studies tended to ignore the macro-level links between severe mental illness, substance misuse and violence while being preoccupied with apparent confounding between these two factors. The choice of mathematical model, the prolonged timescale examined in prospective studies [25, 26] and the reliability of diagnoses in surveys and population case registers may at times have obscured the obvious.

Formulating Causes of Violence from a Psychiatric Perspective

A violent person and their clinical needs cannot readily be formulated from a single defining act. The person's full developmental history of violence may involve many different acts and many different types of violence.

A patient admitted to a secure forensic hospital because of a deliberative, delusionally driven act of serious violence may also have a history of instrumental violence in the course of robberies; the same patient may also have a repetitive history of domestic violence and spousal assault when intoxicated and child abuse at other times; they may display impulsive, expressive acts of interpersonal violence in prisons and hospitals in the context of dominance hierarchies (bullying weaker or less antisocial patients, competing or conspiring with stronger or more antisocial patients). And the same person may have a history of both impulsive non-lethal acts of self-harm to relieve tension and deliberative potentially lethal attempts at suicide.

Each of these patterns of behaviour may in the same person have different biological and psychological processes, social contexts and conscious intentions, though there may also be some uniting factors such as early exposure to violence and recurrent intoxication. Formulation that is intended to produce a plan of care, treatment and structures to reduce the risk of future violence and reduce the seriousness of future violence may have to focus narrowly or be focused selectively on a variety of such problems.

Anger

Anger can be shown to be a proximate cause of violence, for example explaining why some delusions lead to violence on some occasions [27, 28]. Signs of anger and imminent violence include pallor, tachycardia, narrowed attentional range and behaviours including raised voice, staring, grimacing, intrusion into another person's body space, threatening words and preliminary acts of aggression and provocation – pushing, shoving, spitting. Anger, with positive symptoms and personality disorder, can be a strong predictor of violence in hospitals. Anger is particularly proximate to violence with or without any mental illness. In recent research studies, anger emerges as an explanatory mediating factor between persecutory delusions and violence [25, 28–30]. Anger and its manifestations can be taken as a uniting feature for many of the items in short-term risk assessments such as the Dynamic Appraisal of Situational Aggression (DASA) [31] and Brøset Violence Checklist [32, 33].

Anger can be defined as

> an affective state experienced as the motivation to act in ways that warn, intimidate or attack those who are perceived as challenging or threatening. Anger is coupled to and is inseparable from a sensitivity to the perception of challenges or a heightened awareness of threats (irritability). This affective motivation and sensitivity can be subjectively experienced even if no external action occurs. This definition requires little alteration to describe fear. The sensitivity to challenge and threat would be the same, but the affective motivation experienced would instead be to escape, appease, or avoid.[34]

While rages or anger attacks can be described in this way, there is also a rich psychopathological literature describing resentment and prolonged states or grievance and querulousness. There is some limited support in classical psychopathology for anger as the source of paranoid and delusional states.

Of note, the Research Diagnostic Criteria (RDoC) [35] do not refer to anger but deal with 'aggression' under two domains: (1) defensive aggression, which is elicited by a real or perceived threat that leads to a pattern of behaviours directed at terminating the threat. As such, instances of defensive aggression could be considered to belong under the 'responses to acute threat' construct; (2) offensive (proactive) aggression, elicited by competition over resource acquisition or other positive consequences. This form of aggression often arises from differences in social status and dominance.

Fear and anxiety are increasingly related and distinguished through the RDoC approach of relating to neural circuits. RDoC breaks down negative valence symptoms into acute threat (fear), potential threat (anxiety), sustained threat, loss and frustrative non-reward constructs. Anxiety is strongly associated with violence, for example intimate partner violence in both men and women [36]. Anxiety includes categories such as generalised anxiety disorder, panic disorder, social anxiety and post-traumatic stress disorder. Davoren et al. [36] reviewed the relationship between early exposure to witnessing violence, childhood abuse, neglect and insecure attachment and the later relationship with intimate emotionally unstable personality disorder traits such as frantic attempts to avoid abandonment, impulsivity and difficulty controlling anger, which together explained 58.3% of the association between anxiety disorders and intimate partner violence, with intense unstable relationships also significant in women. Anxiety disorders, particularly panic disorder, are strongly associated with alcohol and substance misuse which lead to cycles of intoxication and withdrawal, when rebound symptoms that are more severe than the symptoms originally quelled by the intoxicant are prominent. There is a relationship between panic attacks and rage attacks in unipolar depression which initially appeared possibly related to serotonergic dysfunction, described by Fava et al. [37, 38].

Others have mined a rich but tangled network of neuropharmacological relationships between anxiety disorders, personality disorders, impulsivity, explosive outbursts and self-harm to generate intermittent explosive disorder. This has become more confused by the need to distinguish the relatively objective biological correlates of impulsive angry violence and new operationally defined, overlapping diagnostic entities such as impulsive explosive disorder and disruptive mood dysregulation disorder, as well as attention deficit hyperactivity disorder, antisocial personality disorder, emotionally unstable personality disorder (borderline personality disorder) and schizophrenia. Analysis of the early natural history and co-occurrence of problems is likely the best guide to origins of violence and aggression, since such patterns may become fixed in later life and less clearly related to the biological and environmental factors that gave rise to them. Assessment, identification and specialised treatment of anger in the context of anxiety disorders are critical to reducing burden.

Moral Beliefs, Sentiments and Delusions

Moral beliefs and moral sentiments can have a paradoxical explanatory relationship with violent acts [39]. Although moral beliefs are strongly related in their content to culture and era, there is some evidence for a structural constancy of form across cultures and time. There is some evidence that some delusions may be understood as 'moral delusions' and such delusions are associated with more serious violence, including homicide [40].

According to Haidt, there are five moral domains that can be subdivided into two domains. Individuating domains include care–harm and fairness–injustice. Binding domains include loyalty–betrayal, authority–rebellion and purity sacredness–taboo [41]. Moral beliefs are said to be universal, actionable and punishable. Breaches or affronts to moral behaviour can give rise to angry acts. Ideological and fundamentalist lone actors, terrorist groups and violent political uprisings can all be driven by a sustained and shared moral outrage in which extreme sacrifices are accepted over rational risk–benefit deliberations [42].

Coercive control, spousal assault, child abuse and school bullying may all in some circumstances be related to socialised or unsocialised moral beliefs. Shame inflicted on others through scorn, mockery or 'mobbing' often plays a part in these forms of violence. Moral self-justification for violence should always be treated with scepticism and should not be taken at face value as the true reason or the only reason for a violent act or pattern of actions. Claims for moral justification of a violent act are inevitably also self-justifying.

Amoral Violence

Not all violent actors believe they are acting morally. Egocentric acts may require no moral self-justification. Robberies with violence to fund drug debts and instrumental violence in the course of rape are usually ego-syntonic and do not require even the subjective justification of a sense of entitlement, though such theorising and justifications may be offered after the event.

Cognitive distortions and denials include blaming the victim; rationalising that legal and social prohibitions are mistaken, for example because the act is supposedly legally or morally justified in other cultures or legal systems; or claiming to have acted out of character or not to have been in one's normal state ('I was not myself') [43] – these all represent forms of denial of responsibility.

Simply denying the act itself is often a prudent defence in a criminal process, putting the victim to trial by cross-examination. As a strategy, reserving the option of a late change of plea is a good bet, having seen how the victim bears up under trial by endurance, often with shaming and implied character criticism to discredit the victim. Denial should not be mistaken for a dissociative state, an organic amnesia or concussion. Denial of the act alleged should never in itself be evidence for unfitness to stand trial.

Amnesia for a Criminal Act

Amnesia for a criminal act can arise in some circumstances including (a) the presence of a small number of organic disorders, such as epileptic automatism or hypoglycaemia; (b) a psychotic paramnesia, such as a delusional memory; (c) severe intoxication resulting in an 'alcoholic blackout'; (d) so-called 'crimes of passion'; and (e) malingering [44–47]. Nor is amnesia for a criminal act grounds for a finding of unfitness to stand trial (*R v Podola* [1960]). Amnesia is also never sufficient evidence in itself for lack of capacity to form a criminal intent at the time of a violent act.

False Confessions and Suggestibility

False confessions are more common than is often realised. Miscarriages of justice can arise in such cases. A common factor may be 'source amnesia' or 'memory distrust syndrome' [48, 49] when the source of a piece of information is incorrectly recalled. A classification and system for assessing the reliability of confessions has been described in terms of three established error pathways to false confessions and wrongful convictions: misclassification or bias by investigators and sometimes by psychiatrists; coercion by police interviewers (coerced compliant confessions and coerced internalised confessions); and contamination. According to Dr James McKeith, the best way of preventing miscarriages of justice due to false confession is to ensure that conviction should not be possible based only on a confession that is not corroborated by other independent, objective and reliable factual evidence.

Developmental Factors and Violence

Normal development can be seen as a series of milestones, forks in the road and derailments. These are only metaphors and may not represent any reality. Early developmental delays may progress to global intellectual disability, to patchy focal deficits or to impairments in theory of mind and language manifesting as autistic spectrum disorder.

Attention deficit with or without hyperactivity may be related to patchy cognitive impairments. All of these have been linked to polygenic inheritance and overlap syndromes. Attention deficit hyperactivity disorder (ADHD) can in some cases progress to conduct disorder, though not all conduct disorder arises from ADHD.

Conduct disorder gives rise to functional impairments in school, in the family and in the community. Although behavioural problems including violence may be confined to one of these three domains, typically violence and other behavioural problems emerge in all three settings.

Early-onset substance misuse is difficult to disentangle as cause or effect but is a typical feature of the progression to antisocial personality disorder.

Violence in conduct disorder may be a reflection of early exposure to violence in the home as victim, as witness or both, with the best evidence coming from long-term prospective observational cohort studies [50–53]. Violence may emerge as part of an oppositional-defiant pattern of behaviour. At the risk of over-explanation, oppositional-defiant behaviours often appear in the context of patchy cognitive impairment, frustration, parental difficulties and trauma.

Delinquent and antisocial personality traits including rule-breaking behaviour, deception and fraud, violence, and self-harm may all emerge as part of a transgenerational pattern. Often these traits are found in a young person who is well integrated in a delinquent social group. Gang membership is not necessarily a marker of socialised adaptation. Gang membership selects those who are alienated and unable to participate in mainstream society, and in turn generates psychiatric morbidity through constant tension, fear of other gangs and fear of other gang members [54, 55]. Patterns that emerge over time include adolescent-limited, late-onset and persistent offending [56, 57]. Much less common is the asocial young offender. The early onset of substance misuse can be seen as one of the most parsimonious explanations for the emergence of antisocial and violent behaviour [58].

Family and social roles can come into play: a person suffering from panic disorder and agoraphobia can generate a powerful secondary family structure in which they occupy a position of power and control through dependency. This becomes an important continuing factor for agoraphobia long after panic attacks have become infrequent. Much the same happens in the families of a person with rage attacks. The person need seldom repeat a rage attack to command a secondary family structure in which their minor domestic demands are promptly met. At the same time, a social reputation as a 'hard man' or a champion in the neighbourhood – an honour not to be disrespected – is a further reward that is difficult to relinquish.

Explanations for and Causes of Violence

Distinguishing explanation from cause can be difficult with organic factors naturally claiming precedence, even though they may be remote risks and contributory rather than proximate causes. Social factors play a particularly large role in the processes of labelling and engagement with the youth and criminal justice system. Living in socially deprived and densely populated areas and in areas with poor social cohesion all predispose towards early involvement with social care and criminal justice agencies. Family breakdown, family history of substance misuse and mental illness all form parts of a social milieu that can lead on to conduct disorder, delinquency and long-term engagement with the criminal justice system.

High population density, economic deprivation and lack of social cohesion are all related to recorded rates of crimes of violence, homicide and suicide. The relationship is non-linear with steep increases in violence and suicide above population means for deprivation and population density [3, 59]. Social cohesion can be protective even where economic deprivation is severe [60], with observable effects on use of forensic psychiatry services [61–63].

Intoxication

Intoxication has perhaps the single strongest association with violence [64]. Intoxication is much more than the brief euphoriant effects of psychoactive substances, extending over time into dysphoric states, anxiety, depression, paranoia, withdrawal, confusion and delirium and more prolonged states of psychosis. The early onset of substance misuse is commonly missed unless specific questions are asked. It is the age at first use of each of a series of intoxicants that is most informative, not attempt to date the onset of dependence syndrome. In delinquent populations, first use of tobacco, volatile substances, alcohol and cannabis commonly occurs at around age 12. The newly recognised diagnosis of intermittent explosive disorder was held to precede the onset of substance use disorder in a cross-sectional retrospective survey, but this is complicated by the relationship of this disorder itself to other overlapping diagnostic categories.

Both panic and rage are commonly comorbid with dependence on alcohol, cannabis or benzodiazepines. These give short-term relief of autonomic symptoms, but with chronic use, tolerance may exacerbate the frequency of attacks, probably by lowering the threshold for autonomic reactions and for perception of threat. Substance misuse, by association with rage and panic, acquires in most cultures a double-standard role, a badge of both prestige and shame.

In this context, the relationship of cause and effect between intoxication and withdrawal states on the one hand and on the other hand attention deficit, hyperactivity, conduct disorder, panic, rage, explosive outbursts and expressive impulsive violence may be seen as circular. Drug debts, delinquent and drug-involved peer groups and gangs, acquisitive offending, robbery and instrumental violence follow [55].

The earlier the onset of any use of any intoxicant, the more likely it is that an enduring pattern of polysubstance misuse and dependence will develop, often with a progression from cheap and readily available intoxicants to more expensive and more addictive substances. There may be an overlap between chemical and behavioural 'excessive appetites' [65] that is of relevance when assessing functional mental capacity or for courts when assessing responsibility.

Sedative drugs (alcohol, cannabis, benzodiazepines and their many congeners) all cause short-term cycles of intoxication with impaired perception and judgement (misperception of slights, challenges or provocations), disinhibition (increased sensitivity and irritability) and impaired ability to change cognitive set (inability to accept apology or appeasement); tolerance develops rapidly so that very high doses are taken. In this state, any minor event or misperception can lead to an escalation of aggression and to violence.

While intoxication is usually obvious to the person themselves and to others, withdrawal states occur over longer periods of time and may be more subtle. Depending on the pharmacokinetics and metabolism of the substance or cocktail of substances concerned, a withdrawal state may commence within a few hours or a few days after ingestion; it may last for a few hours or a few days or even months when intoxication has been continuous and heavy, so that down-regulated or sensitised receptor sensitivities need to metabolically readjust. Kraepelin described the complex transitions of acute psychosis often with delirium, followed by a psychosis that can last weeks or months, particularly where multiple drugs have been used ('morphinism and cocainism') for prolonged periods [66, 67] and not the very brief psychotic episodes described for isolated use of amphetamine by Connell, who also recognised prolonged and persistent states due to combined use of methamphetamine and barbiturates [68, 69].

Withdrawal states may represent amplified versions of the opposite state of intoxication. Alcohol and benzodiazepines alleviate tension and anxiety while withdrawal will cause a more intense rebound, with tremulousness, anxiety, panic and rage. Cocaine, amphetamine, mephedrone and other stimulant drugs can give rise to an angry, assertive and domineering mental state with sensitivity and irritability that persists for prolonged periods after acute intoxication. Sensitive and overvalued ideas, illusions and hallucinations may occur at times, though often with partially preserved insight. These prolonged periods of mixed intoxication, withdrawal and occasional confusion were first described by Kraepelin (66, 67).

From a forensic point of view, there may be a more important distinction between intoxicated and unintoxicated states (see *R v Tandy* [1989]) than the debate about the relationship between cannabis psychosis and the subsequent development of a persistent schizophrenia. Case law concerning the admissibility of intoxication, craving or alcohol-induced brain damage as abnormalities of mind for the purpose of a psychiatric defence is often arbitrary and changeable over time. In general, intoxication is not accepted as a mental abnormality on the grounds that it is a foreseeable consequence of a voluntary decision made while sober – at the time of the first drink of the day, for example. The case of *Tandy* sets out the legal reasoning in relation to such matters.

Intoxication may be the habit of a lifetime or a brief interlude of dependence and addiction followed by a lifetime of abstinence. A return to 'controlled drinking' following a period of dependence and addiction is a seductive fiction unsupported by evidence. This should, however, be distinguished from harm reduction.

Harm reduction, the policy of engaging and holding those with dangerous addictions by prescribing safer substitutes, may reduce the risk of virus transmission through shared needles and it may reduce the risk of death due to overdose in the context of lost tolerance. Very few of those enrolled in harm reduction and substitute programmes remain fully abstinent from harmful street drugs. Harm reduction strategies do not necessarily break any pre-existing relationship between intoxication, violence and offending generally, though it is reasonable to be optimistic that there is some benefit.

Cannabis use is associated with violence over the lifetime [58] and all intoxicants increase the risk of violence [23]. Only prolonged abstinence is an acceptable risk management strategy when the pattern of violence is related to intoxication in any way and probably for anyone with a history of violence that is frequent, severe or fatal in nature.

Abnormal Illness Behaviour and Malingering: Dissociation, Dissimulation and Deception

Deception as a personality trait arises as part of the formulation of causes of violence in a number of ways. Habitual deception is part of the syndrome of antisocial personality disorder. It is also part of the syndrome of psychopathic disorder. Deception therefore commonly complicates the psychiatric assessment of patients presenting because of violence. At its most straightforward, defendants may seek to deceive the psychiatrist concerning the context and mental state in which a violent act was perpetrated.

So-called dissociative states in which a patient fabricates physical or psychological symptoms unknown to themselves probably do not exist, or are not useful as a diagnosis [70]. Neurologists preferentially diagnose factitious presentations (conscious and intentional fabrication of symptoms) in healthcare workers as 'hysterical', possibly to avoid the stigma of simulated illness [71].

The distinction between factitious disorder and malingering is also doubtful since both are intentional [72, 73]. Examples include fugues, non-epileptic seizures, 'pseudo-neurology', false memories, group phenomena and many variants. In all of these, the behaviour concerned is only possible if there are intact mental capacities to perceive, remember and recall, form plans and intentions, and carry out complex and purposeful correctly sequenced actions over time. Since 'mind' is legally defined as a collection of capacities, there is no absence of mind and no evidence for impaired functional mental capacities. An inner state can be inferred from external evidence. These abnormal illness behaviours were at one time thought to arise due to complex 'subconscious' processes. Objective evidence of these 'subconscious' processes or 'lack of integration' is always absent or inherently impossible to demonstrate. Modern philosophy of mind dismisses the possibility of such reifications, along with irresistible impulses and square circles [74]. Such phenomena can arise in some cases as iatrogenic artefacts through suggestion and inappropriate advocacy by therapists. Any of these may be invoked as either a cause of violence or as an obstacle to forensic psychiatric assessment.

Factitious disorder is the conscious, intentional fabrication of symptoms and sometimes fabrication of physical signs in order to gain emotional support. Often what is gained is a measure of control over family members and carers. This may be the context in which Freud's nineteenth-century patients sought refuge in non-organic paralyses, aphonias and feints, not only to gain emotional sympathy and support but also to avoid sexual abuse, forced marriages and forced childbearing and to assert some degree of power in a patriarchal world. Asher described the 'Munchhausen' syndrome in which an abnormal personality travels from hospital to hospital claiming a false identity and false medical history while seeking out extreme and sometimes dangerous investigations and interventions. Intact functional mental capacities and intentionality can always be demonstrated in such cases.

A common underlying feature of such cases is a desire to hurt professional carers – doctors, nurses and other professionals who are drawn into systems of deception. A common feature also is that these deceptions cannot be explained by any 'subconscious' process – they are complex planned and intentional acts of deception. Because the mental capacities of understanding, reasoning, planning and executing complex sequences of goal-directed acts are obviously present, there is no 'absence of mind' – no impaired capacity to form a specific intent or impairment of responsibility.

Modern factitious disorder is found in liaison general hospital psychiatry but also in forensic settings, for example in family courts, civil litigation and occasionally child protection cases due to Munchhausen syndrome by proxy [75]. This is a clear example of violence by deception. The deception of members of the caring professions, the weaponising of complaints procedures and the exploitation and dominance of family and other informal carers may under certain circumstances be seen as the intentional harming of others.

Fraud and malingering are distinguished from factitious disorder by the thinnest of differences. In malingering and fraud, the same fabrication of non-organic 'pseudo-symptoms' occurs, in the same capacitous and intentional way and often with the same goal of dominating or controlling family members and exploiting professional and informal carers. But the added element in fraud and malingering is some material gain such as financial reward, including civil damages, avoidance of criminal responsibility and prison, avoidance of military service, avoidance of deportation, or some other material benefit such as access to opiates or benzodiazepines. Forging or altering prescriptions should indicate that the symptoms complained of were unreliable – exaggerated or fabricated to gain an intoxicant. Added features in some cases include a controlling and demanding elicitation of 'confidence' and the ability to play on the naivety, vanity or greed of the 'mark' [76], included here as a caution for the unwary forensic psychiatrist.

Deception is relevant to violence not only because it may intrude into the assessment of psychiatric defences or mitigation but also because it is a core feature of antisocial personality and psychopathic disorder. Fraud and the deliberate gaining of confidence may be a part of an offence of rape. And fraud or deception may be a part of an instrumental violent act in which material gain is the primary goal.

Emotionally Unstable Personality Disorder

Emotionally unstable personality disorder carries within it many characteristics that can give rise to violence. Rapid and intense mood swings may be related to impulsive, emotionally expressive violence. A pattern of unstable relationships can also give rise to violence both as victim and as perpetrator. The repetitive nature of such relationships makes this an important focus for interventions aimed at future prevention.

Both mood swings and unstable relationships typically occur in the context of comorbid substance misuse and withdrawal [77]. This is particularly true of repetitive self-harm. The mounting tension during withdrawal states can be relieved by cutting superficially. It is essential to avoid the use of benzodiazepines and their congeners (zopiclone, gabapentin) as a means of relieving this tension since benzodiazepines are themselves a likely cause and exacerbation.

Serial Violent and Sexual Offenders

Serial violent and sexual offenders who follow fixed patterns of offending behaviour (sadistic killers, serial sex offenders) are rare. Such offending is seldom if ever related to severe mental illness [78].

The origins of paraphilic sexual behaviour are poorly understood, despite many theories. From a forensic psychiatry perspective, what is important is that the propensity or preference is not in itself a problem, a disorder or mental disorder, however sadistic, gruesome or bizarre – the criminal behaviour arises from acting on such propensities in ways that harm others.

There is a narrative description of fantasies that are tentatively tested out in reality, then escalated until acted out, then as the fantasy loses its power to excite, the fantasy is escalated in sensationalism followed by further testing out (offence-parallelling behaviours) and acting out in reality [79]. This may be relevant to some serial offenders but not to the majority, who simply repeat the same fairly crude offending pattern over time.

What is essential is that the preference or propensity does not inevitably or irresistibly lead to acting on the desire or appetite. Formulations based on ideas of weak will or imperious impulses are themselves misconceptions based on the reification of abstractions and mind–body dualism [74].

Bipolar Disorder

Bipolar disorder was thought to be a rare antecedent for violence other than minor and impulsive, irritable acts of violence, often in hospital. The Epidemiological Catchment Area study found evidence of violence also in the community [22].

Schizophrenia and Psychosis

A link exists between schizophrenia and violence in representative population-based samples [80], particularly when not in contact with treatment services [23] and in prospective studies [25], along with an interactive effect with substance misuse [22] and with antisocial personality traits [81, 82]. A recent systematic review and meta-analysis gives a clear account of this relationship [80]. When compared with community controls, there was an increased risk of violence perpetration in men with schizophrenia and other psychoses (pooled odds ratio (OR), 4.5; 95% confidence interval (CI), 3.6–5.6). The risk was also elevated in women (pooled OR, 10.2; 95% CI, 7.1–14.6). Odds of perpetrating sexual offences (OR, 5.1; 95% CI, 3.8–6.8) and homicide (OR, 17.7; 95% CI, 13.9–22.6) were also investigated. Three studies found increased relative risks of arson. Absolute risks of violence perpetration in register-based studies were less than 1 in 20 in women with schizophrenia spectrum disorders and less than 1 in 4 in men over a 35-year period [80]. The pooled odds of violence perpetration in individuals with schizophrenia spectrum disorders without substance misuse comorbidity (n = 11,079) were 3.5 (95% CI, 2.6–4.6; I2= 81%; 95% CI, 68–89) and 9.9 (95% CI, 7.2–13.5) in individuals with schizophrenia spectrum disorders with substance misuse comorbidity (n = 3,586). Odds ratios did not vary by region. In two studies, unaffected family members had higher odds ratios of violence than unaffected community controls, but patients still had elevated odds ratios for violence when compared to their unaffected family members in Sweden (4.2; 95% CI, 3.8–4.5) [83] and in Israel (2.8; 95% CI, 2.5–3.3) [84]. It is essential to be clear about this to give guidance to all mental health practitioners and to patients themselves.

Schizophrenia is a life-shortening illness, particularly in forensic patients [85]. Although there is a greatly increased risk of death by suicide and there is also a greatly increased risk of death by violence, the greatest excess death rate is due to cardiovascular diseases, respiratory diseases and cancers. It follows that reasoning about long-term goals and gains, or even short- to medium-term planning, may seem irrelevant to a person with a foreshortened sense of their own future. Understanding how apparently irrational choices may arise from such altered life prospects is often relevant for all who engage in violent or other offending behaviour for short-term gratification.

Schizophrenia is highly heritable, with many genes of small effect identified. Identified genes include many that code for structural brain elements. Inflammatory hypotheses are also supported. A developmental derailment in late adolescence has been linked to excessive neural pruning or a dysfunction of brain structural maturation. A developmental impairment of functional cognitive ability including social cognition typically occurs before the onset of delusions and hallucinations.

Early onset of cannabis misuse predisposes to later development of schizophrenia. There may be a distinction between those with onset of schizophrenia as part of a developmental progression from conduct disorder and substance misuse through antisocial personality disorder to psychosis. These may have a better prognosis with less cognitive impairment [86, 87].

Schizophrenia is now staged, like cancers, into stage zero: an at-risk mental state; stage one: brief, limited intermittent psychotic episodes; stage two: relapsing and remitting psychotic episodes with recovery between episodes; stage three: relapsing and remitting with a steady decline between episodes; and stage four: a continuous decline in functional capacity, usually with constant symptoms [88].

First presentations with schizophrenia are often due to dangerous or violent behaviour [19], suggesting that positive rather than negative symptoms, and absence of treatment, are related to such behaviour. Of 253 first episodes of schizophrenia, 52 (20%) had behaved in a potentially life-threatening way, and many more were merely abusive or threatening. The dangerous behaviour was definitely linked to delusions or hallucinations in 23. There was a specific intended victim in 75%; mothers and spouses in 56%. These patients were older and had been ill longer than other first-admission schizophrenics. The patients were rarely prosecuted or criminalised due to tolerance for their illness.

Functional impairment in family, work or education and society is increasingly seen as the real handicap in schizophrenia, more so than symptoms. Repeated or habitual violence is probably the most obvious cause of functional impairment in social roles and relationships. However, this may be a circular relationship between cause and effect. Violent behaviour may recur as a dysfunctional way of coping with frustration and anger due to limited ability and alienation.

Hodgins [82] proposes three broad types in schizophrenia: early starters with antisocial behaviour and violence before the onset of psychosis, continuing regardless of mental state and course of illness; late starters who are not antisocial before the onset of psychosis but become violent after the onset of psychosis; and those who have no violent behaviour before or for a decade or more after onset of psychosis, then commit one act of violence, often killing those who care for them.

The complex interrelationship between violence to others, self-harm and suicide may to some extent be mediated by the increased propensity to substance misuse and dependence. However, this is not a full explanation. Schizophrenia is characterised by delusions (fixed false beliefs not amenable to evidence and not culturally shared) and hallucinations (false perceptions experienced in external reality). Typically delusions follow hallucinations but delusions may persist long after hallucinations have remitted with treatment. There is little evidence for command hallucinations as direct causes for violence, when prospective studies are considered [25]. Thought disorder is also typical, and with negative symptoms such as flattening of affect, avolition and 'autistic' preoccupation with an inner world, it may be relevant to impaired capacity to form criminal intentions and to act on these.

There is increasing recognition that neurocognitive impairments and in particular social cognitive impairments may underpin all of these deficits, leading to impulsive violence, for example the less serious acts of expressive violence in hospitals [89]. Delusions in schizophrenia may arise from hallucinations and other abnormal experiences. When abnormal experiences remit spontaneously or with anti-psychotic medication, delusions may resolve, particularly in a person who is relatively cognitively intact. The more cognitively impaired a person is, the more likely it is that delusions may persist [90].

Impaired social cognition is now recognised as a manifestation of schizophrenia. An impaired ability to understand the thoughts, feelings or intentions of others may lead to the misinterpretation of social interactions and situations. This is not the same as autistic spectrum disorder, in which other impairments in social communication and narrowed interests are also present. However, the relationship with callous and unemotional traits and adult psychopathy has given rise to much research. There is some evidence that impaired social cognition is related to expressive violence in forensic hospital patients. Early onset of cannabis misuse predisposes to later development of schizophrenia.

In a series of elegant re-examinations of large prospective databases, Coid and his research group have shown that a rigorous approach to causation can demonstrate that persecutory delusions when accompanied by anger are closely associated with violent acts [8, 25, 29, 30, 91, 92]. Anti-psychotic medication is an effective way of blocking hallucinations in a large proportion of patients. Anti-psychotic medication is also an effective way of preventing the affective arousal and anger which may lead patients to act violently on their delusional beliefs [93–96]. While there may be scruples about the side effects of anti-psychotic medication in relation to weight gain and metabolic syndrome, the effective prevention of anger and violence [97, 98] will generally outweigh such considerations in those with an established history of serious violence while psychotic.

It is useful to consider whether cognitive remediation therapy can ameliorate functional cognitive impairments. Metacognitive therapy may then ameliorate some of the faulty habits of thinking that lead to the formation or persistence of delusional beliefs. Hallucinations and delusions arise from a dysfunctional mental state that is still poorly understood in neurophysiological and neuropsychological terms. An abnormal affective state in which anger and fear may be primary could explain the content of hallucinations and delusions in the same way that elation and sadness can explain the content of secondary delusions in mania and depression.

There are few positive relationships between symptoms and the severity of violence. Moral beliefs and sentiments are characterised by universality (the belief that everyone should share this moral belief), actionability (the sense that it is right to act on a moral belief and wrong to refrain from acting) and punishability [41]. The moral content of the delusion or system of delusions (harm, injustice, betrayal, abuse of power and authority, impurity or taboo acts) may explain the emotional power, actionability and punishability of delusional beliefs [39]. There is some tentative evidence that delusions with a strong moral form and content may relate to severe violence [40].

Delusional Disorder

Delusional disorder occupies a difficult nosological position between personality disorder and schizophrenia. The diagnosis is characterised by what appear to be delusions or overvalued ideas in the absence of hallucinations or obvious thought disorder. The delusions are non-bizarre in content; that is, they concern matters that are possible in the real world. First-rank symptoms such as thought broadcast, thought withdrawal, made acts and third-party auditory hallucinations in external reality are excluded. Delusions of infidelity, poisoning and persecution are typical and are associated with violence.

There is a strong relationship with alcohol misuse and other substance misuse disorders. Persistent complainers, vexatious litigants, threateners and stalkers overlap significantly with delusional disorder (see Chapter 12). All of these behavioural presentations may as easily be explained as arising from long-standing developmental personality traits [99, 100].

Delusional disorder is poorly responsive to anti-psychotic medication. However, anti-psychotic medication may have the beneficial effect of ameliorating the pervasive anger which characterises such patients and leads to violence.

Organic States

Organic psychosis, drug-induced states, delirium and intellectual disability may all be put forward as explanations for violent acts or as mitigation. Organic psychosis may arise in association with epilepsy, particularly left temporal lobe epilepsy. The syndrome is typically a schizophreniform psychosis with delusions and hallucinations. A useful though not definitive feature is the presence in some cases of an aura, often a recurring smell or an intense emotion. There is a strong association also with prolonged rages that appear to be unrelated to any external precipitant, or else are disproportionate to any real or perceived precipitant. People with epilepsy will usually learn that with the onset of an aura, they should sit down somewhere safe to avoid falls, accidents and other consequences.

The same is often true for post-ictal confusional states and even psychoses. Post-ictal psychoses, however, may be associated with prolonged rages and mood-congruent delusions and are difficult to treat since so many anti-psychotic medications are themselves liable to lower the seizure threshold.

Head injuries and the early stages of neurodegenerative disorders such as Huntington's chorea can also give rise to a coarsening of personality with disinhibition of sexual behaviour and violence. This can occur before the onset of obvious neurological signs. Huntington's may progress in some cases to psychosis and eventually to dementia.

Drug-induced states may also produce a schizophreniform psychosis. Much more commonly, however, drug-induced organic and toxic processes cause a delirium in which there is some degree of disorientation in time, place or person and some degree of impairment of short-term memory, and there may be illusions and overvalued ideas or beliefs which resemble hallucinations and delusions but with surprisingly preserved or partial and fluctuating insight – a realisation that the state is not real but arises from the drugs ingested or the condition concerned. Intellectual disability is sometimes associated with disinhibited appetitive behaviour, including sexual behaviours directed at non-consenting others.

Autistic Spectrum Disorder

Autistic spectrum disorder has emerged in recent years as a challenge to conventional nosology and to medico-legal aspects of responsibility, treatment and long-term supervision. Deficits in theory of mind can now be identified as important also in schizophrenia and other disorders.

Autism itself ranges from an aspect of global or patchy intellectual impairment to a disorder characterised by a lack of empathy and lack of emotional reactivity, or more commonly lack of emotional awareness. At this milder, borderline end of the spectrum, the distinction between innate and acquired traits is often difficult to distinguish. Callous, unemotional traits in childhood can arise in some cases from some forms of childhood abuse and neglect, while also arising in relation to some genetic markers.

Anyone can learn to be unemotional and rational in carrying out tasks that would otherwise be too upsetting to attempt or to do efficiently and effectively. Ambulance crew and emergency technicians, emergency department doctors and nurses, police officers and firefighters, and soldiers in wartime all acquire these adaptive abilities to be rational, unemotional, decisive and actively helpful (compassionate) in the presence of the pain and distress of others. A propensity for cruel and callous acts is not in itself evidence for some organic deficit due to a genetic or developmental process. Nor is the intentional exercise of these abilities or disabilities necessarily free of responsibility.

Memes, Media and Murderous Acts

The description of a social contagion or copycat phenomenon for suicides was identified with media amplification as Werther's phenomenon when a suicide described in a popular literary work by Goethe led to a cluster of similar suicides that achieved some media interest. In modern times the role of media in relaying and amplifying such narratives has been noted. There is also an overlap of important risk factors with other causes of premature death, including accidental deaths. This has been referred to as an aetiological continuum of self-destruction from sub-intentional to intentional [101].

Homicide followed by suicide of the perpetrator occurs in about 10% of homicides in some surveys. At a population-ecological level there is a correlation between homicide rates and suicide rates [3], while the risk factors for violence, homicide, self-harm and suicide overlap extensively [102], though this does not imply that the causes overlap to the same extent. Most homicide-suicides are uxoricides (murder of an intimate partner).

Intimate partner violence is recognised as extremely common in representative sampling of populations, although most goes unreported and unrecorded in crime statistics. As children are exposed to such violence as well as being directly victims of violence, abuse and neglect, it is intimate partner violence that most often figures in theories of transgenerational violence, delinquency, substance misuse, educational failure and mental illnesses, particularly affective illnesses. Men are most often reported as the perpetrators, progressing from one violent relationship to another over time. However, men are also victims of intimate partner violence, with some relationships being mutually violent. Men who are violent to their intimate partners are often violent and antisocial in many situations outside the home, often with comorbid antisocial personality and substance misuse. Women account for a significant amount of intimate partner violence. These women are more likely to be violent only in the home. For men and women, the largest representative combined cross-sectional population sample from two household surveys in the UK [36] found 1.6% admitted to having perpetrated violence towards an intimate partner on at least one occasion in the preceding five years. Females were significantly more likely to admit to having perpetrated intimate partner violence than men. Anxiety disorders (such as generalised anxiety disorder, panic disorder, social phobia and post-traumatic stress disorder) alcohol dependence (particularly in men), drug dependence (particularly in women) depression and emotionally unstable personality disorder were all significantly associated with intimate partner violence and in each case the association was stronger in male perpetrators than in female perpetrators.

Antisocial personality disorder was also significantly associated with perpetration of intimate partner violence; however, this association was stronger among female perpetrators than among male perpetrators. Psychosis was not significantly associated with intimate partner violence, though it was indirectly associated through anxiety. Other mental disorders were strongly associated with anxiety disorders, however, so that in this cross-sectional model, even when adjusted for demographic variables, all contributed significantly to intimate partner violence. For the complete sample, the strongest contributory variables to the association between anxiety disorders and intimate partner violence were emotionally unstable personality disorder, which explained 12.9% of the association, antisocial personality disorder, which explained 11% of the association, and alcohol dependence, which explained 9.2% of the association. Each individual emotionally unstable/borderline trait was also significantly associated with anxiety disorders for the complete sample, males and females. Anxiety disorders were significantly associated with intimate partner violence when controlling for each individual borderline trait on univariate analysis for the complete sample. Using multivariate analysis for the total sample, anxiety disorders remained significantly associated with intimate partner violence. Alcohol dependence, antisocial personality disorder, frantic attempts to avoid abandonment, impulsivity and difficulty controlling anger together explained 58.3% of the association between anxiety disorders and intimate partner violence, with unstable, intense relationships also contributing significantly in women [36].

Coercive control is a relatively new category of crime describing a persistent pattern of controlling, coercive and threatening behaviour, including all or some forms of domestic abuse by a partner or ex-partner. While being the victim of coercive control is not a mental illness in itself, it can give rise to low self-esteem, low expectations, depression and anxiety.

Familicide, sometimes called extended suicide, occurs when a parent kills family members, most often their children and spouse, then kills – or attempts to kill – themselves. There is no single psychiatric diagnosis or typical formulation to describe this phenomenon. Media and sometimes coroners and courts may ask forensic psychiatrists for some easy formula to explain these tragic events.

Infanticide, the killing of a child under the age of one year by the child's mother, is a uniquely defined offence. In some jurisdictions the definition includes a reference to breastfeeding or to puerperal psychosis. This offence was shown to have many and various origins ranging from puerperal psychosis through social stigma and lack of social support [103]. A small proportion of those who kill children, whether infants or older, were described as having 'Medea' syndrome and – where the father is the killer – 'reverse Medea'. Of greater concern in modern times has been the killing of children as an end point of cruelty and neglect [104], often in the context of family dysfunction and barriers to care, including structural racism and communication failures. The perpetrators of such crimes are seldom found to have any psychiatric disorder relevant to a psychiatric defence or therapeutic disposal. Complex issues arise when social work, health services and mental health services intersect, exposing mental health and other healthcare professionals to vicarious liability, or at least to criticism (see Chapter 3).

The killing of parents is similarly associated with a range of disorders, but more commonly arises in the course of schizophrenia and may at times be related to delusional misidentification syndromes [105]. This is the most common presentation for patients with schizophrenia without a history of delinquency who commit a single serious act of violence relatively late in the course of their illness.

Mass killing – variously school shootings, mall shootings, college shootings or simple mass shootings are multiple killings at the same time. These are distinguished from spree killings which are killings at two or more locations with almost no time break between murders, sometimes with the less easily defined added requirement for no cooling-off period. These have many of the characteristics of social contagion or media amplification, including lack of a clear psychiatric diagnosis in most cases and the obvious social problem of gun availability [106]. Mullen described a series of five who survived such episodes [107] and characterises them as attempted 'autogenic suicides', merging with the phenomenon of 'suicide by cop' (see later in this section). In an American series of 170 who killed four or more victims, about half communicated or 'leaked' their plans. This was often in the context of counselling or suicidality, suggesting that those who gave advance warning or communication were engaging in a 'cry for help' rather than 'fame seeking' [108, 109]. There has been some interest in characterising the schools where such events take place. There is a growing literature on helping traumatised survivors. One systematic review identified weak associations with mental illness, suicidal ideation, intimate partner violence, socio-economic status, community distress, family life, childhood trauma, current or previous substance abuse, and firearm access. Such destructive motivations may be understood within larger social structures and cultural scripts. Of the possible interventions, gun control is the most obvious and most likely intervention to have large and immediate benefits.

Stealing children is a rare but important problem presented to forensic psychiatrists – it is included here because of the obvious harm to the child and to the parents, as well as the trauma and in some cases violence and murder of the child victim [110–112]. Variants include kidnapping for ransom and terrorism [113, 114] and the taking of a person's own child in the course of a domestic dispute and confrontation [115]. This latter phenomenon is typically a manifestation of a family crisis and threatened separation, often in the context of marital violence, substance misuse and coercive control.

Suicide by cop is a formulation used to explain the behaviour of some mass killers and hostage takers; most commonly, those who provoke a police armed response unit then seek to provoke their own death [116]. Hutson et al. reviewed a large American series of officer-involved shootings and suggest the following criteria: (1) evidence of the individual's suicidal intent, (2) evidence they specifically wanted officers to shoot them, (3) evidence they possessed a lethal weapon or what appeared to be a lethal weapon, and (4) evidence they intentionally escalated the encounter and provoked officers to shoot them. They point out, however, that such cases account for only 11% of a large series of officer-involved shootings in the USA [117]. Mullen described five surviving perpetrators of mass killings as follows: 'They are isolates, often bullied in childhood, who have rarely established themselves in effective work roles as adults. They have personalities marked by suspiciousness, obsessional traits, and grandiosity. They often harbour persecutory beliefs, which may occasionally verge on the delusional' [107]. Of note, however, are the many other social contexts and structural injustices that may complicate officer-involved shootings, particularly the very disproportionate numbers of black and minority-ethnic victims of police shootings in the USA.

Terrorist groups and 'lone wolf' actors are described in Chapter 14. The role of moral reasoning as a binding factor and a motive for commitment to acts that are both violent to others and self-destructive has been interpreted in terms of the 'devoted actor' [42, 118]. It should always be recalled that a delusional belief cannot be explained by cultural factors or context, and if shared by more than an immediate and close group (*folie a deux* or *folie a plus*), it is not a delusion, however extreme or unusual. To pathologise terrorist acts or organised crime activity comes too close to the political misuse of psychiatry [119]. Student protest was at one time also categorised with delinquency and research was published to link protest to family and social factors [120]. False diagnoses such as sluggish schizophrenia (manifesting only as social deviance with opposition to the state), drapetomania (the urge of African-American slaves to run away) and the former pathologisation of homosexuality all represent examples of political misuse of psychiatry. Forensic psychiatrists have a particular responsibility to be alert to this and to prevent it.

Genocide is defined in the United Nations Genocide Convention as any of five 'acts committed with intent to destroy, in whole or in part, a national, ethnic, racial or religious group, as such'. These five acts are: killing members of the group, causing them serious bodily or mental harm, imposing living conditions intended to destroy the group, preventing births, and forcibly transferring children out of the group. Victims are targeted because of their real or perceived membership of a group, not randomly. Incitement to genocide is also defined as a crime. There is a required intent (*mens rea*) consisting of both a general intent and a specific intent.

Hospital violence and bullying: much emphasis is placed on the use of restrictive practices in hospitals including seclusion, restraint and forced medication. These explorations are always incomplete if they do not also discuss the necessity for proportionality when preventing violence by patients against patients and violence by patients against staff [121]. These are not rare events [122]. Much in-patient violence can be characterised as impulsive and emotional. It may be related to positive symptoms of psychosis and also to cognitive impairments [89]. Bullying of patients by patients – including threats, extortion and exploitation – is typically part of a dysfunctional culture of forced in-group loyalty, often related to debt and drug use. Dominance hierarchies and gang cultures may play a part. Although more often researched in prisons and schools, this is a matter for perpetual vigilance in secure hospitals. Forensic psychiatrists and clinicians may be held liable for failing to be aware of or acting to prevent hospital violence and bullying, neglect and other forms of abuse [123, 124].

Court Reports and Medico-legal Expert Opinion Regarding Violent Offenders

The form and ethical context of court reports will be described in Chapters 1 and 16. All expert evidence must be grounded in good science. Unstructured expertise cannot be based only on subjective experience – expertise is always the outcome of education, training and experience [125].

Courts are interested in capacity to form a criminal intent, for example to cause serious harm. Mind is a collection of mental capacities [126, 127]. Mental capacity to form an intent can always be inferred from purposeful actions [74, 128]. When considered in this way, many transiently fashionable defences such as multiple personality [129], dissociation or automatism will obviously be the products of intact mental capacities. True epileptic automatisms consist of rudimentary and confused movements. Sleep automatism represents an example of confused thinking concerning the nature of mental defences with some egregious examples passing into legal precedent [130].

Treatment

Treatment will be covered more extensively in Chapters 7, 8 and 15 on treatment. Risk assessment and risk management is also dealt with in Chapter 6. Risk assessment is relevant here as a means of formulating treatment and long-term risk management. Dangerousness – the product of risk in its narrow sense as the likelihood of an event in a defined time period, and the seriousness of the risk [131, 132] – is one of the most relevant issues when assessing need for therapeutic security.

A null hypothesis here is that most criminal careers end spontaneously with advancing age. This desistence from acquisitive and violent offending may represent delayed maturation, a self-interested decision to avoid future imprisonment or the risks of violent death through gangs and conflict, the opening up of better options and career opportunities in life, the establishment of a successful long-term relationship, and, perhaps most commonly, abstinence from intoxicants. A positive disposition may be central for all of these.

Persistent offending into midlife may arise due to careers in crime or more rarely due to some 'specialist' form of offending such as sexual offending, particularly against children, serial sexual offending for other paraphilic reasons, including sexual sadism, and patterns of domestic familial violence. Androgen deprivation therapy will reduce preoccupation with sexual fantasies and may reduce some sexual offending [133, 134]. While there is some evidence that some forms of motivational work may have some benefit, the use of anti-psychotic medication, particularly in long-acting injection (depot) form, is supported by several studies [93]. This should be a matter for the criminal justice system and not primarily for secure forensic hospitals or forensic psychiatry.

The evidence that long-acting injections of anti-psychotic medication prevent violence and suicide in schizophrenia is among the strongest for therapeutic benefit in psychiatry. The evidence for long-acting injections of anti-psychotic medication extends even to prisoners with histories of violence but without established diagnoses [93, 135]. The added value of metacognitive and cognitive-behavioural therapies has so far not been tested in rigorous, randomised controlled trials of 'treatment as usual' versus treatment as usual plus additional psychological elements.

Given the functional impairments in schizophrenia that persist lifelong when symptoms are controlled or in remission, any long-term risk management plan to prevent future violence should commence with long-term abstinence and long-term adherence to anti-psychotic medication. Beyond that, social supports that provide for housing welfare and security for the future will do most to prevent the stresses that lead to relapse of substance misuse, relapse of acute psychosis and reoffending.

All approaches to treatment will be more successful if the patient enters voluntarily. Involuntary treatment is justified where capacity to give or withhold consent is impaired. But any treatment that is commenced without consent should quickly succeed in engaging the will and preference of the patient if it is to lead to long-term stabilisation and desistence from relapses and reoffending. A central part of motivational work is to offer a better quality of life. Security and two further elements, self-actualisation and self-transcendence, are characteristics of successful models of care.

A history of deception, dissimulation or malingering for any sort of gain or any evidence of unreliability concerning health, history or symptoms should make a psychiatric disposal as a sentencing option equally unreliable. Conditional discharge under supervision following prolonged and successful programmes of treatment in a secure forensic hospital has been repeatedly shown to greatly diminish further violence [136–139]. This is accomplished by continued compulsion regarding medication, usually by long-acting injection, and supported abstinence by means of repeated sampling for intoxicants and where possible for medication blood levels. Typically, transition to the community is gradual and proceeds along steps of social structure and support, monitoring and liberty. However, the levels of supervision and control possible in a secure forensic hospital are not possible in the community and so a progressive series of therapeutic risks are taken in which the responsibility lies with the patient rather than the psychiatrist and team.

Summary

Most violence occurs in the absence of mental illness or mental disorder of any sort. Many violent acts are not related to mental illness, even in those who have concurrent diagnoses of a mental illness. Intoxication, delinquency and social context play large parts in many acts of violence.

Violence is more likely in patients with severe mental illnesses, substance misuse issues, personality disorders, acquired brain injuries and some developmental disorders. These disorders aggregate and there may be interactive effects between them that further increase risk.

Distinguishing between mental disorders, functional capacity to form a criminal intent, free will and responsibility requires an educated and sceptical approach to clinical assessment and formulating expert evidence to assist a court. Populist beliefs that extreme crimes are in themselves evidence of mental disorder should be challenged, not accepted. A true empathic understanding may recognise that apparently self-defeating acts or acts leading to only short-term gratification or reward may be the product of rational choices where there is no long-term expectation of future, delayed benefits (see Table 2.1).

In attempting to formulate the causes of violence in a particular case, the sceptical psychiatrist should go no further than to say that some weak inferential evidence might suggest that in some cases of X, some cases of Y might follow. A psychiatrist should be of more assistance to a court when offering advice on possible treatment than when offering advice on so-called mental defences and degrees of responsibility or guilt.

Forensic psychiatrists should never usurp the role of a jury or legal decision maker by commenting on final issues (truthfulness, guilt or innocence, full or diminished responsibility). Nor should experts attempt to reinterpret the law to suit their own beliefs. When offering opinions about therapeutic disposals to a court, it is essential to be cautious about the prospects for preventing future violence in the medium or long term.

Courts should not look to psychiatrists as the primary preventers of future violence, even in the severely mentally ill. While violence can be reduced in frequency and severity while a patient is detained in a psychiatric hospital where intoxicants and weapons can or should be excluded, and medication adherence can or should be ensured, once in the community, psychiatrists and mental health professionals have less ability to control or prevent violence.

Table 2.1 Empathic understanding and compassionate psychiatry

	Empathy	Compassion
Foreshortened future	No belief in a long-term future	Make no promises. Negotiate agreed goals on short-term basis at first, not medium to longer term
Attachment insecurity	Expects that carers will abandon	Explain and prepare for all intervals in treatment, even short holidays
Pathological dependence [140]	Needs are cloaked by violent maladaptive reactions when progress towards discharge is interpreted as rejection	Always seek fully informed consent. Provide evidence of necessary supports
Sensitivity	Intense sensitivity to perceived slights and unfairness	Make and communicate clear rules regarding boundaries and limits, while also explaining medium- and longer-term pathways to recovery
State-dependent impairments	Intoxication impairs ability to change cognitive set	Never engage when intoxicated – including with benzodiazepines
Deception of self and others	Appeals to entitlement, 'trust me'	Reward factual evidence of progress, not dysfunction
In-group loyalty	Gang culture, subverting therapeutic milieu	Orientate towards 'good authority'; do not personalise or blame an external authority
Denial strategies	Avoiding responsibility by language – passive voice: 'it happened'; minimisation: 'the incident'	Emphasise ownership: 'I did X'; factual description: 'when I killed X'

References

1. Pinker S. *The Better Angels of Our Nature: Why Violence Has Declined*. New York, Viking, 2011.

2. Europe Co. *Dangerous Offenders – Recommendation CM/Rec(2014)3 and Explanatory Report*. Strasbourg, Council of Europe, 2014.

3. Kennedy HG, Iveson RC, Hill O. Violence, homicide and suicide: strong correlation and wide variation across districts. *British Journal of Psychiatry* 1999; 175: 462–6.

4. Beards S, Gayer-Anderson C, Borges S et al. Life events and psychosis: a review and meta-analysis. *Schizophrenia Bulletin* 2013; 39 (4): 740–7.

5. Bebbington P. Causal models and logical inference in epidemiological psychiatry. *British Journal of Psychiatry* 1980; 136: 317–25.

6. Everitt B, Smith A. Interactions in contingency tables: a brief discussion of alternative definitions. *Psychological Medicine* 1979; 9 (3): 581–3.

7. McGuffin P, Katz R, Bebbington P. The Camberwell Collaborative Depression Study. III. Depression and adversity in the

relatives of depressed probands. *British Journal of Psychiatry* 1988; 152: 775–82.

8. Freestone MC, Ullrich S, Coid JW. External trigger factors for violent offending: findings from the U.K. prisoner cohort study. *Criminal Justice and Behavior* 2017; 44 (11): 1389–412.

9. Danese A, Widom CS. Objective and subjective experiences of child maltreatment and their relationships with psychopathology. *Nature Human Behaviour* 2020; 4 (8): 811–18.

10. Häfner H, Boker W, Kohler C. *Crimes of Violence by Mentally Abnormal Offenders: A Psychiatric and Epidemiological Study in the Federal German Republic.* Cambridge, Cambridge University Press, 2011.

11. Broker W, Hafner H. Crime of violence by mentally disordered offenders in Germany. *Psychological Medicine* 1977; 7: 733–6.

12. Gibbens T. *Gewalttaten Geistesgestörter-Eine psychiatrisch-epidemiologische Untersuchung in der Bundes-republik Deutschland (Crimes of Violence by Mentally Disordered Offenders in Germany: A Study in Psychiatric Epidemiology).* Berlin, Springer-Verlag, 1973.

13. Taylor PJ, Gunn J. Violence and psychosis. I. Risk of violence among psychotic men. *British Medical Journal (Clinical Research Edition)* 1984; 288 (6435): 1945–9.

14. Wessely S, Taylor PJ. Madness and crime: criminology versus psychiatry. *Criminal Behaviour and Mental Health* 1991; 1 (3): 193–228.

15. Taylor PJ, Gunn J. Homicides by people with mental illness: myth and reality. *British Journal of Psychiatry* 1999; 174 (1): 9–14.

16. Mullen PE. A reassessment of the link between mental disorder and violent behaviour, and its implications for clinical practice. *Australian & New Zealand Journal of Psychiatry* 1997; 31 (1): 3–11.

17. Wallace C, Mullen PE, Burgess P. Criminal offending in schizophrenia over a 25-year period marked by deinstitutionalization and increasing prevalence of comorbid substance use disorders. *The American Journal of Psychiatry* 2004; 161 (4): 716–27.

18. Golenkov A, Large M, Nielssen O, Tsymbalova A. Forty-year study of rates of homicide by people with schizophrenia and other homicides in the Chuvash Republic of the Russian Federation. *BJPsych Open* 2021; 8 (1): e3.

19. Humphreys MS, Johnstone EC, MacMillan JF, Taylor PJ. Dangerous behaviour preceding first admissions for schizophrenia. *British Journal of Psychiatry* 1992; 161 (4): 501–5.

20. Nielssen O, Large M. Rates of homicide during the first episode of psychosis and after treatment: a systematic review and meta-analysis. *Schizophrenia Bulletin* 2010; 36 (4): 702–12.

21. Nielssen OB, Malhi GS, McGorry PD, Large MM. Overview of violence to self and others during the first episode of psychosis. *The Journal of Clinical Psychiatry* 2012; 73 (5): e580–7.

22. Swanson JW, Holzer CE, 3rd, Ganju VK, Jono RT. Violence and psychiatric disorder in the community: evidence from the Epidemiologic Catchment Area surveys. *Hospital & Community Psychiatry* 1990; 41 (7): 761–70.

23. Swanson J, Estroff S, Swartz M et al. Violence and severe mental disorder in clinical and community populations: the effects of psychotic symptoms, comorbidity, and lack of treatment. *Psychiatry* 1997; 60 (1): 1–22.

24. Link BG, Stueve A. *Psychotic Symptoms and the Violent/Illegal Behavior of Mental Patients Compared to Community Controls.* Violence and Mental Disorder: Developments in Risk Assessment. The John D. and Catherine T. MacArthur Foundation series on mental health and development. Chicago, IL, The University of Chicago Press, 1994, pp. 137–59.

25. Ullrich S, Keers R, Coid JW. Delusions, anger, and serious violence: new findings from the MacArthur Violence Risk Assessment Study. *Schizophrenia Bulletin* 2014; 40 (5): 1174–81.

26. Liu YY, Yang M, Ramsay M, Li XS, Coid JW. A comparison of logistic regression, classification and regression tree, and neural networks models in predicting violent re-offending. *Journal of Quantitative Criminology* 2011; 27 (4): 547–73.

27. Kennedy H, Kemp L, Dyer D. Fear and anger in delusional (paranoid) disorder: The association with violence. *The British Journal of Psychiatry* 1992; 160 (4): 488–92.

28. Ullrich S, Keers R, Shaw J, Doyle M, Coid JW. Acting on delusions: the role of negative affect in the pathway towards serious violence. *The Journal of Forensic Psychiatry & Psychology* 2018; 29 (5): 691–704.

29. Coid JW, Kallis C, Doyle M, Shaw J, Ullrich S. Shifts in positive and negative psychotic symptoms and anger: effects on violence. *Psychological Medicine* 2018; 48 (14): 2428–38.

30. Coid JW, Kallis C, Doyle M, Shaw J, Ullrich S. Identifying causal risk factors for violence among discharged patients. *PLoS One* 2015; 10 (11): e0142493.

31. Griffith JJ, Meyer D, Maguire T, Ogloff JRP, Daffern M. A clinical decision support system to prevent aggression and reduce restrictive practices in a forensic mental health service. *Psychiatric Services* 2021; 72 (8): 885–90.

32. Almvik R, Woods P, Rasmussen K. The Brøset Violence Checklist: sensitivity, specificity, and interrater reliability. *Journal of Interpersonal Violence* 2000; 15 (12): 1284–96.

33. Lockertsen Ø, Varvin S, Færden A, Vatnar SKB. Short-term risk assessments in an acute psychiatric inpatient setting: a re-examination of the Brøset Violence Checklist using repeated measurements – differentiating violence characteristics and gender. *Archives of Psychiatric Nursing* 2021; 35 (1): 17–26.

34. Kennedy HG. Anger and irritability. *British Journal of Psychiatry* 1992; 161: 145–53.

35. Insel TR. The NIMH research domain criteria (RDoC) project: precision medicine for psychiatry. *American Journal of Psychiatry* 2014; 171 (4): 395–7.

36. Davoren M, Kallis C, González RA, Freestone M, Coid JW. Anxiety disorders and intimate partner violence: can the association be explained by coexisting conditions or borderline personality traits? *The Journal of Forensic Psychiatry & Psychology* 2017; 28 (5): 639–58.

37. Fava M, Anderson K, Rosenbaum JF. 'Anger attacks': possible variants of panic and major depressive disorders. *The American Journal of Psychiatry* 1990; 147 (7): 867–70.

38. Fava M, Rosenbaum JF. Anger attacks in depression. Depression and Anxiety 1998; 8 (Suppl. 1): 59–63.

39. O'Reilly K, O'Connell P, Corvin A et al. Moral cognition and homicide amongst forensic patients with schizophrenia and schizoaffective disorder: A cross-sectional cohort study. *Schizophrenia Research* 2018; 193: 468–9.

40. O'Reilly K, O'Connell P, O'Sullivan D et al. Moral cognition, the missing link between psychotic symptoms and acts of violence: a cross-sectional national forensic cohort study. *BMC Psychiatry*. 2019; 19 (1): 408.

41. Haidt J. The new synthesis in moral psychology. *Science* 2007; 316 (5827): 998–1002.

42. Atran S. The devoted actor: unconditional commitment and intractable conflict across cultures. *Current Anthropology* 2016; 57 (S13): S192–S203.

43. Kennedy H, Grubin D. Patterns of denial in sex offenders. *Psychological Medicine* 1992; 22 (1): 191–6.

44. Taylor PJ, Kopelman MD. Amnesia for criminal offences. *Psychological Medicine* 1984; 14 (3): 581–8.

45. Kopelman MD. Amnesia: organic and psychogenic. *British Journal of Psychiatry* 1987; 150 (4): 428–42.

46. Kopelman MD. Psychogenic amnesia. *The Handbook of Memory Disorders* 2002; 2: 451–71.

47. McKay GCM, Kopelman MD. Psychogenic amnesia: when memory complaints are

medically unexplained. *Advances in Psychiatric Treatment* 2009; 15 (2): 152–8.

48. Gudjonsson GH, Kopelman MD, MacKeith JA. Unreliable admissions to homicide: a case of misdiagnosis of amnesia and misuse of abreaction technique. *British Journal of Psychiatry* 1999; 174: 455–9.

49. Gudjonsson G. Memory distrust syndrome, confabulation and false confession. *Cortex* 2017; 87: 156–65.

50. Gonzalez RA, Kallis C, Ullrich S et al. Childhood maltreatment and violence: mediation through psychiatric morbidity. *Child Abuse & Neglect* 2016; 52: 70–84.

51. Kolvin I, Miller FJ, Fleeting M, Kolvin PA. Social and parenting factors affecting criminal-offence rates: findings from the Newcastle Thousand Family Study (1947–1980). *The British Journal of Psychiatry* 1988; 152 (1): 80–90.

52. Farrington DP, Coid JW, Murray J. Family factors in the intergenerational transmission of offending. *Criminal Behaviour and Mental Health* 2009; 19 (2): 109–24.

53. Farrington DP, Gundry G, West DJ. The familial transmission of criminality. *Medicine, Science and the Law* 1975; 15 (3): 177–86.

54. Coid JW, Ullrich S, Keers R et al. Gang membership, violence, and psychiatric morbidity. *The American Journal of Psychiatry* 2013; 170 (9): 985–93.

55. Wood JL, Kallis C, Coid JW. Differentiating gang members, gang affiliates, and violent men on their psychiatric morbidity and traumatic experiences. *Psychiatry* 2017; 80 (3): 221–35.

56. Farrington DP, Ttofi MM, Coid JW. Development of adolescence-limited, late-onset, and persistent offenders from age 8 to age 48. *Aggressive Behavior* 2009; 35 (2): 150–63.

57. Farrington DP, Ttofi MM, Crago RV, Coid JW. Prevalence, frequency, onset, desistance and criminal career duration in

self-reports compared with official records. *Criminal Behaviour and Mental Health* 2014; 24 (4): 241–53.

58. Schoeler T, Theobald D, Pingault JB et al. Continuity of cannabis use and violent offending over the life course. *Psychological Medicine* 2016; 46 (8): 1663–77.

59. Faris REL, Dunham HW. *Mental Disorders in Urban Areas: An Ecological Study of Schizophrenia and Other Psychoses*. Chicago, IL, University of Chicago Press, 1939.

60. O'Neill C, Kelly A, Sinclair H, Kennedy H. Deprivation: different implications for forensic psychiatric need in urban and rural areas. *Social Psychiatry and Psychiatric Epidemiology* 2005; 40 (7): 551–6.

61. Pierzchniak P, Farnham F, Taranto N et al. Assessing the needs of patients in secure settings: a multi-disciplinary approach. *The Journal of Forensic Psychiatry* 1999; 10 (2): 343–54.

62. Coid JW. Socio-economic deprivation and admission rates to secure forensic psychiatry services. *Psychiatric Bulletin* 1998; 22 (5): 294–7.

63. Coid J, Kahtan N, Cook A, Gault S, Jarman B. Predicting admission rates to secure forensic psychiatry services. *Psychological Medicine* 2001; 31 (3): 531.

64. Fazel S, Smith EN, Chang Z, Geddes JR. Risk factors for interpersonal violence: an umbrella review of meta-analyses. *British Journal of Psychiatry* 2018; 213 (4): 609–14.

65. Orford J. *Excessive Appetites: A Psychological View of Addictions*, 2nd ed. New York, John Wiley & Sons Ltd, 2001.

66. Kraepelin E. *Clinical Psychiatry: A Text-Book for Students and Physicians, Abstracted and Adapted from the Seventh German ed. of Kraepelin's 'Lehrbuch der Psychiatrie'*. Bristol, Thoemmes Press, 2002.

67. Kraepelin E. *Lectures on Clinical Psychiatry*. New York, Hafner, 1968.

68. Connell PH. Amphetamine psychosis. *BMJ* 1957; 1 (5018): 582.

69. Connell PH. Drug addiction [abridged]: amphetamine dependence. *Proceedings of the Royal Society of Medicine* 1968; 61 (2): 178–81.

70. Kanaan RA, Carson A, Wessely SC et al. What's so special about conversion disorder? A problem and a proposal for diagnostic classification. *British Journal of Psychiatry* 2010; 196 (6): 427–8.

71. Bass C, Halligan P. Factitious disorders and malingering in relation to functional neurologic disorders. *Handbook of Clinical Neurology* 2016; 139: 509–20.

72. Bass C, Wade DT. Malingering and factitious disorder. *Practical Neurology* 2019; 19 (2): 96–105.

73. Kanaan RAA, Wessely SC. The origins of factitious disorder. *History of the Human Sciences* 2010; 23 (2): 68–85.

74. Kenny A. The psychiatric expert in court. *Psychological Medicine* 1984; 14 (2): 291–302.

75. Parnell TF, Day DO. *Munchausen by Proxy Syndrome: Misunderstood Child Abuse.* New York, SAGE Publications, 1997.

76. Orbach B, Huang L. Con men and their enablers: the anatomy of confidence games. *Social Research: An International Quarterly* 2018; 85 (4): 795–822.

77. Freestone M, Howard R, Coid JW, Ullrich S. Adult antisocial syndrome co-morbid with borderline personality disorder is associated with severe conduct disorder, substance dependence and violent antisociality. *Personal Mental Health* 2013; 7 (1): 11–21.

78. Brittain RP. The sadistic murderer. *Medicine, Science and the Law* 1970; 10 (4): 198–207.

79. MacCulloch MJ, Snowden PR, Wood PJ, Mills HE. Sadistic fantasy, sadistic behaviour and offending. *British Journal of Psychiatry* 1983; 143: 20–9.

80. Whiting D, Gulati G, Geddes JR, Fazel S. Association of schizophrenia spectrum disorders and violence perpetration in adults and adolescents from 15 countries: a systematic review and meta-analysis. *JAMA Psychiatry* 2022; 79 (2): 120–32.

81. Hodgins S, Mednick SA, Brennan PA, Schulsinger F, Engberg M. Mental disorder and crime: evidence from a Danish birth cohort. *Archives of General Psychiatry* 1996; 53 (6): 489–96.

82. Hodgins S. Violent behaviour among people with schizophrenia: a framework for investigations of causes, and effective treatment, and prevention. *Philosophical Transactions of the Royal Society B: Biological Sciences* 2008; 363 (1503): 2505–18.

83. Fazel S, Wolf A, Palm C, Lichtenstein P. Violent crime, suicide, and premature mortality in patients with schizophrenia and related disorders: a 38-year total population study in Sweden. *The Lancet Psychiatry* 2014; 1 (1): 44–54.

84. Fleischman A, Werbeloff N, Yoffe R, Davidson M, Weiser M. Schizophrenia and violent crime: a population-based study. *Psychological Medicine* 2014; 44 (14): 3051–7.

85. Uhrskov Sørensen L, Bengtson S, Lund J, Ibsen M, Långström N. Mortality among male forensic and non-forensic psychiatric patients: matched cohort study of rates, predictors and causes-of-death. *Nordic Journal of Psychiatry* 2020: 1–8.

86. Hodgins S, Piatosa MJ, Schiffer B. Violence among people with schizophrenia: phenotypes and neurobiology. *Neuroscience of Aggression* 2013: 329–68.

87. Flynn D, Smith D, Quirke L, Monks S, Kennedy HG. Ultra high risk of psychosis on committal to a young offender prison: an unrecognised opportunity for early intervention. *BMC Psychiatry* 2012; 12: 100.

88. McGorry PD, Hartmann JA, Spooner R, Nelson B. Beyond the 'at risk mental state' concept: transitioning to transdiagnostic psychiatry. *World Psychiatry: Official Journal of the World Psychiatric Association (WPA)* 2018; 17 (2): 133–42.

89. O'Reilly K, Donohoe G, Coyle C et al. Prospective cohort study of the relationship between neuro-cognition, social cognition and violence in forensic patients with schizophrenia and

schizoaffective disorder. *BMC Psychiatry* 2015; 15: 155.

90. O'Reilly K, O'Connell P, Ryan A et al. Deficit not bias: a quantifiable neuropsychological model of delusions. *Schizophrenia Research* 2020; 222: 496–8. doi: 10.1016/j.schres.2020.05.055.

91. Coid JW, Ullrich S, Bebbington P, Fazel S, Keers R. Paranoid ideation and violence: meta-analysis of individual subject data of 7 population surveys. *Schizophrenia Bulletin* 2016; 42 (4): 907–15.

92. Coid JW, Ullrich S, Kallis C et al. The relationship between delusions and violence: findings from the East London first episode psychosis study. *JAMA Psychiatry* 2013; 70 (5): 465–71.

93. Fazel S, Zetterqvist J, Larsson H, Långström N, Lichtenstein P. Antipsychotics, mood stabilisers, and risk of violent crime. *Lancet* 2014; 384 (9949): 1206–14.

94. Topiwala A, Fazel S. The pharmacological management of violence in schizophrenia: a structured review. *Expert Review of Neurotherapeutics* 2011; 11 (1): 53–63.

95. Witt K, van Dorn R, Fazel S. Risk factors for violence in psychosis: systematic review and meta-regression analysis of 110 studies. *PLoS One* 2013; 8 (2): e55942.

96. Citrome L, Volavka J, Czobor P et al. Effects of clozapine, olanzapine, risperidone, and haloperidol on hostility among patients with schizophrenia. *Psychiatric Services* 2001; 52 (11): 1510–14.

97. Krakowski M, Tural U, Czobor P. The importance of conduct disorder in the treatment of violence in schizophrenia: efficacy of clozapine compared with olanzapine and haloperidol. *American Journal of Psychiatry* 2021; 178 (3): 266–74.

98. Keers R, Ullrich S, Destavola BL, Coid JW. Association of violence with emergence of persecutory delusions in untreated schizophrenia. *The American Journal of Psychiatry* 2014; 171 (3): 332–9.

99. Shepherd M. Morbid jealousy: some clinical and social aspects of a psychiatric symptom. *Journal of Mental Science* 1961; 107 (449): 687–753.

100. Mullen PE. Jealousy: the pathology of passion. *British Journal of Psychiatry* 1991; 158 (5): 593–601.

101. Neeleman J, Wessely S, Wadsworth M. Predictors of suicide, accidental death, and premature natural death in a general-population birth cohort. *Lancet* 1998; 351 (9096): 93–7.

102. Abidin Z, Davoren M, Naughton L et al. Susceptibility (risk and protective) factors for in-patient violence and self-harm: prospective study of structured professional judgement instruments START and SAPROF, DUNDRUM-3 and DUNDRUM-4 in forensic mental health services. *BMC Psychiatry* 2013; 13: 197.

103. D'Orbán PT. Women who kill their children. *The British Journal of Psychiatry* 1979; 134 (6): 560–71.

104. *The Victoria Climbie Inquiry: Report of an Inquiry by Lord Laming.* London, HM Stationery Office, 2003.

105. Carabellese F, Rocca G, Candelli C, Catanesi R. Mental illness, violence and delusional misidentifications: the role of Capgras' syndrome in matricide. *Journal of Forensic and Legal Medicine* 2014; 21: 9–13.

106. Rubens M, Shehadeh N. Gun violence in United States: in search for a solution. *Frontiers in Public Health* 2014; 2: 17.

107. Mullen PE. The autogenic (self-generated) massacre. *Behavioral Sciences & the Law* 2004; 22 (3): 311–23.

108. Peterson J, Erickson G, Knapp K, Densley J. Communication of intent to do harm preceding mass public shootings in the United States, 1966 to 2019. *JAMA Network Open* 2021; 4 (11): e2133073.

109. Meloy JR, O'Toole ME. The concept of leakage in threat assessment. *Behavioral Sciences & the Law* 2011; 29 (4): 513–27.

110. d'Orban P. Child stealing: a typology of female offenders. *The British Journal of Criminology* 1976; 16 (3): 275–81.

111. d'Orbán P. Child stealing and pseudocyesis. *The British Journal of Psychiatry* 1982; 141 (2): 196–8.

112. d'Orbán P, Haydn-Smith P. Men who steal children. *British Medical Journal (Clinical Research Edition)* 1985; 290 (6484): 1784.

113. Phillips EM. Pain, suffering, and humiliation: the systemization of violence in kidnapping for ransom. *Journal of Aggression, Maltreatment & Trauma* 2011; 20 (8): 845–69.

114. Forest JJF. Global trends in kidnapping by terrorist groups. *Global Change, Peace & Security* 2012; 24 (3): 311–30.

115. Kennedy HG, Dyer DE. Parental hostage takers. *British Journal of Psychiatry* 1992; 160: 410–12.

116. Mohandie K, Meloy JR. Clinical and forensic indicators of 'suicide by cop'. *Journal of Forensic Sciences* 2000; 45 (2): 384–9.

117. Hutson HR, Anglin D, Yarbrough J et al. Suicide by cop. *Annals of Emergency Medicine* 1998; 32 (6): 665–9.

118. Atran S, Sheikh H, Gomez A. Devoted actors sacrifice for close comrades and sacred cause. *Proceedings of the National Academy of Sciences of the United States of America* 2014; 111 (50): 17702–3.

119. van Voren R. Ending political abuse of psychiatry: where we are at and what needs to be done. *BJPsych Bulletin* 2016; 40 (1): 30–3.

120. Jessor R, Jessor SL. *Problem Behavior and Psychosocial Development: A Longitudinal Study of Youth.* New York, Academic Press, 1977.

121. Kennedy HG, Mullaney R, McKenna P et al. A tool to evaluate proportionality and necessity in the use of restrictive practices in forensic mental health settings: the DRILL tool (Dundrum restriction, intrusion and liberty ladders). *BMC Psychiatry* 2020; 20 (1): 515.

122. Broderick C, Azizian A, Kornbluh R, Warburton K. Prevalence of physical violence in a forensic psychiatric hospital system during 2011–2013: patient assaults, staff assaults, and repeatedly violent patients. *CNS Spectrums* 2015; 20 (3): 319–30.

123. Fallon P, Bluglass R, Daniels G, Edwards B. *Report of the Committee of Inquiry into the Personality Disorder Unit, Ashworth Special Hospital Volume 1.* London, HM Stationery Office, 1999.

124. Warden J. Ashworth report confirms problems with special hospitals. *BMJ* 1999; 318 (7178): 211.

125. Collins H, Evans R. *Rethinking Expertise.* Chicago, IL, University of Chicago Press, 2008.

126. Kenny A. *Freewill and Responsibility* (Routledge Revivals). London, Taylor & Francis, 2011.

127. Kenny A. *The Metaphysics of Mind.* Oxford, Oxford University Press, 1992.

128. Grounds A. On describing mental states. *British Journal of Medical Psychology* 1987; 60 (4): 305–11.

129. Hacking I. *Rewriting the Soul: Multiple Personalities and the Sciences of Memory.* Princeton, NJ, Princeton University Press, 1995.

130. Broughton RJ. Sleep disorders: disorders of arousal? Enuresis, somnambulism, and nightmares occur in confusional states of arousal, not in 'dreaming sleep'. *Science* 1968; 159 (3819): 1070–8.

131. Shaw S. The dangerousness of dangerousness. *Medicine, Science and the Law* 1973; 13 (4): 269–71.

132. Scott P. Assessing dangerousness in criminals. *British Journal of Psychiatry* 1977; 131 (2): 127–42.

133. Boons L, Jeandarme I, Vervaeke G. Androgen deprivation therapy in pedophilic disorder: exploring the physical, psychological, and sexual effects from a patient's perspective. *The Journal of Sexual Medicine* 2021; 18 (2): 353–62.

134. Thibaut F, Cosyns P, Fedoroff JP et al. The World Federation of Societies of Biological Psychiatry (WFSBP) 2020 guidelines for the pharmacological treatment of paraphilic disorders. *The*

World Journal of Biological Psychiatry 2020; 21 (6): 412–90.

135. Sariaslan A, Leucht S, Zetterqvist J, Lichtenstein P, Fazel S. Associations between individual antipsychotics and the risk of arrests and convictions of violent and other crime: a nationwide within-individual study of 74 925 persons. *Psychological Medicine* 2021: 1–9.

136. Coid J, Hickey N, Kahtan N, Zhang T, Yang M. Patients discharged from medium secure forensic psychiatry services: reconvictions and risk factors. *The British Journal of Psychiatry* 2007; 190 (3): 223–9.

137. Doyle M, Power LA, Coid J et al. Predicting post-discharge community violence in England and Wales using the HCR-20V3. *International Journal of*

Forensic Mental Health 2014; 13 (2): 140–7.

138. Doyle M, Dolan M. Predicting community violence from patients discharged from mental health services. *The British Journal of Psychiatry* 2006; 189 (6): 520–6.

139. Jewell A, Cocks C, Cullen AE, Fahy T, Dean K. Predicting time to recall in patients conditionally released from a secure forensic hospital: a survival analysis. *European Psychiatry* 2018; 49: 1–8.

140. Jamieson L, Taylor PJ, Gibson B. From pathological dependence to healthy independence: an emergent grounded theory of facilitating independent living. *The Grounded Theory Review* 2006; 6 (1): 79–108.

Cases

R v Podola [1960] 1 QB 325, [1959] 3 All ER 418, [1959] 43 Cr App R 220.

R v Tandy [1987] EWCA Crim 5 Case No.: 1067/G2/87; [1989] 1 WLR 350.

Outcomes from the Key Inquiries and the Evolution of Modern Forensic Psychiatry

Kevin Murray

Introduction

The Hippocratic Oath demands confidentiality from medical practitioners. However, forensic psychiatry is the practice of psychiatry in the public arena, 'before the forum'. The evolution of modern forensic psychiatry may be understood in terms of the professional quest for clinical advances, supported by a humane legislative framework, while being subject to occasional critical public scrutiny of specific cases, perhaps to a greater extent than any other branch of medicine. This chapter will signpost the key events and their public examination which have shaped the present practice of forensic psychiatry in the United Kingdom. What follows is broadly but not strictly a decade-by-decade account of the major events and themes.

The 1950s

The 1959 Mental Health Act

Modern forensic psychiatry could be reasonably said to originate in the late 1950s. In 1954 there were about 150,000 patients detained in psychiatric hospitals in England [1]. As psychiatric practice evolved following the introduction of effective pharmacological treatments, and it was recognised that many patients could be managed in the community with appropriate support, the Percy Report [2] laid the foundations for the 1959 Mental Health Act (MHA). This did away with the 'antiquated legislation of the past' [3] which authorised detention for treatment under a number of statutes, some dating back to the nineteenth century: Bluglass [3] provides more details.

The 1959 Act applied only to England and Wales; there was separate legislation in 1960 for Scotland and in 1961 for Northern Ireland. There are important detail differences in the legislation in the different jurisdictions, which are beyond the scope of this review. In terms of the development of forensic psychiatry, there are three areas of particular interest.

Firstly, the 1959 Act simplified sentencing to hospital treatment following conviction for a criminal offence (S 60), with or without restrictions on discharge (S 65). Where this disposal was anticipated, the courts required two medical recommendations, but discretion as to making the order lay with the sentencing judge

> if the court is of opinion, having regard to all the circumstances including the nature of the offence and the character and antecedents of the offender, and to the other available methods of dealing with him, that the most suitable method of disposing of the case is by means of an order under this section, the court may by order authorise his admission to and detention in such hospital as may be specified in the order.

The Act also provided for transfer for treatment for remand and sentenced prisoners (Ss 72, 73) with restrictions on discharge (S 74). These templates have remained essentially unchanged since their introduction: the patients dealt with using such legislation, periodically updated, form the daily workload of forensic psychiatrists.

Secondly, the Act introduced Mental Health Review Tribunals, allowing patients or their nearest relatives to challenge their detention. Although patients on restricted orders were excluded until the 1983 Act, the template was once again established.

Thirdly, the Act ended the separate legislation for mental illness and learning disability, establishing four categories of mental disorder: mental illness, subnormality (in the parlance of the times), severe subnormality and psychopathic disorder. The Act allowed detention for treatment for mental illness and severe subnormality at any age, but for subnormality or psychopathic disorder, detention below 21 was not allowed. The requirement that a disorder must be 'of a nature or degree which warrants detention in hospital for treatment' and that 'it is necessary for the patient's health or safety or for the protection of others', which were set out in Section 26 of the 1959 Act, remain unchanged today, with the addition of the 'appropriate treatment' test. The differential treatment of those diagnosed with psychopathic disorder was to have far-reaching consequences for treatment provision and remains controversial.

The Homicide Act 1957

The Homicide Act received Royal Assent in March 1957. By introducing in England and Wales the verdict of not guilty of murder but guilty of manslaughter on the grounds of diminished responsibility, it established an effective mental condition defence in capital cases which fell short of the insanity threshold, broadly similar to 'culpable homicide' which was long established in Scottish law. This significantly expanded the role of psychiatrists in advising the courts. Dell [4] described how psychiatric evidence and hospital disposals expanded in importance after the 1957 and 1959 Acts became law, then declined somewhat after the effective abolition of the death penalty in 1965 so that judicial execution was no longer the mandatory sentence for those not found insane. The sentence of hospital order, usually with restrictions on discharge, was available for those found guilty of manslaughter in the same way as for any other mentally disordered offender. Ss 37 and 41 provide almost identical powers today.

The 1960s

After the legal changes of the late 1950s, the developments in the 1960s were primarily service-based rather than legislative.

Enoch Powell, Regional Secure Hospital Units and the 'Water Towers' Speech, 1961

The move from asylum to community treatment anticipated in the 1959 Act was mapped out as policy in Enoch Powell's well-known 'Water Towers' speech [5]: 'There they stand, isolated, majestic, imperious, brooded over by the gigantic water-tower and chimney combined . . . the asylums which our forefathers built with such immense solidity to express the notions of their day.' Powell, as minister for health from 1960 to 1963, anticipated the closure of at least half the 150,000 beds in the asylums by the mid-1970s, to be replaced by smaller general hospital units. Powell also commissioned a review of forensic services 'to consider the role of the special hospitals and the classes of patients to be treated in them, having regard to the new mental health law' in recognition that not all patients could be managed in local open-door units. Subsequently the Working Party on the Special Hospitals [6] proposed the development of 'Regional Secure Hospital Units'. Decades were to pass before these came into being.

Broadmoor Hospital had been founded in 1863. At the centenary lunch in 1963 Enoch Powell gave a speech on the standards to which society should aspire in the treatment of the 'mentally afflicted' [7]. Sadly, the planned refurbishment of Broadmoor, which he announced, and the impetus for the proposed regional secure units lost momentum after he resigned in October 1963 at a time of some political turmoil.

Alongside the gradual move away from the asylum to community-based care, it became evident that there were increasing numbers of patients who would be failed by the new service models:

A picture, therefore, emerges of a stage army of hopelessly inadequate chronic psychotics who express their pathology in part by offences against the criminal law, and who as a result, spend a goodly period of their lives being shunted between the prison and the mental hospital systems. It is fair to say that in terms of one system they are reckoned to be incorrigible and in terms of the other incurable [8].

Murder (Abolition of the Death Penalty) Act 1965
The Murder (Abolition of the Death Penalty) Act 1965 was initially a time-limited provision, made permanent in 1969. Theoretically, the death penalty remained available for a miscellany of arcane offences, until the adoption of the European Convention on Human Rights in the Human Rights Act 1998 ended these anomalies. The 1965 Act meant that psychiatrists no longer had to give a view on mental condition defences knowing that rejection of manslaughter would result in the mandatory death sentence, albeit sometimes commuted to life imprisonment by the home secretary, as in 19 of the 48 death sentences passed between the 1957 Homicide Act and the 1965 law [9].

The Parliamentary Estimates Committee, 1968: Overcrowding in the Special Hospitals
The Parliamentary Estimates Committee visited Broadmoor in 1968: they reported that they were 'shocked at the overcrowding there', with 'one day room holding 40 people as a dormitory'. Such shock notwithstanding, there was no further progress on the development of the proposed Regional Secure Hospital Units in the 1960s, with mentally disordered offenders for whom no bed was available being imprisoned instead of receiving treatment. Tidmarsh subsequently [10] described how the annual number of referrals to Special Hospitals almost doubled from 311 in 1961 to 582 in 1973, and how 'Her Majesty's judges feel angry and frustrated when they have to impose inappropriate prison sentences, not in keeping with the spirit of the 1959 Act, on mentally abnormal offenders because there is no vacancy in the "special hospitals"'. The committee also recommended building a further Special Hospital for mentally ill and psychopathic offenders in the north of England to relieve the overcrowding in Broadmoor. Finally, they recommended that the Special

Hospitals provide security equivalent to a category B prison: 30 years later, the Tilt Review [11] achieved this.

Of course, pressure to increase beds for admissions made headlines, rather than increasing efforts to promote throughput by more timely discharge. It is, however, important to understand how difficult it was to transfer Special Hospital patients [12]; between 1961 and 1965, more patients were discharged from the Special Hospitals direct to the community (220) than transferred to less secure services (191).

The 1970s

The Glancy Report 1973 and the Long-Term Challenging Patients

By 1970, no progress had been made on Powell's proposed Regional Secure Hospital Units, another working party was convened. The Glancy Report [13] described some neglected locked wards and some units for patients with 'mental handicap [sic]' in the traditional 'County' hospitals, but no strategic plan for challenging patients. The report once again suggested 1,000 beds in designated secure units for these patients as the asylums were closing. These difficult, treatment-resistant, long-stay patients who did not require Special Hospital security were sometimes referred to as 'Glancy patients' in reports over the next two decades: their care has been increasingly outsourced to the independent sector since the mid-1990s.

Graham Young and the Aarvold Committee, 1972–3

After Glancy's working party had been commissioned but before they had reported, there was the first of a series of moral panics about clinical decision-making. Graham Young had been sent to Broadmoor at the age of 14 in 1962 following the attempted murders of his father, his sister and a friend by poisoning. By 1971 he was considered safe for release and was discharged with the agreement of the Home Office. Without informing those supervising him, he found work with a lens maker, using complex chemical coatings. Over some nine months he poisoned several of his workmates, two of whom died. He was subsequently convicted of two counts of murder and two of attempted murder and sentenced to life imprisonment: Bowden's 1996 account [14] is recommended. The home secretary immediately set up two inquiries. The first, chaired by Sir Carl Aarvold, was to consider the law controlling restricted patients; the second inquiry was chaired by Lord Butler.

The Aarvold Committee's conclusions were generous: 'From our enquiries we are satisfied that the case was dealt with in accordance with the procedures accepted at the time to ensure that proper weight was given to questions of public safety' [15]. An editorial in the *BMJ* also argued against undue panic: 'What is of paramount importance . . . is to see the problem in perspective. The report emphasizes that Young was unique in forensic psychiatric experience and also the fact that there are very few exceptionally difficult cases which might slip through the network of precaution already established.' The same editorial noted that 'Young was the only patient to have committed homicide whilst under active supervision, a remarkable record when one takes into account (as the report points out) that Broadmoor has housed many of the most dangerous and difficult patients in the country' [16].

Aarvold recommended ending fixed-term restriction orders, available under the 1959 Act, as the duration of risk could not be predicted when making the order. He suggested a register of cases identified at sentencing as causing particular concern: this was not taken up. He proposed establishing an Advisory Board to assist the home secretary when requested on proposals for transfer or discharge: this operated until 2003 when possible release of minutes under Freedom of Information legislation led to its abolition. He proposed multidisciplinary case conferences prior to discharge, when all those involved in his care should be comprehensively briefed on the background and risk factors, with information disclosed to family, employers and landlords; the patient would be asked to consent to disclosure, the inference being that refusal to consent would inhibit discharge. Finally, Aarvold argued for the broader involvement of mental health services in the care of 'restricted' patients. This was strongly opposed in the *BMJ* whose lead writer [16] argued that all restricted patients should be admitted to Special Hospitals and discharged direct to specialist hostels: this was, of course, before the advent of medium-secure units (MSUs).

Meanwhile, work had begun on the additional Special Hospital proposed by the Estimates Committee in 1968, adjacent to the existing Moss Side Special Hospital in Maghull, Merseyside. Park Lane Hospital opened as an Advance Unit in 1974 and was fully operational by 1984.

The Butler Committee Reports, 1974 and 1975

The Butler Committee had two objectives: firstly 'to consider to what extent and on what criteria the law should recognise mental disorder or abnormality in a person accused of a criminal offence as a factor affecting his liability to be tried or convicted, and his disposal'; and secondly, 'to consider what, if any, changes were necessary in the powers, procedure and facilities relating to the provision of appropriate treatment, in prison, hospital or the community, for offenders suffering from mental disorder or abnormality, and to their discharge and aftercare'. It was to have a far-reaching impact on the arrangements for secure psychiatric services for the next 25 years.

The committee issued an Interim Report [17] in April 1974 and their full report in October 1975 [18]. The Interim Report is well summarised by Parker [19]. It emphasised the urgent need for 'Regional Secure Hospital Units' to address the 'yawning gap' between what was available in the ordinary NHS services and the Special Hospitals. It noted the pressure to accept Glancy patients into the Special Hospitals and the difficulties in transferring them back to the NHS when progress permitted. It acknowledged courts' difficulties in obtaining beds for mentally disordered offenders, with imprisonment in the absence of any other option, and how prisons also struggled to transfer unwell prisoners. In response to all this, Butler doubled Glancy's proposed 1,000 secure beds to 2,000 to meet the needs of the NHS, the Special Hospitals, the courts and the prisons. The government responded promptly to the Interim Report: within three months they had accepted the immediate need for 1,000 places in regional secure units, to be increased to 2,000 'as and when resources permit' [20], with capital funding identified for these 1,000 beds. This was the single most immediate response to clinical needs in the period this review covers.

In their substantive report, October 1975, the Butler Committee were disappointed that no progress had been made in establishing the new units, and noted the reluctance of some regions to accept these were needed. Even where the need was accepted, the allocated capital funds were not always used for these units. Cohen [21] tracked the £5.2 million allocated in 1976–7: 25% went to offset general overspends and two thirds were carried over to 1977–8.

Butler deliberated at length on the treatment of psychopathic disorder, anticipating in turn the Reed Review, the Fallon Report, the Dangerous and Severe Personality Disorder (DSPD) literature and the Lord Chief Justice in *Vowles*. Butler was sceptical regarding treatment in hospital for those so diagnosed. Instead, he proposed designated prison treatment units, with a new renewable and reviewable prison sentence, for offences which would not otherwise warrant a life sentence but where the offender was identified as higher risk. Although this was rejected at the time, it anticipated the Indeterminate sentence for Public Protection (IPP) available from 2005 to 2012, since replaced by the determinate sentence with an extended licence. Butler suggested retaining the category of psychopathy in the Act for selected cases where the prospects for treatment were thought to be good. To improve the assessment of difficult cases, interim hospital orders were proposed, allowing up to six months in hospital before any final recommendation for a hospital order.

Undoubtedly, the major achievement of the Butler Committee was to ensure that the long-proposed programme for regional secure units finally went ahead.

The Carstairs Escapes and Homicides, 1976

On 30 November 1976 Robert Mone and Thomas McCulloch succeeded in a carefully planned escape from the Scottish State Hospital, Carstairs. In less than 5 hours they had killed another patient and a member of staff, scaled the perimeter fence and stopped a passing police car, killing one policeman and injuring a second. They were apprehended just over the English border 70 miles away.

Following their arrest, the two men were remanded in custody, convicted of the murders and sentenced to life imprisonment, neither ever returning to hospital. The Scottish prison authorities were left with two very difficult prisoners who never returned to Carstairs.

A public inquiry [22] recommended more robust management systems for the hospital and increased security. The report makes uncomfortable reading. Arguably, the development of integrated regional forensic services in Scotland was delayed substantially by these events, so that when, in 2006, Glasgow finally opened a regional secure unit, it was one of the last large urban centres in western Europe to do so.

Rampton: The Secret Hospital (1979) and the Boynton Report (1980)

Following the change of government in May 1979, the new minister Patrick Jenkin was scarcely into office before being given a preview of the Yorkshire television film *Rampton, the Secret Hospital* to be broadcast on 22 May. This showed the routine and severe mistreatment of patients. The minister immediately set up a review team under Sir John Boynton and referred the allegations of ill-treatment to the police. A number of nurses were prosecuted and some convicted; also, 'without conspicuous publicity, some medical staff were removed or relocated' [23].

Boynton [24] reported in November 1980: the *Lancet* [25] described the bleak, humiliating and institutionalising structure of the patients' day: 11 hours locked in rooms overnight without any personal belongings; woken at 8.00 am; beds stripped and searched; empty chamber pots in the sluice; collect day clothes from the store and change in the main corridor, under observation; meals eaten in silence; 'anyone wishing to smoke has to light his cigarette on the wall lighter in the corridor, then wait on the threshold of the room and ask "Please may I come in Sir"'. Bowden's critical summary is also illuminating [26].

Boynton made over 200 recommendations including setting up an independent inspectorate for all institutions responsible for detained patients (subsequently the Mental Health Act Commission), accelerating discharge where appropriate (122 of the 900 patients were awaiting discharge), introducing individualised treatment programmes and establishing an effective local management team led by the medical director, the chief nurse and an administrator, providing local authority and leadership replacing that provided by default by the Prison Officers Association (POA). The report was also critical of the professional and cultural isolation of the hospital. These themes were to be revisited in subsequent critical reports on the Special Hospitals over the next 30 years.

1980s

The Early Years of the Medium-Secure Units Programme

By the early 1980s there was real progress in the introduction of regional (later termed medium) secure hospital units. Most started with interim units in converted locked wards upgraded with airlock entrances, secure exercise areas and toughened windows: these included the Rainford Unit for Liverpool in 1976, the Prestwich Unit for Manchester and the Lyndhurst Unit for Hampshire in 1977, followed by the Bethlem Royal Hospital unit in 1980. Treasaden [27] summarised the early years of the programme, and in the same book Bluglass [28] describes its further development.

At the same time the Royal College of Psychiatrists provided a view on secure facilities generally [29] and on Special Hospitals in particular [30]. Neither report was particularly influential: to a large extent the first report reiterated Butler's support for a mixed economy of high- and medium-secure services; the second was criticised for offering little leadership after the Boynton Report [31].

The Trial of Peter Sutcliffe, 1981 – Or Psychiatry on Trial?

In January 1981 Peter Sutcliffe was arrested and charged with 13 counts of murder and 7 counts of attempted murder between 1976 and 1980. Before his trial it was confirmed that he had no previous contact with psychiatric services: this was not a case where 'opportunities were missed'. In relation to the future of forensic psychiatry, the most important issue was the manner in which his trial was conducted. He was assessed by four very experienced forensic psychiatrists, one of whom reflected later: 'Many observers have commented that the psychiatrists were naive and gullible, unaware of the fact that all the psychiatrists interviewed Mr Sutcliffe believing that they were going to obtain a typical history of Brittain's sadistic killer [32], but after much soul-searching, found they could not avoid the diagnosis of schizophrenia' [33].

Having interviewed the prosecution psychiatrists, the attorney general, who led for the prosecution, accepted that pleas of not guilty to the murders but guilty to manslaughter on grounds of diminished responsibility were appropriate. When the case opened at the Old Bailey on 29 April 1981, the judge set aside this acceptance, deciding that the issue should go to a jury. As Kay commented, in relation to the subsequent cross-examinations, 'The pressures on the doctors were such that the judge, on more than one occasion, told the psychiatrists that they themselves were not on trial. However . . . no one in the court, least of all the psychiatrists, believed that . . .. If Mr Sutcliffe could not be hanged, then those attempting to give him a defence should be' [34]. Similarly, McCulloch commented, 'on subsequent reflection ... the only way to prosecute the case was to discredit the medical evidence' [34].

The 1983 Mental Health Act

Revisions to the 1959 Act had been proposed by the Butler and Aarvold reports in the mid-1970s, in 'A Human Condition', the influential two-part critique by Larry Gostin on behalf of MIND [35], and in the November 1978 White Paper 'A Review of the Mental Health Act 1959' [36]. These proposals were eventually enacted in the 1983 Act. Bluglass [37] provides a comprehensive guide to the 1978 draft and the subsequent legislation as it was enacted [38].

There were a number of important changes for forensic psychiatry. The 1983 Act updated the language of the 1959 Act concerning categories of mental disorder, substituting 'mental impairment' for 'mental subnormality'. In order to detain those categorised as psychopathically disordered or mentally impaired, but not those categorised as mentally ill or severely mentally impaired, doctors must assert that treatment would 'be likely to alleviate or prevent deterioration of (the patient's) condition' (S3), so that hospitals could not detain the untreatable. This subsequently became a major point of dispute in mental health tribunals, where patients who refused to participate in any therapy argued that treatment was neither 'alleviating nor preventing deterioration' in their condition. The Act expanded the powers of the Courts, to remand for reports (S 35), for treatment (S 36), on an interim hospital order (S 38), and to summon information on the availability of beds (S 39), but not to order that a bed be made available.

Over the decade before the 1983 Act there was considerable debate about consent to treatment for detained patients. In 1973 the minister asserted to Parliament that detention for treatment under the 1959 Act authorised any treatment prescribed by the detained patient's consultant, although seeking consent if the patient was able to consent was good practice [39]. Gostin [35] had challenged this assumption, proposing that any treatment to be given to a hospital 'resident' unable or unwilling to give consent should be reviewed by a local independent body, the 'Committee on the Rights and Responsibilities of Staff and Residents of Psychiatric Hospitals' (p. 116). Particular concern attached to 'suspect' treatments 'which involves surgery, electro-convulsive therapy or the use of experimental drugs or procedures' [40]. The 1983 Act's consent to treatment provisions, Ss 56–64, including the Second Opinion Approved Doctor (SOAD) arrangements provided by the Mental Health Act Commission (MHAC), emerged from this debate.

Tribunals' powers (Ss 65–79) were extended to include jurisdiction over restricted patients, S 41 and S 49: this followed the 1981 case at the *ECHR of X v United Kingdom*, which established that compliance with Art 5.4 required that a tribunal must have the power to discharge a detained patient even if they had previously offended violently, and in the face of political objection [41].

S 121 of the Act established the MHAC as an independent monitoring body concerned with the conditions and treatment of patients detained under the Act and their rights. Its remit was to visit services, meet patients and ensure that legal rights were upheld; to investigate complaints where appropriate; to appoint second-opinion doctors to review proposed treatment plans for incapacitous or non-consenting detained patients; to monitor the Code of Practice; and to publish a biennial report.

Progress in Service Provision

By 1984 Park Lane Hospital had fully opened, providing 370 beds in 17 wards. There were plans to rebuild Broadmoor but the project was suspended after the first phase because of cost over-runs. The MSU programme gathered pace, with the replacement of the interim units from the 1970s with the first wave of permanent units. Snowden [42] described the 460 beds open in permanent units by June 1988, still less than half Butler's initial 1,000 beds. He also noted that the first permanent unit to open, the Hutton Unit in Middlesbrough, was about to be remodelled to correct 'design faults': almost all of the early units have been subject to major redesign as the challenges of managing this patient group emerged.

The Health Advisory Service Report on Broadmoor (1989) and Jimmy Savile's Appointment

The Hospital Advisory Service, later renamed the Health Advisory Service, was established in 1969 to advise the secretary of state. It periodically visited the Special Hospitals, including visiting Broadmoor in the early 1970s; that report was never published. In 1988 their highly critical report [43] led to the removal of then medical director and the institution of a system of general management across the four Special Hospitals (Moss Side and Park Lane were at the time separate hospitals). Their criticisms echoed Boynton, albeit they were not quite so severe. Their report described discussions between management and staff, represented by the Prison Officers Association (POA), that were focussed more on conditions of service than on therapeutic advances. The regime was overly custodial and security was cited as the reason for the POA's 'defensive isolationist negotiating ploy' [44]. There were difficulties in recruiting doctors and nurses. The report was particularly critical of the limited contact between male and female patients: 'the effective suppression of heterosexual activity has created the situation where homosexuality is implicitly tolerated by the staff'.

The minister for health, Edwina Currie, responded by instituting a major change in the management of the Special Hospitals: previously local management had been in the hands of the troika of medical director, chief nurse and hospital administrator. Kaye and Franey [45] describe the tortuous accountability arrangements at that time, with the Special Hospitals Service Board taking major policy decisions but with no means of implementing them, and the local management having the responsibility for implementation. Instead, the Special Hospitals Service Authority was introduced, and for Broadmoor in addition a Task Force chaired by a senior civil servant but including

> the television personality Mr Jimmy Savile; Mrs Edwina Currie, the junior health minister, [who] believes that he will encourage change in what the (Hospital) Advisory Service describes as a 'philosophy and ethos established and nurtured for over 100 years . . . [and] largely impervious to liberalisation.' Mrs Currie said last week: 'Under Jimmy Savile's guidance, shifts in attitude and pattern of delivery of service have already been achieved. He is an amazing man and has my full confidence' [46].

Mrs Currie was later to row back on that ringing endorsement [47].

The 2014 Inquiry into Jimmy Savile's behaviour at Broadmoor [48] concluded that he had sexually assaulted at least five and probably more individuals, including both staff and patients, during his period of association with Broadmoor which dated back to the 1960s when he first volunteered at the hospital, and ended finally in the early 2000s. He had most control while chairing the Task Force in the late 1980s. The report notes that his abusive behaviour at Broadmoor was less extensive than at other hospitals, and emphasises the importance of robust systems of management where patients are vulnerable patients, and that celebrity is not a reason to breach protective systems.

1990s

In terms of lasting impact on the provision of forensic services, the 1990s were probably the decade which had the greatest significance.

Home Office Circular 66/90

In September 1990, the Home Office issued Circular 66/90 [49], promoting diversion for mentally disordered offenders to more appropriate care and treatment. This arguably represents the high-water mark in seeking to provide a mental health pathway for mentally disordered offenders, which was to be significantly eroded in subsequent years.

The Reed Committee, 1991–4

Fifteen years after the Butler Report, the 'Steering Committee' of a 'Review of Health and Social Services for Mentally Disordered Offenders' was established under the chairmanship of Dr John Reed, a former consultant psychiatrist. The committee published a series of consultation papers [50], followed by their definitive and wide-ranging reports [51] comprising: an overall summary (1992); service needs (1993); finance, staffing and training (1993); the academic and research base (1993); special issues and differing needs (1993); high-security and related psychiatric provision (1994); and services for people with psychopathic disorder (1994).

Reed's guiding principles were 'that care should be provided on the basis of individual need, as far as possible in the community, near to the patient's home, at the level of security justified by the patient's dangerousness, and with the aim of maximising rehabilitation and the prospect of independent living' [52]. Reed's focus was on the great mass of mentally disordered offenders who commit low-level crimes and revolve through the courts, prisons and local services to no great advantage. He emphasised the value of local arrangements for assessment at the point of arrest, for court diversion schemes and for specialised bail facilities, as proposed by Circular 66/90. Older, larger hospitals should not close until newer community-based services were available. The NHS should provide psychiatric services in prisons, as well as general medical care, with additional staff recruited to achieve this. Reed also supported the expansion of academic forensic psychiatry as a discipline, and the 1990s and 2000s were certainly the high-water mark of academic forensic psychiatry in the UK, with more than a dozen professorial chairs in England, as well as academic departments in Scotland, Wales and outside the UK in Dublin: more than half of those in England have since fallen vacant.

Reed considered how to approach problematic cases where it was unclear whether hospital or prison was more appropriate. He supported the introduction of a hybrid order 'reserved for those cases where there was substantial doubt over whether the offender would benefit from hospital treatment' [53]. After much debate [54], this was introduced as S 45A of the 1983 Act, amended by the Crime (Sentences) Act 1997, applicable only to those diagnosed as psychopathically disordered.

Reed supported expanding the medium-secure programme from 635 beds available in 1992, still well short of Butler's 1975 target, to 1,500 beds, with no further reduction in the high-secure estate before then. When the final summary report was published, Chiswick was generous: 'The Reed report has profound implications for the government, patients, doctors, and managers . . . . The report is impressive because it is comprehensive . . . (forensic) patients should not be disadvantaged by their status as offenders' [55].

Arguably, the series of scandals from the early 1990s diverted attention from Reed's aspirations to the more immediate deficiencies of services and risk to the public from untreated or inadequately treated offenders.

The Blom-Cooper Report, 1992

The Committee of Inquiry into Complaints about Ashworth Hospital [56] was set up in April 1991 under the chairmanship of Louis Blom-Cooper QC following concern about the death of a patient in 1988 and other allegations, once again reported in a television programme. Its remit was extended to include allegations of ill-treatment of four further patients, two of whom had died, and also into how a number of specific complaints were managed and the broader working of the complaints system and linked management systems, including the police and hospital advisory committee. The report was published in July 1992. The committee made serious criticisms of the management of the hospital, the disengagement of senior professionals and the anti-therapeutic ward milieu in which denigration of patients was routine. It catalogued abuse of patients without consequence for the abusers. The unit general manager, the director of medical services and the director of nursing services were removed from their posts.

The Inquiry made 90 recommendations, covering the allegations of mistreatment, the role of MHAC in the investigation of complaints, dealing with racism and homophobia, and the use of seclusion. The Ashworth Task Force was instituted to implement the action plan. This was to prove far from straightforward.

Christopher Clunis, Jonathan Zito, the Ritchie Report and the Care Programme Approach

On 17 December 1992 Christopher Clunis fatally stabbed Jonathan Zito at Finsbury Park underground station. The incident received only limited initial media attention. However, on New Year's Eve 1992, a young man also suffering from schizophrenia climbed into the lions' enclosure at London Zoo and was seriously injured. His family were friends with Marjorie Wallace, an experienced mental health campaigner, who was able to mobilise media attention and was invited to meet the secretary of state for health, Virginia Bottomley, within the week. Mrs Bottomley went on to announce a review of the arrangements for care in the community the same month [57].

Christopher Clunis pleaded guilty to manslaughter on 28 June 1993. The court heard evidence of his long and unsatisfactory contact with mental health services across London and of his violence and use of weapons. He was sentenced to a restricted hospital order. Jonathan Zito's widow Jayne was interviewed extensively by the press and asserted firmly that both her late husband and Christopher Clunis had been let down by the failure to provide adequate and assertive community care. 'Somebody is responsible for murdering my Jon . . .. If someone had taken care of Mr Clunis, my husband Jon would have been here with me today' [58].

Although the government initially resisted calls for any wider-ranging inquiry, on 1 July 1993 a further high-profile case reached court. Michael Buchanan pleaded guilty to the manslaughter of a retired policeman, Frederick Graver. Mr Buchanan also had a history of poorly managed mental health problems and had been discharged from hospital less than three weeks before the homicide. Public pressure grew and on 22 July the Department of Health announced there would be a barrister-led independent inquiry into the Clunis case.

The Ritchie Inquiry reported in February 1994. It traced 'a catalogue of failure and missed opportunity', yet deliberately did not identify one person or service for particular blame [59]. There was no oversight of Christopher Clunis' needs or any meaningful transfer of information between successive services: each contact was treated as a discrete event. Police reluctance to prosecute someone known to be mentally ill resulted in poor recording of his violence, which was often omitted or poorly documented in hospital discharge summaries, in line with the prevailing ethos of not acknowledging the propensity for violence of those with psychosis, particularly that complicated by drug misuse. On the day of the report's publication, Jayne Zito was reported to be 'holding Virginia Bottomley personally responsible for her husband's death' [60].

Probably the most significant legacy of the Clunis case was the strengthening of the Care Programme Approach (CPA) with the requirement that care coordinators take continuing responsibility for the care of patients subject to CPA unless they are transferred to another service or until such care is no longer regarded as necessary. CPA had been introduced in 1991 to improve and better structure the management of patients with severe mental illness discharged into the community. It followed on from the Spokes Inquiry [61] into the murder of a psychiatric social worker by one of her mentally ill clients and the Griffiths review of care in the community [62]. Simpson [63] gives a helpful summary of the background and weakness of the policy.

The Death of Orville Blackwood and Two Other Patients: 'Big, Black and Dangerous' Report, 1993

Alongside the concerns about inadequate community care, the Special Hospital Service Authority (SHSA) commissioned a review into the circumstances surrounding the deaths of three patients at Broadmoor Hospital between 1984 and 1991. The Inquiry [64] was chaired by Herschel Prins, an eminent criminologist. It described a culture of racism at the hospital: 'The experience of Afro-Caribbean inner-city youngsters is not fully understood by Eurocentric psychiatry and those who work in the psychiatric system. It is important that differences are recognised and catered for.' The report was subtitled 'Big, Black and Dangerous', words used by staff to describe the three patients. All three died in seclusion having been restrained and injected with high doses of anti-psychotics. The report recommended increased caution in the use of such prescribing and was followed shortly afterwards by the advice from the Royal College of Psychiatrists [65]. The Inquiry team anticipated that their recommendations would meet opposition and offered to revisit the hospital in 12 months to review progress (p. 77). It seems that the SHSA did not respond to this suggestion [66].

The hazards of extended physical restraint and the impact of racism on the experience of patients and staff were further illustrated in the Inquiry into the death of David 'Rocky'

Bennett, a Jamaican man detained at the Norvic Clinic MSU in Norwich [67]. He died during an episode of extended physical restraint, not involving injected medication, in October 1998. The Inquiry's recommendation to limit the duration of prone restraint was not accepted as such but has influenced teaching and practice of the prevention and management of violence and aggression.

Her Majesty's Chief Inspector of Prisons Concerns

When Lord Woolf was investigating the Strangeways disturbances, he invited the chief inspector of prisons, Judge Stephen Tumim, to contribute. Judge Tumim had been appointed by Home Secretary Douglas Hurd in 1987. In the 1990s his reports became increasingly critical of conditions in prison, particularly for the mentally ill. His contract was not renewed, as was usual, by the then home secretary Michael Howard, in 1995. Instead he appointed Sir David Ramsbotham, a former senior soldier. However, he in turn was equally critical of prison conditions, arguing forcibly for equality of access to NHS facilities for the mentally disordered [68]. His contract was similarly allowed to lapse in 2001. However, the pressure successive chief inspectors brought to bear contributed to the commissioning of the most comprehensive assessment of the treatment needs of prisoners. In 1998, the Office for National Statistics reported on prisoners' psychiatric morbidity [69]. They found that up to 90% of prisoners had a diagnosable mental health problem, including drug and alcohol dependency and personality disorder in this wide definition; that 70% had two or more conditions; and that the prevalence rates for functional psychosis in the previous year were 7% for males sentenced, 10% for males on remand and 14% for female prisoners. These astounding findings received less attention than they deserved because of other events which overshadowed them, but which also pushed forensic mental health up the national agenda.

The Fallon Report, 1999

On 25 September 1996 Stephen Daggett, a patient on Lawrence Ward in the Personality Disorder Unit (PDU) at Ashworth Hospital, absconded while on a shopping trip into Liverpool: he took with him his bankbooks, a passport and a driving licence, none of which he should have had. He fled to Amsterdam, from where he negotiated his return to Ashworth subject to publicising his concerns about the management of the PDU. He returned to the hospital on 8 October; he was debriefed and produced a 60-page document entitled 'My Concerns'.

> He ... painted a picture of a ward where a small coterie of patients had succeeded in thoroughly undermining the Patient Care Team. He alleged that pornography, drugs and alcohol were freely available; that patients were running businesses, which was against hospital policy; that a child had been put at risk of abuse at the hands of paedophiles; that the security of the ward was severely compromised; and that a number of staff were corrupt [70].

He was transferred to Rampton shortly after his return. Between October 1996 and February 1997 the number of those aware of his allegations slowly grew until they eventually reached senior management at Ashworth and the MHAC, who had been given a copy of 'My Concerns' by Daggett at Rampton. On 6 February the then secretary of state for health

Stephen Dorrell was informed of the allegations: he announced the establishment of an independent Inquiry the following day.

The Fallon Report [70] was published in January 1999. It presents a picture of failed management of a service where the risk of patients subverting the system was highest. The greatest concerns attached to the unsupervised visits of the young girl to a ward where she was clearly at risk of abuse. Drugs and hard-core pornographic videos were available, duplicated and sold by patients. Staff had ceded control for decision-making to more assertive patients. The local Patient Care Team, as the ward clinical team were known, chose to disregard policies with which they disagreed and there were inadequate senior managerial controls to pick this up. There was a culture at a senior level of suppression of bad news. The Inquiry team discussed whether the earlier Blom-Cooper review had contributed to these events: they were critical of the accelerated introduction across the whole hospital of the more liberal/therapeutic regime: 'We have no doubt that the application of the recommendations of the Blom-Cooper Report across the whole campus of Ashworth Hospital, without regard to the different regimes needed by the different sub-groups of patients, was a fundamental error which created complex managerial problems rather than an enlightened solution' (70, 2.1.22). They emphasised the difference in needs between primarily personality disordered offender patients and those with a primary diagnosis of mental illness, and made very specific comments about the treatment pro-grammes and ward arrangements for the personality disorder groups.

In total Fallon made 58 recommendations, covering lines of accountability for clinical teams and managers, development and implementation of policies, national provision for primarily personality disordered offenders, legislation, child protection, security arrange-ments, and most conspicuously that Ashworth Hospital should close as soon as alternative arrangements might be made for those detained there: 'we are convinced that the system in its present form is rotten and unsustainable, and trying to sustain it will only make matters worse' (70, 7.3.24). This recommendation was immediately rejected by the secretary of state.

The report was generally received well: most unusually, the *Psychiatric Bulletin* for August 1999 included a series of articles on the Inquiry, including an acknowledgement on behalf of the Royal College of Psychiatrists [71] of the professional failings in the context of the historic difficulties high-secure hospitals had faced and an acceptance from the consultant body at Ashworth of the need to improve [72].

It is hard to overstate the lasting impact of the Fallon and subsequent Tilt reports in the high-secure services. Most immediately, arrangements were set in place to merge the three high-secure hospitals with nearby specialist mental health trusts who were already experi-enced in provision of forensic care at medium-secure level: so Ashworth became part of Merseycare Trust, Broadmoor became part of West London NHS Trust and Rampton became part of Nottinghamshire Healthcare NHS Trust. The consequent integration into more outward-facing NHS services has probably achieved more in terms of combatting the professional isolation and raising clinical standards than any other high-secure services initiative over the period of this review. The full report remains essential reading for senior forensic clinicians and managers more than 20 years on.

The Tilt Report, 2000

One of Fallon's recommendations was that 'an independent review of all aspects of physical security at Ashworth Hospital take place and be repeated at regular intervals'

(70, 2.21.16). When Frank Dobson, the secretary of state for health, reported Fallon's conclusion to the House of Commons on 12 January 1999, he extended this review across the high-secure estate [73]. The chair was Sir Richard Tilt, former director general of the Prison Service. The other committee members were drawn from the prison service, an NHS Trust manager and a senior civil servant as secretary to the review team [11]. Perhaps the absence of clinical involvement contributed to the hostile reception the review received when it was published in February 2000, despite the panel having spent significant time at each high-secure hospital and meeting with staff representatives there [74].

Tilt made 86 recommendations, dealing primarily with physical and procedural security. Many of these were welcome: 'Additional funding, which should be used in the first instance to facilitate the movement of patients no longer needing high security care, should be provided over the next 3 years', an aspiration unfulfilled since Powell 40 years earlier, thereby allowing the high-security hospitals to focus on care for those who could not be safely managed in any less secure setting. Perimeter security was to be improved to prison category B standard to make escape very difficult: Tilt noted that the number of escapes from within the secure perimeters had reduced, with none in the five years prior to his report but seven in the five years prior to that. Tilt argued for greater unescorted movement for patients within the more secure perimeters: this proved more difficult to achieve. The anachronistic dormitories at Broadmoor and Rampton were to close. Other recommendations had less clinical face value: the establishment of a register of the highest-risk patients, for example, so that in early 2007, 23% of Broadmoor patients, 31% of Ashworth patients and 46% of Rampton patients were categorised as 'high risk', rendering the concept increasingly meaningless [75]. Tilt also suggested that 'the feasibility of locking the rooms at night of all patients on admission and intensive care wards, and all "high risk" patients, should be examined': the English high-secure hospitals had all moved to 24-hour unlock in the early 1990s, and this recommendation was particularly controversial. Finally, Tilt set out the basis for the expanded safety and security directions which still, largely unchanged, continue to determine much clinical practice in high-security hospitals: dealing with, among other matters, searching patients and staff, managing mail and telephone calls, checking external security, and, most contentiously, access to contemporary information technology (i.e. computers and the internet). These also provide a statutory basis for such practices and provide fair processes for appeal and review [76]. This gave patients in high-secure hospitals equivalent protection of rights to those held by prisoners under the Prison Rules.

Exworthy and Gunn [74] criticised Tilt's failure to emphasise the importance of relational security, contrasting his approach with previous inquiries into prison disturbances, although arguably relational security should be a basic expectation in a hospital. They were also concerned that the prison approach might damage morale and recruitment at institutions which had taken a battering over the previous decade, and that the emphasis on security would be detrimental to patients transferring from high- to medium-secure services. In practice, however, recruitment improved in the 2000s after remuneration was improved, and the development of longer-stay medium-secure services allowed the high-security hospitals to substantially reduce in size over the next two decades, with reduction in length of stay [77]. What Tilt achieved was to ensure that security could be relied on, if not taken for granted, in the public mind: if someone was sent to a high-secure hospital having been convicted of the most serious offences, then they would not escape. In addition, the perimeters are now secure and drugs and alcohol do not enter, in contrast to the situation described on Lawrence Ward. The issue of the denial of access to twenty-first-century technology remains unresolved.

Michael Stone and the Dangerous and Severe Personality Disorder Programme

In October 1998, while the Fallon Inquiry was underway, Michael Stone was convicted of the July 1997 murder of Lin Russell and one of her daughters and the attempted murder of a second daughter. The police investigation had made little headway until a re-enactment on the television programme *Crimewatch* in July 1998, which prompted a psychiatrist from the Trevor Gibbens MSU in Maidstone to alert them to the similarity between the e-fit of the suspect and his patient, Michael Stone. He was convicted of two counts of murder and attempted murder and sentenced to life imprisonment.

On 15 February 1999 the then home secretary Jack Straw announced 'a number of legal changes intended to better protect the public from dangerous people in our society ... with new legal powers for the indeterminate but reviewable detention of dangerous personality disordered individuals' who did not satisfy the existing 'treatability' test [78]. Thus the DSPD programme was conceived, although Maden suggested that 'the true motivation was not a single case but longstanding frustration within government at the refusal of psychiatrists to address the problem of high-risk offenders with personality disorder. The profession was seen as cynically hiding behind the "treatability" clause ... to avoid responsibility for dangerous and difficult patients' [79]. The Department of Health (2003) initiative on personality disorder was part of the same programme [80].

The entry criteria for the programme were that individuals:

(1) were more likely than not to offend within five years, causing serious physical or psychological harm from which recovery would be difficult or impossible;
(2) had significant personality disorder; and
(3) had an offending risk that was functionally linked to the personality disorder [81].

The treatment programmes were delivered in two category A prisons, Frankland and Whitemoor, and two high-secure hospitals, Broadmoor and Rampton. Substantial funds were provided for both capital and revenue, like the Butler programme a generation earlier. The programme attracted controversy about the diagnostic reliability [82] and the predictability of risk [83]. Ultimately, the hospital programmes were not considered to provide value for money and were discontinued – Broadmoor in 2012, Rampton some years later. The prison programmes evolved into the Offenders with Personality Disorder (OPD) programme [84, 85]. Tyrer et al. [86] provide a balanced overview of the successes and failures of the programme. However, the fundamental clinical ambivalence about committing to treat those with severe personality disorder, still evident in the refusal of some MSUs to admit such patients, and the judicial apprehension about sentencing committing such offenders to hospital rather than prison [87], remain unresolved.

2000s

Homicide Inquiries and Their Impact

In the first decade of the twenty-first century public concern focussed more on medium-secure and local services than on high security, with reports on homicide by patients known to mental health services and receiving follow-up care, such as Robinson et al. [88]. When those homicides took place following the escape of a patient from a secure setting, the concern was amplified [89]. For clinicians trying to deliver safe, high-quality services with limited resources, such inquiries could be very threatening [90]: exhaustive critical analysis with the benefit of hindsight could usually identify aspects of care which were suboptimal, albeit rarely demonstrating any causal link with the tragic outcome. Although the Zito Trust maintained a focus on the needs of patients [91], inquiries could be seen by the families of the victim as fault-finding exercises – following the language of Health Service Guidance 94/ 27, 'when something goes wrong' rather than opportunities for learning and service improvement. The pain of the bereaved families is acknowledged in the preface to almost every report, and in the accounts documented by the Hundred Families group [92]. It is far from clear, however, that the inquisitorial approach has led to improved care and reducing risk, or whether by lowering morale and harming recruitment into services it has had the opposite effect. Crichton [93] gives a well-balanced overview. The National Confidential Inquiry into Suicide and Homicide (NCISH) [94] undertook a thematic review of such reports and aggregated their findings into 15 headings, on CPA policy and implementation, on risk assessment, on granting leave and so on: such well-grounded analysis unfortunately makes fewer headlines than the homicide reports themselves. Encouragingly, the most recent National Confidential Inquiry into Suicide and Homicide data suggests that homicides by patients known to mental health services in the 12 months prior to the homicide have reduced from 58 annually between 2007 and 2011 to 44 annually from 2012 to 2017 [95].

Strengthening the Role of Capacity in Mental Health Law 1: *Re C*, Bournewood and the Mental Capacity Act 2005

The 2000s saw a clash of competing narratives in the context of revising mental health legislation. On one side, there was public concern about discharged mentally ill patients who were non-compliant with treatment who then relapsed and acted dangerously, as described in so many homicide inquiries.

However, there was also a call to treat patients with mental disorder in exactly the same manner as patients offered treatment for physical disorders, which had grown since the case of *Re C* [96] and the Bournewood case. C was a patient in Broadmoor in 1994 who developed gangrene, in addition to his schizophrenic illness. He objected to the doctor's proposal to amputate: his solicitor supported his objection which was ultimately upheld by the court, which determined that notwithstanding his schizophrenia, he had the ability to decide to risk his physical health and die with two legs rather than live with one. Consultant forensic psychiatrist Professor Nigel Eastman was instructed by C's solicitors and, building on earlier work by Applebaum and Grisso [97], formulated the test of capacity as the ability to understand, retain and use information provided to make a decision, and to communicate that decision, which became the bedrock of capacity assessments for the subsequent 25 years.

The 1997 Bournewood case [98] concerned a man with profound learning difficulties who attended a local day hospital and had thence been admitted to another hospital on an informal basis because of concerns about his disturbed behaviour. Although he was said to be compliant with admission, his carers objected that inability to give consent did not constitute agreement to informal admission. The case was heard at successive courts up to the European Court of Human Rights. The concerns of the carers were upheld, requiring legislation to cover the deprivation of liberty for those unable to consent: the result was the Mental Capacity Act 2005.

Strengthening the Role of Capacity in Mental Health Law 2: The 2007 Mental Health Act – Coercive or Capacity Based?

Against this backdrop, the Department of Health commissioned a review of the 1983 MHA by an expert committee chaired by Professor Genevra Richardson; this reported in July 1999 [99]. Grounds [100] described the report as impressive, avoiding discrimination against those with mental disorder and balancing compulsion to accept treatment with entitlement to treatment of a high standard. However, the Green Paper which was published alongside the Richardson Report was 'harsher in tone and less liberal' [100], emphasising safety rather than reciprocal access to high standards when detained. The subsequent White Paper, 'Reforming the Mental Health Act' (Department of Health 2000), was 'a profoundly illiberal document' [100], quite at odds with the capacity-based approach advocated by, for example, Szmukler and Holloway [101]. A draft Bill was published in 2002 and, having noted the comments, a further draft in September 2004. Full details of this tortuous process are set out in the 2005 Joint Parliamentary Report [102], which details the shortcomings of the proposed legislation. These 2004 proposals met with no more support than the earlier ones, with unresolved divisions between those prioritising the public safety agenda and more assertive treatment and those prioritising capacity and autonomy ahead of coercion. Ultimately the government chose a less ambitions path; see Hansard, 23 March 2006 [103]: 'An Act to amend the Mental Health Act 1983'.

The main changes were that the four categories of mental disorder introduced in the 1959 Act were abolished and replaced by the single category 'mental disorder'; the 'treatability test' for detention for mental impairment and psychopathic disorder, which was central to the Michael Stone case, was weakened, with 'appropriate treatment was available' instead of 'treatment would alleviate or prevent deterioration'; and finally the powers for supervised treatment in the community were introduced. The introduction of the single category of mental disorder had the effect of making S 45A 'hybrid order' disposals available for all diagnoses, rather than only for psychopathic disorder. Thus, instead of Reed's intention to encourage clinicians to offer treatment to those who might simply have been sentenced to prison, a prison sentence with initial treatment in hospital became an available disposal for the mentally ill [104]. This was quite a different proposition, and one which was to be expanded further by the Court of Appeal in the case of *Vowles*.

The Francis Report, 2009: Homicide in Broadmoor

On 2 December 2002 Richard Loudwell killed Joan Smythe, age 82, in her home in Rainham, Kent. He was admitted to Broadmoor on remand in January 2004. On 22 April 2004 he pleaded guilty to manslaughter on the grounds of diminished responsibility [105]. He was due to return to court for sentence the following week. Peter Bryan was admitted to Broadmoor on 15 April 2004 [106]. He had previously killed a woman with whom he had argued about being dismissed from his job, and been sent to Rampton in 1993 [107]. He subsequently transferred to the John Howard Centre MSU in east London in 2001, and was discharged to community follow-up the following year. In March 2004 he killed and mutilated the body of a fellow community mental health patient, within a very few hours of leaving the open psychiatric ward where he had been an informal patient for the previous week. He was referred to Broadmoor for urgent admission while on remand. He was managed in seclusion for the first four days after admission because of concerns regarding the level of risk he posed, and the absence of signs of risk prior to the second homicide. On Sunday evening, 25 April, three days after Richard Loudwell's guilty plea to manslaughter, Peter Bryan severely assaulted him in an area of the ward out of sight of the nursing office; Richard Loudwell never recovered consciousness and died six weeks later. On 15 March 2005 Peter Bryan pleaded guilty to two counts of manslaughter on the grounds of diminished responsibility. He was sentenced to life imprisonment and returned to Broadmoor, detained under Ss 47/49 as a transferred prisoner.

Homicide is a rare but not unknown event in high-secure hospitals [108]. The coincidence in this instance of the circumstances of Richard Loudwell's offence, Peter Bryan's previous offences, particularly the gruesome nature of his second homicide, and a fatal assault occurring in Broadmoor attracted considerable public attention. The three separate inquiries referenced above each looked at one of the homicides. The Francis Inquiry into events at Broadmoor was rightly the most critical, particularly of the failure to prevent the bullying Richard Loudwell was subject to after he spoke about his offence to other patients, and of the wider managerial oversight of the services. With the Francis Report arriving alongside a critical Care Quality Commission report [109], change at the most senior level in the Trust was inevitable [110].

2010s

Night-Time Confinement and Long-Term Segregation in High-Secure Hospitals

The possibility of night-time confinement (NTC) for high-risk patients and those on admission or intensive care wards envisaged by Tilt was implemented throughout the hospital-based dangerous severe personality disorder (DSPD) services from their inception, albeit hardly ever implemented outside these services: it was asserted that the cost-savings were necessary to support their richer daytime therapeutic regime. However, as part of the cost-reduction programmes following the introduction of austerity regimes, in 2011 the three English high-security hospitals committed to the general introduction of NTC, providing patients had access to a nurse call system and in-room toilets. Clinical imperatives could, in individual cases, override the general move to NTC where a clinical need precluded locking the door. The rationale was that in an era of diminishing resources, it was better to concentrate staffing in daytime with more interaction with patients, not at night when most patients were asleep. Despite protests from the forensic faculty of the Royal College of Psychiatrists, and concern but not opposition from the Care Quality Commission, NTC was introduced gradually from 2012 with surprisingly little opposition from patients.

NTC was most easily introduced at Ashworth, the most modern of the three hospitals; it was also straightforward to introduce at Rampton except the last villa wards until these closed in 2016. In Broadmoor the majority of patients were accommodated in nineteenth-century buildings which fell below the standard required for NTC until the opening of the new hospital in December 2019. However, the Trust Board acceded to requests from the patients not to move to NTC in the new hospital rehabilitation wards, at least for the present. The situation is therefore that NTC is implemented for all patients at two of the high-security hospitals and for approximately half of the patients at the third.

NTC remains controversial: the February 2019 *Psychiatric Bulletin* includes three articles discussing the practice [111, 112, 113]. The practice was also criticised by the European Committee for the Prevention of Torture (CPT) [114]: 'Para 139. The CPT continues to believe that the systematic locking-in of patients at night, which amounts to ten hours of de facto seclusion, is not acceptable in a care establishment provided there are sufficient staff . . .. The CPT recommends that the United Kingdom authorities . . . review the use of night-time confinement.' In response the UK government has committed to a review, the outcome of which is awaited. The practice of NTC continues as a matter of routine in other high-security hospitals, notably in Carstairs. To date there have been no proposals for NTC in MSUs, either in the NHS or in the independent sector: it is unclear why the same financial constraints do not lead to the same outcomes in these services, which operate in the same trusts as Ashworth, Broadmoor and Rampton, or whether the lower-security needs of patient in MSUs would mean this must be disproportionate.

The CPT also criticised the extent and operation of long-term segregation (LTS) in the high-security hospitals, suggesting that for a number of patients it was unnecessary, that the management of patients during LTS was anti-therapeutic and that the practice was inadequately underpinned by policy and the MHA Code of Practice, and should have a statutory basis, as is the case for NTC in the Safety and Security Directions [115].

Outcomes from Forensic Care and the *R v Vowles* Decision, 2011

Over the greater part of the period under review, the task for forensic psychiatrists has been to identify those offenders with mental health problems and arrange effective individual treatment programmes to meet their needs and thereby promote both health gain and public safety. The evidence suggests that these objectives were successfully achieved. The Home Office *Statistical Bulletin* series until 2004 included tables detailing the actual and expected reconviction rates for violent and sexual offences committed by released conditionally discharged patients and a matched sample of released prisoners for the first two years post-release. The 2004 *Bulletin* [116] shows that, from 1987 to 2002, of the 2,139 patients conditionally discharged for the first time, 24 committed a serious violent or sexual offence, a rate of approximately 1%. The rate for matched released prisoners was 11%; that is, the public were some 10 times safer when treatment, including follow-up, was provided on a restricted hospital order rather than a prison sentence and release to standard aftercare. Changes in collecting post-release data mean that such comparisons are no longer available [117]. Recently Fazel and colleagues published a meta-analysis of international outcomes following discharge from secure hospitals [118]. They conclude that

> compared with reoffending rates for general prisoners matched by age, forensic patients had lower rates of repeat offending . . .. [Specifically] we compared reoffending in individuals with violent index offences, and with prisoners with longer sentences as comparators, and we also investigated rates of violent reoffending and compared such rates with prisoners. Even with these comparisons, rates of repeat offending were lower in forensic patients.

Given this evidence, the approach taken by the Lord Chief Justice in *Vowles* [119] is all the more perplexing. The background to the case is not material, but the Lord Chief Justice used it to revise the approach to be taken in considering sentencing for mentally disordered offenders. Peay [120] provides a very helpful analysis:

> Following Vowles, the pure therapeutic approach looks to take second place to a mixed precautionary punitive approach . . .. When they were first introduced the s.45A orders created a disposal option for offenders suffering from psychopathic disorder, where a judge had already rejected a recommendation for a s.37/41 order because of an offender's high culpability for the offence or because of the serious risk the offender posed to the public . . .. The order both encouraged psychiatrists to have a therapeutic go with the difficult to treat psychopathic offenders, and retained a cautious and flexible approach to release . . .. The decision in Vowles arguably turns this on its head. The judgment asserts that where medical practitioners suggest that an offender is suffering from mental disorder, and where the offending is wholly or in significant part attributable to the mental disorder, and treatment is available, and a hospital order may be the appropriate way of dealing with the case, then the courts should first consider using a s.45A order. Only once that has been rejected should they consider the s.37 or s.37/41 order. Yet, if the offending was wholly or in significant part attributable to the mental disorder that would seemingly imply that culpability was low or absent.

It is reassuring to note that subsequent decisions appear to row back slightly from the approach advocated in Vowles, such as *Edwards* at para. 12:

> A level of misunderstanding of the guidance offered in Vowles appears to have arisen . . .. Section 45A and the judgment in Vowles do not provide a 'default' setting of imprisonment . . .. The sentencing judge should first consider if a hospital order may be appropriate under section 37 (2) (a). If so, before making such an order, the court must consider all the powers at its disposal including a s.45A order ... because a disposal under section 45A includes a penal element and the court must have 'sound reasons' for departing from the usual course of imposing a sentence with a penal element. Sound reasons may include the nature of the offence and the limited nature of any penal element (if imposed) and the fact that the offending was very substantially (albeit not wholly) attributable to the offender's illness [121].

Time will tell how far the pendulum will swing back.

Proposals for Reform of the MHA (Again): Wessely, 2018

The final area to discuss in this survey is the most recent proposal for reform of the MHA, going once again over the ground described ahead of the 1959, 1983 and 2007 reforms. Professor Sir Simon Wessely, recent president of the Royal College of Psychiatrists, was invited to lead the review [122]. His report was subtitled 'Increasing Choice, Reducing Compulsion'. He sets out four guiding principles:

- choice and autonomy – ensuring service users' views and choices are respected
- least restriction – ensuring legal powers are used in the least restrictive way
- therapeutic benefit – ensuring patients are supported to get better, so they can be discharged from the Act
- the person as an individual – ensuring patients are viewed and treated as rounded individuals.

Quite rightly, these are framed to improve the care and experience of the great number of patients who are provided for in more general psychiatric services. Innovations proposed include greater opportunity for patients to express treatment preferences with statutory Advance Choice Documents (ACDs) to be taken into account if compulsory care is unavoidable; earlier access to Second Opinion Approved Doctors; care and treatment plans (C&TPs) to be jointly developed; and so on. Wessely also foresees the fusion of mental health and mental capacity legislation in due course, but not yet: referring to the Richardson Expert Committee's work in 1998, he says, 'I hope that she will feel that we are at last achieving some of the objectives that she wished for almost 20 years ago' (p. 8).

In terms of forensic psychiatry, relatively little is said in the 2018 review, although the general principles outlined as the framework for the review apply equally to those detained under Part III of the Act. The proposals are more about detail than principle: allowing magistrates to remand to hospital for assessment and treatment at an earlier stage in their proceedings; promoting diversion in general and reducing or abolishing the remand to custody in the absence of any other place of safety; speeding up transfers from custody to secure hospital places (these last two critically dependent on the availability of beds); no extension of the MHA to authorise treatment in prison; delegation of authority to Responsible Clinicians for transfer and leave of absence for most restricted patients, with the Ministry of Justice having an override power for selected higher-risk patients; promoting absolute discharge decisions by tribunals so that conditional discharge status does not remain in place unnecessarily; and perhaps most intriguingly, bringing together the tribunal and the Parole Board to jointly consider release for post-tariff transferred prisoners. It remains to be seen how far these recommendations progress into the eventual Green Paper: almost two years on, this is not yet in sight.

Conclusion

What, if any, conclusions may be drawn from this survey? Some problems, notably psychopathy, are not obviously nearer a solution. Attempted legal revisions may founder on the mutually exclusive objectives of promoting capacity and autonomy, and enforcing compliance with community follow-up. There have been fewer high-profile investigations either into community tragedies or into in-patient scandals, and the racism which was described, for example, in Blom-Cooper and in Prins may be less prevalent. There is a dearth of good follow-up studies generally, and particularly on the obesity epidemic patients are experiencing. Ultimately, it seems we continue to work towards higher clinical standards and more choice for our patients, only to be periodically derailed when things go wrong. When Harold Macmillan became prime minister, he was asked what would determine his government's course. He replied: 'Events, dear boy, events.' As a forensic psychiatrist, it's hard to disagree.

References

1. Gunn J, Taylor P. *Forensic Psychiatry: Clinical, Legal and Ethical Issues*. London, Butterworth Heineman, 1993.

2. Percy E. *The Royal Commission on the Law Relating to Mental Illness and Mental Deficiency*. The Percy Report. Cmnd 16. London, HMSO, 1957.

3. Bluglass R, Bowden P (eds) *Principles and Practice of Forensic Psychiatry*. London, Churchill Livingstone, 1990, p. 1173.

4. Dell S. *Murder into Manslaughter*. Maudsley Monographs 27. Oxford: Oxford University Press, 1984.

5. Opening address, National Association for Mental Health Conference, 9 March 1961: http://enochpowell.info/wp-content/uploads/Speeches/1957-1961.pdf, p. 38.

6. Ministry of Health. Special Hospitals: Report of a Working Party (the Emery Report). London, HMSO, 1961.

7. Speech at Broadmoor Centenary Lunch, 26 June 1963. http://enochpowell.info/wp-content/uploads/Speeches/1962-1963.pdf, p. 44.

8. Rollin H. The care of the mentally abnormal offender and the protection of the public. *Journal of Medical Ethics* 1976; 2: 157–62.

9. Gordon H. *Broadmoor: An Inside Story.* London, Psychology News Press, 2011.

10. Tidmarsh D. Secure hospital units. *BMJ* 1974: 286.

11. Tilt R, Perry B, Martin C et al. Report of the Review of Security at the High Security Hospitals, Department of Health, 2000.

12. Tennant G, Parker E, McGrath PG, Street D. Male admissions to the English Special Hospitals: 1961–1965 – a demographic survey. *BJPsych* 1980; 136: 181–90.

13. Report on Security in NHS Psychiatric Hospitals. London, DHSS, 1973 (the Glancy Report).

14. Bowden P. Graham Young: The St Albans poisoner. *Criminal Behaviour and Mental Health*, 1996 Supplement: 17–24.

15. Home Office. *Report on the Review of Procedures for the Discharge and Supervision of Psychiatric Patients Subject to Special Restrictions.* Cmnd 5191. London, HMSO, 1973.

16. Anon. Editorial: dangerous patients. *BMJ* 1973; 1: 247.

17. Interim Report of the Committee on Mentally Abnormal Offenders. Cmnd 5698. London, Home Office and Department of Health and Social Security, 1974.

18. Report of the Committee on Mentally Abnormal Offenders. Cmnd 6244. London, HMSO, 1975.

19. Parker E. The development of secure provision. In Gostin E (ed.) *Secure Provision.* London, Tavistock, 1985.

20. Department of Health HSC (IS) 61, July 1974.

21. Cohen R. Where did the money go? *Health and Social Service Journal*, 30 September 1977.

22. State Hospital, Carstairs: Report of Public Local Inquiry into Circumstances Surrounding the Escape of Two Patients on 30 November 1976 and into Security and other arrangements at the Hospital. Edinburgh, HMSO, 1977.

23. Mawson D. A doctor's view. In Kaye C and Franey A (eds) *Managing High Secure Care.* London, Jessica Kingsley, 1998.

24. Department of Health and Social Security. *Report of the Review of Rampton Hospital: The Boynton Report.* Cmnd. 8073. London, HMSO, 1980.

25. *Lancet.* Commentary from Westminster. 1980; 316: 1094–5.

26. Bowden P. *Psychiatric Bulletin of the Royal College of Psychiatrists* 1981; 5 (1): 15–16.

27. Treasaden IH. Current practice in regional interim secure units. In Gostin L (ed.) *Secure Provision.* London, Tavistock, 1985.

28. Bluglass R. The development of regional secure units. In Gostin L (ed.) *Secure Provision.* London, Tavistock, 1985.

29. Royal College of Psychiatrists. *Secure Facilities for Psychiatric Patients: A Comprehensive Policy.* London, RCPsych, 1980.

30. Royal College of Psychiatrists. *The Future of the Special Hospitals.* London, RCPsych, 1983.

31. Bowden P. *Bulletin of the Royal College of Psychiatrists* 1983; 8 (3): 54.

32. Brittain R. The sadistic murderer. *Medicine, Science and the Law* 1970; 10: 198–207.

33. Kay T. Book review: *Voices from an Evil God* by Barbara Jones. *Journal of Forensic Psychiatry* 1993; 4 (2): 380–5.

34. MacCulloch M. Letter: the trial of Peter Sutcliff. *Journal of Forensic Psychiatry* 1993; 4 (3): 583–9.

35. Gostin L. *A Human Condition.* London, Mind, 1975.

36. *A Review of the Mental Health Act 1959.* Cmnd 7320: London, HMSO, 1978.

37. Bluglass R. Review of the Mental Health Act, 1959: A summary of the White Paper. *Bulletin of the Royal College of Psychiatrists* 1978; 2 (11): 192–6.

38. Bluglass R. The Mental Health Act 1983. In Bluglass R and Bowden P (eds) *Principles and Practice of Forensic Psychiatry.* London, Churchill Livingstone, 1989.

39. Hansard. HC Debs. Ser 5. 849 (23 January 1973), 77.

40. Hilton C. Changes between the 1959 and 1983 Mental Health Acts (England & Wales), with particular reference to consent to treatment for electroconvulsive therapy. *History of Psychiatry* 2007; 18 (2): 217–29.

41. *X v The United Kingdom* – 7215/75 [1981] ECHR 6 (5 November 1981). www.bailii.org/eu/cases/ECHR/1981/6.html.

42. Snowden P. Regional secure units and forensic services. In Bluglass R and Bowden P (eds) *Principles and Practice of Forensic Psychiatry.* London, Churchill Livingstone, 1989, p. 1383.

43. Health Advisory Service. *Health Advisory Service Report on Broadmoor Hospital.* London, Health Advisory Service, 1988.

44. Edwina Currie, minister for health, quoted in *BMJ*, 26 November 1988, p. 1357.

45. Kaye C, Franey, F. The inheritance. In Kaye C and Franey A (eds) *Managing High Secure Care.* London, Jessica Kingsley, 1998, pp. 44–5.

46. Smith R. Broadmoor slammed, reforms proposed. *British Medical Journal* 1988; 297: 1357.

47. Edwina Currie voices regrets over Jimmy Savile after inquiry criticism. *The Guardian*, 26 June 2014.

48. Kirkup B. *Jimmy Savile Investigation: Broadmoor Hospital Report to the West London Mental Health NHS Trust and the Department of Health.* London, Department of Health, 2014.

49. Baxter R. Provision for mentally disordered offenders. Home Office Circular 66/90, 3 September 1990, MNP/90 1/55/8. www.cps.gov.uk/sites/default/files/documents/legal_guidance/Home%2520Office%2520Circular%252066%252090.pdf.

50. Department of Health, Home Office. *Review of Health and Social Services for Mentally Disordered Offenders and Others Requiring Similar Services.* London, Department of Health, Home Office, 1991.

51. Department of Health. *Review of Health and Social Services for Mentally Disordered Offenders and Others Requiring Similar Services.* London, Department of Health, 1993.

52. *Review of Health and Social Services for Mentally Disordered Offenders and Others Requiring Similar Services.* Final Summary Report. Cmnd 2088. London, HMSO, 1992.

53. Reed J. *Review of Health and Social Services for Mentally Disordered Offenders and Others Requiring Similar Services.* Working Group on Psychopathic Disorder. London, HMSO, 1994.

54. Eastman N. Hybrid justice: Proposals for the mentally disordered in the crime (sentences) bill – The ethical, legal and health service cost implications. *Psychiatric Bulletin* 1997; 21: 129–31.

55. Chiswick D. Reed report on mentally disordered offenders. *BMJ* 1992; 305 (6867): 1448–9.

56. Blom-Cooper Sir L. et al. *Report of the Committee of Inquiry into Complaints about Ashworth Hospital*, Cmnd 2028, vols 1 and 2 (Chairman: Sir Louis Blom-Cooper). London, HMSO, 1992.

57. Sulitzeanu-Kenan R. *Mental State of Inquiry: Tragedy, Policy and Accountability in the Case of the Ritchie Inquiry.* Washington, DC, American Society for Public Administration, 2008.

58. Zito J, reported in *Daily Mail*, 29 June 1993.

59. Ritchie J, Dick D, Lingham R. *The Report of the Inquiry into the Care and Treatment of Christopher Clunis.* London, HMSO, 1994, p. 105.

60. *Guardian*, 25 February 1994.

61. Department of Health and Social Security. *Report of the Committee of Inquiry into the Care and Aftercare of Sharon Campbell.* London, HMSO, 1988.

62. Griffiths R. *Community Care: Agenda for Action.* London, HMSO, 1988.

63. Simpson A, Bowers L, Miller C. The history of the Care Programme Approach in England: Where did it go wrong? *Journal of Mental Health* 2003; 12 (5): 489–504.

64. *Report of the Committee of Inquiry into the Death at Broadmoor Hospital of Orville Blackwood and a Review of the Deaths of Two Other Afro-Caribbean Patients: 'Big, Black and Dangerous?'* London, Special Hospitals Service Authority, 1993.

65. Royal College of Psychiatrists. *Consensus Statement on the Use of High Dose Antipsychotic Medication* (Council Report CR26). London, Royal College of Psychiatrists, 1993.

66. Kaye C, Franey A. Inquiries and inspections. In Kaye C and Franey A (eds) *Managing High Secure Care.* London, Jessica Kingsley, 1998, p. 237.

67. *Independent Inquiry into the Death of David Bennett.* Norfolk, Suffolk and Cambridgeshire Strategic Health Authority, 2004.

68. Ramsbotham D. *Patient or Prisoner? A Discussion Paper for HM Chief Inspector of Prisons.* London, The Home Office, 1996.

69. Singleton N, Meltzer H, Gatward R et al. *Psychiatric Morbidity among Prisoners: Summary Report.* Office for National Statistics, on behalf of the Department of Health. London, HMSO, 1998.

70. Fallon P, Bluglass R, Edwards B, Daniels G. *Report of the Committee of Inquiry into the Personality Disorder Unit, Ashworth Special Hospital* (the Fallon Report). London, HMSO, 1999, p. 193.

71. Report of the Committee of Inquiry into the Personality Disorder Unit, Ashworth Special Hospital: Comments of the Royal College of Psychiatrists. *Psychiatric Bulletin* 1999; 23: 452–4.

72. Response to the Fallon Inquiry: From the Ashworth Hospital medical staff. *Psychiatric Bulletin* 1999; 23: 461–2.

73. Hansard HC. Deb. 12 January 1999, vol. 323, cc. 107–23.

74. Exworthy T, Gunn J. Taking another tilt at high security hospitals. *BJPsych* 2003; 182: 469–71.

75. Murray K. Data presented at Broadmoor seminar on high risk patients, November 2009.

76. The High Security Psychiatric Services (Arrangements for Safety and Security) Directions, 2019.

77. Murray K. The high security hospitals: Ashworth, Broadmoor and Rampton Hospitals. In Puri B and Treasaden I (eds) *Forensic Psychiatry: Fundamentals and Clinical Practice.* London: CRC Press, 2017.

78. Hansard HC. Deb. 15 February 1999, vol. 325, cc. 601–14.

79. Maden A. Dangerous and severe personality disorder: Antecedents and origins. *British Journal of Psychiatry* 2007; 190 (Suppl. 49): S8–S11.

80. National Institute for Mental Health in England. *Personality Disorder: No Longer a Diagnosis of Exclusion.* National Institute for Mental Health for England (NIMH(E)), 2003.

81. Department of Health and the Home Office. *Managing Dangerous People with Severe Personality Disorder.* Proposals for Policy Development, 1999.

82. Moran P. Dangerous severe personality disorder: Bad tidings from the UK. *International Journal of Social Psychiatry* 2002; 48 (1): 6–10.

83. Szmukler G. Violence risk prediction in practice. *British Journal of Psychiatry* 2001; 178: 84–8.

84. Craissati J, Minoudis P, Shaw J et al. *Working with Personality Disordered Offenders: A Practitioners Guide.* London, Ministry of Justice, 2011.

85. National Offender Management Service (NOMS). *The Offender Personality Disorder Strategy,* 2015.

86. Tyrer P, Duggan C, Cooper S et al. *Medicine, Science & the Law* 2010; 50: 95–9.

87. *R v LV; R (LV) v SSJ* [2015] EWCA Crim 45, [2015] EWCA Civ 56.

88. Robinson R, Coleman K, Sensky T, Walker M. *The Independent Review into the Care and Treatment of Mr Anthony Hardy*. London, North Central London Strategic Health Authority, 2005.

89. Robinson, R, Fenwick J, Wood S. *The Independent Inquiry into the Care and Treatment of John Barrett*. London, South West London Strategic Health Authority, 2006.

90. Salter M. Serious incident inquiries: A survival kit for psychiatrists. *Psychiatric Bulletin* 2003; 27: 245–7.

91. Shepperd D. *Learning the Lessons* (2nd ed.). London, Zito Trust, 1996.

92. www.hundredfamilies.org.

93. Crichton J. A review of published independent inquiries in England into psychiatric patient homicides, 1995–2010. *Journal of Forensic Psychiatry and Psychology* 2011; 22: 761–89.

94. National Confidential Inquiry into Suicide and Homicide by People with Mental Illness. *Independent Homicide Investigations*. University of Manchester, 2008.

95. National Confidential Inquiry into Suicide and Homicide annual report, England Northern Ireland Scotland and Wales, 2019. University of Manchester.

96. *Re C (Adult: Refusal of Medical Treatment)* [1994] 1 All ER 819, [1994] 1 WLR 290 (H.C.).

97. Appelbaum PS, Grisso T. Assessing patients' capacities to consent to treatment. *The New England Journal of Medicine* 1988; 319 (25): 1635–8.

98. *HL v UK* (2004) – App no 45508/99; 40 EHRR 761.

99. Department of Health. *Report of the Expert Committee: Review of the Mental Health Act 1983*. London, Department of Health, 1999.

100. Grounds A. Reforming the Mental Health Act. *BJPsych* 2001; 179: 387–9.

101. Szmukler G, Holloway F. Maudsley Discussion Paper no. 10. *Mental Health Law: Discrimination or Protection?* London, South London and Maudsley NHS Trust, 2000.

102. HL Paper 79-1; HC 95-1. House of Lords, House of Commons. London, HMSO, 23 March 2005.

103. Hansard, 23 March 2006, Column 27WS.

104. Delmage E, Exworthy T, Blackwood NJ. The 'Hybrid Order': origins and usage. *The Journal of Forensic Psychiatry & Psychology* 2015; 26 (3): 325–36.

105. Harbour A, Needham BH, Bolter L. *Independent Inquiry into the Care and Treatment of Richard Loudwell*. Medway Primary Care Trust and Medway Council, March 2006.

106. Francis, R, Baird J, Daniels G. *Independent Inquiry into the Care and Treatment of Peter Bryan and Richard Loudwell: A report for NHS London*. NHS London, September 2009.

107. Mishcon J, Exworthy T, Lindsey M. *Independent Inquiry into the Care and Treatment of Peter Bryan: Part One. A Report for NHS London*. NHS London, September 2009.

108 Gordon H, Oyebode O, Minne C. Death by homicide in Special Hospitals. *Journal of Forensic Psychiatry* 1997; 8 (3): 602–19.

109. *Care Quality Commission: Investigation into West London Mental Health NHS Trust*. Care Quality Commission, July 2009.

110. Eaton L. Commissioners publish highly critical reports on mental health services. *British Medical Journal* 2009. https://doi.org/10.1136/bmj.b2978.

111. Silva E, Shepherd A. Tick, tock, lock: night-time confinement in high security – history, practice, ethics and practicalities. *BJPsych Bulletin* 2019; 43 (1): 1–3. doi: https://doi.org/10.1192/bjb.2018.80.

112. Thomson L. Night-time confinement and the practice of realistic medicine. *BJPsych Bulletin* 2019; 43 (1): 32–4. doi: https://doi.org/10.1192/bjb.2018.83.

113. Szmukler G. Night-time confinement is an unacceptable hospital practice. *BJPsych Bulletin* 2019; 43 (1): 35–7. https://doi.org/10.1192/bjb.2018.82.

114. European Committee for the Prevention of Torture and Inhuman or Degrading Treatment or Punishment. *Report to the Government of the United Kingdom on the Visit to the United Kingdom (CPT).* Strasbourg, Council of Europe, 2017.

115. *The High Security Psychiatric Services (Arrangements for Safety and Security) Directions.* London, Department of Health and Social Care, 2019.

116. Ly L, Foster S. *Home Office Statistical Bulletin 22/05: Statistics of Mentally Disordered Offenders.* ISSN 1358–510X. London, the Home Office, 2004.

117. *Ministry of Justice Statistics Bulletin: Statistics of Mentally Disordered Offenders 2008 England and Wales.* London, Ministry of Justice, 2008.

118. Fazel S, Fimińska Z, Cocks C, Coid J. Patient outcomes following discharge from secure psychiatric hospitals: Systematic review and meta-analysis. *BJPsych* 2016; 208 (1). https://dx.doi.org/10.1192%2Fbjp.bp.114.149997.

119. *Vowles and others* [2015] EWCA Crim 45.

120. Peay J. Responsibility, culpability and the sentencing of mentally disordered offenders: objectives in conflict. *Criminal Law Review* 2016; 3: 152–64. http://eprints.lse.ac.uk/64221.

121. *R v Edwards* [2018] EWCA Crim 595.

122. *Modernising the Mental Health Act: Increasing Choice, Reducing Compulsion.* Final report of the Independent Review of the Mental Health Act 1983, December 2018.

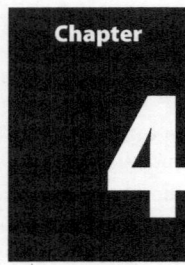

Prison Psychiatry

Ian Cumming

Introduction

To those outside the walls, prisons are poorly understood; the perception of prison is often derived from common culture and even well-researched documentaries fail to fully describe the environment.

Prisons date back to before concepts of justice and existed in ancient Greek and biblical times. The presence of mental illness and mental disorder in prison is a universal given transcending time and geography. As such, they are appropriate places for a psychiatrist to work, though not to everyone's taste, and many find the challenges difficult and at times without compromise, particularly in the delicate balance between mental health and security [1, 2, 3].

With the gradual development of more devolved and specialist services in psychiatry, prisons potentially remain one of the last places where a psychiatrist can experience the broadest range of mental disorder. The clinician can experience the full gamut of conditions from acute and chronic mental illness to anxiety, depression, personality disorder, learning disability, neurodevelopmental disorders, alcohol and substance misuse, and many others. Prisoners are one of the most disadvantaged groups and as such small changes can make an enormous difference. Prisons are thus a rich environment and offer a psychiatrist the opportunity to develop and hone diagnostic skills and communicate with a wide range of care and custodial partners [4].

This chapter seeks to provide clinicians a better understanding of prisons and overcome many of the myths and misconceptions, hopefully with the objective of making the environment more attractive and interesting for future psychiatrists who may be seeking a challenge or a change in direction.

The clinician may ask what prisons are for; are they for rehabilitation and reformation, are they or should they be a source of labour, are they for deterrence or are they for punishment [5]? In reality, prisons have oscillated between the extremes of punishment and rehabilitation depending on the state of the existing government and what is believed attractive to the public; thus, when government needs to show a hand strong in justice, they become places more for punishment – seen, for example, in the late 1970s when the UK government of the day announced a manifesto promise of the 'Short Sharp Shock'.

With similar crime rates, some countries imprison far more than others [6]. The USA has a prison population of 737/100,000 population, Russia 615 and Japan 62; England and Wales at 148/100,000 has one of the highest rates per 100,000 in western Europe . For many, the role of prison is to simply incapacitate and remove individuals who pose a risk from society. However, there have been more enlightened times when there was a greater focus on rehabilitation. The current state of prisons in any country is best understood by its history, economy, religion, government, case law and policy, as well as by tragedy, notoriety and dilemma.

A Brief History of Prisons

The term 'jail' is derived from the term 'gaol' – still used in the term 'gaoler', which itself is derived from the Latin term *cavus*, meaning 'a hollow', from which came the term *cavea*, meaning dungeon or cage. In the UK, we utilise the term 'prison' as a generic term for a custodial environment. Outside of the UK, for instance in the USA, the term 'jail' is for those on remand pending trial and prison is for those convicted and sentenced, with the two populations being kept apart and distinct.

In England, William the Conqueror sought to impose royal authority with the construction of the Tower of London in the year 1078, the first royal prison and built to hold the king's enemies. There were other similar ventures to hold private enemies, but it was not until Henry II (1154–89) through the Assizes of Clarendon that sheriffs were ordered to build jails in each county to hold those accused of felonies until they could be tried. Debt was a key reason but over time more and more offences were added, such as vagrancy and moral offences. Jails also had a history of charging fees to allow the prisoner more comfort.

Edward VI in 1553 gave the Palace of Bridewell to the City of London to be used as a prison for petty offences. The Palace of Bridewell had been a pioneering experiment operating under a Royal Charter with a court of governors to meet and manage the institution – they would appoint, among others, physicians, nurses and surgeons. The Act of 1609 saw them introduced into every county.

Population management has been a key driver of prisons in any country. Evolving from the concept of exile, the UK government sought to remove offenders by transportation to the colonies. John Howard, who had earlier been captured and imprisoned by French privateers, was appointed sheriff of Bedfordshire and was instructed to inspect prisons in the county. He later expanded his inspection across England and into Europe. He found the prisons in a poor state, with many unable to leave as they were unable to pay the gaoler's fee for their upkeep, which had to be settled before they could get out of prison. As a result, those found innocent of a felony could be found guilty of debt if they could not pay the fee.

After presenting the matter to a select committee, he produced a detailed document, 'The State of the Prisons in 1777' [7]. The document included plans for improvement. He applied to the county justices to provide the keeper with a regular wage and contributed to the end of prisoners being held many to a room, moving towards single cells. He also identified the presence of mentally ill people in Bridewell. It was from John Howard that an independent system of inspection was established and from where the later Prison Inspectorate evolved. Predating this had been the establishment of the Prison Medical Service in 1774; as a national service, it was the longest-standing health service until its demise at the end of the twentieth century.

Following the American War of Independence in 1776, the loss of colonies in the USA meant that there was nowhere for prisoners to be transported to, so the Penitentiary Act of 1779 saw the establishment of state prisons and the use of prison hulks to manage the population by holding prisoners on ships. Living conditions in the hulks were harsh, with high mortality rates and ill health prevalent. Although they were only meant to be used temporarily, use of hulks continued until the last was decommissioned in the 1860s. Transportation resumed with the deportation of prisoners to Australia in 1787.

During the eighteenth century there was increasing recognition of mentally disordered offenders. The implementation of the Criminal Lunatics Act in 1800 saw the defence of not guilty by reason of insanity, with prisoners being detained at His Majesty's pleasure. The County Asylum Act of 1808 encouraged the building of county lunatic asylums and the Lunacy Act of 1845 made the establishment of these compulsory to help remove the mentally ill from prisons and workhouses.

Medical knowledge about mental health began to increase. As the numbers of mentally disordered prisoners increased combined with the criminally insane in county asylums, an asylum for the criminally insane was established first in Ireland at Dundrum (1850), then at Broadmoor, which opened in 1863.

There were attempts to localise those with a mental disorder. The mentally ill at Dartmoor were transferred to Millbank Penitentiary in 1864, and in 1897 Parkhurst prison took on the role of holding those unfit for ordinary prisons due to a mental instability other than insanity.

The early nineteenth century saw a shift towards harsh environments and punishment. Sir Edmund Du Cane (HMP Wormwood Scrubs is located on a road in London that bears his name) implemented unpleasant environments with the use of treadmills and cranks that prisoners would have to turn to obtain food (the term 'screw' comes from the process of prison officers increasing the tension of the crank to make it harder).

Doctors had a role in determining who could be exempt from hard labour and also determined the minimum diet to sustain life. With recognition that being exposed to other prisoners might cause further offending, prisons were run silently for a period. In Pentonville prisoners were housed separately; there was recognition that using such a system led to a marked increase in the 'rate of lunacy'.

The early part of the twentieth century saw a focus upon mental conditions in prisons with more interest in psychotherapy, eventually leading to therapeutic communities for those with shell shock. The idea that therapeutic environments could work with psychopathy led to the creation of therapeutic prisons such as HMP Grendon in 1962.

The creation of the National Health Service (NHS) in 1948 did not incorporate prisons, which remained separate with healthcare managed by the Prison Medical Service. The latter part of the twentieth century saw more interest and penetration by mental health services into prisons, usually in the form of discreet sessions between a local mental health provider and the prison. Later the seminal document 'Patient or Prisoner' (1996) identified that health in prisons was being left behind, with difficulties in retention and recruitment of staff. This in turn led to the publication in 1999 of 'The Future Organisation of Prison Healthcare'. Eventually the NHS began to take over responsibility for prison healthcare in 2003, with budgetary responsibility also transferred to the NHS.

Current Status (UK)

Against a background of various incarnations, prisons in the UK are now subsumed within His Majesty's Prison and Probation Service (HMPPS). At the time of writing, there are 117 prisons in England and Wales. The majority are run by HMPPS with a small number run by private companies, notably G4S, Sodexo and Serco. Government spending has decreased since 2009/10, with some reversal in the trend recently.

The prison population remains at a high level and hovers between 80,000 and 85,000. The proportion who are women was 17% in 1900, 2% in the late 1960s and around 5% now. The number of older prisoners has risen by 25% since 2016. Prisons can be categorised in many ways such as local, high-security, training, resettlement, open, closed, female, male and young offender, as well as other secure environments such as removal centres or detention centres.

Most cities will have a local remand prison; they are usually busy and have a high turnover. Prisoners are classified as either in category D (the lowest), C, B or A – the latter is itself further subdivided into standard, high and exceptional. There are a small number of high-security prisons (previously known as dispersal prisons) which hold these higher-risk prisoners (usually determined at the point of conviction) – that is, Category A. There are often no more than one or two exceptional-risk prisoners at any one time in England and Wales and there are considerable implications in moving such prisoners to court and other establishments.

Healthcare is a basic right for prisoners. Although not all prisons have a healthcare unit, the right of access is ensured. Prison healthcare is categorised as:

Type 1: daytime cover, generally part-time staff.

Type 2: daytime/24-hour cover, generally by full-time staff but no in-patient facilities.

Type 3: healthcare centre with 24-hour nurse cover, usually with in-patient facilities.

Type 4: the same as Type 3 but with a national or regional assessment area for use by other prisons.

Incidence and Prevalence of Mental Disorder

There is considerable literature on the relationship between mental disorder and crime at all levels. A common assumption is that mentally ill persons accumulate in prisons due to failures of 'care in the community' and 'closing the asylums'. Although these factors might have some relevance, mentally ill prisoners have always been in prison and are a feature in any prison throughout the world and through time.

The prison population and its management continues to be an issue for England and Wales and many other countries. There are many factors which influence this, such as rising crime in a recession but also changes in sentencing.

In general, it would be best to consider that issues which may be relevant in the routes into prison for those with a mental disorder are a combination of the following factors:

- General – those of crime in general.
- Specific: nature of condition on offence, such as a delusion causing an individual to attack another or ongoing illness poorly responsive to treatment.
- Comorbid: homelessness, lack/breakdown of supporting relationships, illegal drug use, alcohol use, financial difficulties, personality disorder and so on.
- Service provision issues.

Individuals with mental illness and other mental disorders often have a greater range of comorbid issues which might have an impact on offending. The final factor of service provision will not be universal but in some prisons and parts of the country it may be very relevant. Psychiatrists who work in prison will be familiar with situations in which patients have not been able to access services or have been excluded for one reason or another. Mental health services in the community have become more and more specialised and these can be difficult to navigate, sometimes with exclusion criteria that pass patients on to another service. The factors listed above can also be relevant to the route out of custody and, after return to the community, reintegration back into existing services.

Worldwide Studies

Although there are considerable geographical variations in rates of imprisonment per 100,000 across the world, the rates of mental disorder are broadly similar. Fazel and Danesh reviewed 62 surveys of prison studies across 12 countries covering around 22,790 prisoners [8]. This found, among men, rates of psychosis at 3.7%, major depression at 10% and those with a personality disorder at 65%. This review has been repeated on a number of occasions with no improvement [9, 10, 11].

UK Studies

The UK's research has been largely dominated by two main studies. The first was conducted in two parts by Gunn, Maden et al. in 1991 and 1995 which examined the sentenced and remand prison population, respectively [12, 13]. In 1998 the Office of National Statistics (ONS) published its own survey of psychiatric morbidity [14]. The Gunn and Maden studies were major pieces of work in which mental health practitioners directly interviewed a representative and randomly chosen sample of prisoners across prisons in England and Wales. In addition to these interviews, they utilised medical records, discipline records, interviews with prison staff, notes and reports from NHS hospitals and data on previous convictions. In the remand study both interviewers were psychiatrists. These two studies' findings are set out in Tables 4.1 and 4.2.

In addition to establishing a diagnosis, both studies made recommendations for treatment options of the individuals interviewed, which included hospital transfer. It was felt that there should be clear policies for the management of mental disorder. This was directed to the Prison Medical Service (who were the providers of medical care in prisons at that time), asking when this should be taken over by the NHS and importantly emphasising that this should apply to all forms of mental disorder and not just mental illness/psychosis. The study asked for explicit standards or thresholds as to when those with psychosis should be transferred out. It also recommended that standards of care for those who remain in prison should be equivalent to the NHS.

This study made the direct recommendation that the solution to mentally disordered offenders in prison with mental illness was in the NHS and that equivalence within the prison system was needed. These two themes continued to haunt and overshadow future policy directions.

The issue of mentally ill prisoners links to the other particular issue of why the Mental Health Act does not and has not applied within a prison setting, and whether this has a bearing upon the levels of mental illness within prisons. Thus, it would be reasonable to assume that some of the mentally ill prisoners were ill because of a lack of insight and a refusal to take treatment, but what proportion does this apply to and would the instigation of the Mental Health Act in prison cause any change in the absolute numbers of mentally ill prisoners?

The later ONS study ('Psychiatric Morbidity among Prisoners in England and Wales', Tables 4.3 and 4.4) was conducted in the aftermath of the Gunn and Maden studies and commissioned by the Department of Health in 1997 to gather baseline data and inform later policy decisions [14]. It included all prisons in England and Wales and attempted to estimate psychiatric morbidity; it was not clear why this was necessary as the earlier Gunn

Table 4.1 Prevalence of mental disorder in the remand population

	Adult males (%)	Male youths (%)	Women (%)
All psychosis	5.9	1.9	4.5
Schizophrenia	5.5	1.9	3.3
Schizoaffective	0.2	0	0.4
Bipolar	0.2	0	0.8
Neuroses	28.1	18.9	43.7
Neurotic disorders	19.1	15.0	27.4
Adjustment disorders	9.0	3.9	16.3
Personality disorders	11.0	11.7	15.5
Substance misuse (all)	39.0	36.4	41.6
Alcohol	15.6	13.6	8.2
Organic	0.7	1.5	1.6
Mental retardation	0.2	2.0	2.4
Uncertain diagnosis	1.5	0.5	2.9

Note: The term 'neuroses' combine neurotic disorders (depressive episodes, anxiety disorders and post-traumatic stress disorder) with adjustment disorders.

Table 4.2 Prevalence of mental disorder in the sentenced population

	Adult males (%)	Male youths (%)	Women (%)
All psychosis	2.4	0.2	1.1
Schizophrenia	1.5	0.2	1.1
Affective	0.5	0	0
Paranoid	0.4	0	0
Neuroses	5.2	4.5	13.2
Neurotic disorders	3.6	3.0	7.7
Adjustment disorders	1.6	1.5	5.5
Personality disorders	7.3	11.4	8.4
Substance misuse (all)	20.1	15.8	28.9
Alcohol	8.6	8.7	4.4
Organic	0.9	0.5	2.6
Mental retardation	0.4	0.2	2.2
Uncertain diagnosis	1.3	0.5	1.8

Table 4.3 ONS study – personality disorder

	Male remand (%)	Male sentenced (%)	Female (%)
Personality disorder (all)	78	64	50
Antisocial	63	49	31
Antisocial (only)	28	30	11
Antisocial (and other)	35	20	20
Paranoid	29	20	16
Borderline	23	14	20
Avoidant	14	7	11

and Maden studies had themselves been commissioned by the Home Office Research and Planning Unit on behalf of the Prison Directorate of Health Care – this perhaps hints at the divide that existed between the Home Office (Department of Justice) and the Department of Health at that time. The later ONS study also replicated an earlier design that had been used outside of prison [15].

In contrast to the Gunn and Maden studies, the ONS study aimed to interview 1,200 remand prisoners (1 in 8 of those in prison), 1,200 sentenced prisoners (1 in 34 of those in prison) and 800 female prisoners (1 in 3 of those in prison). Of the total of 3,563 selected, 3,142 (88%) were interviewed (called a lay interview). Every fifth person was selected for a follow-up interview and of these 76% (or 505 in number) were interviewed again (called a clinical interview).

The later clinical interview generated most notably data about personality disorder and utilised the SCID (structured clinical interview for *DSM* 4). This showed that the prevalence of any personality disorder was 78% for male remand prisoners, 64% for sentenced prisoners and 50% for female prisoners.

Neurotic disorders in the week prior to interview were assessed in the lay interviews using the CIS-R (clinical interview schedule – revised). It is to be noted that this is different from the Gunn and Maden studies of neurotic conditions. It was conducted by non-clinical staff and involved 14 sections to determine the presence of a particular neurotic symptom in the past month. A positive response leads on to a further enquiry, giving a more detailed assessment of the symptom in the previous week.

The various symptoms include (but note that these do not equate to a diagnosis) sleep problems, worry, fatigue, depression, irritability, depressive ideas, concentration/forgetfulness, anxiety, obsessions, somatic symptoms, compulsions, phobias, worry about physical health and panic. The findings were again far higher than the general population and in most cases double. It was noted that remand prisoners had roughly double the incidence of sentenced prisoners.

One particular aspect of this study and indeed many others is the validity of such tools within a prison population. Does a prisoner who is depressed at being in prison have the same depression that might be felt in the community after a loss? Ill health in prison also has a different currency. While many tools that have been well validated in the community are used in a prison, there are few if any tools which have originated from and been validated in a prison setting. As an example, in general patients come to see psychiatrists in the

Table 4.4 ONS study – neurotic disorders

	Male remand	Male sentenced	Female remand	Female sentenced	Male household	Female household
	Proportion of population with a score of 2+ on each symptom					
Sleep problems	67	54	81	62	21	28
Worry	58	42	67	58	17	23
Fatigue	46	35	64	57	21	33
Depression	56	33	64	51	8	11
Irritability	43	35	51	43	19	25
Depressive ideas	38	20	57	39	7	11
Concentration	34	23	53	38	6	10
Anxiety	33	21	42	32	8	11
Obsessions	30	22	35	24	7	12
Somatic symptoms	24	16	40	30	5	10
Compulsions	24	15	25	18	5	8
Phobias	20	13	31	22	3	7
Worry over physical health	22	16	25	23	4	5
Panic	18	8	26	15	2	3

community because a symptom is troubling them, and we as clinicians typically accept that this is the case and our formulation proceeds. In a prison setting we notice an underlying doubt as to why they might have such a symptom. Research tools are often poorly geared for deception.

The ONS study also examined psychotic and affective disorders (Table 4.5) and recognised that this was far more problematic for lay interviewers. These were interviewed in the later clinical interviews by psychiatrists – the same sample followed up for the assessment of personality disorder. The clinicians were trained to carry out interviews using SCAN 1.0 (schedules for clinical assessments in neuropsychiatry) which was programmed onto a laptop computer. One of the components for assessing psychosis was the PSE10 (present state examination).

The study looked at the relationship between various questions in the lay interview and the results of the SCAN interview and built up a model of what clusters of factors are highly correlated with positive cases of psychotic psychopathology. This model was then applied to the remaining sample to provide an estimate of the likely prevalence of psychoses among the sample as a whole. These are outlined in Table 4.6.

The studies also examined substance misuse, self-harm and intellectual functioning for completeness and to allow comparison with the Gunn and Maden studies. These are summarised in Tables 4.7 and 4.8.

Table 4.5 Prevalence of functional psychosis (from clinical interviews)

	Male remand	Male sentenced	Female
	Proportion of population (%) in past year		
Schizophrenia	2	1	3
Other non-organic psychotic disorders	7	4	10
Any schizophrenic or delusional disorder	9	6	13
Manic episode	1	1	1
Severe or recurrent depression +psychosis	1		1
Any affective psychosis	2	1	2
Any functional psychosis	10	7	14

Table 4.6 Proportion of respondents likely to have a psychotic disorder

	Lay interviews (%)	Clinical interviews (%)
Male remand	9	10
Male sentenced	4	7
Female remand	21	14
Female sentenced	10	

Table 4.7 Prevalence of self-harm

	Male remand	Male sentenced	Female remand	Female sentenced
	Cumulative percentage of the population			
Suicidal thoughts				
Past week	12	4	23	8
Past year	35	20	50	34
Lifetime	46	37	59	52
Suicide attempts				
Past week	2	0	2	1
Past year	15	7	27	16
Lifetime	27	20	44	37
Self-harm (not suicide attempt) during current prison term	5	7	9	10

Table 4.8 Prevalence of drug dependence

	Male remand	Male sentenced	Female remand	Female sentenced
	Proportion of population (%) in year prior to entering prison			
Any drug dependence	51	43	54	41

Overall UK Study Findings

Both studies highlighted that between 5% and 10% of the remand population has a psychosis, and roughly half that prevalence in the sentenced population. There are high levels of substance misuse, alcohol misuse, self-harm, adjustment disorders, neurotic disorders and personality disorder. It is to be noted that in terms of the latter, the later ONS study showed considerably higher levels of personality disorder with, for example, in the male remand population there being 11% in the Gunn and Maden study and 78% in the ONS study. This reflects that the ONS study used a tool specific for the purpose, though there are some confounding issues when applying such a tool in a prison population where criminality is one parameter in establishing the diagnosis.

In addition to high morbidity there is the turnover or churn rate, with several times the population of a prison entering and leaving through the year [17–21]. This presents considerable challenges in identifying and delivering care. Certain populations have even higher levels of mental disorder [22–25] including young offenders and elderly prisoners. Immigration and removal centres are another such example. In 2013 [26, 27] and 2021 [28], the Royal College of Psychiatrists issued a position statement about such centres and identified high levels of depression, post-traumatic stress disorder, anxiety and suicidal ideation. There are many possible reasons, including high levels of stressful events such as torture and detention in their own country or during transit, as well as separation from family and isolation. The propensity to deteriorate and relive previous detention is considerable.

Historically, mental health services had been invited into prisons to provide specialist input. The generalist nature of the Prison Medical Service meant that this was largely with a focus on mental illness and issues which were more challenging and beyond the abilities of the medical services within the prison. With the dissolution of the Prison Medical Service, delivery of mental healthcare passed to the NHS, though psychiatry has largely continued to focus upon mental illness with limited capacity and the desire to address the much larger and more complex group with personality disorder and substance misuse who do not fall into this category.

With the recognition of high levels of morbidity in the prison population, it was soon apparent that there was a paucity of understanding as to how such levels could be managed and how services should be profiled. Forensic psychiatry in the UK continued to keep prisons at a distance and only since the move of provision and funding to the NHS have services become interested in working in such environments.

Court Diversion

This is a fitting point to look briefly at how mentally disordered offenders have arrived in prison and what their experience will be as they pass through the criminal justice system [29, 30]. Perhaps surprisingly, there is sometimes a poor understanding of the pathway into and through prison – particularly the mechanics of the criminal justice system and how this impacts on the mentally ill.

In any forensic psychiatry service, the majority of patients will be either going through or have come through the criminal justice service [31, 32]. At the time of writing, mental health services have penetrated various parts of the criminal justice pathway. They can be found within street triage services, in police stations [33–36], at the magistrate court, at some of the crown courts and in prisons [37–39]. As the type of patient is effectively the same, it would seem likely that these roles and services will evolve into a single entity [40].

Why do we have court diversion? At its simplest, the recognition that there were many people in prison with a mental disorder and the presence of their illness acted as an impediment to processes for leaving custody, for example getting bail. There was also a recognition that moving from prison to hospital as a prisoner meant that they required by default a higher level of security than if they were admitted to hospital from the community. These factors, combined with the simplistic view that there was a link between the high levels of mentally disordered offenders and the large prison population, have underpinned the development of court liaison and diversion services.

In many respects, moving those charged with offences out of the criminal justice service to health services is nothing new – Part III of the Mental Health Act has many options for effecting such a movement. The key aspect of court diversion and liaison was to implement this as early as possible.

The idea of court liaison and diversion in England and Wales had been promoted by the Home Office in 1990. The original court diversion services were piloted in around 1989; these were essentially local initiatives between health and courts, often championed by individuals [41–43]. The idea was further supported by the 1992 Reed Report [44–45] which recommended a nationwide provision of properly resourced schemes. By the time of the later Bradley Review (itself commissioned to look at mentally disordered offenders caught up in custodial settings), services continued to develop and embrace other parts of the criminal justice pathway such as the crown court, but the provision was ad hoc, locally variable, often without funding and operating vastly different models [46].

The impact and effect of court diversion and liaison services has been considerably researched. There had often been a lack of clarity about what they provided and how many were in operation. It was also unclear as to how effective they were. Lord Bradley in 2009 had been asked to conduct an independent review to determine to what extent offenders with mental health problems or learning disabilities could be diverted from prison to other services and what were the barriers to such diversion. The initial focus was on the organisation and effectiveness of court diversion and liaison schemes, though the report extended into the whole of the offender pathway.

Bradley recommended through the National Programme Board for England and Wales the development of a national model of criminal justice mental health teams and to include it within the standard NHS Contract for mental health and learning disabilities services on a non-mandated basis. Bradley also recommended screening and assessment in the police station. Earlier studies [47] had shown that services at the police station did not duplicate what went on in the court but tended to identify more minor offences, and allowed signposting to local services and might contribute to reducing more serious offending later, though there was no actual evidence that this was so. To better understand how such services work, it is worth pausing to clarify the criminal justice trajectory and where mental health services work.

Arrest to Police Custody

Even before arrest, street triage services are increasingly being developed. These provide on-the-spot advice to police when they encounter people who may have a mental health problem. This might be in the form of advice but overall seeks to allow an officer to make better decisions [48].

After an individual commits an offence, they are often arrested and taken to the police station. Here they will be searched and have details taken. Normally after a short period they will be questioned and possibly charged. Until the point of charging, mental health services can interface in a number of ways. Assuming that the arrested person has a mental health problem, the first challenge facing the police is whether the individual is fit to be interviewed and also medically and psychiatrically fit to be detained.

This is the more familiar face of visiting police stations, where typically at the request of the forensic medical examiner mental health services, appropriate adults and social workers will be called in to assist. It is within this time period that civil sections of the Mental Health Act might come into play and the patient may be admitted to hospital. The police are obliged under section C of the Police and Criminal Evidence Act 1984 (PACE), if they have information or suspicion of mental health issues, to treat the person accordingly. An appropriate adult should support the person during the process and they should have appropriate clinical attention as soon as reasonably practicable. Appropriate adults are best considered as those people who have mental health experience, although in their absence a relative can be considered.

Mental health services are increasingly present in police stations [49–50]. The criminal justice mental health worker will aim to work with the police in assessing individuals, providing guidance as well as developing pathways out of custody such as a Mental Health Act assessment [51].

Police Custody to Magistrates' Court

In common law jurisdictions, criminal cases are tried in an adversarial process in which a prosecutor presents evidence of the crime and a defence lawyer rebuts this. A judge ensures fair process. In other legal traditions, the judge takes a more active, inquisitorial role.

After an individual is charged, the next decision facing the police is whether an accused can be granted police bail before going to the magistrates' court or whether they should be held overnight to face court the next day. It is at magistrates' courts that patients may encounter court diversion services which are now commonplace within many courts in England and Wales. The presence of a mental health issue might in certain situations be a disadvantage in achieving bail with the fear that their mental health condition will impact upon their reliability.

At a number of points and usually when they attend court, defendants have an opportunity to be granted bail. This will normally be put forward to the judge by their solicitor and may be opposed by the Crown Prosecution Service (CPS) lawyer. There are many reasons why bail may not be granted. In essence, the court needs to be confident that the defendant will appear again, will not commit offences and will not intimidate witnesses, and sometimes that they are not a risk to themselves or others. The defendant may lack the capacity to consent to bail conditions and may refuse bail conditions due to delusions or impaired judgement. An address is also a requirement, which can be difficult if the offence is towards someone who they live with or nearby a victim. Our patients are sometimes affected by this and one should consider whether the nature of their condition might mean that they fail to attend.

Magistrates' and crown courts are the main but not the only part of the court service and not the only place at which mentally ill patients might appear. There are also county courts, high courts and others. His Majesty's Courts Service (HMCS) came into formal existence in April 2005 and now administers all but the lower tribunals (Figure 4.1).

At a magistrates' court there are two different types of magistrate. The vast majority of magistrates in England and Wales are lay members of the public, sometimes known as justices of the peace. These magistrates are responsible for handling over 95% of all criminal cases in England and Wales. They represent the ideal of having members of the community involved in legal issues and reflect community values and as such are mixed in gender, age, ethnicity and so on whenever possible to bring a broad experience of life to the bench. They are not legally trained, are unpaid and sit typically in groups of three. Two are also permissible but a single magistrate is not; they sit with a legally qualified clerk. Magistrates cannot sentence for longer than 6 months or 12 months in the case of consecutive cases.

There are in addition what used to be called stipendiary magistrates. These are professional lawyers who act as magistrates for a fee (a stipend). A large proportion work in city centres such as London. They tend to be far more efficient and productive than the lay magistrates. Since 2000, stipendiary magistrates have been known as district judges (magistrates' courts). District judges hear criminal cases, youth cases and some civil proceedings

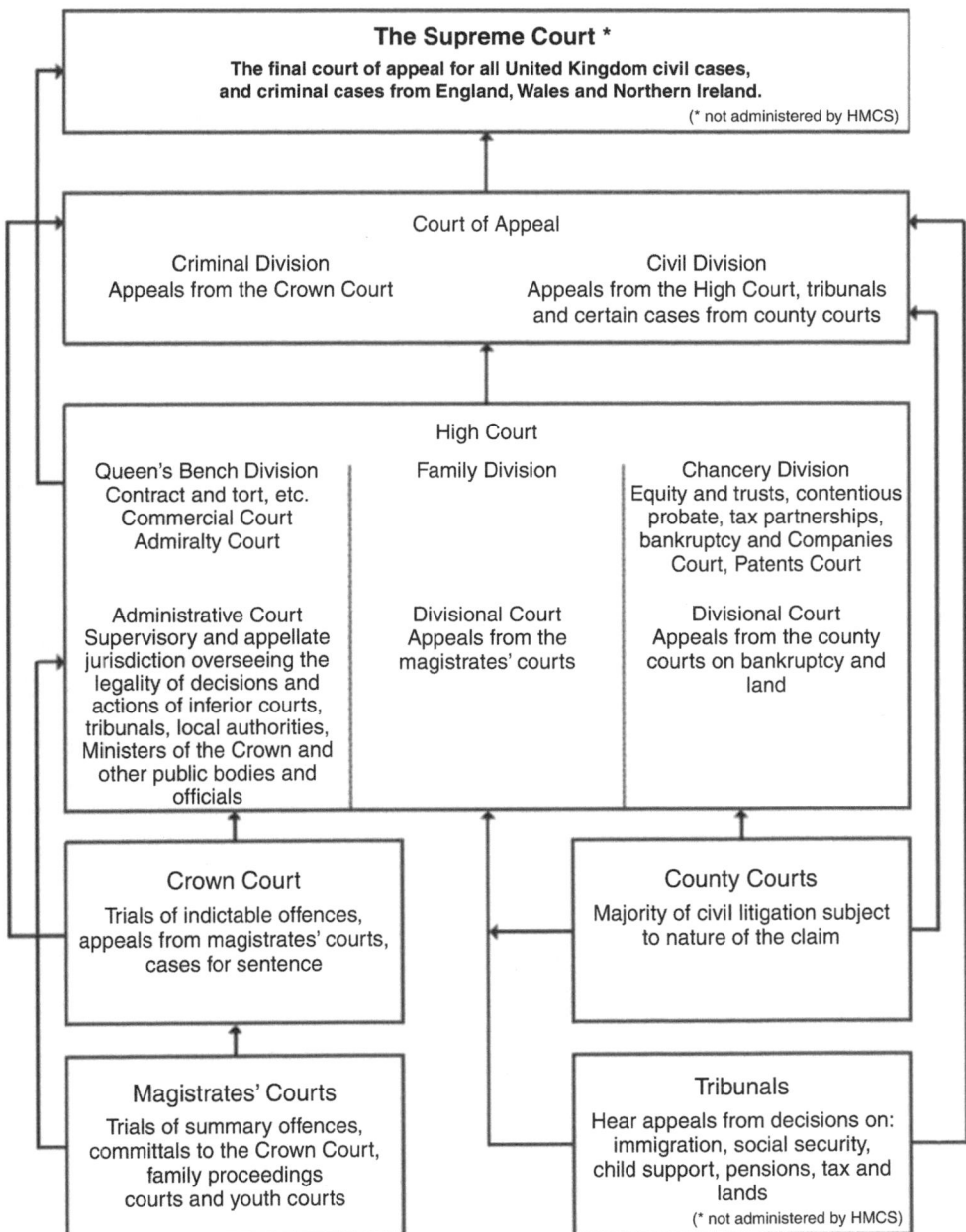

The Supreme Court *
The final court of appeal for all United Kingdom civil cases, and criminal cases from England, Wales and Northern Ireland.
(* not administered by HMCS)

Court of Appeal

Criminal Division
Appeals from the Crown Court

Civil Division
Appeals from the High Court, tribunals and certain cases from county courts

High Court

Queen's Bench Division
Contract and tort, etc.
Commercial Court
Admiralty Court

Family Division

Chancery Division
Equity and trusts, contentious probate, tax partnerships, bankruptcy and Companies Court, Patents Court

Administrative Court
Supervisory and appellate jurisdiction overseeing the legality of decisions and actions of inferior courts, tribunals, local authorities, Ministers of the Crown and other public bodies and officials

Divisional Court
Appeals from the magistrates' courts

Divisional Court
Appeals from the county courts on bankruptcy and land

Crown Court

Trials of indictable offences, appeals from magistrates' courts, cases for sentence

County Courts

Majority of civil litigation subject to nature of the claim

Magistrates' Courts

Trials of summary offences, committals to the Crown Court, family proceedings courts and youth courts

Tribunals

Hear appeals from decisions on: immigration, social security, child support, pensions, tax and lands
(* not administered by HMCS)

Figure 4.1 Court structure of His Majesty's Courts Service. Diagram reproduced from His Majesty's Courts Service – Structure of HMCS. Crown copyright.

and can be authorised to hear cases in the family proceedings courts. Some are authorised to deal with extradition proceedings and terrorist cases. District judges are also authorised to sit as prison adjudicators and usually hear cases alone.

There are in the main three types of offences: indictable, summary and offences triable each way. Indictable offences are those that cannot be dealt with at the magistrates' court and must be sent to the crown court. Summary offences are dealt with at the magistrates' court. The third category can be dealt with at either. This will usually occur if the defendant pleads not guilty and elects for a trial at crown court. Alternatively, it might occur if, for instance, the defendant has a considerable history of offending and is beyond the sentencing powers of the magistrates' court (i.e. it is felt that they require a longer sentence than can be provided by the magistrates' court). Magistrates can only sentence defendants to a maximum of 18 months. The distinction between the two is not always obvious.

At the court, quite a lot happens. The issues are essentially about entering a plea, bail and sentencing directions; that is, deciding when and where the defendant can be sentenced. Let us assume that the defendant is sent to the crown court or 'committed'.

Crown Court: Committal to Conviction

After the defendant is committed to the crown court, there is often some time before the case is heard and dealt with. The crown court deals with more serious criminal cases such as murder, rape or robbery, some of which are on appeal or referred from magistrates' courts.

Trials are heard by a judge and a 12-person jury. Members of the public are selected for jury service or may have to go to court as witnesses. The crown court is based at 77 centres across England and Wales. It deals with cases transferred from the magistrates' courts. It also hears appeals against decisions of magistrates' courts and deals with cases sent for sentence from magistrates' courts.

The crown court system in England and Wales was only established in 1956 and took over from the old quarter and assize sessions. The current court system in England and Wales is the result of almost 1,000 years of evolution, with Henry II establishing a jury of 12 local knights in the twelfth century. Today there are many thousand judicial officeholders in England and Wales (this includes many part-time, high court and district judges), with the most senior judge being the Lord Chief Justice.

Crown court trials are typically conducted by a mixture of circuit judges, recorders and high court judges. There are around 600 circuit judges in England and Wales and they specifically hear criminal or civil cases. They must be lawyers who have held a right of audience for at least 10 years. They are appointed by the king following a fair and open competition administered by the Judicial Appointments Commission. When hearing criminal cases, they wear a red sash over their left shoulder. They are referred to as 'your honour'. Recorders are fee-paid part-time judges, often working as the first step on the judicial ladder to appointment to the circuit bench. They tend to handle less complex or serious matters coming before the court. There are about 106 high court judges (criminal jurisdiction) in England and Wales. They hear the most serious and sensitive cases in the crown court. They usually sit in London but also travel to major court centres around the country. They are given the prefix 'the honourable' and referred to as Mr/Mrs Justice *surname* and called 'my lord' in court.

Individuals are called to become part of a jury by means of a jury summons. They are selected at random by computer from the electoral register. It is a public duty and there are only a few situations in which one might be excused. These include being on bail and currently or having in the past suffered from a mental health problem (such as being in hospital or under a guardianship order). Jury duty can be deferred once.

In contrast to a magistrates' court, crown courts are far more formal and theatrical. They tend to take far longer with each case and additionally entail considerable cost in laying on appearances, trials and so on. The latter is to be stressed because any psychiatric issue which impinges on courts leads to pressure on the public purse. Typically, a murder case can take up to a year between arrest and sentencing at the crown court. The main issue is the length of time that the court is required to find for a trial. For serious offences or those that involve multiple defendants, a large window of time is required, and this is often difficult to find, hence the long delay before those cases come to court. Minor or less complex cases require a smaller window of time and hence tend to come to trial sooner.

These issues are important as mental health services often fail to understand that, like any other government organisation, the court service has priorities which have consequences if they are not met. Both magistrates' and crown courts are regularly aware of how often mental health issues impact upon the progression of cases through the court.

After committal to crown court, the next date is a plea and case management hearing. During this time the CPS puts together the case against the defendant and this is given to the defendant and their lawyers. After looking at this, the defendant will (usually after discussion with their lawyers) make a decision as to whether to plead guilty or not guilty.

It is also in this period that decisions about fitness to plead are central and considered. This is often the reason behind psychiatrists' involvement at this point. Psychiatrists are employed by both the defence and prosecution to consider this in appropriate cases.

Assuming that the defendant is fit to plead and stand trial, a defendant will be asked for their plea. If they plead guilty, they will move forwards to conviction. If they plead not guilty, they will move ahead to a trial before a jury. The trial process is quite complex and full of terminology. In essence, at the beginning of the trial a jury is first selected or 'voir dire' (which means 'to speak the truth').

It is important to note that in common law jurisdictions the criminal justice process in the courts is also known as an 'adversarial' system. This means that two sides argue the issue out in front of a jury who decides guilt or otherwise. However, other countries have different systems and include an 'inquisitorial' system of law. An inquisitorial system is a legal system where the court or a part of the court is actively involved in determining the facts of the case, as opposed to an adversarial system where the role of the court is solely that of an impartial referee between parties. Inquisitorial systems are used in most countries in Europe and Latin America. This is also the type of system found in a coroner's court.

At the beginning of the trial the defendant is asked once more for their plea. The prosecution then presents its case against the defendant. Witnesses are called and give 'evidence in chief' before being cross-examined by the defence. After the prosecution concludes its case, the defence then starts its own case. Here, once more, witnesses are called and give evidence in chief before being cross-examined – this time by the prosecution. After the case concludes, each side gives closing speeches before the judge gives a summing up. The judge is there to make sure that the law is carried out correctly. This includes clarifying points of law, explaining these to the jury and helping to prevent miscarriages of justice. It is at this point that the jury retire and then later return; it is desirable that there is a unanimous finding but sometimes judges will accept a specified majority verdict. Let us assume that the defendant is found guilty: what happens next?

Crown Court: Conviction to Sentencing

There is quite often a period between conviction and the next step, sentencing, which is also the prerogative of the judge. This is sometimes called JR or judge's remand/respite. This is another period where psychiatrists interface. Here, mental health issues are considered and often put forward in the form of psychiatric reports. This represents one of the main routes for mentally disordered offenders out of the criminal justice system.

A sentence needs to:

1. Protect the public.
2. Punish the offender fairly and appropriately.
3. Encourage the offender to make amends for their crime.
4. Contribute to crime reduction by stopping reoffending.

The courts can impose four levels of sentence, depending on the seriousness of the offence:

- discharges
- fines
- community sentences
- imprisonment.

Fines are the most common option used by the courts. Community sentences can include 'restorative justice' – making amends directly to the victims of crime. The most severe punishment, imprisonment, is generally only used for the most serious offences.

If a crime is an imprisonable offence, it will have a maximum term laid down by Parliament. Judges and magistrates are also given sentencing guidelines – designed to provide consistency throughout the criminal justice process. There are also fixed minimum sentences for some serious repeat offenders. In recent decades sentencing has become very complex and taxes judges considerably. Custodial sentences can be seen as determinate – that is, fixed and specific – or indeterminate such as a life sentence.

The Mental Health Act in Prison

The Mental Health Act does not apply in prisons. The Mental Health Act is specific in its application to a hospital and so excludes prisons. It is unclear why prisons are excluded or why this was not reconsidered when the Act was revised in 2007, or indeed if any consideration was ever given to this. It seems likely that this reflects concerns around using the Mental Health Act as a form of social control of prisoners. There may also have been a fear that cheap and unregulated prisons would be used to warehouse the mentally ill instead of providing expensive, secure forensic hospitals.

Would the Mental Health Act make a difference in a prison? In some respects, it would allow the treatment of patients without insight. In the author's experience, this is likely to be a small proportion. It would have an effect on maintaining that group of patients/prisoners whose condition fluctuates, but again this is a small group.

Mental Health Services in Prison

In reality, as applies to many aspects of health, there are many different designs and no clear concepts as to what a service should consist of or what level of resource is required to meet the needs of the prison population. There is no reason to consider that any one model of care in a prison is superior and there are many different models through Europe and other parts of the world [52–56]. Although we now have a system commissioned by the NHS and managed by various providers, in many countries the commissioning and delivery of health services remains the responsibility of correctional prison services, with some having dedicated mental health hospitals within prisons where patients can be treated under compulsion [57–60].

In this author's view, the largest limit on the design and development of prison mental health services has been the funding envelope and what can be delivered within it. This means more marginalisation of psychiatrists, as they are usually the costliest component of a service. Mental health, though important, is of course only one aspect of health needs in prison. A provider might have to deliver primary care, substance misuse and alcohol services, public health, dentistry, radiological and optometry, and treatment for chronic health conditions, as well as balancing a service which incorporates doctors, nurses and many other allied health professions. Additionally, prisons vary enormously in their needs, with the highest level of need in busy city remand prisons as compared to an open prison or one which caters for sentenced prisoners serving long sentences. As a consequence, there is not one design which fits all prisons.

In addition to a wide need and a rich variety of conditions, the psychiatrist in prison also has to contend with further barriers to care such as working without a Mental Health Act and, when a patient needs to be transferred and treated outside of prison, navigating complicated pathways to care. It is worth noting that mental health is not necessarily the responsibility of local commissioners. A person with a heart condition can be seen by a cardiologist in a local hospital, while in the UK a person with a mental illness has to go to the area responsible for mental healthcare and at the right level of security.

The last two decades have seen an increased penetration of mental health services into prisons in the UK; at the same time, the commissioning and competitive tendering for health services has driven costs down with many discontinuities in service providers and, many would assume, a loss of quality [61]. Prisons in busy city areas often had large 'inpatient' areas – parts of the prison reserved for the mentally ill and physically infirm, de facto hospitals but without the regulatory structures for hospitals in the community. The 1990s and early 2010s saw a reduction in the provision of these – they were costly and so there was a shift towards managing prisoners in the main prison as much as possible, with some prisons even dispensing with in-patient units. Prisoners were supported in the main prison by 'in-reach' services and day centres. However, studies [62] have shown that of those with a major mental disorder, only 35% had been assessed by in-reach mental health teams and this was more likely if they had an acute psychosis.

Mental illness in prison is detected by a variety of routes and any service should have a good range of strategies to try and identify and prioritise mental illness [63–69]. Mental illness is not always obvious; many prisoners hide their mental illness either because of lack of insight or fear of stigma and the belief that they are perceived as vulnerable. Sometimes prison mental health services are made aware of a patient from community services or through court diversion, but this is not a given, and relevant systems need to be developed to improve detection rates. Forrester [70] found that around 25% of those with mental illness will be detected for the first time in prison. In reality, low referral rates are never an issue and a greater difficulty is meeting the need. Systematic screening at reception in remand prison can be a successful strategy, though as for all such processes it requires a well-resourced follow-through service that leads to health gains [35].

Mental health practitioners in prison often have to decide where to locate a mentally disordered prisoner in terms of their risk to themselves or others. In-patient units, when available, are not always the best option and with the right support many acutely unwell patients can be managed in the main prison. The mental health practitioner will also have to consider the issues of safety to other prisoners as much as to themselves. Some will need to be managed in the healthcare centre. It is wrongly assumed that an 'in-patient unit' is similar to a ward in a psychiatric hospital. This is not the case and usually they are simply another area where there is more monitoring. It is often here that many of the people who will be transferred to hospital are located.

A key concern for many years has been the delay of transferring prisoners to hospital from prison [71]. It would be simplistic to generalise and propose that all mentally ill prisoners should be in a hospital. Firstly, the capacity does not exist; secondly, the financial burden is too great; and finally, having a mental illness should not automatically equate to avoiding justice or punishment. For some, they are only in prison for a short time and there would not be a rationale to try and effect a transfer even if this could be achieved.

In general, patients transferred to hospital fall into three groups:

- those who are acutely ill who require treatment
- those who are complex and require assessment and diagnosis that cannot be delivered in a prison (e.g. for court)
- those who are chronically vulnerable due to a mental illness.

The process is complicated but recent years have seen more effort to speed up the process of transfer, which in the past had seen significant delays. In reality, patients fall above or below a threshold which is dynamic. There are a plentiful range of mechanisms to move a prisoner from prison to hospital at all stages of the criminal justice pathway from the point of arrest to the person who is a sentenced prisoner; in essence, these are either through the court or through the Ministry of Justice.

What about those who have mental health needs but are below the threshold for transfer to a hospital? There needs to be a shift from seeing the mental health morbidity of this group as a burden to an opportunity. With a recognition of the links between health and crime, the ability to make small changes to a large group has the potential to have a large impact on the overall incidence of crime in the community. Apart from a very small number, the vast majority of prisoners return to the area they came from. Some are without access to healthcare, substance misuse services and mental health services. The problems facing the offender in the resettlement process are enormous and many are linked. The offender faces poor physical and mental health, homelessness, unemployment and poverty, as well as resuming and repairing relationships. Matters are compounded with short sentences and the unpredictability of release and health needs. Continuity of care is a major difficulty in the transit between the community and prison and vice versa [72–76].

Hunger Strikes

For any practitioner in prison, it will not be long before they meet a prisoner who begins to refuse food and/or fluids. The World Health Organization ('Health in Prisons: A WHO

Guide to the Essentials in Prison Health') has outlined some of the reasons or motivations behind prisoners who stop eating:

- religious issues
- somatic problems
- mental disorders
- protest fasting.

The latter two are likely to be the areas where the mental health clinician becomes involved. Those entering prison have many rights taken away from them such as not being able to wear their own clothes (or only a certain type), loss of money and loss of identity with the imposition of a prison number. They cannot vote, they have restricted access to communication and media, and they exist in a state of powerlessness; there are a limited number of ways to express protest or effect change.

Although fasting is a commonplace human experience, stopping food and fluids can have a powerful effect for a prisoner when they feel they are not being listened to. In the early 1920s suffragettes used hunger striking as a political tool in their efforts to secure votes for women, and this became a frequent practice for those imprisoned. The management at the time was force feeding – eventually the government passed the Prisoners Temporary Discharge for Ill Health Act in 1913 (known as the Cat and Mouse Act), allowing their temporary release.

Suffragettes were not the only body to employ a hunger strike. Irish nationalists went on hunger strikes at around the same time and continued into the 1980s. In 1961, the Suicide Act changed the law so that suicide was no longer illegal. At the time there was no specific prison rule which justified force feeding, though the prison medical officer felt obliged to preserve life. In July 1974 the home secretary made a statement in relation to IRA prisoners in HMP Brixton who were on hunger strike with the comment, 'the doctor's obligation is to the ethics of his profession and to his duty at common law. He is not required as a matter of prison practice to feed a prisoner artificially against the prisoner's will'.

This led to a change in management as well as discussion within the medical profession and internationally, leading to the World Medical Association declaring in 1975 that artificial feeding should not be forced on capacitous patients. This has underpinned practice since then and in 1981 it saw the death by hunger strike of 10 Irish Republican prisoners in Long Kesh Prison.

It is worth pausing to consider some ambiguity here. A doctor in prison can allow and monitor a prisoner who wishes to die by hunger strike but this would not apply if the same patient who had capacity decided to hang themselves in front of staff [77, 78]. In 1994, Rosemary Wool, the then director of healthcare for prisons, issued a document, 'Food Refusal, Advance Directives and Mental Capacity', that outlined how capacity should be assessed and restated a court judgment (*The Home Department v Robb*) that declaring food and fluid refusal is not attempted suicide, and so healthcare staff would not be aiding and abetting a prisoner by letting it happen.

The majority of those embarking on a hunger strike have a motive and frequently only last a matter of hours or days. Certain populations seem to show more such behaviour as seen in higher levels in detention centres, often a consequence of uncertainty about their future.

The first step for a psychiatrist is nearly always finding a motive or aim. Assessing for the presence of a mental disorder and/or its effect on capacity is imperative. Accepting that the morbidity of mental disorder in prisons is high, the latter has greater weight. The clinician will need to balance difficult issues and tackle dilemmas, particularly if the patient has issued instructions about not being resuscitated or given advanced directives. Although the occurrence of a hunger strike is encountered reasonably often, death is rare – however, this should not make the clinician complacent.

Death from dry fasting (no food or fluids) commonly occurs in 4 to 10 days and usually due to issues with cardiac rhythms. If the patient only takes in water in whatever form, normally a healthy person without any comorbidity can survive a hunger strike for 75 to 80 days. Some undertaking such a process may prolong the duration by the intake of vitamins, trace minerals and perhaps small amounts of food which may allow a patient to survive a number of months.

In addition to assessing capacity, the wish to hunger strike should be assessed frequently, if not daily, and conducted privately. It is important to involve the wider establishment in discussion while respecting any confidentiality. Monitoring (if the patient permits) is essential. In the event of a prisoner who decides to end their hunger strike, refeeding should be cautious [79] – glycaemia triggers insulin secretion which itself starts the movement of electrolytes and fluids across cell membranes. Rapid changes can be lethal. Additionally, glucose intake can precipitate Wernicke's encephalopathy.

Suicide, Self-Harm and Violence

It is beyond the scope of this chapter to comprehensively cover self-harm, suicide and violence but it must be recognised that all are a reality of life in prison [80]. Prisons are no longer complacent about these issues and there are considerable energies devoted to collating data as well as management and prevention.

Recent data from 2020 show astonishingly high levels of self-harm in UK prisons, which are increasing. There were 19,702 incidents of self-harm in 2004 and 63,328 in 2019. Although data collection is an issue, taking account of population changes saw the rate per 1,000 prisoners increase from 264 to 764. Self-harm is particularly prevalent in female establishments [81]; the rate for men in 2019 was 650 per 1,000 compared to 3,130 per 1,000 for women.

The most common method of self-harm in prison is cutting and scratching in both men and women. Documents from the HMPPS reporting system provide considerable detail on when self-harm is likely to occur with a recognition that self-harm is highest in the first 90 days. Although the vast majority occur in a normal location, certain areas such as segregation and healthcare are recognised as greater-risk areas. The figures are of course skewed and thus a small number of individuals can account for high levels – thus, in 2019, 390 men and 116 women had over 20 self-harm incidents in a year [82, 83].

Deaths in custody (from all sources) have also increased from 146 per year in 2000 to 300 in 2019. Self-inflicted death has remained largely static from 81 to 84 per year in 2000 and 2019, respectively, with a surge to 124 in 2016. What is clear is that the rate is many times higher than outside of prison [84, 85] and this tends to reflect the morbidity of the group, particularly substance misuse [86–88], as well as the adversity of the environment.

Management of risk such as self-harm in prison is through the ACCT (Assessment Care Custody and Teamwork) document. This is a document which is raised by any member of staff and seeks to describe, monitor and manage the risk, particularly important when prisoners move around an establishment or go between establishments. The document is subject to formal and regularly documented review. Accepting that self-harm and suicide has remained static, it is debatable how much of an impact it has made.

There are other bodies which have monitored and researched deaths in custody which the reader should access. Historically, one of the key considerations is whether the group who go on to take their own lives are the same as those who self-harm. Although previous self-harm is found in a good proportion of those who take their own lives, are the issues the same?

An insight into the toxicity of the environment (and thus its impact on mental health) can be seen in the levels of violence. In the year ending December 2019 there were 28,113 prisoner-on-prisoner assaults and 9,995 assaults on staff. Serious assaults occurred at a level of 3,813 serious assault incidents, with 2,921 being prisoner-on-prisoner and 952 serious assaults on staff.

Drug Use

There are many reasons why drug use in prisons is unwelcome, not least due to debt, violence and the effects on mental health, including deaths by overdose and suicides while intoxicated [86–88]. Elsewhere in the chapter (Tables 4.1, 4.2 and 4.8) is a review of the morbidity of drug and alcohol use in prisoners. It is not surprising to find that the use of illegal drugs in prisons is a major issue. The Ministry of Justice and other agencies have often found that the prisons with the highest levels of instability have the highest incidence of positive random tests. Prisons are not uninformed on the issues and go to great lengths to combat their traffic into prisons. In the main, the three routes are through goods, staff and relatives/visitors. As at airports, prisons are usually trying to keep up with trends and new tactics, seen, for example, with the use of drones.

Although a small proportion make their own alcohol – sometimes called hooch – illegal drugs are the main challenge. For some time, the key drugs were heroin and cannabis. Drugs such as cocaine, crack and amphetamines are uncommon in England and Wales but the prevalent drugs change rapidly over time and from place to place. Some of the earlier research highlighted that cannabis users might shift to heroin as the cannabis remains detectable in urine for a much longer period than heroin. Heroin concentration and quality tends to be of a low level, and this has been seen when prisoners leave prison and overdose due to using a higher quality following a loss of tolerance in prison.

The last few years have been plagued by the rise of synthetic drugs or novel psychoactive substances (NPS). These appeared for the first time in the UK in around 2008; many were attracted to their easy availability to the extent they could be obtained through mail order and websites. They produced many of the effects of illegal drugs but as they were engineered, they did not fall under the Misuse of Drugs Act 1971. They are often not detected by routine testing. In reality, the drugs continued to morph and were branded for other purposes such as not for human consumption or as bath salts.

In 2016, they were criminalised and for a period the stock made its way onto the streets, where they continue to be a problem. Prisons have faced similar challenges and they remain a major issue in prisons and are very difficult to police. NPS can be broadly grouped into synthetic cannabinoids, depressants, stimulants and hallucinogens. Spice is the name given to a synthetic cannabinoid; originally leaves and other matter were sprayed with the active compound. To avoid detection in the prison estate, letters and cards are sprayed, allowed to dry and then sent into prison using the normal post. It is difficult to detect and unlike cannabis has a much more unpredictable effect on people, particularly in terms of mental health. A particularly severe psychosis with prolonged effects can be produced [89–92]. Prisoners use spice as it is affordable and is easily accessed to the extent that the use is now twice the level of cannabis.

Conclusions

This chapter has sought to provide clinicians with a better understanding of prisons and overcome many of the myths and misconceptions, with the objective of making the environment more attractive and interesting for future psychiatrists. In addition to a wide need and a rich variety of conditions, the psychiatrist in prison must contend with barriers to care such as working without a Mental Health Act and, when a patient needs to be transferred and treated outside of prison, navigating complicated pathways to care. Mental disorder is prevalent in all prison systems. Pathways into prison may be related to general factors, specific factors such as delusions and comorbidities and complications of mental illness such as homelessness and breakdown of relationships, as well as service provision issues.

Following surveys of prison psychiatric morbidity, the prevailing policy has been to divert prisoners in need of hospital care out of prisons. Court diversion models can focus on any point in the pathway from community to the criminal justice system. In prison, specialist mental health services are needed to address the high levels of morbidity due to self-harm, drug use, suicide, self-harm, hunger strikes and many other manifestations of developmental problems and traumatic experiences.

References

1. Recommendation CM/Rec(2012)5 of the Committee of Ministers to Member States on the European Code of Ethics for Prison Staff.

2. Recommendation Rec(2006)2 of the Committee of Ministers to Member States on the European Prison Rules. https://rm .coe.int/european-prison-rules-978-92-87 1-5982-3/16806ab9ae.

3. United Nations Office on Drugs and Crime. United Nations Standard Minimum Rules for the Treatment of Prisoners (the Nelson Mandela Rules). A/ RES/70/175. (2015) General Assembly, Vienna, Justice Section, UNDOC. www.un .org/en/events/mandeladay/mandela_ rules.shtml.

4. Wilson S, Cummin I. The history of prison psychiatry. In Wilson S, Cummin I (eds) *Psychiatry in Prisons: A Comprehensive Handbook*. London, Jessica Kingsley Publishers, 2010.

5. Walker N. *Why Punish?* Oxford, Oxford University Press, 1991.

6. Fair H, Walmsley R. World prison population list. 13th ed., 2021; 5. www.pri sonstudies.org/sites/default/files/resource s/downloads/world_prison_population_ list_13th_edition.pdf.

7. Howard J. *The State of the Prisons (1777–1784)*. London, J. M. Dent & Sons, 1929.

8. Fazel S, Danesh J. Serious mental disorder in 23000 prisoners: a systematic review of 62 surveys. *Lancet* 2002; 359 (9306): 545–50.

9. Fazel S, Seewald K. Severe mental illness in 33,588 prisoners worldwide: systematic review and meta-regression analysis. *British Journal of Psychiatry* 2012; 200 (5): 364–73.

10. Baranyi G, Scholl C, Fazel S et al. Severe mental illness and substance use disorders in prisoners in low-income and middle-income countries: a systematic review and meta-analysis of prevalence studies. *Lancet Global Health* 2019; 7 (4): e461–e471.

11. McKenzie N, Forrester A. Editorial: mental health in correctional and criminal justice systems (CCJS) – exploring how diagnosis, treatment and cultural differences impact pathway through the CCJS. *Frontiers in Psychiatry* 2023; 14: 1293060.

12. Gunn J, Maden A, Swinton M. *Mentally Disordered Prisoners*. London, Home Office, 1991.

13. Maden A, Taylor CJA, Brooke D et al. *Mental Disorder in Remand Prisoners*. London, Home Office, 1995.

14. Singleton N, Meltzer H, Gatward R. *Psychiatric Morbidity Among Prisoners in England and Wales.* London, Office for National Statistics, 1998.

15. Meltzer H, Gill B, Petticrew M. *The Prevalence of Psychiatric Morbidity Among Adults Aged 16–64, Living in Private Households in Great Britain.* London, Office of Population Censuses and Surveys, 1995.

16. Birmingham L, Mason D, Grubin D. Prevalence of mental disorder in remand prisoners: consecutive case study. *British Medical Journal* 1996; 313 (7071): 1521–4.

17. Birmingham L, Mason D, Grubin D. A follow-up study of mentally disordered men remanded to prison. *Criminal Behaviour and Mental Health* 1998; 8: 202–13.

18. Parsons S, Walker L, Grubin D. Prevalence of mental disorder in female remand prisons. *Journal of Forensic Psychiatry* 2001; 12: 194–202.

19. Wright B, Duffy D, Curtin K et al. Psychiatric morbidity among women prisoners newly committed and amongst remanded and sentenced women in the Irish prison system. *Irish Journal of Psychological Medicine* 2006; 23 (2): 47–53.

20. Curtin K, Monks S, Wright B et al. Psychiatric morbidity in male remanded and sentenced committals to Irish prisons. *Irish Journal of Psychological Medicine* 2009; 26 (4): 169–73.

21. Kennedy HG, Monks S, Curtin K et al. Psychiatric morbidity in sentenced, remanded and newly committed prisoners, 2004. www.academia.edu/1048 9242/Mental_Illness_in_Irish_Prisoners_ Psychiatric_Morbidity_in_Sentenced_Re manded_and_Newly_Committed_Prison ers_Contents.

22. Fazel S, Doll H, Långström N. Mental disorders among adolescents in juvenile detention and correctional facilities: a systematic review and metaregression analysis of 25 surveys. *Journal of the American Academy of Child and Adolescent Psychiatry* 2008; 47 (9): 1010–19.

23. Flynn D, Smith D, Quirke L, Monks S, Kennedy HG. Ultra high risk of psychosis on committal to a young offender prison: an unrecognised opportunity for early intervention. *BMC Psychiatry* 2012; 12: 100.

24. Fazel S, Hope T, O'Donnell I, Jacoby R. Hidden psychiatric morbidity in elderly prisoners. *British Journal of Psychiatry* 2001; 179: 535–9.

25. Davoren M, Fitzpatrick M, Caddow F et al. Older men and older women remand prisoners: mental illness, physical illness, offending patterns and needs. *International Psychogeriatrics* 2015; 27 (5): 747–55.

26. Working Group on the Mental Health of Asylum Seekers and Refugees of the Royal College of Psychiatrists. Detention of people with mental disorders in Immigration Removal Centres. Medical Justice, 2013.

27. Royal College of Psychiatrists. Position Statement PS07/16: Definition of torture in the context of immigration detention policy, 2016. www.rcpsych.ac.uk/pdf/P S07_2016.pd.

28. Royal College of Psychiatrists. Position Statement PS02/21. Detention of people with mental disorders in immigration removal centres (IRCs), 2021.

29. Forrester A, Hopkin G. Mental health in the criminal justice system: a pathways approach to service and research design. *Criminal Behaviour and Mental Health* 2019; 29: 207–17.

30. National Institute for Health and Care Excellence. Health of people in the criminal justice system NICE pathways, 2019.

31. Shaw J, Creed F, Price J, Huxley P, Tomenson B. Prevalence and detection of serious psychiatric disorder in defendants attending court. *Lancet* 1999; 353 (9158): 1053–6.

32. Brown P, Bakolis I, Appiah-Kusi E et al. Prevalence of mental disorders in defendants at criminal court. *BJPsych Open* 2022; 8 (3): e92.

33. Samele C, McKinnon I, Brown P et al. The prevalence of mental illness and unmet needs of police custody detainees. *Criminal Behaviour and Mental Health* 2021; 31 (2): 80–95.

34. McKenna B, Furness T, Brown S et al. Police and clinician diversion of people in mental health crisis from the Emergency Department: a trend analysis and cross comparison study. *BMC Emergency Medicine* 2015; 15: 14.

35. Simpson AIF, Gerritsen C, Maheandiran M. A systematic review of reviews of correctional mental health services using the STAIR framework. *Frontiers in Psychiatry* 2022; 12: 747202.

36. Chaplin E, McCarthy J, Marshall-Tate K et al. A realist evaluation of an enhanced court-based liaison and diversion service for defendants with neurodevelopmental disorders. *Criminal Behaviour and Mental Health* 2023. doi: 10.1002/cbm.2315.

37. Pakes F, Winstone J. A site visit survey of 101 mental health liaison and diversion schemes in England. *The Journal of Forensic Psychiatry & Psychology* 2010; 21: 873–86. doi: 10.1080/14789949.2010.511241.

38. Birmingham L. Diversion from custody. *Advances in Psychiatric Treatment* 2001; 7: 198–207. doi: 10.1192/apt.7.3.198.

39. James D. Court diversion at 10 years: can it work, does it work and has it a future? *The Journal of Forensic Psychiatry & Psychology* 1999; 10: 507–24.

40. Pierzchniak P, Purchase N, Kennedy H. Liaison between prison, court and psychiatric services. *Health Trends* 1997; 29: 26–29.

41. Joseph PL, Potter M. Mentally disordered homeless offenders: diversion from custody. *Health Trends* 1990; 22 (2): 51–3.

42. Joseph PL, Potter M. Diversion from custody. I: Psychiatric assessment at the magistrates' court. *British Journal of Psychiatry* 1993; 162: 325–30. doi: 10.1192/bjp.162.3.325.

43. Joseph PL, Potter M. Diversion from custody. II: Effect on hospital and prison resources. *British Journal of Psychiatry* 1993; 162: 330–4.

44. Reed J. *Review of Health and Social Services for Mentally Disordered Offenders and Others Requiring Similar Services: Final Summary Report.* London, Her Majesty's Stationery Office, 1992.

45. Chiswick D. Reed report on mentally disordered offenders. *British Medical Journal* 1992; 305 (6867): 1448–9.

46. Bradley K. *The Bradley Report: Lord Bradley's Review of People with Mental Health Problems or Learning Disabilities in the Criminal Justice System.* London, Department of Health, 2009.

47. James D. Court diversion at 10 years: can it work, does it work and has it a future? *The Journal of Forensic Psychiatry & Psychology* 1999; 10: 507–24.

48. Keown P, French J, Gibson G et al. Too much detention? Street triage and detentions under Section 136 Mental Health Act in the North-East of England: a descriptive study of the effects of a street triage intervention. *BMJ Open.* 2016; 6 (11): e011837.

49. McKinnon I, Grubin DJ. Health screening in police custody. *Journal of Forensic and Legal Medicine* 2010; 17 (4): 209–12.

50. Samele C, McKinnon I, Brown P et al. The prevalence of mental illness and unmet needs of police custody detainees. *Criminal Behaviour and Mental Health* 2021; 31 (2): 80–95.

51. McKinnon IG, Thomas SD, Noga HL, Senior J. Police custody health care: a review of health morbidity, models of care and innovations within police custody in the UK, with international comparisons. *Risk Management and Healthcare Policy* 2016; 9: 213–26.

52. HG Kennedy. Models of care in forensic psychiatry. *BJPsych Advances* 2022; 28 (1).

53. Forrester A, Exworthy T, Olumoroti O et al. Variations in prison mental health services in England and Wales. *International Journal of Law and Psychiatry* 2013; 36 (3–4): 326–32.

54. Shepherd A, Hewson T, Hard J, Green R, Shaw J. Equivalence, justice, injustice: health and social care decision making in relation to prison populations. *Frontiers in Sociology* 2021; 6: 649837.

55. Ismail N, de Viggiani N. How do policymakers interpret and implement the

principle of equivalence with regard to prison health? A qualitative study among key policymakers in England. *Journal of Medical Ethics* 2018; 44 (11): 746–50.

56. McKenna B, Skipworth J, Tapsell R et al. Impact of an assertive community treatment model of care on the treatment of prisoners with a serious mental illness. *Australasian Psychiatry* 2018; 26 (3): 285–9.

57. Felthous AR, Bloom JD. Jail-based competency restoration. *Journal of the American Academy of Psychiatry and the Law* 2018; 46 (3): 364–72.

58. Moncany AH, Blanchet M, Duchêne L, Malinowski C, de Ranchin R. Psychiatric care in specially equipped hospital units. *Soins* 2022; 67 (870–1): 40–4.

59. Tomlin J, Lega I, Braun P et al. Forensic mental health in Europe: some key figures. *Social Psychiatry and Psychiatric Epidemiology* 2021; 56 (1): 109–17.

60. Salize HJ, Dressing H, Fangerau H et al. Highly varying concepts and capacities of forensic mental health services across the European Union. *Frontiers in Public Health* 2023; 11: 1095743. doi: 10.1007/s00127-020-01909-6.

61. Lennox C, Leonard S, Senior J et al. Conducting randomized controlled trials of complex interventions in prisons: a Sisyphean task?. *Frontiers in Psychiatry* 2022; 13: 839958.

62. Senior J, Shaw J, Hassan L et al. An evaluation of the reception screening process used in prisons in England and Wales. Report to Offender Health, Department of Health. Offender Health Research Network, 2009.

63. Iqbal MU, Byrne O, Kennedy HG, Davoren M. Admissions to the National Forensic Mental Health Service, Central Mental Hospital Dundrum, before, during and after the COVID-19 pandemic: changes in the need for security and urgency of need for admission. *European Psychiatry* 2023; 66 (S1): S60–S61. doi: 10.1192/j.eurpsy.2023.216.

64. Simpson A, Brinded P, Fairley N, Laidlaw T, Malcolm F. Does ethnicity affect need for mental health service among New Zealand

prisoners? *Australian and New Zealand Journal of Psychiatry* 2003; 37 (6): 728–34. doi: 10.1080/j.1440-1614.2003.01260.x.

65. Grubin D, Carson D, Parsons S. Report on new prison reception health screening arrangements: the results of a pilot study in 10 prisons. University of Newcastle, 2002.

66. Evans C, Brinded P, Simpson A, Frampton C, Mulder R. Validation of brief screening tools for mental disorders among New Zealand prisoners. *Psychiatric Services* 2010; 61: 923–38. doi: 10.1176/ps.2010.61.9.923.

67. Martin M, Colman I, Simpson A, McKenzie K. Mental health screening tools in correctional institutions: a systematic review. *BMC Psychiatry* 2013; 13: 275. doi: 10.1186/1471-244X-13-275.

68. Flynn G, O'Neill C, Kennedy HG. DUNDRUM-2: prospective validation of a structured professional judgment instrument assessing priority for admission from the waiting list for a forensic mental health hospital. *BMC Research Notes* 2011; 4: 10.

69. Jeandarme I, Habets P, Kennedy H. Structured versus unstructured judgment: DUNDRUM-1 compared to court decisions. *International Journal of Law and Psychiatry* 2019; 64: 205–10.

70. Forrester A, Till A, Simpson A, Shaw J. Mental illness and the provision of mental health services in prisons. *British Medical Bulletin* 2018; 127 (1): 101–9.

71. Pierzchniak P, Purchase N, Kennedy H. Liaison between prison, court and psychiatric services. *Health Trends* 1997; 29 (1): 26–9.

72. Byng R, Lennox C, Kirkpatrick T et al. Development and evaluation of a collaborative care intervention for male prison leavers with mental health problems: the Engager research programme. *Programme Grants for Applied Research* 2022; 10 (8).

73. Hopkin G, Evans-Lacko S, Forrester A, Shaw J, Thornicroft G. Interventions at the transition from prison to the community for prisoners with mental illness: a systematic review. *Administration and*

Policy in Mental Health and Mental Health Services Research 2018; 45: 623–34.

74. McKenna B, Skipworth J, Tapsell R et al. A prison mental health in-reach model informed by assertive community treatment principles: evaluation of its impact on planning during the pre-release period, community mental health service engagement and reoffending. *Criminal Behaviour and Mental Health* 2015; 25 (5): 429–39.

75. Smith D, Harnett S, Flanagan A et al. Beyond the walls: an evaluation of a pre-release planning (PReP) programme for sentenced mentally disordered offenders. *Frontiers in Psychiatry* 2018; 9: 549.

76. Shaw J, Conover S, Herman D et al. *Critical Time Intervention for Severely Mentally Ill Prisoners (CrISP): A Randomised Controlled Trial.* Southampton, NIHR Journals Library, 2017.

77. Brockman B. Food refusal in prisoners: a communication or a method of self-killing? The role of the psychiatrist and resulting ethical challenges. *Journal of Medical Ethics* 1999; 25 (6): 451–6.

78. Wynia M, Cho EH, Naples-Mitchell J. The ethics of caring for detained people on hunger strike. *Annals of Internal Medicine* 2022; 175 (5): 732–4.

79. Eichelberger M, Joray ML, Perrig M, Bodmer M, Stanga Z. Management of patients during hunger strike and refeeding phase. *Nutrition* 2014; 30 (11–12): 1372–8.

80. Favril L, Shaw J, Fazel S. Prevalence and risk factors for suicide attempts in prison. *Clinical Psychology Review* 2022; 102190.

81. Walker T, Shaw J, Gibb J et al. 2020. Lessons learnt from the narratives of women who self-harm in prison. *Crisis* 2021; 42 (4): 255–62.

82. Zhong S, Senior M, Yu R et al. Risk factors for suicide in prisons: a systematic review and meta-analysis. *The Lancet Public Health* 2021; 6 (3): e164–74.

83. Favril L, Yu R, Hawton K, Fazel S. Risk factors for self-harm in prison: a systematic review and meta-analysis. *The Lancet Psychiatry* 2020; 7 (8): 682–91.

84. Shaw J, Appleby L, Baker D. *Safer Prisons: A National Study of Prison Suicides 1999–2000 by the National Confidential Inquiry into Suicides and Homicides by People with Mental Illness.* London, Department of Health, 2003.

85. Fazel S, Grann M, Kling B, Hawton K. Prison suicide in 12 countries: an ecological study of 861 suicides during 2003–2007. *Social Psychiatry and Psychiatric Epidemiology* 2011; 46: 191–5.

86. World Health Organization (WHO). Preventing overdose deaths in the criminal justice system, 2014. www.euro.who.int/__data/assets/pdf_file/0020/114914/Preventing-overdose-deaths-in-the-criminal-justice-system.pdf.

87. Vaughan AD, Zabkiewicz DM, Verdun-Jones SN. In custody deaths of men related to mental illness and substance use: a cross-sectional analysis of administrative records in Ontario, Canada. *Journal of Forensic and Legal Medicine* 2017; 48: 1–8.

88. Iqtidar M, Sharma K, Mullaney R et al. Deaths in custody in the Irish prison service: 5-year retrospective study of drug toxicology and unnatural deaths. *BJPsych Open* 2018; 4 (5): 401–3.

89. Yeruva RR, Mekala HM, Sidhu M, Lippmann S. Synthetic cannabinoids – 'spice' – can induce a psychosis: a brief review. *Innovations in Clinical Neuroscience* 2019; 16 (1–2): 31.

90. Shalit N, Barzilay R, Shoval G et al. Characteristics of synthetic cannabinoid and cannabis users admitted to a psychiatric hospital: a comparative study. *Journal of Clinical Psychiatry* 2016; 77 (8): e989–e995.

91. Bloomfield MA, Ashok AH, Volkow ND et al. The effects of Delta9-tetrahydrocannabinol on the dopamine system. *Nature* 2016; 539 (7629): 369–77.

92. D'Souza DC, Radhakrishnan R, Sherif M et al. Cannabinoids and psychosis. *Current Pharmaceutical Design* 2016; 22 (42): 6380–91.

Legal Issues and Expertise in Forensic Psychiatry

Penelope Brown and Richard Latham

Psychiatrists, alongside other medical experts, have a role in applying clinical and scientific expertise in legal contexts. The courts use expert evidence when dealing with matters outside the knowledge of the layperson, in particular the judge and jury. Forensic psychiatry training has a particular focus on the care and treatment of offenders with mental disorder. Forensic psychiatry practitioners are expected to have not only specialised knowledge of mental disorder but also detailed knowledge of the relevant legal issues and justice systems [1]. It is crucial that psychiatrists acting as expert witnesses understand the nature of the legal issues in order to function competently at court. This chapter outlines the role of the psychiatrist as an expert witness and summarises legal issues on which forensic psychiatrists are asked to comment in criminal settings, namely fitness to plead, mental health defences and sentencing.

Doctors As Experts

Expert witnesses are used, and have been for centuries, in diverse disciplines by courts and the role of the forensic psychiatrist as an expert witness has crystallised over time. The law has long recognised issues such as lunacy and insanity, but it was not until 1760 in the case of Earl Ferrers,[1] the last peer of the realm to be hanged for the murder of his steward, that medical expert testimony was called to provide a general definition of insanity. The novelty of medical testimony limited the weight of the evidence of the doctor in *Ferrers* [2]. However, towards the latter part of the eighteenth century, medical testimony on mental health issues become more widely accepted in criminal cases in England. This in turn has led to a complex and fluctuating relationship between the legal and medical professions, not least because the two do not speak the same language.

At the turn of the nineteenth century, before forensic psychiatrists existed as a separate professional group, medical witnesses were often treated by the courts with suspicion and even rudeness [3]. As stated by Mr Justice Field in 1888:[2] 'When trial by medical men comes into vogue, well and good; but so long as trial by jury is the law of the land, I will not allow a medical man to be substituted for the jury.' The controversy continues as to whether expert testimony should provide an opinion on questions which the jury are sworn to try (the ultimate issue).

While it became widely accepted that the existence of insanity at court ought never be decided without medical evidence, the role of the medical expert was originally limited to facts upon which the jury would form an opinion on the ultimate issue. However, in recent

---

[1] *R v Ferrers* (1760) 19 State Trials 886.
[2] *Hitchens* (1888). Taunton Assizes, Field J, Somerset County Herald, 18 February, 8.

years the development of more nuanced mental health defences such as diminished responsibility has called into question the ability of the jury to understand the mental health issues and reach informed decisions. The role of the expert has in turn widened to not only comment on facts but to also give opinions which can, in some circumstances, include an opinion on the ultimate issue [4].

What Is an Expert?

In law, the term 'expert' derives its meaning from the common law of a number of jurisdictions [5]. The evidence of an expert is admissible if it assists the court with information which is likely to be outside the experience and knowledge of judge and/or jury.[3] Determining whether the individual offering an opinion is an expert is based on whether that person has undergone sufficient training or study to warrant the status of expert or whether they have acquired their expertise by experience. Experts must only give evidence on matters within their expertise, and when they do they should rely on information which is part of a recognised body of knowledge or experience,[4] although formal qualifications to be an expert witness are not deemed necessary.[5] This might be controversial as the study and understanding of mental health conditions evolves and organisation of this understanding does not happen immediately. Minority or controversial opinions will, however, be allowed if the expert has sufficient training.[6]

It is important for medical witnesses to recognise whether they are acting as an expert witness or professional witness. Professional witnesses are also referred to as witnesses of fact. They will generally have been directly involved in the management of the patient, or have had some professional involvement with the other parties involved. This could be a patient under their care who is accused of a crime or the victim of an alleged offence. According to guidance from the Academy of Medical Royal Colleges, a professional witness is expected to provide evidence of their clinical findings, observations and actions. Witnesses of fact must limit evidence as far as possible to what is recorded or remembered and should not speculate or venture to give opinion. Being a witness of fact is generally a requirement rather than a matter of choice. It is usually a matter of choice for a doctor to act as an expert. The expert will be instructed by solicitors, or other parties, including the court, if they are willing to accept instruction to assist in the case. A key expectation of an expert witness is impartiality and their duty is to the court. It is crucial that they are not influenced by the party who instructs them.

It is generally advised that, other than in highly exceptional circumstances, expert witnesses will not be personally involved with the patient in the case, and must declare any potential conflicts of interest [6]. However, guidance from the UK Royal College of Psychiatrists notes that in highly specialist fields such as forensic psychiatry, this guidance can be difficult to adhere to, either for practical reasons or because the law effectively requires such evidence (e.g. when the psychiatrist is asked to comment on whether hospital-based disposal is appropriate and confirm availability of a bed in a specialist unit [5]). Practitioners should be familiar with the law, practice and professional guidelines in

---

[3] *R v Turner* [1975] QB 834.
[4] *The Queen v Bonython* [1984] SASR 45, adopted into common law in England and Wales by the Court of Appeal (e.g. G [2004] EWCA Crim 1240, para. 15).
[5] For example, *Silverlock* [1894] 2 QB 766 and *Hodges* [2003] EWCA Crim 290.
[6] *Robb* [1991] 93 Cr App R 16.

the country where they work to ensure they are acting appropriately when taking on combined roles of expert and clinical roles [7]. Where psychiatrists find themselves performing dual roles, they must be sensitive to differences between their legal and clinical obligations. Particular caution is needed around information sharing, bias and conflict of interest, and the impact on the therapeutic relationship.

Responsibility As an Expert Witness

Expert witnesses are subject to rules and guidance in terms of their responsibilities (e.g. in terms of disclosing information) or the structure of their reports. It is important that anyone embarking on acting as an expert witness becomes familiar with any rules within that jurisdiction. In the UK, the Criminal Procedure Rules 2020 (Part 19) outline what is expected in an expert report, as summarised in Box 5.1.

There is a need for any doctor to recognise that in acting as an expert witness they are working in a different setting to the hospital or out-patient clinic. In clinical practice all information is relevant, but information becomes evidence when acting as an expert witness and therefore subject to 'rules of evidence' such as admissibility. Experts should seek consent from the patient prior to undertaking any work on a report and consider principles of confidentiality. Information not relevant to the purposes of the report should not be

---

Box 5.1 Content of expert report (Criminal Procedure Rules 2020 Rule 19.4)

a. Detail qualifications, relevant experience and accreditation

b. Detail any literature or other information relied on in making the report

c. Include a statement setting out the substance of all facts given to the expert which are material to the opinions expressed in the report, or upon which those opinions are based

d. Make clear which of the facts stated in the report are within the expert's own knowledge

e. Where the expert has based an opinion or inference on a representation of fact or opinion made by another person for the purposes of criminal proceedings

   i. identify the person who made that representation to that expert

   ii. give the qualifications, relevant experience and any accreditation of that person

   iii. certify that that person had personal knowledge of the matters stated in that representation

f. Where there is a range of opinion on the matters dealt with in the report

   i. summarise the range of opinion, and

   ii. give reasons for the expert's own opinion

g. If the expert is not able to give his/her opinion without qualification, state the qualification

h. Include such information as the court may need to decide whether the expert's opinion is sufficiently reliable to be admissible as evidence

i. Contain a summary of the conclusions reached

j. Contain a statement that the expert understands an expert's duty to the court, and has complied and will continue to comply with that duty; and

k. Contain the same declaration of truth as a witness statement

disclosed [1]. Experts must also demonstrate how they have reached their opinion; there must be evidence of reasoning.

Acting as an expert witness is not without risk. Failure in discharging duties can undermine the profession as a whole and have devastating consequences for the individual clinician. There are a number of examples of experts being publicly criticised or even struck off their professional register for professional misconduct. Perhaps the biggest risk for an expert is acting outside their expertise.[7] Doctors in training should only undertake expert witness work under the supervision of an appropriately qualified senior colleague, who should be aware of their own responsibility for the report's accuracy and reliability [5]. The trainees experience and level of training should be made clear in the report, as should the name and experience of their supervisor.

Assessment in Legal Proceedings

Before embarking on an assessment, it is very important that there is a clear understanding of the questions (or instructions) you are being asked to address. Without this, there is a risk of evidence being of no use or addressing matters that should be avoided by the expert. The letter of instruction ensures that both the instructing party and the expert share an understanding of what is expected.

The main components of clinical assessment of a defendant or client are not discussed in detail here because of the overlap with ordinary clinical assessment. Consent for the clinical assessment should include informing the interviewee of the purpose of the assessment, the different nature of confidentiality and the fact that, as an expert witness, your professional duty is primarily to the court (although you do not dispense with all duties to them).

The preparation of a report (Box 5.1) will involve using other information and the expert should, as far as is practical, have this other information before conducting any assessment. Consent from the interviewee is usually required to access additional information. Written notes made during the assessment may become important later in the legal process and should be kept securely. It is helpful if written notes highlight where quotes are verbatim. Personal information gathered and recorded should be stored in accordance with data protection laws.

Preparing a Report and Giving Evidence

In most cases, oral evidence is not required of the expert, therefore it is important that the written report communicates the expert's findings and opinion without the need for additional explanation. Model report templates are available, but it is up to the expert to decide how to present their report. Some experts summarise their findings at the top of the report, but it is important to ensure the body of the report delineates how opinions are reached. It is also important to separate facts from opinions, and to always cite any information which came from other sources. Many experts start with an introduction, followed by background to the case and issues to be addressed, investigation of the facts and assumed facts, interview with the defendant, opinion, and recommendations.

---

[7] See, for example, *Pool v General Medical Council* [2014] EWHC 3791 (Admin).

Box 5.1 summarises the court's expectations for the report. Other tips include:
- write for the 'intelligent layperson'; any clinical terms or jargon should be clearly explained
- be accurate and comprehensive but also brief
- number paragraphs and pages so it is easy to navigate if oral evidence is required
- use headings and sub-headings
- ensure the report is clearly dated and signed
- include the writer's qualifications and expertise
- include a front page with the name of the court, case number (if available) and name of the case
- avoid being critical of other experts but explain any areas of disagreement.

In adversarial legal systems, opposing sides conduct their own investigations and use witnesses to bring out information. It is important to be aware that an expert witness can be called to give oral evidence in court by any party; that is, if the expert was instructed to prepare a report by the prosecution, it is possible for the defence to call the witness to give oral evidence to clarify their findings. Before giving oral evidence, all witnesses are asked to take the oath (to swear to tell the truth according to their religion) or affirm (promise to tell the truth). If called by the defence, the witness will undergo an initial 'examination-in-chief' in which they are asked questions by that counsel. This is followed by 'cross-examination' by the opposing counsel, and then a re-examination by the defence. The judge can also ask questions. During cross-examination it is likely that you will be challenged, on your opinion and sometimes on your expertise. It is important to remain calm and not become argumentative or defensive. Often there is a conference with the instructing party prior to the hearing in which the barristers will test the expert's opinion and give an indication of questions that are likely to be asked. If the expert has changed their opinion since writing the report, this should be made known to the instructing party.

Tips for giving evidence include:
- be prepared: re-familiarise yourself with your report and any other reports you may be asked to comment on
- consider how you will describe your role and qualifications, as this is usually the first thing you will be asked. Ensure to include evidence that you are appropriately qualified to give evidence (e.g. that you are approved under section 12 of the Mental Health Act (MHA) in England and Wales)
- sit through the evidence of other expert witnesses if you can
- arrive in good time and ensure you have your papers in order, to avoid fumbling on the witness stand
- be aware how to address the court (check with those instructing you)
- face whoever is asking questions, but when answering ensure you face the jury (or the judge if there is no jury present)
- do not rush your answers: it is better to pause and take your time
- if unsure of the question, ask for clarification
- keep answers brief and to the point, and explain any medical terms or jargon
- do not be afraid to point out if something is not within your expertise or that you do not know the answer to a question.

Common Issues to Be Addressed by Expert Psychiatric Witnesses

Mental disorder is over-represented in all stages of the criminal justice system, including in defendants as they attend court [8]. All mental disorders can impact the accused's ability to participate in their trial, the legal defences available to them and sentencing options for the court. In some cases, defendants with mental disorder require diversion away from the criminal justice system for hospital treatment. This could be at the time of arrest, before or during their trial, or once the case is dealt with and the court needs to decide on an appropriate disposal. There are several issues on which psychiatric expert witnesses are asked to assist the court when an individual with mental disorder is undergoing trial, which are separated in the next subsection in terms of issues relating to mental state at the time of the trial and mental state at the time of the offence. Sentencing and disposal options for these issues are also considered.

Psychiatric Issues at Trial: Fitness to Plead and Effective Participation

'Fitness to plead' concerns a defendant's legal capacities at the time of their criminal trial. It differs from the concept of criminal responsibility and other psychiatric defences described next in that it concerns the mental state of the accused at the time of the trial rather than at the time the alleged offence was committed. A defendant can be fit to plead in court even if they lacked criminal responsibility or were insane at the time of the offence, and vice versa. There is also a possibility that a defendant is both unfit to plead and not criminally responsible for the act committed, although what happens in such cases can be legally complex.

The right to a fair trial is a fundamental human right established in many jurisdictions. According to the European Convention on Human Rights[8] (ECHR) Article 6, 'everyone is entitled to a fair and public hearing'[9] following a criminal charge. However, an individual with a mental disorder might not be capable of participating fully and effectively in the trial process, for example by being unable to assist counsel or understand the charge or the pleas available to them. They might make decisions relating to the trial, such as pleading guilty when they are in fact innocent, that are not in their interests and that they would not have made had they been free from mental disorder. This can lead to unjust verdicts and, at worst, imprisonment for an offence which they did not in fact commit.

Dealing with mentally disordered defendants in criminal trials has been an issue since the Kings Courts were developed in Norman England and the defendant was required to answer 'guilty' or 'not guilty' to the indictment. Those who did not speak were said to 'stand mute'. The jury was called on to establish whether this was due to a mental impairment ('mute by the visitation of God' [9]) or 'mute of malice' (essentially malingering). The latter were subjected to *peine forte et dure* – being starved and crushed under heavy stones (or

---

[8] The full title is the Convention for the Protection of Human Rights and Fundamental Freedoms 1950.

[9] European Convention on Human Rights, Art. 6 (1): 'In the determination of his civil rights and obligations or of any criminal charge against him, everyone is entitled to a fair and public hearing within a reasonable time by an independent and impartial tribunal established by law. Judgement shall be pronounced publicly but the press and public may be excluded from all or part of the trial in the interest of morals, public order or national security in a democratic society, where the interests of juveniles or the protection of the private life of the parties so require, or the extent strictly necessary in the opinion of the court in special circumstances where publicity would prejudice the interests of justice.'

'pressed') until they decided to enter a plea [10]. Those found mute by visitation were spared punishment [11].

It was not until the nineteenth century that a test for fitness to plead was formalised in the 1837 case of Pritchard,[10] a deaf mute indicted for bestiality [12]. He did not enter a plea and was initially found to be mute by visitation by the jury. However, when later asked to answer to the charge, he signed to indicate 'not guilty'. The judge, Baron Alderson, asked the jury to decide whether Pritchard was 'sane or not' and identified three elements required to be fit to plead:

> First, whether the prisoner is mute of malice or not; secondly, whether he can plead to the indictment or not; thirdly, whether he is of sufficient intellect to comprehend the course of proceedings on the trial, so as to make a proper defence – to know that he might challenge any of you to whom he may object – and to comprehend the details of the evidence.

Access to legal counsel was not routinely available until later that century, and was not considered in *Pritchard*. However, this issue was raised in the 1853 case of *Davies*,[11] who was found unfit to plead due to lacking the ability to properly instruct counsel on account of mental illness.

Despite his ability to read and write suggesting he was not, in the legal language of the day, 'an idiot', Pritchard was found unfit and indefinitely detained in prison. At that time there was no requirement for medical evidence to support a finding of unfitness. This was first recommended in 1925 but only became part of legal procedures in 1991 in the Criminal Procedure (Insanity and Unfitness to Plead) Act. The procedures for finding a defendant unfit to plead have since evolved, as described in what follows.

In parallel to the law on fitness to plead, the concept of 'effective participation' has been considered in the high court as a requirement for a trial to be fair according to ECHR Article 6, especially in trials concerning children and other vulnerable defendants. This holds that defendants must not only be physically present in their trials but also play an active role and have reasonable opportunity to make the relevant representations [13]. It recognises that vulnerable defendants and children need to be treated carefully in court and may require reasonable adjustments and additional support in order to take part in their trials.[12]

The Legal Tests

The current legal test for fitness to plead varies across jurisdictions (Box 5.2), but in England and Wales, as well as Northern Ireland, it remains very much based on the original Pritchard Criteria. This has been a source of significant criticism in recent years as the test is thought to focus too much on intellectual and communicative abilities without giving due consideration to the decision-making capacity of the defendants (which is more explicitly considered in the Dusky test to consider 'competence to stand trial' in the USA and 'fitness for trial' in Scotland), in particular whether they can 'use and weigh' information to make proper decisions such as acting in one's best interests [14]. It has been submitted that this is one reason for very low numbers of defendants being found unfit to plead in these countries. The Law Commission of England and Wales [15], alongside the

---

[10] *R v Pritchard* (1836) 7 C & P 303. [11] *R v Davies* (1853) 3 Car. & K. 328.
[12] See, for example, *Stanford v UK* (ECHR, 23 February 1994), App no. 16757/90 and *T and V v UK* [2000], 30 EHRR 121.

Box 5.2 Unfitness to plead tests in common law jurisdictions: UK, USA and Australia

England and Wales and Northern Ireland (Pritchard Criteria, as laid out in *R v Marcantonio* [2016] EWCA Crim 14)

A person is unfit to plead if on the balance of probabilities any one of these is beyond their capability:

1. Understand the charges
2. Decide whether to plead guilty or not
3. Exercise the right to challenge jurors
4. Instruct solicitors and counsel
5. Follow the course of proceedings
6. Give evidence in one's own defence

Scotland (as laid out in the Criminal Procedure (Scotland) Act 1995 and the Criminal Justice and Licensing (Scotland) Act 2010)

A person is unfit for trial if it is established on the balance of probabilities that the person is incapable, by reason of a mental or physical condition, of participating effectively in a trial . . . [with] regard to the ability of the person to

1. understand the nature of the charge,
2. understand the requirement to tender a plea to the charge and the effect of such a plea,
3. understand the purpose of, and follow the course of, the trial,
4. understand the evidence that may be given against the person,
5. instruct and otherwise communicate with the person's legal representative, and
6. any other factor which the court considers relevant.

Ireland (as laid out in The Criminal Law (Insanity) Act 2006 Revised)

An accused person shall be deemed unfit to be tried if he or she is unable by reason of mental disorder to understand the nature or course of the proceedings so as to:

(a)   plead to the charge,
(b)   instruct a legal representative,
(c)   in the case of an indictable offence which may be tried summarily, elect for a trial by jury,
(d)   make a proper defence,
(e)   in the case of a trial by jury, challenge a juror to whom he or she might wish to object, or
(f)   understand the evidence.

Australia (as laid out in the Presser test (*R v Presser* VR 451958))

To be fit to plead an accused must have sufficient mental or intellectual capacity to understand the proceedings and to make an adequate defence, according to the following abilities:

1. an understanding of the nature of the charges;
2. an understanding of the nature of the court proceedings;
3. the ability to challenge jurors;
4. the ability to understand the evidence;

5. the ability to decide what defence to offer; and
6. the ability to explain his or her version of the facts to counsel and the court.

United States of America (as laid out in *Dusky v United States* [1960] 362 US 402; 80 SCt, 788)

Competence to stand trial considers whether the defendant has:

1. sufficient present ability to consult with his lawyer with a reasonable degree of rational understanding – and
2. whether he has a rational as well as factual understanding of the proceedings against him

Northern Ireland Law Commission [16], have proposed a new test which explicitly considers the defendant's decision-making abilities, but at the time of writing this has not been incorporated into law.

The Legal Procedures

The procedure for finding an individual unfit to plead varies across jurisdictions. Here we describe the procedure in England and Wales, where it is outlined in statute in the Criminal Procedure (Insanity) Act 1964, amended by the Criminal Procedure (Insanity and Unfitness to Plead) Act 1991. The issue of unfitness can be raised by the prosecution or defence, and the court was also able to raise the issue even if the defendant enters a plea.[13] The issue must be raised as soon as it arises but can be postponed until the opening of the case for the defence. Once the issue has been raised, the defendant undergoes assessment by a psychiatrist. 'Substantial' medical evidence is required to support a finding of unfitness, which must come from at least two medical practitioners, of whom at least one must be duly approved (i.e. approved under s12 MHA in England and Wales).

It is ultimately for the judge to determine whether the defendant is fit or not, guided by the expert psychiatric evidence. If the defendant is found fit, the trial will proceed. If found unfit, the trial can be postponed for the defendant to undergo treatment or in some cases an application can be made to stay the proceedings. In England and Wales, the case often proceeds to a 'trial of the facts', in which a jury is called upon to determine whether the accused did the act or omission charged. This is not a criminal trial as such, and does not result in a conviction. The trial of facts purely considers the *actus reus* and not the *mens rea*, and is a subject of significant controversy.

If the jury find the defendant did not do the act or omission of which they were charged, the defendant is acquitted. However, if the defendant is found to have done the act on the trial of facts, there are three disposal options to the court, namely:

– a hospital order
– a supervision order
– an absolute discharge order.

If the offence is murder, the judge must impose a hospital order with restrictions.

---

[13] *R v Vent (James Robert)* [1936] 25 Cr App R 55.

Clinical Issues and Fitness to Plead

Studies have found that when defendants are assessed for fitness to plead, the professionals involved are inconsistent in their application of the legal criteria and often use arbitrary criteria or base their assessments on diagnosis alone [17, 18]. If asked to consider fitness to plead, the assessing psychiatrist must be familiar with the legal test in the jurisdiction where the case is being heard. An assessment is carried out and an opinion on whether the criteria are met must be given. This is often done based on clinical assessment alone, although standardised measures for assessing fitness to plead and competence to stand trial have been developed for use in both research and clinico-legal settings [19]. The legal threshold for unfitness is high, and case law has found even individuals with significant mental illness and delusional beliefs can fulfil the criteria to be fit.[14] Amnesia for the offence (a phenomenon often seen even in serious offences) is not grounds for unfitness.[15]

While fitness to plead is not the same as a test for mental capacity, it is important to consider ways in which defendants can be supported so as to be able to participate in their trials, rather than simply diverted from court. This is especially true in light of the United Nations Convention on the Rights of Persons with Disabilities which emphasises the need to 'recognize that persons with disabilities enjoy legal capacity on an equal basis with others in all aspects of life' (Article 12[2]) and 'take appropriate measures to provide access by persons with disabilities to the support they may require in exercising their legal capacity' (Article 12[3]). In line with the law and procedures on effective participation at court, consideration should be given as to whether defendants would benefit from a registered intermediary to support with communication needs, or reasonable adjustments such as Ground Rules hearings (agreed simplification of language used at court), shorter sitting sessions and frequent breaks, attending via videolink, or providing psychological support or treatment to reduce the stress and anxiety around the trial [20].

Psychiatric Issues at the Time of the Offence: Mental Disorder Defences

Criminal law incorporates tests which rely on psychiatric or psychological findings being used to determine the degree of criminal responsibility a person bears. These mental disorder defences are sometimes total – resulting in findings of not guilty – or partial – resulting in a finding of guilt for a lesser offence. Psychiatric evidence may be relevant to other defences or justifications, even if they are not explicitly 'mental disorder defences' or justifications. Psychiatric evidence may also be relevant to the question of capacity to have formed the intent to have committed the offence, not strictly speaking a defence.

Conviction for most crimes requires that two elements are proved beyond reasonable doubt: the act itself (*actus reus*) and the mental or fault element (*mens rea*). Most mental disorder defences tend to map to the *mens rea* element. *Mens rea* can be understood as the state of mind necessary for the act to amount to a criminal offence. In legal terms, this is frequently in terms of intention but may incorporate recklessness or simply knowledge of specific matters. Some crimes are only proven if there is not only a basic intention to act but also an intention to cause specific consequences (specific intent). Recklessness and negligence are related concepts, with recklessness describing a subjective foreseeability of harmful consequences and negligence applying an objective test of being able to foresee consequences.

---

[14] See, for example, *R v Berry (John)* [1978] 66 Cr App R 156 and *R v Robertson* [1968] 1 W.L.R 1767.
[15] *R v Podola* [1960] 1 Q.B. 325.

Mental disorder defences in common law jurisdictions (such as all those considered here) are sometimes contained in one Act of Parliament but have often evolved over decades or centuries of legal judgments and remain purely 'common law tests'. For the purpose of this chapter, each defence or justification is described including, where relevant, the procedure for deciding whether it applies and who must prove it and then some discussion of how mental health evidence may (and may not) be used or be relevant. The jurisdictions are England and Wales (E&W), Northern Ireland (NI), Ireland (Republic of Ireland) and Scotland.

Insanity or Not Criminally Responsible Because of Mental Disorder

Insanity is a defence to any crime and results in a finding of *not guilty by reason of insanity*. In Scotland, there has been modernisation of the language (and the test) and the *special defence* refers to a person who is *not criminally responsible*. There remains, in some jurisdictions, a finding of guilty but insane rather than not guilty (this was previously the outcome in Ireland). The insanity defence continues to be criticised (particularly in E&W), not just because of its outdated language and formulation but also because of the threshold being so high for a finding of insanity [21].

The Legal Tests

In E&W, the *M'Naghten* case provides the common law test for the defence of insanity: 'At the time of the committing of the act, the party accused was labouring under such a *defect of reason*, from *disease of the mind*, as not to know the *nature and quality of the act* he was doing, or, if he did know it, that he *did not know what he was doing was wrong*.'

Defect of reason does not include other aspects of mental functioning and emphasises the cognitive basis of the insanity test and the high threshold required for a finding of insanity. An (irresistible) impulsive or emotionally driven or uncontrollable act would not be sufficient even if the person believed they had no choice but to act in the way they did.[16]

Disease of the mind, however, is more broadly defined legally than might be assumed medically. Epilepsy, arteriosclerosis and hyperglycaemia can, in a legal sense, all be diseases of the mind in addition to psychiatrically defined conditions.

The nature and quality of an act refers to the physical actions of what the person does. It basic terms, someone must not know what they are doing for this part of the test to be satisfied. Knowing that something is wrong has been clarified as meaning legally – as opposed to just morally – wrong.[17]

In Ireland, the test for not guilty by reason of insanity is contained in statute:[18]

> the accused was suffering at the time from a mental disorder, and the mental disorder was such that the accused ought not to be held responsible for the act alleged by reason of the fact that he or she – i) did not know the nature and quality of the act, or ii) did not know that what he or she was doing was wrong, or iii) was unable to refrain from committing the act.

This test includes in point (iii) an irresistible impulse notion, and probably represents a lower threshold than when compared with the E&W test.

---

16 *R v Keal* [2022] EWCA Crim 341.   17 *R v Windle* [1952] 2QB 826.
18 Criminal Law (Insanity) Act 2006.

In Scotland, insanity is not the term used but the 'special defence' is the equivalent test and has been defined in statute:[19] 'A person is not criminally responsible for conduct constituting an offence, and is to be acquitted of the offence, if the person was at the time of the conduct unable by reason of mental disorder to appreciate the nature or wrongfulness of the conduct.' The law excludes personality disorder where it is 'characterised solely or principally by abnormally aggressive or seriously irresponsible conduct'. The Scottish test arguably sets a lower threshold by use of the word *appreciate* as compared with *know*.

In NI, an insane person is defined[20] as 'a person who suffers from mental abnormality which prevents him a) from appreciating what he is doing; or b) from appreciating that what he is doing is either wrong or contrary to law; or from controlling his own conduct'. As with Ireland, there is an implied irresistible impulse part to the defence and, like Scotland, the word *appreciate* rather than *know* is used.

The Legal Procedures

In these four jurisdictions, the ultimate question of insanity is for the jury. The burden is on the defence to prove insanity on the balance of probabilities. Medical evidence is required from at least one qualified mental health professional in each of the four jurisdictions, but the jury are never bound to accept the medical evidence.

The expectation following a finding of insanity is often that treatment in hospital will follow. In Ireland this is the only option described legally but requires certification by a consultant psychiatrist. In E&W there are two other options: a supervision order (a community order which may incorporate a requirement to cooperate with medical treatment) or absolute discharge. In Scotland the orders are similar but the language different (compulsion rather than hospital order and supervision and treatment order rather than supervision order).

Clinical Issues and Insanity

Insanity, despite the nuanced differences that have evolved, remains a high-threshold test with psychosis being the primary mental disorder likely to open the possibility of an insanity defence. The test is almost always focussed on cognition, whether 'knowing' or 'appreciating' wrongness or the nature of actions. This tends to exclude mental disorders where emotional regulation or extreme emotional states are the primary symptom types. The exceptions are those jurisdictions which appear to allow a route to a verdict of insanity that incorporates the inability to inhibit an irresistible impulse and the test becomes not solely cognitive but also volitional.

The 'knowledge of *legal* wrongness' criterion excludes the defence in many cases because while mental disorder may have a significant effect on the perceived moral justification for an action, it is a much higher threshold for a mental state to lead to an inability to know that something is illegal.

The clinical issue that is almost inevitably excluded in most jurisdictions is 'simple' intoxication. NI is the exception to this rule, however. Complexity arises in many cases where the relationship between any substance use, and other mental disorder may be complex. If alcohol has caused neurocognitive changes, then insanity may be available. If chronic use of cannabis has resulted in the development of schizophrenia, then the role of

---

[19] Criminal Procedure (Scotland) Act 1995. [20] Criminal Justice Act (Northern Ireland) 1966.

the cannabis (probably) does not matter. Where the issue is a substance-induced psychosis, then the issue may be more complex and courts may be forced to embrace this complexity and decide the ultimate question.

Automatism

If a person has *no* control over their actions during an altered state of consciousness, then this is an automatism and there is no crime. Automatism is a legal defence which frequently causes confusion because of the awkward relationship between the legal notion of automatism and the medical understanding of automatic behaviours, in for example, epilepsy. There is also a confusing relationship with insanity.

The confusion comes into focus when the distinction between insane and non-insane automatism is considered. Insane automatism results in a finding of not guilty by reason of insanity. If the finding is non-insane automatism, then there is acquittal. The distinction between the two is not a medical distinction and rests on the cause of the automatism – and whether it is internal/intrinsic or external/extrinsic. In many cases, when the legal term automatism is used, it is a reference to non-insane automatism. Non-insane automatism arises when the cause is external. This might be a physical or psychological blow or drugs. Insane automatisms have an internal cause. This might be a mental disorder but might include physical conditions causing mental state abnormalities.

An archetypal example highlighting the confusion is where the cause of the automatism is glycaemic control. An abnormal mental state causing an automatism, arising from hypoglycaemia caused by administration of insulin would lead to a finding of non-insane automatism because the cause is external (the insulin) even though the diabetes itself would be considered internal. This was the successful argument in the cases of Quick[21] (an assault by a nurse on a patient) and Bingham (theft of a can of coke and some sandwiches). However, albeit theoretical, if the hypoglycaemia was caused by an insulin-secreting tumour, it may be considered an intrinsic cause and therefore lead to a finding of insane automatism [22]. This theory may, however, be undermined if the interpretation was that the tumour was 'extrinsic to the mind'. Whatever the likely finding in this example, the distinction remains confusing and incongruous.

The Legal Tests

There is no statutory test for automatism, and it has been defined by cases in different jurisdictions.[22,23] There have been several judgments considering the issue of different causes of mental abnormality and whether they could lead to insane or non-insane automatism.

In *R v Kemp*,[24] the defendant attacked his partner. The defence was based on the suggestion that arteriosclerosis was the cause of an unconscious state leading to the violence. The judge (correctly) directed the jury that the proper consideration was insanity (insane automatism). In *R v Sullivan*,[25] the defendant kicked someone in the head during an epileptic seizure. Again, this could only be an insane automatism. In *R v Hennessy*,[26] a diabetic man in a state of hyperglycaemia attempted to rely on (non-insane) automatism but again insanity was the correct defence. In *R v Burgess*,[27] sleepwalking was considered as

---

[21] *R v Quick* [1973] 3 WLR 26. [22] *Bratty v Attorney General for Northern Ireland* [1963] AC 386. [23] *Ross v H.M. Advocate* [1991] ScotHC HCJAC_2. [24] *R v Kemp* [1957] 1 QB 399. [25] *R v Sullivan* [1984] AC 156. [26] *R v Hennessy* [1989] 1 WLR 287. [27] *R v Burgess* [1991] 2 QB 92.

the cause of the defendant hitting a friend with a bottle. The internal cause was a form of insanity (insane automatism).

In *R v T*[28] the defendant had been raped three days prior to an offence of armed robbery and was later diagnosed with post-traumatic stress disorder (PTSD). It was argued that the rape was an external factor which had caused the automatism and despite the fact that PTSD is a disease of the mind, a non-insane automatism was determined to be a possible verdict for the jury.

In Scotland, there is no recognition of insane automatism, although (non-insane) automatism requires an external factor causing loss of reason that must not be self-induced and could not be foreseen; and a resulting 'total alienation of reason' amounting to complete loss of self-control, demonstrated by expert medical evidence. In Ireland there has been recognition of the insane/non-insane distinction, but it is only non-insane automatism that has been accepted as a defence.

The Legal Procedures

The question of automatism is considered first by the judge. If there is evidence for the jury to consider it, then the judge will direct the jury as to whether it is insane or non-insane automatism that they must consider. Insane automatism is considered, as with insanity on the balance of probabilities, and the burden is on the defence to prove it. However, if the jury consider a non-insane automatism, then the burden falls to the prosecution to prove beyond reasonable doubt that it was not automatism.

In *R v Roach*[29] the complex question of a combination of internal and external factors arose and it was left to the jury to conclude whether the external factors were the cause and therefore whether it was a non-insane automatism. Roach had a diagnosis of personality disorder, was facing trial for wounding with intent to cause grievous bodily harm (GBH) and the psychiatric evidence was contested but included opinions that this was a psychogenic automatism arising from personality disorder.

Clinical Issues in Automatism

Psychiatrists might be instructed to consider a wide range of mental disorders in association with automatism but the high threshold for automatism makes many of these instructions somewhat speculative. Disinhibition, impaired self-control and voluntary intoxication will likely fail as justifying a finding of automatism. The more likely successful cause of automatism is a neurological or neuropsychiatric disorder; for example, epilepsy, sleep disorders or concussion. There is therefore a need for caution when psychiatrists provide opinions in these cases and probably a need for experts from other disciplines in many cases.

Diminished Responsibility

Introduction

Diminished responsibility is only a partial defence to murder with a conviction for manslaughter (or culpable homicide in Scotland) following a successful defence. It can only be raised by the defence. Although each of the jurisdictions here have diminished

---

[28] *R v T* [1990] Crim LR 256. [29] *R v Roach* [2001] EWCA Crim 2698.

responsibility, it is not available in every common law jurisdiction. Where it does not exist, there is often an insanity defence which has been formulated to allow a lower threshold.

The Legal Tests

In E&W and NI[30] the test for diminished responsibility is highly structured: A defendant, D, is not to be convicted of murder, but only manslaughter, if D was suffering from an

- *abnormality of mental functioning* which:
- arose from a *recognised medical condition* and substantially impaired D's ability to:

  - *understand* the nature of D's conduct; or
  - *form a rational judgement*; or
  - *exercise self-control*

- and which *provides an explanation* for D's acts and omissions in doing or being a party to the killing; meaning that it *caused, or was a significant contributory factor in causing*, D to carry out the killing.

In Scotland the test is also found in statute:[31]

A person who would otherwise be convicted of murder is instead to be convicted of culpable homicide on grounds of diminished responsibility if the person's ability to determine or control conduct for which the person would otherwise be convicted of murder was, at the time of the conduct, *substantially impaired* by reason of *abnormality of mind* [mental disorder including psychopathy which was previously excluded].

In Ireland, diminished responsibility is a statutory defence[32] formulated in the following way:

Where a person is tried for murder and the jury or, as the case may be, the Special Criminal Court finds that the person –

(a) did the act alleged,

(b) was at the time suffering from a mental disorder, and

(c) the mental disorder was not such as to justify finding him or her not guilty by reason of insanity, but was such as *to diminish substantially his or her responsibility for the act*,

the jury or court, as the case may be, shall find the person not guilty of that offence but guilty of manslaughter on the ground of diminished responsibility.

The Legal Procedures

The procedural route to diminished responsibility is the same in all these jurisdictions in that the defence must prove on the balance of probabilities that the defence applies. The prosecution will, if medical evidence is unanimous, consider accepting a guilty plea to manslaughter (unlike in a case of insanity where the decision must be made by the jury) but where the issue is tried, then there will inevitably be medical evidence. Expert evidence is commonly heard on the issue of diminished responsibility because of the medical nature of

---

[30] Coroners and Justice Act 2009.   [31] Criminal Procedure (Scotland) Act 1995.
[32] Criminal Law (Insanity) Act 2006.

the law but the jury may still reject even unanimous medical evidence if the issue is put to them. If, however, the medical evidence is unequivocal, reputable and uncontradicted,[33] then the charge of murder should be withdrawn from the jury.

The word *substantial* was considered in the case of *R v Golds*[34] in relation to the E&W test. The word should be left for the jury to interpret, but if they ask for guidance, then they are directed that it means weighty and not, as argued in the Supreme Court, more than trivial.

If diminished responsibility is successful and the outcome is manslaughter or culpable homicide, then sentencing options vary from immediate discharge to (discretionary) life imprisonment, although in many cases a hospital order will be made.

Clinical Issues in Diminished Responsibility

No mental disorder is excluded from being the basis of a successful diminished responsibility defence but there is a tendency towards psychosis being the most common basis of the partial defence.

Intoxication with alcohol has been considered[35] and excluded as a 'recognised medical condition' in English law. In similar terms a substance-induced psychosis is also unlikely to be considered, at least legally, a medical condition or mental disorder.[36]

Adjustment disorder was accepted as the basis of diminished responsibility in *R v Blackman*[37] and Asperger syndrome in *R v Reynolds*.[38] Personality disorder is not excluded from any of these jurisdictions and paranoid personality disorder was allowed in *R v Martin*.[39] Battered woman syndrome, pre-menstrual syndrome and post-natal depression have also been allowed.

Dependence on substances leads to a complex situation and has not been visited in higher courts since 2009 (before the test was reformed in E&W and NI). The law has created a clinically impossible situation of trying to first determine if the substance was taken (effectively) involuntarily because of the addiction and to also determine whether it is any involuntarily taken substance (when compared with what has been taken voluntarily) that has induced the abnormal mental state. Guidance (in *R v Stewart*) assists by posing questions that seem more grounded in clinical language and include questions of severity of dependence (alcohol in this case), degree of control over taking the substance, the capability of abstinence, patterns of substance use and the extent to which ordinary decision-making seemed to have been maintained despite the substance use.[40]

Where there is mental disorder and substance use then there is another – arguably impossible – clinical task which is to try and explain whether the mental disorder (and resulting abnormality) alone would be sufficient basis for diminished responsibility. In effect, the clinical task is to provide an opinion and separate those aspects of the mental state caused by substances from those aspects caused by other mental disorder. Ultimately, the jury will be asked to decide.

---

[33] *R v Brennan* [2014] EWCA Crim 2387.   [34] *R v Golds* [2016] UKSC 61.
[35] *R v Dowds* [2012] EWCA Crim 281.   [36] *R v Lindo* [2016] EWCA Crim 1940.
[37] *R v Blackman* [2017] EWCA Crim 190.   [38] *R v Reynolds* [2004] EWCA Crim 1834.
[39] *R v Martin* [2001] EWCA Crim 2245.   [40] *R v Stewart* [2009] 1 WLR 2507.

Mental Disorder and Its Application to Other Legal Issues
Infanticide

Introduction

Infanticide is both a crime in its own right and a defence (E&W, NI and Ireland). A woman who kills a child up to 12 months can be charged with infanticide rather than another homicide offence in these jurisdictions. However, it is also a partial defence resulting in a finding of manslaughter. In Scotland, the conviction in similar circumstances would be culpable homicide by reason of diminished responsibility (there is no specific infanticide crime or defence). Confusingly, the partial defence of diminished responsibility could also be relevant if the charge had been murder in E&W, NI or Ireland.

The Legal Tests

In E&W, NI and Ireland the test is in statute and infanticide applies where 'the balance of her mind was disturbed by reason of her not having fully recovered from the effect of giving birth to the child or by reason of the effect of lactation consequent upon the birth of the child'. Lactation is no longer a relevant factor and in Ireland legislation has specifically substituted 'by reason of the effect of lactation' with 'by reason of a mental disorder'.

The Legal Procedures

In E&W, NI and Ireland the defence, if raised, must be disproven by the prosecution beyond reasonable doubt. If the charge is infanticide, then the other aspects of murder do not need to be proven including the requirement of an intention to kill or cause serious harm.

If the outcome is a conviction for manslaughter, infanticide or culpable homicide, then sentencing options are diverse, although they can include community sentences with supervision. There is the possibility in a case where an infant has been killed of a combination of insanity, infanticide and diminished responsibility all being considered.

Clinical Issues in Infanticide

Infanticide poses some specific difficulty because it adopts a legal approach to mental abnormality which is unique: 'balance of mind'. Puerperal psychosis or depression may be a straightforward clinical issue to deal with. Adjustment disorders, extreme stress and difficulties bonding with a child might be incorporated into the question of whether the balance of mind is affected. The emphasis, in giving opinions, should be on changes in mental state arising from the birth of the child and, if possible, an explanation of how childbirth has led to the changes. Diagnosis may not be so important (as, for example, it is in diminished responsibility) because the test does not rely on a legal description implying diagnosis is necessary. The effect of the birth does not have to be the only reason for the disturbance if it is 'an operative or substantial cause' (R v Tunstill),[41] which is an important legal judgment in terms of the expression of clinical opinions and emphasises the need to give clear opinions on the relationship between the childbirth and any mental abnormality.

---

[41] *R v Tunstill* [2018] EWCA Crim 1696.

Loss of Control and Provocation

Introduction

Provocation developed as a partial defence to murder – by recognising 'human frailty' – when there was 'loss of mastery over the mind in response to things said or done'. Today, as with diminished responsibility, it is a partial defence resulting in a conviction for manslaughter (culpable homicide in Scotland). In E&W and NI the term 'provocation' has been replaced by 'loss of control' following an attempt to modernise the partial defence. Modernisation seems essential when the origins of the defence are men killing women because of infidelity (now usually excluded as a trigger).

The Legal Tests

In E&W and NI there is a statutory test:[42]

A defendant, D, is not to be convicted of murder (but only manslaughter) if:

- D's acts and omissions resulted from *D's loss of control* (which need not be sudden);
- the loss of self-control had *a qualifying trigger* (fear of serious violence and/or acts or words that constitute circumstances of an extremely grave character and give a justifiable sense of being seriously wronged);
- a person of D's sex and age, with a normal degree of tolerance and self- restraint, and *in the circumstances of D*, might have reacted in the same or a similar way to D; and
- D did not act in a considered desire for revenge.

The Ireland test is a common law test and is based on there having been a sudden and temporary loss of self-control which would have caused such a loss of self-control in any reasonable person. Temporary has been interpreted as meaning the defendant must act before they had regained their composure.

The law in Scotland has evolved in common law and is made out when there is a loss of self-control and a reasonably proportionate relationship between the provocation and the response. There are two ways in which someone might be provoked: when they have been assaulted 'and there has been substantial provocation' or when someone has discovered that their partner has been unfaithful. There is no normal/reasonable person test.

In the E&W/NI statute there is specific exclusion of sexual infidelity justifiably creating the sense of being seriously wronged. It can, however, be taken into account alongside other issues if it is relevant to the totality of the facts (*R v Clinton*).[43] If the defendant has incited the trigger, to create an excuse, then they cannot rely on loss of control.

The jurisdictions which rely on a test based on the reasonable person ('in the circumstances of') comparator is problematic because of difficulty interpreting the extent to which the specific characteristics of the defendant should be taken into account when making this comparison. For example, is the comparison with someone just of the same age and sex, or should it incorporate other factors including mental conditions, personality traits and so on? The statutory test in E&W and NI makes reference to the comparison being with someone in the 'circumstances of D'. The extent of those circumstances can create uncertainty which may be passed onto psychiatrists asked to provide reports.

---

[42] Coroners and Justice Act 2009.   [43] *R v Clinton* [2012] EWCA Crim 2.

The Legal Procedures

The first stage in court, for the consideration of loss of control, to be put to a jury is that the defence provide enough evidence so that a jury might reasonably find loss of control or provocation. Once that is established, then the burden falls to the prosecution to prove beyond reasonable doubt that it is not loss of control or provocation. This, in effect, reverses the burden that exists for diminished responsibility.

Clinical Issues in Loss of Control/Provocation

The existence of a defence reflecting inability to control anger is perhaps controversial and may encourage the notion that in some people, in some circumstances, killing someone is an understandable response. Provocation was and remains very controversial because it is seen to favour men. Abused women who suffered years of abuse and who killed because of cumulative provocation were not able to argue provocation because, archetypally, the killing was not because of a sudden loss of control. Suddenness is not a part of the E&W/NI statutory defence now.

Psychiatric evidence is not accepted on whether the person did in fact lose control, but mental disorder or other characteristics may be relevant to the question of whether someone was more likely to react because of their own characteristics or circumstances. Psychiatric evidence may also be relevant when explaining why another person's actions or words constitute a trigger for this person. For example, a situation where a defendant who was sexually abused as a child is particularly susceptible to a sexual advance being perceived as threatening. The childhood sexual abuse may not have led to a mental disorder diagnosis, but the psychological impact may have had an effect on their perception of a trigger, and might properly be the subject of expert evidence.

Other mental characteristics may be relevant to consideration of loss of control including personality traits, depressive symptoms and other post-traumatic symptoms. In E&W/NI the mental characteristics (within the legal notion of circumstances) must do more than have a bearing on the defendant's general capacity for tolerance and self-restraint.

There is the possibility that the same mental symptoms are relevant to both diminished responsibility and loss of control, albeit for different reasons. Theoretically, justifications such as self-defence could also be put to a jury simultaneously so that the complex situation for the jury is to consider three separate issues, albeit they are likely to be asked to consider them in sequence rather than simultaneously. In simple terms, diminished responsibility is based on the mental condition of the defendant, something internal, whereas loss of control/provocation is based on something external. There is, of course, a complex merging of the two in many, if not most, cases.

Capacity to Have Formed the Requisite Intent

Introduction

The *mens rea* for a specific crime is often expressed in the form of an intention (but may also include recklessness, negligence, knowledge and reasonable or mistaken belief). There is a necessary separation in law of the capacity to have formed an intention from the intention itself. The reality is that this can be complex, but it is only the 'capacity to have formed intent' that a psychiatrist may comment on.

Legal Context

Crimes are sometimes distinguished in terms of severity by whether they are accompanied by an intention; for example, wounding or causing GBH with intent (to cause GBH) as compared with wounding (or inflicting GBH) without a specific intent to do so. Crimes of *basic* intent require that someone intends their actions, whereas others require not only that the actions are intended but that specific consequences are also intended: crimes of *specific* intent. This distinction between crimes of basic and specific intent is not always crystal clear.

The intent or mental element of a crime may be described in detail in law or not, so that there is considerable interpretation allowed. Whatever the mental element – whether intention or not – it is relevant when the issue for a psychiatrist is whether a defendant was likely to have had the mental capacity to have formed that intent.

Clinical Issues When Assessing Incapacity to Have Formed Intent

There is no easy test that applies to all questions of intention. The psychiatrist has to ensure that they understand what the necessary mental element (for the crime) is before embarking on addressing the question of whether they had the capacity to have formed that intention. For example, in the example of GBH above, the question posed may be whether the defendant was likely to have had the mental capacity to have formed the intention to cause GBH. If the clinical scenario is delusions, then there will be a need to map the clinical symptoms onto an opinion relating to why they would or would not have been able to form the intention to cause serious harm. If they did not have the capacity to form the mental element, then there is no crime, but in this example in English law there may be an alternative charge of GBH (without intent) so the ultimate outcome is not acquittal but conviction for a lesser offence.

Intoxication is not allowed, as a matter of common law, to be a defence to any crime except where it plays on the mental capacity of the defendant to have formed the requisite intent (albeit only crimes of specific intent). The bar, however, is set high so that the intoxicated intent is still intent. Lack of memory is not enough to demonstrate that a defendant could not have formed an intention.

In some cases, the *mens rea* may not be based on intention but on a reasonable belief. For example, in a case of rape the defendant must have reasonably believed that there was consent. A psychiatrist may be asked to comment on the effect of mental symptoms on the capacity to have formed that reasonable belief.

Duress by Threats or Circumstances (or Coercion or Necessity)

There are several ways in which someone may be found not guilty of a crime which only tenuously relate to mental conditions. Successfully arguing duress – a defence (as a result of threats or circumstances) – results in acquittal.

The essence of duress by *threats* (coercion) is that the defendant's will is overwhelmed by threats. For example, where a defendant's family is threatened with death, there must be no way to avoid the harm that has been caused if duress is successful. In Scotland, the threats must be accompanied by an immediate danger of violence.

Duress by *circumstances* (necessity) is where someone commits an offence to avoid death or serious harm. The defence of duress contains a question of whether the person making the argument can be said to have been below 'reasonable firmness' (in resisting the threat or coercion). This may incorporate consideration of psychiatric evidence as a characteristic relevant to their firmness but not to whether they were, in fact, coerced or acting out of necessity. As with many defences, drugs or alcohol and their effects will provide no basis for the defence. Which mental disorders may be considered relevant is confusing. For example, PTSD has been accepted but personality traits are probably excluded (*R v Emery*).[44]

Self-Defence and Other Justifications

As well as defences, there are some 'justifications' for offences which mean that actions that would be unlawful are not crimes. The most commonly know is self-defence, with defending another person, preventing an offence, apprehending an offender and preventing serious damage to property making up the rest.

Self-defence and other justifications are, in most jurisdictions, made up of a combination of common law and statute. In the four jurisdictions referenced in this chapter there are subtle differences, but generally all contain some form of the justifications described. Justifications require that someone's actions must have been based on necessity. If, for example, there was an alternative course of action to using violence, then necessity may be difficult to demonstrate. The reasonableness of someone's actions in these justifications is judged in an objective way. However, the circumstances in which someone acted are considered subjectively. If there is sufficient evidence offered by a defendant to justify their actions, then the prosecution must prove that the justification does not apply (beyond reasonable doubt).

The relevance of mental health evidence in the cases where a justification is proposed is limited. If someone is, for example, experiencing psychosis which means they believe honestly that they are defending themselves, then the question for the court should be one of insanity, not self-defence. The rationale is that a person with psychosis who acts violently in these circumstances would, if justifying their actions by self-defence, be acquitted, whereas the person found not guilty by reason of insanity could be admitted to hospital for treatment.

References

1. Völlm BA, Clarke M, Herrando VT et al. European Psychiatric Association (EPA) guidance on forensic psychiatry: evidence based assessment and treatment of mentally disordered offenders. *European Psychiatry* 2018; 51: 58–73.

2. Barber S. R V Earl Ferrers (1760): the trial that saved England from revolution? 2017. http://dx.doi.org/10.2139/ssrn.3414681.

3. Rollin HR. Psychiatry in Britain 100 years ago. *British Journal of Psychiatry* 2003; 183: 292–8.

4. Hallett N. Psychiatric evidence in diminished responsibility. *The Journal of Criminal Law* 2018; 82 (6): 442–56.

5. Rix K, Eastman N, Adshead G. *Responsibilities of Psychiatrists Who Provide Expert Opinion to Courts and Tribunals*. The Royal College of Psychiatrists, 2015.

6. Academy of Medical Royal Colleges. *Acting as an Expert or Professional Witness: Guidance for Healthcare Professionals*, 2019. www.aomrc.org.uk/reports-guidance/acting-as-an-expert-or-professional-witness-guidance-for-healthcare-professionals.

7. Pham T, Taylor P. *The Roles of Forensic Psychiatrists and Psychologists: Professional Experts, Service Providers, Therapists, or All Things for All People?* New York, Springer, 2018.

---

[44] *R v Emery* [1993] 14 Cr App R.

8. Brown P, Bakolis I, Appiah-Kusi E et al. Prevalence of mental disorder in defendants at criminal court. *BJPsych Open* 2022; 8 (3): e92.

9. Grubin D. What constitutes fitness to plead. *Criminal Law Review* 1993: 748–58.

10. Hale M, Emlyn S. *Historia Placitorum Coronae: The History of the Pleas of the Crown*. Philadelphia, PA, Robert H. Small, 1847.

11. Brown P. Unfitness to plead in England and Wales: historical development and contemporary dilemmas. *Medicine, Science and the Law* 2019; 59 (3): 187–96.

12. Loughnan A. *Manifest Madness: Mental Incapacity in the Criminal Law*. Oxford, Oxford University Press, 2012.

13. Exworthy T. Commentary: UK perspective on competency to stand trial. *Journal of the American Academy of Psychiatry and the Law* 2006; 34 (4): 466–71.

14. Vassall-Adams G, Scott-Moncrieff L. Capacity and fitness to plead: The yawning gap. *Counsel* 2006: 14–16.

15. Law Commission of England and Wales. *Unfitness to Plead – Volume 1: Report (law com. No 364)*. London, The Stationery Office, 2016.

16. Northern Ireland Law Commission. *Report: Unfitness to Plead*. Northern Ireland Law Commission, 2013.

17. Mackay R, Kearns G. An upturn in unfitness to plead? Disability in relation to the trial under the 1991 Act. *Criminal Law Review* 2000: 532–46.

18. Mudathikundan F, Chao O, Forrester A. Mental health and fitness to plead proposals in England and Wales. *International Journal of Law and Psychiatry* 2014; 37 (2): 135–41.

19. Brown P, Stahl D, Appiah-Kusi E et al. Fitness to plead: Development and validation of a standardised assessment instrument. *PloS One* 2018; 13 (4): e0194332.

20. Henderson E. 'A very valuable tool': judges, advocates and intermediaries discuss the intermediary system in England and Wales. *The International Journal of Evidence & Proof* 2015; 19 (3): 154–71.

21. Law Commission of England and Wales. *Criminal Liability: Insanity and Automatism*. A Discussion Paper. London, The Stationery Office, 2013.

22. Fenwick P. Automatism, medicine and the law. *Psychological Medicine Monograph Supplement* 1990; 17: 1–27. doi: 10.1017/s0264180100000758.

Expertise, Structured Professional Judgement and Risk Assessment

Mary Davoren and Harry Kennedy

Violence Risk Assessment and the Evolution of Structured Professional Judgement

No one can predict the future with accuracy. Yet doctors in all disciplines are required to make projections about the future. A diagnosis is, among other things, a means of identifying the most likely future course of an illness or disorder. A diagnosis may carry with it a prognosis that is benign, disabling or fatal. The diagnosis and prognosis will also largely influence the approach to treatment. A benign prognosis will imply a relaxed approach to treatment, while a disabling or potentially fatal prognosis will lead towards a more intensive, intrusive and challenging intervention, provided the evidence is strong and reliable for diagnosis, prognosis and treatment effectiveness. Forensic psychiatry sits squarely within this form and process.

The origins of the concept of probability are surprisingly recent, starting with fifteenth-century banking and shipping insurance for Mediterranean trade [1], the nineteenth-century suicide statistics of Durkheim and the twentieth-century mental illness and urban statistics of the Chicago school [2].

Medical Expertise and Risk

Forensic psychiatric services have a dual role: to treat mental disorder and reduce the risk of violent recidivism due to mental disorder [3]. There are many patients with mental illnesses that are difficult to treat, including treatment-resistant schizophrenia and other psychoses, complex organic brain pathologies and complex personality disorders attending general and more specialist mental health services in every country and jurisdiction. Schizophrenia and similar psychoses are life-shortening illnesses, more so for those in forensic psychiatry services due to the most severe and treatment-resistant illnesses [4]. It is the risk of serious violence that brings patients to forensic mental health services and to the attention of consultant forensic psychiatrists. Violence and violent behaviour is an unmet treatment need for patients leading to admission to secure forensic mental health settings [5]. An accurate and realistic approach to violence risk assessment and management is required from doctors practising forensic psychiatry. Therefore, a clear and thorough understanding of violence risk assessment and management, including the use of structured professional judgement instruments such as the Historical-Clinical-Risk for Violence-20 (HCR-20), is vital for all forensic psychiatrists.

Doctors are held to a standard of expertise when exercising professional judgement within their scope of practice. This is obtained through education, training by established experts and experience. The standard required should be in keeping with the standard of other practitioners of like experience and should be reasonable. Arriving at a diagnosis, offering a prognosis and recommending treatment combine qualitative and quantitative judgements. They should be accurate, effective and reliable but they cannot be perfect. An expert opinion and professional expertise have technical meanings. Experts by experience can share their personal experience. Interactional experts acquire knowledge of the vocabulary and context of the subject through regular interaction with expert practitioners. Examples of interactional experts include managers, lawyers and journalists. Interactional experts acquire a limited breadth and finite depth of knowledge of the subject. Expert practitioners are contributory experts, capable of contributing to that body of knowledge and skill through innovation. Only contributory experts can teach and train. Those expert practitioners who teach, train and expand their specialty through research should also have interactional skills, to reflect and to communicate [6]. There is a virtuous cycle linking research and development, teaching and training [7].

The recognition of an expert witness by the courts [8–10] is not the prime purpose of this chapter, though the expertise and expert judgement dealt with here are the basis expected by the courts when seeking expert opinions.

Unstructured professional judgement concerning diagnosis has been refined by means of operationalised diagnostic criteria. Unstructured professional judgement regarding treatment is increasingly held to the highest standards of scientific evidence using random-ised controlled trials and meta-analyses.

Prognosis arises from the prospective observation of outcomes. Epidemiologists and actuaries provide statistical methods in which attempts are made to fit a mathematical or statistical 'model' to real-world systems using methods such as regression analysis and survival curves. It should always be kept in mind that these are at best approximations and can never be sufficient in themselves to establish causal relationships. For this, some additional level of scientific explanation is required.

Bradford Hill set out rigorous methods for distinguishing between risk factors, con-founding factors and what might be true causal factors. At a time when social factors and health-related behaviours were first recognised as interacting with biological factors in the causation of disease, the epidemiological approach in psychiatry was widely accepted and has influenced concepts of risk [11].

Violence Risk

Violence risk is defined as the high likelihood of a further very serious violent or sexual offence against persons. Violence risk assessment is the process by which risk is understood: it examines the nature, seriousness and pattern of offences; it identifies the characteristics of the offenders and the circumstances that contribute to it; it informs appropriate decision-making and action with the aim of reducing risk [12].

Critiques of Violence Risk Assessment

Early studies of unstructured professional judgement concerning the prediction of violence in the mentally ill demonstrated poor predictive accuracy. Actuarial approaches appeared to perform better. Early approaches to the structuring of risk assessment emphasised the need to ground the assessment in theory. The distinction between fixed or historical risk factors and dynamic factors that are state dependent and amenable to change has gained the widest acceptance. Other approaches, however, include distinguishing between remote and proximate factors, intrinsic and extrinsic factors, biological and social factors, life events and difficulties that are independent of the person or dependent on the person themselves.

All risk assessment, whether unstructured, actuarial or structured, is vulnerable to the criticism that it may over predict risk and harm [13, 14]. In practice, structured professional judgement risk assessments are, like actuarial risk assessments, validated in prospective studies comparing a summative score with subsequent outcomes. The use of the receiver operating characteristic area under the curve statistic is designed to minimise the effect of population base rates [15]. An outcome with a very low population incidence rate such as homicide (approximately 1/100,000 persons per annum) will have a high false positive rate. Other forms of violence will have much higher base rates and lower false positive rates [16]. All recommendations for treatment, for example antihypertensives to prevent stroke or oral hypoglycaemics to prevent complications of diabetes, allow for a false positive rate or 'number needed to treat to prevent one adverse event' of about 5 to 1. Approximately five people might be treated for high blood pressure to prevent one stroke, for example. It can tentatively be calculated that the false positive rate for general violence using modern structured professional judgement risk assessments is of the order of 5 to 1 [16]. This is justifiable when social and therapeutic supports and interventions are offered on the basis of the assessment and when the intervention has a known effectiveness. Deprivation of liberty on this basis would be less easy to justify. However, an inescapable problem in population studies is that the largest number of adverse outcomes such as violence or suicide will occur among those thought to be at low risk – because the low-risk cases will be so numerous compared to high-risk cases [14]. Risk assessment has therefore not been adopted in community-based or tier 2 services. Risk assessment is widely used in forensic psychiatry services because probability in these populations is much higher, with few low risk cases. A further criticism of violence risk assessment is the failure to distinguish in the validation studies and in subsequent use between serious violence and less serious harm, between deliberative or instrumental violence and expressive or impulsive violence [17], between violence against identifiable or foreseeable victims and random or unforeseen victims, and violence that occurs in the context of delusions, hallucinations, intoxication, anger or fear, moral imperatives and egocentric gratification.

Form and Content

It is important to note that violence risk assessment instruments are only as useful as the detail that they contain, when used to identify treatment needs and management plans. These instruments must be completed by trained professionals and it is essential they contain a very high level of detail. It is of little use to read an HCR-20 violence risk assessment where the clinician has documented a series of over-arching vague statements in each domain. For example, under item H1 in HCR-20 (the item entitled H1: History of violence) a statement such as 'patient has a history of interpersonal violence and violence against property' should be avoided. Rather, each individual incident, including dates, detail of the incident and the circumstances, must be documented carefully and thoroughly and in chronological order. This is certainly time consuming but is necessary and appropriate given that in many cases the risk of violence towards others may be a reason why the patient is detained in hospital against their wishes and because violence is likely a key target for treatment. In addition to updating the current and future items, the history of violence section should be updated at each patient case conference to include any new incidents which took place over the period under review. This should include all incidents of violence towards staff members and fellow patients in the in-patient setting. Care must be taken to obtain collateral information from family members and others to ensure that violence which may not have resulted in charges or convictions is included as this will also need to be addressed in treatment and therapy sessions.

Risk Assessment

Risk assessment is used here primarily as a means of understanding how medical expertise in psychiatry is used to generate violence risk management plans and expert evidence in court. The use of risk assessment and structured professional judgement instruments always requires formal training and adherence to the handbook of the instrument in question, in order to ensure fidelity.

Some require specific professional training or higher training before eligibility for training in the use of the instrument. Without this, nothing is gained from the use of any such instrument. The formal process of compiling a structured professional judgement instrument, the inferences that can be drawn from it and projections regarding the future cannot be derived from validation studies if the instrument has not been used correctly as validated. In this chapter the reader is expected to obtain or to have obtained such formal training.

Origins of Modern Assessment of Risk of Violence

In 1981 John Monahan [18] reviewed the clinical prediction of violent behaviour in the context of legal requirements for evidence on prediction of dangerous and violent behaviour. Having outlined why accurate prediction is impossible, and why prediction may violate civil liberties and undermine the helping role of mental health professions, he went on to list the problem of base rates – a low-base-rate, rare event will generate a lot of false positives. He then distinguished between statistical data combined statistically in actuarial tables; statistical data combined clinically – when a clinician makes a prediction after looking at test scores; clinical data combined statistically – when probabilities of violence are attached to diagnoses or other qualities or categories; and clinical data combined clinically – an unstructured judgement. He concluded reluctantly that there may be circumstances in which prediction is both empirically possible and ethically appropriate.

Assessing Risk of Violence in Psychiatry

Early in the development of psychiatric assessments of risks of violence, Dietz [19] writing in 1985 set out a precise and demanding account of what a risk assessment might be. Clinical crime prediction had three purposes: injury control, the protection of potential victims; paternalism, the protection of the individual from the consequences of their potential criminal actions; and self-protection, the elimination of personal responsibility and legal liability of the clinician for deleterious consequences of negligent predictive errors. This could be summarised as a conditional projection with great precision. Dietz focussed on the prevention of 'intolerable crimes'. He started with first-rank predictors, by which he meant a list of actual 'intolerable crimes' with a future probability of 50%; second-rank predictors had a probability of committing an intolerable crime of 10 to 50% and a false positive rate of 1 to 10 for every true positive; third-rank predictors would carry a probability of committing an intolerable crime that is at least twice the population rate but still less than 10%. In retrospect, most modern risk assessment inventories and instruments are made up of these third-rank items, which are mostly statistical predictors at a level better than chance – but not a lot better. Also of note, most of Dietz's first- and second-rank predictors would today be included in triage assessment instruments that focus on seriousness of outcomes rather than probability (true risk) such as the DUNDRUM-1 [3, 20, 21]. A clinical service constructed around the assessment of risk and seriousness of risk was said to meet the 'forensic sound barrier' or limit of predictive uncertainty [22, 23].

Expertise and Professional Judgement

The weakness of unstructured professional judgement concerning risk of violence has been used as a straw-man argument to some extent. Professional and clinical judgement is never unstructured, although the term should be replaced by expert clinical judgement [24, 25]. A medical assessment proceeds from observations to findings, from findings to facets or clusters of findings of potential clinical significance representing interim hypotheses, then to diagnoses that subsume and explain the levels below. While novices may proceed by hypothesis and induction (backward-directed reasoning), experts can use forward-directed reasoning. Forward-directed reasoning is characterised by a chain of inferences from data towards an incremental refinement of hypotheses resulting in a diagnostic solution. Forward reasoning is strongly correlated with accuracy in experts. Novices and intermediate students tend to employ a form of backward reasoning such as the hypothetico-deductive method. Experts progress from data to refined hypotheses and on to diagnostic solutions because of their highly structured and well-developed pattern recognition capabilities. These schema-driven expert cognitive processes can, however, be error prone in the absence of an expert knowledge base [25–27]. Interactional experts and experts by experience often fail to realise this vulnerability to error unless assisted [28].

Taking an oral history, interviewing informants and reviewing notes is followed by observation and examination. All history-taking and all assessment of mental state should follow a structure that is consistent but also flexible and responsive to the patient and the flow of the examination and interview. Following a diagnostic formulation, a prognosis may be communicated concerning the future and treatment will then be recommended. This process can be summarised as a fact-gathering phase: a phase of investigation guided by a differential diagnosis and projections about the future (prognosis). These projections or conjectures that derive from an educated eye and the active listening of a well-primed ear are the origins of all clinical science and ultimately all medical science including 'wet lab' work.

All assessment, diagnosis and treatment planning is structured according to professional expertise. These are of necessity organised according to levels of complexity, expertise and responsibility. Tier 1 assessments and interventions are basic and uncomplicated tasks that can be completed by any recent graduate; tier 2 tasks can be completed with minimal further training by use of a handbook, guidebook or algorithm; tier 3 requires formal training in the task at hand, often reserved to a professional with specific specialist skills and experience; and tier 4 assessments and interventions are complex at a level that cannot be completed by using 'off-the-shelf' formulations, instruments and intervention programmes – a highly individualised and nuanced assessment and treatment plan is required, provided by the highest level of expertise (contributory expertise) in which some degree of innovation and individualisation is required, though always built upon existing knowledge and experience, on structured assessments chosen for the purpose and interventions known to be effective in similar presentations and contexts. At this level, expert professional judgement at the highest level is 'unstructured', though scaffolded and supported by the use of structured professional judgement instruments, and by scientific and clinical education, training and experience.

Diagnosis As Structured Professional Expertise

Modern psychiatry originates in observation and so-called unstructured professional judgement. A cognitive process moves from observation to diagnosis, then prognosis and treatment. Randomised controlled trials have precedence in treatment but not in diagnosis or prognosis. Here, prospective observational whole-cohort studies take precedence. Meta-analysis enables the results of multiple randomised controlled trials to be pooled achieving better statistical power. However, the meta-analysis of prospective observational cohort studies or cross-sectional case register data does not necessarily generate more reliable results. Pooling good studies and poor studies merely dilutes the good studies; regional differences and variations may be real and pooling them describes a non-existent average.

The foundations of modern psychiatry originate in unstructured professional judgement: the process of careful clinical observation and compiling of case series. Kraepelin's distinction between affective and nonaffective psychosis [29] remains controversial [30] but is of enormous clinical utility. Kraepelin's description of 'morphinism and cocainism' [29, 31] rings true in the modern era of novel psychoactive substances and polysubstance misuse. Kraepelin also described morbid jealousy. Shepherd's description of morbid jealousy was built on painstaking description of more than 70 case vignettes [32]. Shepherd's sceptical approach to diagnosis in relation to this symptom or syndrome fits well with the modern interest in transdiagnostic and personalised approaches [33]; Brittain's [34] description of the sadistic murderer and the subsequent tabulation of cases and formulation by McCulloch and Snowden [35] follow the same pattern. Mullen's descriptions of morbid jealousy [36], stalkers, threateners and vexatious litigants [37] in Chapter 12 of this volume work in the same forward-directed way. The early twentieth-century essays of Lewis [38], Shepherd and Mullen follow a consistent structure, starting with a review of the linguistic origins of the subject's terminology, then a review of the development of the existing literature including the emergence of different schools before progressing to a modern understanding, at times a synthesis, at other times dismissing the topic itself before recommending future directions. A late twentieth-century development of this method involved compiling vignettes as raw material [39, 40], and later still attempting to use vignettes as the basis for some form of classification or mechanistic understanding [35].

Robins and Guze [41] suggested five criteria or postulates for validating diagnosis: clinical description, laboratory tests, delimitation, follow-up studies and family data, where the goal was specifying prognosis. These might be adapted to the validation of risk assessment instruments and other similar tools. Operational diagnostic criteria emerged from the need for better prognosis but even more so from the need for better inter-rater reliability [42]. The research diagnostic criteria [43] and World Health Organization international classification of diseases were designed to enable research that had validity across countries [44]. These criteria evolved interactively with structured or semi-structured diagnostic interviews such as the present state examination [42], schedules for clinical assessment in neuropsychiatry (SCAN) [45] and schedule for affective disorders and schizophrenia [46, 47], in an evolving progression [48–50] that is not always more rigorous [51]. The best of these include elements of disease staging and progression, taking account of functional impairments as well as symptoms. However, the most widely used instruments are more limited [50]. Case registry data seldom employs diagnostic interviews or operationalised diagnostic criteria but has a certain real-world validity which is itself limited. The use of these operationalised diagnostic criteria and structured diagnostic interviews represents an important advance in the reliability of psychiatric diagnosis and prognosis. Operationalised diagnostic criteria have been criticised because of the lack of transparency in their origins, because of a tendency over time towards splitting entities into multiple categories that may be singular though variable, and in some cases because of the reification (the error of believing that giving a thing a name makes it real) of entities that may not exist at all [52]. The naming of a natural category has no effect on the category, but the naming of a human category may have a 'looping' effect that changes the person labelled or the category itself [53, 54]. Scientific research can raise a human kind to the more solid grounding of a natural, biological kind [53].

Bias and Fairness 1

Classification systems and risk assessments run the risk of appearing to be long lists of pejorative and negative descriptions. There is a real risk of racist bias, Eurocentric bias, gender bias and other forms of structural violence from unexamined assumptions, leading to unexamined processes such as admission triage, risk assessment or discharge decisions.

For this reason, evidence-based instruments are put forward as having the real advantage of being able to limit inherent discrimination. Whether this is achieved in practice has been closely examined for diagnostic instruments but less so for risk assessment instruments.

Qualitative research has been put forward as a means of minimising the a priori assumptions of researchers. However, the very small convenience samples of self-selected interviewees employed in most qualitative research and the inevitable heuristic bias of the qualitative researcher who interprets transcriptions make such methods essentially subjective. Delphi methods may be marginally more open, provided the experts consulted have relevant experience as well as expertise. The emphasis on consensus in iterative Delphi methods may, however, dampen originality when drafting new measurement instruments.

New approaches to data mining from unselected databanks cannot be regarded as free of a priori assumptions since the contents of such data banks – the patients and their data – have been selected by some process of custom and practice. Fairness has numerous definitions when applied to risk assessment instruments and structured professional judgement generally (sensitivity fairness, error rate balance, calibration, predictive parity, statistical parity) [55–57].

All such instruments carry the risk that having been drafted and validated for a 'typical' or majority population, they may carry an inherent bias against minority groups. At least one study failed to substantiate evidence of bias [57]. Unstructured assessments such as triage for admission to secure forensic hospitals identify an excess of admissions from some ethnic minorities but no evidence that this is disproportionate to need [58, 59]. This suggests that a marker of fairness would be to extend the use of objective criteria through the use of structured professional judgement instruments. The possibility remains that risk assessments might have a bias that disadvantages migrant, first nations, ethnic minority and culturally and linguistically diverse groups. This may be addressed in Canada by means of a *Gladue* report specifically addressing such matters. These may be a model for good practice more generally. *Gladue* reports provide insights into an Indigenous person's unique circumstances that may have led to their offending as well as community-based options for rehabilitation. There may be value in augmenting the risk evaluation with culturally relevant *Gladue*-style considerations identified by relevant Indigenous people [56, 57, 60, 61].

Expertise

Collins and Evans [6] provide a system for defining, examining and recognising the social and linguistic culture of expertise. Ubiquitous expertise is universal and includes a huge body of tacit knowledge – things you know how to do without being able to explain how you do them. Examples include fluency in the natural language of each society, moral sensibility and political discrimination.

Next come dispositions – personal qualities such as linguistic fluency or interactive ability and analytic flair or reflective ability. Specialist expertise divides into ubiquitous tacit knowledge and specialist tacit knowledge. Ubiquitous tacit knowledge includes general knowledge such as sport or popular music. Acquiring this depends on extensive ubiquitous expertise – knowledge of language and social custom and practice. Specialist tacit knowledge is acquired through immersion and is essential for specialist expertise [62]. The highest level is contributory expertise: what is required to do an activity with competence. Just below this is interactional expertise: the ability to master the knowledge of a specialist domain in the absence of practical competence.

Meta-expertise divides into external or transmuted expertise and internal expertise. External transmuted expertise is the domain of judges [63]. This is transmuted because the judge uses social discrimination to produce technical discrimination. Judges do not possess the expertise in question but make judgements about experts who do possess it. They do so by judging the expert's demeanour, the internal consistency of their opinions and meta-criteria outlined below.

Internal non-transmuted meta-expertise is based on having one level or another of the expertise being judged. Technical connoisseurship resembles the expertise of art critics or music journalists who are not themselves artists or musicians. Skilful discrimination occurs when one specialist judges another. This can be an expert judging another who is more expert (upwards discrimination), equally expert or less expert (downward discrimination). Collins and Evans argue that only downward discrimination is reliable, with the other directions leading to wrong impressions of reliability or irresolvable disputes.

Referred expertise is the use of an expertise learned in one domain to make judgements about another domain. Examples include appointing an expert in one scientific domain to manage a project in another. Meta-criteria are used by non-experts to judge between experts when they do not have access to other forms of expertise. These include checking the qualifications of experts, checking the expert's track record of success and assessing the expert's experience. Experience is held to be the best guide [6].

Contributory Expertise

Contributory expertise is acquired according to one theory, by five stages leading to internalisation [64]. This system closely matches the traditional apprenticeship approach in medicine [65]. The five stages are novice, advanced beginner, competence, proficiency, expertise and mastery.

Novices [66] learn to follow explicit rules in an effortful way, unresponsive to changes in context, through laboured problem solving. Advanced beginners respond to some aspects of change and context. Competence commences when specific features of the situation are recognised and responses becomes more intuitive than calculating. Proficiency is marked by the ability to recognise and respond to whole-problem situations 'holistically', though still with some conscious choice and analysis before making decisions [67]. Mastery or expertise is the fifth stage. Complete contexts are unselfconsciously recognised and performance is related to them in a fluid way using cues that need not be articulated because they have been internalised. If articulated, they might not correspond, or might even contradict the rules explained to novices. An essential aspect of contributory expertise is the ability to improvise and innovate – to contribute new knowledge and skills, thereby expanding the field.

In this system, the deliberative decision-making of Kahneman [68] and the skilful intuitions of Gigerenzer [69] are compatible [62, 70, 71]. Collins and Evans point out that the ability of a contributory expert to expand their subject is also a matter of interactive ability, a generalised skill in communication, a disposition that can also be passed from generation to generation. Reflective ability is a further generalisable skill that is not essential for contributory expertise but can be taught and should be essential for the roles of analyst, teacher, trainer and leader.

Interactional Expertise

Interactional expertise is expertise in the language of a specialism in the absence of expertise in its practice [6]. While contributory expertise requires formal knowledge – rules, formulae, facts – it also requires informal or tacit knowledge which is acquired through immersion and consists of rules that are more difficult to express explicitly but are known through their expression in action [72]. It is easy for those who have internalised the rules and become enculturated into the form of life that expresses them to see when they have been broken. The language of the subject is often learned by managers, journalists and lawyers who then may overestimate their expertise. Contributory experts have usually little difficulty in recognising these interactional experts who lack the essential tacit knowledge of the practitioner. Interactional experts have their own contributory expertise that consists of interactive ability and reflective ability. For this reason, the contributory expert who can also interact, communicate and reflect should have a special role within the domain of expertise. Non-contributory experts who are limited to interactional expertise have an essentially parasitic relationship with contributory experts and cannot sustain their fluency in the subject without continued frequent interaction with contributory experts.

Collins and Evans have interesting things to say about 'fake doctors' and other imposters, who can appear very convincing due to a combination of language skills (acquiring interactional expertise) and confidence [73, 74]. When they are found out, it is usually because of some deficit in basic technical knowledge or skill.

Training and Practice Effects

As outlined earlier, the skills of the professional who uses a structured professional judgement instrument as a step in the process of risk assessment require formal training and adherence to that training. In areas other than psychiatry, a minimum number of complex procedures must be completed to achieve acceptable outcomes per procedure [75-77], and a further regular number of new cases is required to maintain competence at the individual and at the institutional level, for example in surgery and obstetrics [78-82]. This results in benefits measured in mortality and side effects even when adjusted for case mix for example in obstetrics [83, 84]. Forensic psychiatry is a third- or fourth-tier service and can be expected to require the same processes of volume to maintain competencies and standards. It has been shown that training improves inter-rater reliability in the use of triage instruments [85] and risk instruments. Writing about the skills and effectiveness of psychotherapists, the essential role of systematic, ongoing formal feedback is emphasised as a means of renewing deliberative practice. This in turn leads to a determination of baseline levels of effectiveness including skills and strengths that need improvement. This feedback can feel challenging and hard. It is not inherently enjoyable or immediately rewarding. Its absence, however, can lead to arrested development as an expert practitioner [86].

Predictive Validity

Numerous reviews of the predictive validity of risk assessments conclude that the evidence for predictive validity is often weak. In a review of evidence for assessments and interventions in forensic psychiatry generally [87, 88], the reviewers found many gaps. In a systematic review of risk and outcome measures [89], Shinkfield et al. [89] were able to identify both risk assessment instruments and outcome measures specific to forensic practice that were supported by good evidence.

Statistical validation for actuarial instruments commenced with compiling lists of risk factors validated against outcomes using basic statistical tests such as Chi-squared, t-tests or analysis of variance. At a subsequent stage, correlation coefficients were used. Actuarial checklists [90] were validated in much the same way, with items added either according to a weighting factor (proper linear models) or reduced to simple scores 'absent' or 'present' summated (improper linear models). The next step in validation was suggested by Mossman, noting that the statistical validation of laboratory tests according to sensitivity and specificity should be applied also to instruments for assessing the risk of violence [15]. With this came a recognition that for very rare events (a low population base rate), all but the most exact tests would have a high false positive rate [13]. This was used as an argument against risk assessment in a debate that is now largely superseded by greater understanding of how and when such instruments should be used. The next phase in validation studies placed emphasis on content validity. The view that risk assessment instruments should be regarded as means of identifying targets for treatment and risk management is vulnerable to the criticism that many risk factors are either remote or indirect, in effect confounding items arising from co-linearity [91].

Coid et al. [92] applied a lagged model to a prospective cohort study of 409 male and female patients discharged from medium-secure forensic hospitals in England and Wales to the community. Measures were taken at baseline pre-discharge, 6 and 12 months after discharge. Outcomes were ascertained using a structured interview, the MacArthur community violence instrument and police-recorded crimes. Eight items of the HCR-20v3 and four SAPROF (Structured Assessment of PROtective Factors for violence risk) items did not predict violent behaviour better than chance. In re-analyses considering temporal proximity of risk or protective factors and subsequent violence as outcome, risk was elevated due to violent ideation (odds ratio (OR) 6.98), instability (OR 5.41) and poor coping-stress

(OR 8.35). All three risk factors were explanatory variables which drove the association with violent outcome. Self-control (OR 0.13) conveyed protective effects and explained the association of other protective factors with violence. Different factors appear to predict violence in other populations, for example non-clinical representative samples of women in the community [93]. It does not follow that a structured professional judgement instrument consisting of a range of risk factors is incorrect, only that different risk factors may be relevant for different groups in different geographic and social situations. Coid's group has drawn attention also to the complexities of modelling risks and causes when relationships are non-linear [94] and very time dependent. In these circumstances the choice of mathematical model used can have too large an effect on the result [95].

Validation Standards

Standards for risk assessment, including a system for rating the quality and reliability of risk assessment instruments and a format for a risk assessment and risk management report for courts prior to sentencing, have been set out in a series of guidance notes by the Risk Management Authority of Scotland in the Risk Assessment Tools Evaluation Directory (RATED) [96]. In its fourth edition, this sets out a system for rating tools:

> practitioners can use with confidence validated tools that possess a robust validation history and empirical grounding. These tend to be tools that have also evidenced sufficient inter-rater reliability (the degree in which two or more assessors consistently rate items within a tool), specificity (the ability of a test to classify when an individual does not possess a particular characteristic), sensitivity (the extent to which an instrument can correctly classify when an individual possesses a particular characteristic) and predictive accuracy (ability to distinguish between certain populations, such as those who reoffend and those who do not) in identifying individuals at risk of re-offending.

The 'robust validation history and empirical grounding' refers to [96]:

> Empirical grounding in sound theoretical evidence and extensive scientific findings observed in prior research. Greater weight is attached to studies by authors who are independent of the authors of the tool; studies published in peer reviewed journals; more recent studies; independently funded studies; studies relevant to the population concerned, for example within the same language, culture, model of care and in some cases legal structure; relevant to a defined target population; larger studies are preferred to smaller studies; and studies with a defined focus such as inter rater reliability, statistically significant predictive power, usefulness, sensitivity and specificity.

Inter-rater reliability is the degree to which two or more assessors are consistent in their ratings when using the same risk assessment tool. Intra-class correlation or Kappa coefficients are relevant measures. Without evidence of reliability, the performance of an assessment tool cannot be replicated and validation cannot be attained. Even if a tool has predictive validity, its usefulness will be undermined if it is applied inconsistently by different practitioners.

Validation history requires two or more independent papers written by different authors and published in peer-reviewed journals. Papers demonstrate predictive validity of the tool or its practical usefulness (clinical utility to enable the practitioner to undertake a risk formulation and risk management planning) for the assessment and management of risk of harm to others. This includes:

- general predictive validity, demonstrating that the tool distinguishes between recidivist and non-recidivist groups. This is typically measured using the receiver operating characteristic
- applicability of the tool for female offenders
- applicability of the tool for ethnic minorities
- applicability of the tool for mental disabilities including mental disorders or learning disabilities or both.

While the Risk Management Authority of Scotland is a carefully managed body driven by public policy that is transparent, other claims to authority should be considered critically. Editors' groups have a legitimate basis for publishing guidelines on the form and structure of research articles, ethical standards and statistical standards. Anyone may compose a set of standards. Following Feinstein, clinometrics has developed to measure patient-reported outcome measures [97, 98]. The COSMIN group is an ad hoc collective that has published standards for the validation of measurement instruments [99]. They set out as their principles that it is usually a bad idea to develop a new measurement instrument; that objective measurements are not better than subjective measures; that Cronbach's alpha has nothing to do with validity; and why they say valid instruments do not exist. Each of these statements is playfully incorrect when applied to outcome measures and should not be taken seriously when measurement-based care is a means of improving objective outcomes in forensic psychiatry [100]. It will be necessary to devise new measurement instruments where none currently exists, though it is usually better to carry out a local validation of an internationally established instrument; objective measurements are always better than subjective measures, at least in clinical settings such as forensic psychiatry where objective outcomes matter; Cronbach's alpha measure of internal consistency, along with measures of inter-rater reliability, is important for measures of reliable and meaningful change [101]; valid instruments do exist, provided the thing measured is a measurable quantity and not a post-modern literary or semantic artefact. The COSMIN standards also insist on a qualitative source for content that is at odds with the values of scientific processes in literature review and they insist on factor analysis. Factor analysis is itself a highly artefactual method that will always produce the number of factors set by the initial parameters. In research it is better to take a critical view of different statistical and mathematical modelling methods to seek robustness [95].

Local Validation

In addition to broadening the range of measures to be used when assessing the validity and utility of a measurement instrument, the value of local validation should go beyond checking inter-rater reliability.

Reliable and Meaningful Change

Clinically significant change is defined as the extent to which therapy moves someone outside the range of the dysfunctional population or within the range of the functional population. A reliable change (RC) index can be calculated based on both statistical reliability and clinical significance to determine whether the magnitude of change for a given patient is statistically reliable [102, 103]. This has been further developed by the Evidence Based Medicine centre into a system for calculating reliable and clinically significant change [101] comprising two elements. 'Reliable change' asks: has the patient changed sufficiently to be confident that the change is beyond that which could be attributed to measurement error? 'Clinically significant change' asks how the end state of the patient compares with the scores observed in socially and clinically meaningful comparison groups. A web calculator is available for local validation studies [104]. A notable advance in the design of structured professional judgement instruments in forensic psychiatry has been the introduction of meaningful units of measurement, specifically relating to levels of therapeutic security, first suggested by Eastman [105], then by Shaw [106] and others [107, 108], and used variously to assess triage needs [3, 21, 109], admission to high, medium or low security, treatment programme completion [110–114] and forensic recovery [115–117], and readiness to move to a less secure setting, notably in the DUNDRUM (Dangerousness Understanding Recovery and Urgency Manual) Toolkit.

Unstructured Violence Risk Assessment

The first generation of risk assessment consisted of unstructured clinical or unstructured professional judgement. This consisted of individual doctors or professionals drawing on their expertise, scientific training, clinical training and experience to give an estimate of risk, typically noting a patient to be at high, medium or low risk of a particular outcome. However, unstructured clinical judgement was shown to have very poor consistency and reliability in decision-making. When unstructured professional judgement was applied to the study of violence, the lack of a scientific grounding in evidence and good method quickly emerged [90, 118]. Predicting violence in the context of mental illness is not the same as predicting survival and treatment response in other areas of medicine. In some settings, such as general adult psychiatry or child and adolescent mental health settings, where the risk of a serious violent outcome is generally low, this type of risk assessment could potentially be tolerated. In forensic mental health settings where patients have a history of serious violent behaviour and may be detained in hospital on the basis of the risk of violence they pose when unwell, such an unscientific approach is inadequate.

Actuarial Risk Assessment

The second generation of risk assessments began with the development of actuarial instruments. These consisted of a checklist of factors, statistically associated with the outcome in question, for example items that are statistically associated with a risk of violence. The aim of these instruments was to list and check the presence or absence of each risk factor, combine them in weighted scores according to an algorithm and produce a risk prediction score for the individual patient. A particular patient might be estimated to have a 40% chance of engaging in violence in the next five years.

They appeared to be a step forward in transparency from unstructured judgement, insofar as they were derived from evidence and had a statistical method, but such a statement is of limited clinical use to a psychiatrist. Should a doctor detain a patient on the basis of a 40% chance of violence? They also do not allow any role for the experience of the clinician assessing the patient to take a view on the risk decision. Actuarial risk assessments could be shown to have better predictive accuracy than the unstructured professional judgements of the day. However, the scores they generated were less reliable when used in different populations from the validation sample; a checklist might omit some factor unique to a particular patient; and the risk factors included were not necessarily causal, since remote, indirect or even confounding factors could still be better than random predictors. These cannot be relied on when formulating treatment, though they may have some relevance to risk mitigation or risk management. A recent case has been made for using actuarial check lists by non-clinicians as a means of screening out low risk cases.

Structured Professional Judgement: The HCR-20

The development of the HCR-20 heralded the third generation of violence risk assessment instruments [119, 120]. The HCR-20 combined the factors which were statistically associated with risk of violence with the clinician's judgement. Typically, a list of risk factors, each of which is supported by evidence from the research literature, is given an operational definition and equally weighted, scoring in the form absent, possible/partial, present (0,1,2 for research purposes). Rather than adding up a score as in an actuarial instrument, a final professional judgement (low risk, medium risk, high risk) is arrived at having considered the list of defined items. The aim was to structure the clinical judgement of the forensic psychiatrist, to ensure no relevant items were missed while still allowing the clinician the freedom to make the final decision. Structured professional judgement was introduced to build on the advances of actuarial checklist approaches while compensating for some of its deficiencies. The object is to improve inter-rater reliability, to improve consistency between professionals and to provide evidence for the predictive accuracy of the judgement. It is very useful as a method of providing teaching and training in the exercise of professional judgement.

An early advantage of this approach and this instrument was the publication of a manual for interventions to reduce and manage risk, linked to the HCR-20 [121]. The HCR-20 violence risk assessment is internationally validated and is used routinely in forensic mental health settings worldwide. It is considered the 'industry standard' at this time. The HCR-20 and similar instruments provide assessments of risk that are usually validated over a period of 6 to 12 months. The handbooks for these instruments typically recommend that multiple sources of information improve accuracy and validity of the assessment. Many recommend that the assessment should be completed by a multidisciplinary team, though the evidence that this improves accuracy and validity is sparse. In the interests of patient engagement in the process, co-production of a risk assessment has attracted attention. One study of co-produced risk assessment, however, showed that it had no predictive validity [122, 123]. Self-rating, however, can be a valuable exercise in patient engagement and risk management. Recent studies have questioned the extent to which the dynamic sub-scales of these instruments are actually responsive to change [124].

The HCR-20 violence risk assessment led to the development of many other structured professional judgement risk assessment instruments. Variants closely modelled on the original provide assessment instruments for specific risks such as sex offending, domestic violence and spousal assault and stalking. These included the Sexual Violence Risk-20 (SVR-20), Risk for Sexual Violence Protocol (RSVP) for assessing risk of sexual violence, shorter-term violence risk assessments such as START (short-term assessment of risk and treatability) and assessments of protective factors against committing acts of violence, for example SAPROF. The Female Additional Manual (FAM) for HCR-20 is designed to address issues of violence risk that may be more commonly found in female populations [125] and there are risk assessments designed specifically for young people such as SAPROF-Youth and

SAVRY (Structured Assessment of Violence Risk in Youth). There is a growing emphasis on the importance of formulation at the end of a structured assessment, on specifying the conditions within which structured professional judgement is dependent and on considering protective factors and resilience as well as risk factors and vulnerabilities.

Protective Factors

The prediction of violence in adolescence introduced protective factors and this has been extended into instruments specifically assessing protective and resilience factors. A risk factor increases the probability of harm under defined conditions and within a defined time period. A protective factor is not merely the absence of risk. A protective factor should be shown statistically to interact with risk factors to make harm less likely even when risk factors are present [126, 127].

Short-Term Risk Assessments

Very short-term assessments of imminent risk have proved popular when anticipating, de-escalating and managing imminent violence in in-patient settings. The Brøset [128, 129] and dynamic appraisal of situational aggression (DASA) [130, 131] are typically carried out by nursing staff once or twice a day at the beginning or end of a shift. These are based on observable behaviours. Because these are behaviours that are antecedent to violence, proximate to acts of violence and explanatory, these could more accurately be described as causal assessments. The statistical validation of repeated measures requires a more complex approach than the simple area under the curve [132, 133]. An added validation question concerns the extent to which these assessments result in actual reductions in in-patient violence [130, 134]. These are discussed further in Chapter 9.

Suicide Risk Assessment

It is notable that there are very few well-validated actuarial or structured professional judgement instruments for the assessment of risk of suicide. The Suicide Risk Assessment and Management Manual (SRAMM) developed from community psychiatry services in Glasgow, Scotland aimed to model on the HCR-20 methodology while identifying risk factors associated with suicide [135, 136]. It has some international validation [137]. Of greater practical value has been the demonstration that most assessment instruments for violence also predict risk of self-harm and suicide [138, 139], with the START laying a particular claim to this use [140]. However, risk assessment for deliberate self-harm and suicide remains in the early stages at this time.

Other Uses of Structured Professional Judgement Instruments in Forensic Settings

Violence risk assessment is not the only important decision that needs to be taken by consultant forensic psychiatrists. Decisions such as which level of therapeutic security to admit a patient to, or decisions regarding a patients' readiness for moves to less secure placements, are complex and important. They are often the decisions which matter most to patients and their families, as well as being vital for meeting patients' needs but also balancing beds and resources in healthcare systems, where resources are universally finite

[141, 142]. Given that the development of structured professional judgement instruments led to improved consistency, reliability and transparency in decision-making regarding violence risk assessment, it was therefore only a matter of time before the same methodology was applied to these other vital decisions.

Needs Assessments

The origins of needs assessment can be traced back to the programmed closure of asylums with re-provision of mental health services in communities. The evaluation of this large-scale multiannual programme gave rise to John Wing's social behavioural schedule [44, 143] and that in turn gave rise first to the HoNOS (health of the nation outcome scale) family of assessment inventories [144] and then to the Camberwell assessment of need (CAN) family of instruments [145]. A notable feature of these instruments in their general form is that the published validation studies emphasise inter-rater reliability and test–re-test reliability but seldom consider predictive or criterion validity, in a domain where goals and criteria for outcomes are seldom defined.

Drafting individual care plans should start with a list of needs for health, welfare and quality of life. Similarly, planning a model of care requires an aggregated needs assessment for all patients using the service. At the individual level, needs assessment should reflect goals such as reducing the risk of violence as well as more general goals related to mental health, global function and welfare. At the service level this would produce an aggregated needs assessment in which specialist goals (need for therapeutic security, need for specialist treatment programs, need for structured community after-care) are combined with more general mental health and quality-of-life needs and goals.

Structured Assessment of Need for Secure Care

During the 1990s a series of projects examined the extent to which patients in high or medium security continued to need detention at that level or could more easily be moved to less secure places or the community. Initially these relied on expert panels who were presented with a mixture of vignettes and standard measures of risk and need [106, 146–149]. This work led to the need for agreed definitions of high, medium or low therapeutic security [141]. These definitions were framed in terms of physical (environmental), procedural and relational security [150]. This work in turn identified a distinction between triage admission criteria [3, 20, 21, 109, 151, 152] and evidence that a patient was ready to move to less secure places or the community [112–115]. Those requiring treatment to reduce or manage dangerous behaviour may require a therapeutically safe and secure setting in which such treatment can be delivered. There is evidence that those admitted to a level of therapeutic security less than their assessed need are likely to fail in treatment owing to violence and disruptive behaviour in hospital [153].

Triage criteria, deciding what level of therapeutic security is appropriate on admission, are quite distinct from risk assessment and should not necessarily correlate with measures of risk [20]. The seriousness of risk if at large in the community, the need for specialist treatments and the management of violent or disruptive behaviour within the hospital are common factors in a series of such assessment tools. The emergence of these criteria in turn led to the development of structured professional judgement instruments to guide decision-makers, notably in the DUNDRUM Toolkit.

Structured Assessment of Treatment Response and Forensic Recovery

Forensic patients progress from higher to lower levels of therapeutic security as they progress in treatment and show evidence of recovery in a forensic context [110, 111, 115, 117, 153]. There is some evidence that dynamic measures of risk of violence change over the course of an admission to a secure forensic hospital. However, there is also evidence that these measures are poorly responsive to change in longer-term patients [124]. There is good evidence that those who move from high to medium security or who are discharged to the community are less likely to be recalled if they have lower scores on dynamic risk [154–157].

A difficulty arises if attempts are made to construct individual care plans based on the item content of structured risk assessments [92]. There is little evidence about which elements of a treatment plan are effective in reducing risk of violence and reducing the seriousness of risk. A treatment plan based on remote or indirect risk factors may do nothing more than address confounding factors. As far as possible, a treatment plan should be based on causal factors. Although much attention is paid to risk formulation, relatively little is known about causal formulation. The best evidence for what works suggests that treatment should be multimodal [158], treatment should be more prolonged and more frequent [159] and treatment response should be continuously monitored [100]. Successful treatment completion depends on progressing through stages of engagement, cycles of change, personal recovery, personal needs and social or cultural needs. Each of these can be operationalised.

There is good evidence that those who score higher on a measure of need for therapeutic security (DUNDRUM-1 triage security scale) will require longer lengths of stay [114, 160]. Those misplaced at a lower level of therapeutic security than they require appear less likely to complete treatment successfully, due to violent and disruptive behaviour in hospital [153]. There is also evidence that changes in a measure of multimodal treatment completion (DUNDRUM-3 programme completion) mediate changes in a measure of dynamic risk of violence [161]. This is in keeping with evidence that changes in a measure of multimodal programme completion predict moves to less secure places and predict conditional discharge to the community [111, 112, 115, 117].

Recovery in a forensic setting emphasises working alliance and cooperation between clinicians and patients. The emphasis in a measure of recovery in a forensic setting (the DUNDRUM-4 forensic recovery sale) is also on objective aspects, for example stability, reliable use of leave, attitudes relevant to risk, media profile and also subjective aspects such as hope [112, 115].

Leave from a secure hospital: Readiness for leave from a secure hospital is an essential and often decisive first step in preparation for a move to a community placement. A risk assessment such as the HCR-20 has repeatedly been shown to predict success or failure when moved to a less secure place or conditionally discharged. For the antecedent step of leave, the risk assessment must be used in the context of a judgement support framework such as a hospital-wide leave panel or a decision-making structure such as an independent review by a minister or a legal review board (see Chapter 7). The factors most relevant to success or failure of leave are local community ties such as family or intimate relationships who are supportive of treatment adherence, good working alliance and interpersonal trust in clinicians (a bilateral relationship) and concordance, and successful completion of core treatments in mental health, substance misuse, specific offending behaviours and criminogenic need, and a motivational structure based on quality of life, self-actualisation (the ability to express oneself and one's identity in satisfying ways) and self-transcendence [115] (the sense of belonging and making a valued contribution). Of note, these factors, derived from the clinician rated and self-rated versions of DUNDRUM-3 and DUNDRUM-4, are predominantly positive and protective, while the majority of risk assessments concerning leave list negative predictors [162–171].

Conditional discharge: Decisions by mental health review boards and tribunals represent a perfect example of the use of structured professional judgement assessments and opinions for presentation to a legally independent and responsible judgement support framework, this being more of a decision-making structure than a support framework. A study of the content of psychiatric reports to review boards showed convergence with the content of risk assessments such as the HCR-20, though in practice this is not what was presented [172, 173].

In a series of studies a structured professional judgement instrument, DUNDRUM-3, for measuring treatment completion in units of meaningful change, calibrated or tethered to definitions matching moves from high to medium security, medium to low security, and low security to the community, can be shown to have predictive validity in an English high-secure hospital [117], an Irish integrated secure hospital [111, 112, 115] and cross-sectional studies in other jurisdictions [113, 114, 174]. An instrument for measuring forensic recovery the DUNDRUM-4, callibrated in the same units of meaningful change had the same predictive validities. A patient self-report version correlated with the staff ratings but did not have predictive validity. The difference between staff-rated and patient-rated scores tended to converge as treatment progressed, yielding a measure of concordance, which was predictive of moves to less secure places and conditional discharge [115]. Like measures of need for levels of therapeutic security that are also measured in units of meaningful difference or change, it is notable that these measures have not only good internal consistency and inter-rater reliability when used by trained clinicians but also predictive validity for hard outcomes such as moves to less secure places and conditional discharge, even across jurisdictions, service models, languages and cultures. This suggests that the clinical needs and service model responses have common features that predominate over legal and administrative differences. This should not be surprising since legal and administrative structures and processes are in most cases designed to facilitate treatment, recovery and the prevention of violence.

Functional Mental Capacity

The assessment of functional mental capacity to give or withhold consent to treatment is the paradigm for a series of expert opinions sought by courts and legislation from psychiatrists and particularly from forensic psychiatrists. Examples include fitness for interview by the police, fitness to stand trial and plead to a charge, insanity and diminished responsibility, and in civil law, the capacity to marry, testamentary capacity, capacity to enter into a contract, capacity to consent to research and as many other such functions as a court may wish to define [175, 176].

Each of these has in common that the courts or legislation set out a requirement for psychiatric expertise and in some cases psychiatric responsibility concerning a legally defined function. Typically there will be a statutory or common law definition of a test concerning the abilities of the patient in relation to the decision or function in question. A psychiatrist recognised by the court as an expert or recognised in statute as competent will be required to carry out an assessment, draft a report and opinion, sign a certificate or present for oral evidence and cross-examination.

The form and content of the legally defined test sets the structure for the psychiatrist's assessment and opinion. This is in the most literal sense a structured professional opinion. It would be more accurate not to use the term structured professional judgement since judgement is the prerogative of the court; experts advise, courts decide, we as experts are guests in their house [8].

In legal custom and practice, functional mental capacity tests have replaced status tests and outcome tests in much the same way that structured professional judgement has replaced unstructured assessment and actuarial checklists. Some status tests remain, for example 'child' defined by age or 'licensed', for example to drive a car or to practise medicine or the law. Outcome tests are denigrated by lawyers as merely tests of whether the patient agrees with the doctor (a lawyer's definition of insight). While an unwise or self-defeating decision cannot be taken as evidence of legal incapacity to make a decision, protecting the vulnerable from the consequences of this dysfunctional decision-making (e.g. to prevent violence) requires some independent evidence that their ability to make a competent decision is impaired.

Functional capacity tests will be defined in specific terms by statute or by the court according to the matter in hand. Typically this begins with a diagnostic step requiring evidence of a legally defined mental disorder. New Zealand and Scotland have attempted to abandon this step. This creates a gap in the chain of causal reasoning and makes malingering easier. There follows a test which for practical purposes will set out a series of tests, for example the Pritchard criteria concerning fitness to plead or the M'Naghten criteria in relation to legal insanity.

The use of functional mental capacity tests defined by law turns on a number of legal assumptions. The first and most remote from medical, psychiatric reality is the legal principle that any particular functional incapacity is not closely tied to the severity of a mental disorder. The second legal assumption is that all such tests are independent of each other. Neither of these are borne out by research on patients in forensic settings. The more severe the mental illness as measured objectively, the more likely a patient is to lack mental capacities in a number of functional areas. Patients who lack one functional mental capacity are likely to lack other functional mental capacities [177].

Psychiatrists do not take a uniform approach to the various assessments of functional mental capacity and may be subject to heuristic biases leading to errors [178]. Physicians' assessments of competence to consent to treatment are often subjective and inconsistent [179, 180]. The need for a structured professional judgement instrument to improve adherence to criteria, consistency, reliability and reviewability follows from this [181].

Drawing on cumulative jurisprudence, Grisso and Appelbaum [182, 183] analysed the interaction between expert evidence and judgements of the higher courts. The MacArthur Competence Assessment for Treatment (MacCAT-T) [184] and MacArthur Competence Assessment for Fitness to Plead (MacCAT-FP) [185] and related structured professional judgement tools conceptualised a generalisable approach to the mental capacities required for any specific decision as comprising understanding, reasoning (comparative and consequential) and appreciation, and the ability to communicate a decision [186, 187]. There may, however, be other mental capacities relevant to decision-making in other mental disorders. Difficulties due to volitional impairment have been described in those with anorexia nervosa, substance dependence and habitual self-harm [188] but are questionable from the point of view of philosophy of mind [8, 189, 190]. It has been suggested that these represent an important further domain of mental capacity. Volitional impairments can be cognitive or evaluative disabilities with either contributing to difficulties in decision-making [191]. An evaluative disability has greater coherence and may arise from a mismatch between externally observed 'fact' and subjective view, which may be measured by the 'appreciation' sub-scales of the MacCAT-T and MacCAT-FP [188]. This may tentatively be related to insight [192–196] or anosognosia, understood at different levels of emergence. Similarly, financial capacity in schizophrenia and serious mental illness has been conceptualised into nine domains [197], but others have compared competence assessments in other domains [198] and found the four-domain approach [182] to be relevant [177, 199, 200].

The mental capacity to use material information to arrive at a decision is most often impaired in psychosis by the inability to believe the information due to delusions. Other impairments of functional mental capacity to make a decision can arise when a person is unable to exert their will, whether because of delusions, lack of motivation or susceptibility to influence due to the disability [201]. In these cases, the delusional belief or impulse can be distinguished from merely eccentric but competent choices and behaviours because the underlying diagnosis provides a link in a causal chain of explanation leading from disease to impaired neurocognitive capacity to fixed false belief and so to the inability to believe the information given or to use it to arrive at a decision. From a medical perspective, without a diagnostic step in the process, eccentric or self-defeating decisions or actions could easily be mistaken for incapacity [177, 199, 200].

While the structural unity, robustness and medico-legal origins of the assessment of understanding, reasoning, appreciation and communicating a decision have 'reach' (the ability to be extended into new areas of legal decision-making), the courts will always be concerned to return to the unique formula of each separate functional capacity – the test for fitness to stand trial may look completely different from the test for testamentary capacity, even though both can be reduced to tests of understanding, reasoning and appreciation and communication of a decision.

Structured professional judgement tools such as the various MacArthur competence assessment tools will yield a score which does not define a threshold for capacity or incapacity, as they are not measured in units of meaningful change. A very simple decision-making task or a decision that carries consequences of little importance will require only very basic levels of mental capacity. A task of greater complexity or a decision with more serious, life-changing consequences will require a much higher level of decision-making capacity. This moveable threshold is itself properly a matter for a court to decide unless some concrete guidance is given in statute form. For research purposes, studies often take the unstructured expert judgement of a senior psychiatrist as standard, using a legal definition or threshold [202]. A more objective research threshold is to take the inability to express a choice or decision in the face of increasing complexity as the standard or threshold [177].

The MacCAT-T [184, 186] measures understanding, reasoning, appreciation and the ability to communicate a decision in relation to proposed treatment. Each patient is given individual information on their disorder including symptoms and diagnosis. They are then informed about the nature, benefits and risks of three treatment options, for example no medication, the recommendation of the treating physician or the patient's own choice. For each of the three options, two positive and two negative pieces of information are given: 12 items of information in total. The information disclosed is given in short sentences composed of words of high lexical frequency and simple syntax, to minimise the cognitive and memory demands imposed by the task [203]. The framing of information regarding risks uses both verbal and numerical information [204–206]. The information disclosed is confined to health matters and does not include any information that could be interpreted as an inducement or coercive, such as promises of privileges or earlier release. The patient is then asked to choose one of the three and to explain their choice. For each option, understanding is examined by asking the patient to retell the information in their own words. Reasoning is assessed using questions that examine whether the patient can grasp the consequences of their decision for or against a treatment in their daily lives and whether they can draw comparisons between options. For appreciation, patients are asked if they can relate the information to themselves, acknowledge the specified disorder disclosed to them as their diagnosis at the beginning of the interview and also if they can see a benefit for themselves in the proposed treatment. In a study that compared the legal requirement for full disclosures of all material information with the cognitive burden of increasing information, patients were then given two extra positive and negative pieces of information about each of the three options (12 extra items of information). This resulted in a significantly increased number of patients becoming incapable of expressing a choice [199].

A further problem that arises is the difficulty of completing complex question and answer assessments such as the MacArthur instruments. Typically 60% of patients in a general psychiatric or forensic setting are found to lack functional capacity to consent to treatment, but in a forensic setting, only 60% are willing or able to be assessed, often because the severity of their mental illness prevents them from participating in a prolonged interview. Less demanding rating processes may therefore offer a more successful form of assessment [181]. In practice, psychiatrists called upon to assess capacity to give or withhold consent where the patient is too disturbed to take part in a full interview can nonetheless assess functional mental capacities relevant to the legal task, having regard to all the sources of information available, including attempted or fragmentary interviews, observation, information from key workers, relatives, notes and investigations – including, where possible, psychological assessments. In addressing the legally defined structure of the test, the four abilities – understanding, reasoning, appreciating and communicating a decision – having regard to the ability to believe information material to the decision will help form the structure of the expert opinion.

Fitness to plead and to stand trial should be relatively easy to standardise as a structured professional judgement instrument, although the minor variations of jurisdictional rules, custom and practice even within the USA prompt reluctance and an assertion of uniqueness in each assessment [207]. The MacCAT-FP has been validated for use in England [185], based on a tool developed in the USA [208]. A vignette is read to the patient and questions are then asked to elicit the individual's ability to understand the information given, to reason about the information and to appreciate the relevance of the information to their own situation. It yields scores for three mental capacities: understanding, reasoning and appreciation, relevant to the patient's impending trial, and also the ability to communicate a decision. Other approaches have also been instrumentalised [209], including simplified versions of the four capacities test [181].

Fitness for interview: Similar instruments exist for assessing fitness for interview by the police, including the ability to understand a notification of rights and to exercise those rights [210, 211], showing a general lack of reliability, at least when used as simple scores.

Insanity and its legal variants in different jurisdictions including diminished responsibility has been reviewed and found to be a variable assessment, despite apparently clear legal criteria [212–214]. In practice, there is a much higher degree of agreement between experts than disagreement, with a legal view that a public trial is better than a consensus among experts that deprives the jury of its discretion [8, 215]. An approach based on volitional capacity as an element of the psychiatric defence is of some interest as an addition to the more usual four capacities approach to support, structure and guide the insanity assessment across different jurisdictions, in order to improve the reliability and consistency of such evaluations [216–218]. This clinical approach to the exercise of expert opinion stands in counterbalance with the legal view that all such assessments are predominated by variable legal and jurisdictional issues and the uniqueness of each case [219].

Malingering: There is no structured professional judgement instrument for the assessment of malingering, though there are several psychological assessment instruments [220]. The interaction of dissociation, dissimulation and deception in the assessment of violent behaviour has been described in Chapter 2. Insofar as any psychiatrist presents in court to give evidence and be cross-examined, an awareness of the possibility of deception is essential. Malingering in the face of a long prison sentence is rational and self-interested, though also egocentric and antisocial. Courts and juries are in almost all cases sceptical of psychiatric defences that serve to avoid responsibility. In one famous interchange, this was laid bare:

> MR X , cross-examining for the prosecution: 'Prison officers have told us that six days before you first saw [the defendant] he had said: "I'm going to do a long time in prison, 30 years or more, unless I can convince people here that I'm mad. Then I'll do 10 years in the loony bin." What do you make of that Dr Y, in the context of your evidence?'

> DR Y: 'I think it is a very straightforward decision to make. Is this man pretending to be mad, and has he duped me and my colleagues, or am I, from my clinical examination, right in saying that he is a paranoid schizophrenic? As far as I can see in this particular case, either he is a competent actor, or I am an inefficient psychiatrist.'

> MR JUSTICE Z: 'This is not for any of us to decide, it is for the jury.'

Deception is relevant to expert opinion when giving evidence concerning violence, not only because it may intrude into the assessment of psychiatric defences or mitigation but also because it is a core feature of antisocial and psychopathic disorder. Fraud and the deliberate gaining of confidence may be a part of an offence of rape. And fraud or deception may be a part of an instrumental violent act in which material gain is the primary goal. Any evidence of fraud or deception should cast substantial doubt on any psychiatric defence or mitigation. Mounting or supporting a psychiatric defence or finding of unfitness to stand trial in the face of clear evidence of fraud, deception or any unreliability concerning symptoms or medical history is itself an unreliable expert opinion and will appear biased. It is an opinion built on sand.

Any psychiatrist who presents as an expert in court must be willing to accept that it is possible that they may have been deceived by the person they assessed. No psychiatrist should express an opinion regarding the truthfulness or credibility of the person assessed, though reliability may be commented on. And no opinion should be defended even in the teeth of new contradictory evidence.

When giving expert evidence regarding violence and mental disorder, the obligation to assist the court and to be truthful under oath includes an obligation to avoid advocacy for any fee payer or for a patient. There is an obligation to be scientifically sceptical. An expert should not accept uncritically any information that cannot be confirmed from a second source or that might be inherently self-serving. No expert can give evidence as to truthfulness – that is exclusively a matter for the court to decide. Any expert can be deceived. It is always necessary to acknowledge this and therefore to avoid statements regarding credibility. Reliability may, however, be relevant and should always be considered.

When assessing with a view to a court report concerning a psychiatric defence to a charge of violence or harm to others, the following signs may be noted:

Three positive features for reliability and treatability: Documented pre-existing diagnosis, symptoms and findings that are typical and relevant to the offence; crime is out of character (not simply a continuation of antisocial personality disorder); first witnessed statements and police interviews, first clinical examination are abnormal and relevant (loosely adapted from Fenwick [221]).

Three negative features for reliability and treatability: No history of fraud for gain and the offence is not simply acquisitive, exploitive or dishonest; no health-related unreliability, fabrication, deception, concealment or obstruction; no use of false complaints, ad hominem arguments or threats against witnesses, clinicians or experts.

Judgement Support Frameworks

As a structural means of ensuring evidence-based decision-making that is objective, unbiased and balances risks and therapeutic gains, while also balancing the best interests of the patient and the public interest and safety, it is useful to process significant decisions regarding risk and detention through a second level of governance. Discharge from a secure forensic hospital is commonly decided by a legal panel; leave is often reserved by statute to a minister on the recommendation of a clinical director or governance structure; courts will decide whether to send to a high-, medium- or low-secure hospital. All of these judgement support frameworks and decision makers benefit from expert evidence that is structured and supported by the use of the risk assessment, triage and treatment completion instruments described here.

Summary

Risk has been taken as a paradigm for structured professional judgement. A thorough understanding of the nature of expertise in psychiatry and in the courts is necessary for the practice of forensic psychiatry. The process of both teaching and acquiring clinical expertise is considered both from first principles and in relation to topics such as the use of structured professional judgement instruments and judgement support frameworks. These extend to all aspects of practice including triage and needs assessment, leave, conditional discharge, treatment programme completion, forensic recovery, a range of functional mental capacities, legal defences and reliability.

References

1. Hacking I. *The Emergence of Probability: A Philosophical Study of Early Ideas about Probability, Induction and Statistical Inference.* Cambridge: Cambridge University Press, 2006.

2. Faris REL, Dunham HW. *Mental Disorders in Urban Areas: An Ecological Study of Schizophrenia and Other Psychoses.* Chicago, IL University of Chicago Press, 1939.

3. Williams HK, Senanayke M, Ross CC, Bates R, Davoren M. Security needs among patients referred for high secure care in Broadmoor Hospital England. *BJPsych Open* 2020; 6 (4): e55.

4. Uhrskov Sørensen L, Bengtson S, Lund J, Ibsen M, Långström N. Mortality among male forensic and non-forensic psychiatric patients: matched cohort study of rates, predictors and causes-of-death. *Nordic Journal of Psychiatry* 2020: 1–8.

5. Maden T. *Treating Violence: A Guide to Risk Management in Mental Health.* Oxford: Oxford University Press, 2007.

6. Collins H, Evans R. *Rethinking Expertise.* Chicago, IL: University of Chicago Press, 2008.

7. Kennedy HG, Simpson A, Haque Q. Perspective on excellence in forensic mental health services: what we can learn from oncology and other medical services. *Frontiers in Psychiatry* 2019; 10: 733.

8. Kenny A. The psychiatric expert in court. *Psychological Medicine* 1984; 14 (2): 291–302.

9. Grounds A. The psychiatrist in court. *British Journal of Hospital Medicine* 1985; 34 (1): 55–8.

10. Rix K, Mynors-Wallis L, Craven C. *Rix's Expert Psychiatric Evidence.* 2nd ed. Cambridge, Cambridge University Press, 2020.

11. Hill AB. The environment and disease: association or causation? *Proceedings of the Royal Society of Medicine* 1965; 58 (5): 295–300.

12. Council of Europe. *Dangerous Offenders – Recommendation CM/Rec(2014)3 and Explanatory Report.* Strasbourg, Council of Europe, 2014.

13. Mossman D. Critique of pure risk assessment or, Kant meets Tarasoff. *University of Cincinnati Law Review* 2006; 75: 523.

14. Szmukler G, Everitt B, Leese M. Risk assessment and receiver operating characteristic curves. *Psychological Medicine* 2012; 42 (5): 895–8.

15. Mossman D. Assessing predictions of violence: being accurate about accuracy. *Journal of Consulting and Clinical Psychology* 1994; 62 (4): 783.

16. Kennedy H. Risk assessment is inseparable from risk management: comment on Szmuckler (*Psychiatric Bulletin*, 2000, 24, 6–10). *Psychiatric Bulletin* 2001; 25 (6): 208–11.

17. Tyrer P, Cooper S, Herbert E et al. The Quantification of Violence Scale: a simple method of recording significant violence. *International Journal of Social Psychiatry* 2007; 53 (6): 485–97.

18. Monahan J. *The Clinical Prediction of Violent Behavior.* U.S. Department of Health and Human Services, Public Health Service, Alcohol, Drug Abuse, and Mental Health Administration. Bethesda, MD, National Institute of Mental Health, 1981.

19. Dietz PE. Hypothetical criteria for the prediction of individual criminality. In C. D. Webster and S. J. Hucker (eds) *Dangerousness: Probability and Prediction, Psychiatry and Public Policy.* Cambridge, Cambridge University Press, 1985, pp. 87–102.

20. Flynn G, O'Neill C, McInerney C, Kennedy HG. The DUNDRUM-1 structured professional judgment for triage to appropriate levels of therapeutic security: retrospective-cohort validation study. *BMC Psychiatry* 2011; 11: 43.

21. Freestone M, Bull D, Brown R et al. Triage, decision-making and follow-up of patients referred to a UK forensic service: validation

of the DUNDRUM toolkit. *BMC Psychiatry* 2015; 15: 239.

22. Menzies R, Webster C, Sepejak D. Hitting the forensic sound barrier: predictions of dangerousness in a pre-trial psychiatric clinic. In C. D Webster and S. J. Hucker (eds) *Dangerousness: Probability and Prediction, Psychiatry and Public Policy.* Cambridge, Cambridge University Press, 1985, pp. 115–43.

23. Menzies R, Webster CD, McMain S, Staley S, Scaglione R. The dimensions of dangerousness revisited. *Law and Human Behavior* 1994; 18 (1): 1–28.

24. Groen GJ, Patel VL. Medical problem solving: some questionable assumptions. 1985; 19.

25. Patel VL, Kaufman DR, Magder SA. The acquisition of medical expertise in complex dynamic environments. In A Ericsson (ed.) *The Road to Excellence: The Acquisition of Expert Performance in the Arts and Sciences, Sports and Games.* Hillsdale, NJ, Lawrence Erlbaum Publishers, 1996, pp. 127–65.

26. Groen GJ, Patel VL. Medical problem solving: some questionable assumptions. *Medical Education* 1985; 19.

27. Patel VL, Cohen TA, Murarka T et al. Recovery at the edge of error: debunking the myth of the infallible expert. *Journal of Biomedical Informatics* 2011; 44 (3): 413–24.

28. Slaughter LA, Keselman A, Kushniruk A, Patel VL. A framework for capturing the interactions between layperson' understanding of disease, information gathering behaviors, and actions taken during an epidemic. *Journal of Biomedical Informatics* 2005; 38: 298–313.

29. Kraepelin E. *Clinical Psychiatry: A Text-Book for Students and Physicians, Abstracted and Adapted from the Seventh German ed. of Kraepelin's 'Lehrbuch der Psychiatrie'.* Bristol, Thoemmes Press, 2002.

30. Griesinger W. *Mental Pathology and Therapeutics*: W. Wood & Company, 1882.

31. Kraepelin E. *Lectures on Clinical Psychiatry.* New York, Hafner Pub. Co., 1968.

32. Shepherd M. Morbid jealousy: some clinical and social aspects of a psychiatric symptom. *Journal of Mental Science* 1961; 107 (449): 687–753.

33. McGorry PD, Hartmann JA, Spooner R, Nelson B. Beyond the 'at risk mental state' concept: transitioning to transdiagnostic psychiatry. *World Psychiatry: Official Journal of the World Psychiatric Association (WPA)* 2018; 17 (2): 133–42.

34. Brittain RP. The sadistic murderer. *Medicine, Science and the Law* 1970; 10 (4): 198–207.

35. MacCulloch MJ, Snowden PR, Wood PJ, Mills HE. Sadistic fantasy, sadistic behaviour and offending. *British Journal of Psychiatry* 1983; 143: 20–9.

36. Mullen PE. Jealousy: the pathology of passion. *British Journal of Psychiatry* 1991; 158 (5): 593–601.

37. Mullen PE, Lester G. Vexatious litigants and unusually persistent complainants and petitioners: from querulous paranoia to querulous behaviour. *Behavioral Sciences & the Law* 2006; 24 (3): 333–49.

38. Lewis A. Psychopathic personality: a most elusive category. *Psychological Medicine* 1974; 4 (2): 133–40.

39. Dietz PE, Hazelwood RR, Warren J. The sexually sadistic criminal and his offenses. *Bulletin of the American Academy of Psychiatry and the Law* 1990; 18 (2): 163–78.

40. Hazelwood RR, Dietz PE, Warren J. The criminal sexual sadist. *FBI Law Enforcement Bulletin* 1992; 61: 12.

41. Robins E, Guze SB. Establishment of diagnostic validity in psychiatric illness: its application to schizophrenia. *American Journal of Psychiatry* 1970; 126 (7): 983–7.

42. Wing JK, Birley J, Cooper J, Graham P, Isaacs A. Reliability of a procedure for measuring and classifying 'present psychiatric state'. *The British Journal of Psychiatry* 1967; 113 (498): 499–515.

43. Spitzer RL, Endicott J, Robins E. Research diagnostic criteria: rationale and reliability. *Archives of General Psychiatry* 1978; 35 (6): 773–82.

44. Wing J. *Epidemiologically-Based Mental Health Needs Assessments: Review of Research on Psychiatric Disorders (ICD-10, F2-F6)*. London, Royal College of Psychiatrists, Research Unit, 1992.

45. Wing J. SCAN and the PSE tradition. *Social Psychiatry and Psychiatric Epidemiology* 1996; 31 (2): 50–4.

46. Spitzer R, Endicott J. *Schedule for Affective Disorders and Schizophrenia (SADS) 3*. New York, Biometric Research, New York State Psychiatric Institute, 1977.

47. Endicott J, Spitzer RL. A diagnostic interview: the schedule for affective disorders and schizophrenia. *Archives of General Psychiatry* 1978; 35 (7): 837–44.

48. Spitzer RL, Williams JB, Gibbon M, First MB. *User's Guide for the Structured Clinical Interview for DSM-III-R: SCID*. Washington, DC, American Psychiatric Association, 1990.

49. First M, Spitzer R, Gibbon M, Williams J. *Structured Clinical Interview for DSM-IV Axis I Disorders (SCID-I) s, Clinician Version, Administration Booklet*. Arlington, VA, American Psychiatric Publishing Inc., 2012.

50. Spitzer RL, Williams JB, Gibbon M, First MB. The structured clinical interview for DSM-III-R (SCID): I: history, rationale, and description. *Archives of General Psychiatry* 1992; 49 (8): 624–9.

51. Kendler KS, Spitzer RL, Williams JB. Psychotic disorders in DSM-III-R. *The American Journal of Psychiatry* 1989; 146 (8): 953–62.

52. Hacking I. Lost in the forest. *London Review of Books* 2013; 35 (15): 7–8.

53. Hacking I (ed.). Kinds of people: moving targets. *Proceedings: British Academy*. Oxford, Oxford University Press, 2007.

54. Hacking I. Degeneracy, criminal behavior, and looping. *Genetics and Criminal Behavior* 2001: 141–68.

55. Ashford LJ, Spivak BL, Shepherd SM. Racial fairness in violence risk instruments: a review of the literature. *Psychology, Crime & Law* 2021: 1–31.

56. Venner S, Sivasubramaniam D, Luebbers S, Shepherd SM. Cross-cultural reliability and rater bias in forensic risk assessment: a review of the literature. *Psychology, Crime & Law* 2021; 27 (2): 105–21.

57. Venner S, Sivasubramaniam D, Luebbers S, Shepherd SM. Exploring rater cultural bias in forensic risk assessment. *International Journal of Forensic Mental Health* 2021; 20 (3): 213–26.

58. Coid J, Kahtan N, Gault S, Jarman B. Ethnic differences in admissions to secure forensic psychiatry services. *The British Journal of Psychiatry* 2000; 177 (3): 241–7.

59. Coid JW, Kirkbride JB, Barker D et al. Raised incidence rates of all psychoses among migrant groups: findings from the East London first episode psychosis study. *Archives of General Psychiatry* 2008; 65 (11): 1250–8.

60. Shepherd SM, Anthony T. Popping the cultural bubble of violence risk assessment tools. *The Journal of Forensic Psychiatry & Psychology* 2018; 29 (2): 211–20.

61. Shepherd S. Criminal engagement and Australian culturally and linguistically diverse populations: challenges and implications for forensic risk assessment. *Psychiatry, Psychology and Law* 2016; 23 (2): 256–74.

62. Patel VL, Arocha JF, Kaufman DR. Expertise and tacit knowledge in medicine. In Horvath RJSJA (ed.) *Tacit Knowledge in Professional Practice: Researcher and Practitioner Perspectives*. New York, Lawrence Erlbaum Associates Publishers, 1999, pp. 75–99.

63. Posner RA. *How Judges Think*. Cambridge, MA, Harvard University Press, 2010.

64. Dreyfus SE. The five-stage model of adult skill acquisition. *Bulletin of Science, Technology & Society* 2004; 24 (3): 177–81.

65. Coughlin LD, Patel VL. Processing of critical information by physicians and medical students. *Journal of Medical Education* 1987; 62 (10): 818–28.

66. Arocha JF, Patel VL. Novice diagnostic reasoning in medicine: accounting for

evidence. *The Journal of the Learning Sciences* 1995; 4: 355–84.

67. Patel VL, Kaufman DR, Magder SA. The acquisition of medical expertise in complex dynamic environments. In Ericsson A (ed.) *The Road to Excellence: The Acquisition of Expert Performance in the Arts and Sciences, Sports and Games.* Hillsdale, NJ, Lawrence Erlbaum Publishers, 1996, pp. 127–65.

68. Kahneman D. A perspective on judgment and choice: mapping bounded rationality. *American Psychologist* 2003; 58 (9): 697.

69. Donner-Banzhoff N, Seidel J, Sikeler AM et al. The phenomenology of the diagnostic process: a primary care-based survey. *Medical Decision Making* 2017; 37 (1): 27–34.

70. Carroll A. Good (or bad) vibrations: clinical intuition in violence risk assessment. *Advances in Psychiatric Treatment* 2012; 18 (6): 447–56.

71. Kahneman D, Klein G. Conditions for intuitive expertise: a failure to disagree. *American Psychologist* 2009; 64 (6): 515.

72. Collins H. *Tacit and Explicit Knowledge.* Chicago, IL, University of Chicago Press, 2010.

73. Hanoch Y, Wood S. The scams among us: who falls prey and why. *Current Directions in Psychological Science* 2021; 30 (3): 260–6.

74. Orbach B, Huang L. Con men and their enablers: the anatomy of confidence games. *Social Research: An International Quarterly* 2018; 85 (4): 795–822.

75. Gordon TA, Burleyson GP, Tielsch JM, Cameron JL. The effects of regionalization on cost and outcome for one general high-risk surgical procedure. *Annals of Surgery* 1995; 221 (1): 43.

76. Tseng JF, Pisters PW, Lee JE et al. The learning curve in pancreatic surgery. *Surgery* 2007; 141 (4): 456–63.

77. Schmidt CM, Turrini O, Parikh P et al. Effect of hospital volume, surgeon experience, and surgeon volume on patient outcomes after pancreaticoduodenectomy: a single-institution experience. *Archives of Surgery* 2010; 145 (7): 634–40.

78. Amato L, Colais P, Davoli M et al. Volume and health outcomes: evidence from systematic reviews and from evaluation of Italian hospital data. *Epidemiologia e prevenzione* 2013; 37 (2–3 Suppl. 2): 1–100.

79. Amato L, Fusco D, Acampora A et al. Volume and health outcomes: evidence from systematic reviews and from evaluation of Italian hospital data. *Epidemiologia e prevenzione* 2017; 41 (5–6 Suppl. 2): 1–128.

80. Lee B, Kim K, Park Y, Lim MC, Bristow RE. Impact of hospital care volume on clinical outcomes of laparoscopic radical hysterectomy for cervical cancer: a systematic review and meta-analysis. *Medicine* 2018; 97 (49).

81. Ananth C, Lavery J, Friedman A, Wapner R, Wright J. Serious maternal complications in relation to severe pre-eclampsia: a retrospective cohort study of the impact of hospital volume. *BJOG: An International Journal of Obstetrics & Gynaecology* 2017; 124 (8): 1246–53.

82. Hata T, Motoi F, Ishida M et al. Effect of hospital volume on surgical outcomes after pancreaticoduodenectomy. *Annals of Surgery* 2016; 263 (4): 664–72.

83. Hehir MP, Ananth CV, Wright JD et al. Severe maternal morbidity and comorbid risk in hospitals performing< 1000 deliveries per year. *American Journal of Obstetrics and Gynecology* 2017; 216 (2): 179. e1–e12.

84. Friedman AM, Ananth CV, Huang Y, D'Alton ME, Wright JD. Hospital delivery volume, severe obstetrical morbidity, and failure to rescue. *American Journal of Obstetrics and Gynecology* 2016; 215 (6): 795. e1–e14.

85. Habets P, Jeandarme I, Kennedy HG. Determining security level in forensic psychiatry: a tug of war between the DUNDRUM toolkit and the HoNOS-Secure. *Psychology Crime & Law* 2020: 1–19.

86. Rousmaniere T, Goodyear RK, Miller SD, Wampold BE. *The Cycle of Excellence: Using Deliberate Practice to Improve*

Supervision and Training. New York, John Wiley & Sons, 2017.

87. Howner K, Andiné P, Bertilsson G et al. Mapping systematic reviews on forensic psychiatric care: a systematic review identifying knowledge gaps. Frontiers in Psychiatry 2018; 9: 452.

88. Howner K, Hofvander B, Tapp J. Editorial: what works for forensic psychiatric patients: from treatment evaluations to short and long-term outcomes. *Frontiers in Psychiatry* 2020; 11 (1254).

89. Shinkfield G, Ogloff J. A review and analysis of routine outcome measures for forensic mental health services. *International Journal of Forensic Mental Health* 2014; 13 (3): 252–71.

90. Meehl PE. *Clinical vs. Statistical Prediction*. Minneapolis, MN, University of Minnesota Press, 1954.

91. Coid JW, Yang M, Ullrich S et al. Most items in structured risk assessment instruments do not predict violence. *The Journal of Forensic Psychiatry & Psychology* 2011; 22 (1): 3–21.

92. Coid JW, Kallis C, Doyle M, Shaw J, Ullrich S. Identifying causal risk factors for violence among discharged patients. *PLoS One* 2015; 10 (11): e0142493.

93. Yang M, Wong SC, Coid JW. Violence, mental health and violence risk factors among community women: an epidemiological study based on two national household surveys in the UK. *BMC Public Health* 2013; 13: 1020.

94. Yang M, Coid JW, Pan H. Multilevel generalized linear models for modelling age-related gender difference in violent behaviour and associated factors in the general household population. *International Journal of Methods in Psychiatric Research* 2005; 14 (3): 130–45.

95. Liu Y-y, Yang M, Ramsay MS, Li XS, Coid JW. A comparison of logistic regression, classification and regression tree, and neural networks models in predicting violent re-offending. *Journal of Quantitative Criminology* 2011; 27: 547–73.

96. Risk Management Authority. *Risk Assessment Tools Evaluation Directory (RATED)*. Paisley, Scotland, Risk Management Authority (RMA), 2019.

97. Feinstein AR. An additional basic science for clinical medicine: IV. The development of clinimetrics. *Annals of Internal Medicine* 1983; 99 (6): 843–8.

98. Fava GA, Tomba E, Sonino N. Clinimetrics: the science of clinical measurements. *International Journal of Clinical Practice* 2012; 66 (1): 11–15.

99. De Vet HC, Terwee CB, Mokkink LB, Knol DL. *Measurement in Medicine: A Practical Guide*. Cambridge, Cambridge University Press, 2011.

100. Glancy G, Choptiany M, Jones R, Chatterjee S. Measurement-based care in forensic psychiatry. *International Journal of Law and Psychiatry* 2021; 74: 101650.

101. Evans C, Margison F, Barkham M. The contribution of reliable and clinically significant change methods to evidence-based mental health. *Evidence Based Mental Health* 1998; 1 (3): 70–2.

102. Jacobson NS, Truax P. Clinical significance: a statistical approach to defining meaningful change in psychotherapy research. *Journal of Consulting and Clinical Psychology* 1991; 59 (1): 12–19.

103. Jacobson NS, Follette WC, Revenstorf D. Psychotherapy outcome research: methods for reporting variability and evaluating clinical significance. *Behavior Therapy* 1984; 15 (4): 336–52.

104. Evans C. Reliable and clinically significant change, 1998. www.psyctc.org/stats/rcsc.htm.

105. Eastman N, Bellamy S. Admission Criteria to Secure Psychiatric Care: ACeSS Schedule (unpublished paper for South Thames Regional Office of NHS Executive and High Security Psychiatric Services Commissioning Board). London, St George's Hospital Medical School, 1998.

106. Shaw J, Davies J, Morey H. An assessment of the security, dependency and treatment

needs of all patients in secure services in a UK health region. *The Journal of Forensic Psychiatry* 2001; 12 (3): 610–37.

107. Dickens G, Sugarman P, Picchioni M, Long C. HoNOS-Secure: tracking risk and recovery for men in secure care. *The British Journal of Forensic Practice* 2010; 12 (4): 36–46.

108. Collins M, Davies S. The Security Needs Assessment Profile: a multidimensional approach to measuring security needs. *International Journal of Forensic Mental Health* 2005; 4 (1): 39–52.

109. Habets P, Jeandarme I, Kennedy HG. Applicability of the DUNDRUM-1 in a forensic Belgium setting. *Journal of Forensic Practice* 2019; 21 (1): 85–94.

110. O'Dwyer S, Davoren M, Abidin Z et al. The DUNDRUM Quartet: validation of structured professional judgement instruments DUNDRUM-3 assessment of programme completion and DUNDRUM-4 assessment of recovery in forensic mental health services. *BMC Research Notes* 2011; 4: 229.

111. Davoren M, O'Dwyer S, Abidin Z et al. Prospective in-patient cohort study of moves between levels of therapeutic security: the DUNDRUM-1 triage security, DUNDRUM-3 programme completion and DUNDRUM-4 recovery scales and the HCR-20. *BMC Psychiatry* 2012; 12: 80.

112. Davoren M, Abidin Z, Naughton L et al. Prospective study of factors influencing conditional discharge from a forensic hospital: the DUNDRUM-3 programme completion and DUNDRUM-4 recovery structured professional judgement instruments and risk. *BMC Psychiatry* 2013; 13: 185.

113. Adams J, Thomas SD, Mackinnon T, Eggleton D. The risks, needs and stages of recovery of a complete forensic patient cohort in an Australian state. *BMC Psychiatry* 2018; 18 (1): 35.

114. Eckert M, Schel SH, Kennedy HG, Bulten BH. Patient characteristics related to length of stay in Dutch forensic psychiatric care. *The Journal of Forensic Psychiatry & Psychology* 2017; 28 (6): 863–80.

115. Davoren M, Hennessy S, Conway C, Marrinan S, Gill P, Kennedy HG. Recovery and concordance in a secure forensic psychiatry hospital – the self rated DUNDRUM-3 programme completion and DUNDRUM-4 recovery scales. *BMC Psychiatry* 2015; 15: 61.

116. Kennedy HG, Davoren M, O'Flynn P, O'Sullivan OP. How to measure progress in forensic care. In Birgit Vollm PB (ed.) *Long-Term Forensic Psychiatric Care: Clinical, Ethical and Legal Challenges.* Cham, Springer, 2019, pp. 103–21.

117. McCullough S, Stanley C, Smith H et al. Outcome measures of risk and recovery in Broadmoor High Secure Forensic Hospital: stratification of care pathways and moves to medium secure hospitals. *BJPsych Open* 2020; 6 (4): e74.

118. Grove WM, Meehl PE. Comparative efficiency of informal (subjective, impressionistic) and formal (mechanical, algorithmic) prediction procedures: The clinical–statistical controversy. *Psychology, Public Policy, and Law* 1996; 2 (2): 293.

119. Webster C, Douglas K, Eaves D, Hart S. HCR-20: Assessing risk for violence (Version 2). Burnaby, Mental Health, Law, and Policy Institute, Simon Fraser University, 1997.

120. Douglas KS, Hart SD, Webster CD, Belfrage H. *HCR-20V3: Assessing Risk for Violence: User Guide.* Burnaby, Mental Health, Law, and Policy Institute, Simon Fraser University, 2013.

121. Douglas K, Webster C, Hart S, Eaves D, Ogloff J. *HCR-20-Violence Risk Management Companion Guide.* Burnaby, Mental Health, Law and Policy Institute, Simon Fraser University, 2001.

122. Troquete NA, van den Brink RH, Beintema H et al. Risk assessment and shared care planning in out-patient forensic psychiatry: cluster randomised controlled trial. *British Journal of Psychiatry* 2013; 202 (5): 365–71.

123. van den Brink RH, Troquete NA, Beintema H et al. Risk assessment by client and case manager for shared decision making in outpatient forensic psychiatry. *BMC Psychiatry* 2015; 15: 120.

124. O'Shea LE, Dickens GL. The HCR-20 as a measure of reliable and clinically significant change in violence risk among secure psychiatric inpatients. *Comprehensive Psychiatry* 2015; 62: 132–40.

125. Strand SJM, Selenius H. Assessing risk for inpatient physical violence in a female forensic psychiatric sample: comparing HCR-20v2 with the Female Additional Manual to the HCR-20v2. *Nordic Journal of Psychiatry* 2019; 73 (4–5): 248–56.

126. Rutter M. Resilience in the face of adversity: protective factors and resistance to psychiatric disorder. *The British Journal of Psychiatry* 1985; 147 (6): 598–611.

127. Rutter M. Psychosocial resilience and protective mechanisms. In Rolf J, Masten AS, Cicchetti D, Nuechterlein KH and Weintraub S (eds) *Risk and Protective Factors in the Development of Psychopathology*. Cambridge, Cambridge University Press, 1990.

128. Lockertsen Ø, Varvin S, Færden A, Vatnar SKB. Short-term risk assessments in an acute psychiatric inpatient setting: a re-examination of the Brøset Violence Checklist using repeated measurements – differentiating violence characteristics and gender. *Archives of Psychiatric Nursing* 2021; 35 (1): 17–26.

129. Almvik R, Woods P, Rasmussen K. The Brøset Violence Checklist: sensitivity, specificity, and interrater reliability. *Journal of Interpersonal Violence* 2000; 15 (12): 1284–96.

130. Maguire T, Daffern M, Bowe SJ, McKenna B. Evaluating the impact of an electronic application of the Dynamic Appraisal of Situational Aggression with an embedded Aggression Prevention Protocol on aggression and restrictive interventions on a forensic mental health unit. *International Journal of Mental Health Nursing* 2019; 28 (5): 1186–97.

131. Ogloff JR, Daffern M. The dynamic appraisal of situational aggression: an instrument to assess risk for imminent aggression in psychiatric inpatients. *Behavioral Sciences & the Law* 2006; 24 (6): 799–813.

132. Maguire T, Daffern M, Bowe SJ, McKenna B. Predicting aggressive behaviour in acute forensic mental health units: a re-examination of the dynamic appraisal of situational aggression's predictive validity. *International Journal of Mental Health Nursing* 2017; 26 (5): 472–81.

133. Kennedy HG, Mullaney R, McKenna P et al. A tool to evaluate proportionality and necessity in the use of restrictive practices in forensic mental health settings: the DRILL tool (Dundrum restriction, intrusion and liberty ladders). *BMC Psychiatry* 2020; 20 (1): 515.

134. Griffith JJ, Meyer D, Maguire T, Ogloff JRP, Daffern M. A clinical decision support system to prevent aggression and reduce restrictive practices in a forensic mental health service. *Psychiatric Services* 2021; 72 (8): 885–90.

135. Ijaz A, Papaconstantinou A, O'Neill H, Kennedy HG. The Suicide Risk Assessment and Management Manual (S-RAMM) validation study 1. *Irish Journal of Psychological Medicine* 2009; 26 (2): 54–8.

136. Fagan J, Ijaz A, Papaconstantinou A et al. The Suicide Risk Assessment and Management Manual (S-RAMM) validation study II. *Irish Journal of Psychological Medicine* 2009; 26 (3): 107–13.

137. SanSegundo MS, Ferrer-Cascales R, Bellido JH et al. Prediction of violence, suicide behaviors and suicide ideation in a sample of institutionalized offenders with schizophrenia and other psychosis. *Frontiers in Psychology* 2018; 9: 1385.

138. Abidin Z, Davoren M, Naughton L et al. Susceptibility (risk and protective) factors for in-patient violence and self-harm: prospective study of structured professional judgement instruments START and SAPROF, DUNDRUM-3 and

DUNDRUM-4 in forensic mental health services. *BMC Psychiatry* 2013; 13: 197.

139. O'Shea LE, Picchioni MM, Mason FL, Sugarman PA, Dickens GL. Predictive validity of the HCR-20 for inpatient self-harm. *Comprehensive Psychiatry* 2014; 55 (8): 1937–49.

140. Nicholls TL, Brink J, Desmarais SL, Webster CD, Martin M-L. The Short-Term Assessment of Risk and Treatability (START): a prospective validation study in a forensic psychiatric sample. *Assessment* 2006; 13 (3): 313–27.

141. Kennedy H. Therapeutic uses of security: mapping forensic mental health services by stratifying risk. *Advances in Psychiatric Treatment* 2002; 8 (6): 433–43.

142. Kennedy HG. Models of care in forensic psychiatry. *BJPsych Advances* 2021: 1–14.

143. Wing JK, Brown GW. Social treatment of chronic schizophrenia: a comparative survey of three mental hospitals. *Journal of Mental Science* 1961; 107 (450): 847–61.

144. James M, Painter J, Buckingham B, Stewart MW. A review and update of the Health of the Nation Outcome Scales (HoNOS). *BJPsych Bulletin* 2018; 42 (2): 63–8.

145. Phelan M, Slade M, Thornicroft G et al. The Camberwell Assessment of Need: the validity and reliability of an instrument to assess the needs of people with severe mental illness. *British Journal of Psychiatry* 1995; 167 (5): 589–95.

146. Pierzchniak P, Farnham F, Taranto Nd et al. Assessing the needs of patients in secure settings: a multi-disciplinary approach. *The Journal of Forensic Psychiatry* 1999; 10 (2): 343–54.

147. Harty M-A, Shaw J, Thomas S et al. The security, clinical and social needs of patients in high security psychiatric hospitals in England. *The Journal of Forensic Psychiatry & Psychology* 2004; 15 (2): 208–21.

148. Shaw J, McKenna J, Snowden P et al. The North-West Region. I: Clinical features and placement needs of patients detained in Special Hospitals. *Journal of Forensic Psychiatry* 1994; 5 (1): 93–105.

149. Shaw J, McKenna J, Snowden P et al. Clinical features and placement needs of all North West Region patients currently in Special Hospital. *Journal of Forensic Psychiatry* 1994; 5: 93–106.

150. Kaye C, Franey A. *Managing High Security Psychiatric Care*. New York, Jessica Kingsley, 1998.

151. Cohen A, Eastman N. *Assessing Forensic Mental Health Need: Policy, Theory and Research*. London, RCPsych Publications, 2000.

152. Flynn G, O'Neill C, Kennedy HG. DUNDRUM-2: prospective validation of a structured professional judgment instrument assessing priority for admission from the waiting list for a forensic mental health hospital. *BMC Research Notes* 2011; 4: 230.

153. Jeandarme I, Habets P, O'Reilly K, Kennedy HG. Is non-completion of treatment related to security need? *Criminal Behaviour and Mental Health* 2021; 31 (5): 321–30.

154. Dolan M, Khawaja A. The HCR-20 and post-discharge outcome in male patients discharged from medium security in the UK. *Aggressive Behavior: Official Journal of the International Society for Research on Aggression* 2004; 30 (6): 469–83.

155. Doyle M, Power LA, Coid J et al. Predicting post-discharge community violence in England and Wales using the HCR-20V3. *International Journal of Forensic Mental Health* 2014; 13 (2): 140–7.

156. Jewell A, Dean K, Fahy T, Cullen AE. Predictors of Mental Health Review Tribunal (MHRT) outcome in a forensic inpatient population: a prospective cohort study. *BMC Psychiatry* 2017; 17 (1): 25.

157. Vitacco MJ, Tabernik HE, Zavodny D, Bailey K, Waggoner C. Projecting risk: the importance of the HCR-20 risk management scale in predicting outcomes with forensic patients. *Behavioral Sciences & the Law* 2016; 34 (2–3): 308–20.

158. McGuire J. A review of effective interventions for reducing aggression and violence. *Philosophical Transactions of the Royal Society of London Series B, Biological Sciences* 2008; 363 (1503): 2577–97.

159. Wampold BE. How important are the common factors in psychotherapy? An update. *World Psychiatry: Official Journal of the World Psychiatric Association (WPA)* 2015; 14 (3): 270–7.

160. Davoren M, Byrne O, O'Connell P et al. Factors affecting length of stay in forensic hospital setting: need for therapeutic security and course of admission. *BMC Psychiatry* 2015; 15: 301.

161. O'Reilly K, Donohoe G, Coyle C et al. Prospective cohort study of the relationship between neuro-cognition, social cognition and violence in forensic patients with schizophrenia and schizoaffective disorder. *BMC Psychiatry* 2015; 15 (1): 155–.

162. Campagnolo D, Furimsky I, Chaimowitz G. Abscorsion from forensic psychiatric institutions: a review of the literature. *International Journal of Risk and Recovery* 2019; 2 (2): 36–50.

163. Chaplin E, Hearn D, Ndegwa D, Norman P, Hammond N. Developing the leave/abscond risk assessment (LARA) from the absconding literature: an aide to risk management in secure services. *Advances in Mental Health and Intellectual Disabilities* 2012; 6 (6): 280–90.

164. Cullen AE, Jewell A, Tully J et al. A prospective cohort study of abscorsion incidents in forensic psychiatric settings: can we identify those at high-risk? *PLoS One* 2015; 10 (9): e0138819.

165. Hilterman EL, Philipse MW, de Graaf ND. Assessment of offending during leave: development of the Leave Risk Assessment in a sample of Dutch forensic psychiatric patients. *International Journal of Forensic Mental Health* 2011; 10 (3): 233–43.

166. Lyall M, Bartlett A. Decision making in medium security: can he have leave? *The Journal of Forensic Psychiatry & Psychology* 2010; 21 (6): 887–901.

167. Mezey G, Durkin C, Dodge L, White S. Never ever? Characteristics, outcomes and motivations of patients who abscond or escape: a 5-year review of escapes and absconds from two medium and low secure forensic units. *Criminal Behaviour and Mental Health* 2015; 25 (5): 440–50.

168. Mohan D, Jamieson E, Taylor PJ. The use of trial leave for restricted special hospital patients. *Criminal Behaviour and Mental Health* 2001; 11 (1): 55–62.

169. Scott R, Goel V, Neillie D, Stedman T, Meehan T. Unauthorised absences from leave from an Australian security hospital. *Australasian Psychiatry* 2014; 22 (2): 170–3.

170. Sklenarova H, Neutze J, Kretschmer T, Nitschke J. Granting leave to patients in bavarian forensic-psychiatric hospitals: a survey to describe the current process and develop guidelines. *Frontiers in Psychiatry* 2020; 11: 287.

171. Watson TM, Choo L. Understanding and reducing unauthorized leaves of absence from forensic mental health settings: a literature review. *The Journal of Forensic Psychiatry & Psychology* 2020: 1–17.

172. Côté G, Crocker AG, Nicholls TL, Seto MC. Risk assessment instruments in clinical practice. *The Canadian Journal of Psychiatry* 2012; 57 (4): 238–44.

173. Crocker AG, Nicholls TL, Charette Y, Seto MC. Dynamic and static factors associated with discharge dispositions: the national trajectory project of individuals found Not Criminally Responsible on Account of Mental Disorder (NCRMD) in Canada. *Behavioral Sciences & the Law* 2014; 32 (5): 577–95.

174. Wharewera-Mika J, Cooper E, Wiki N et al. The appropriateness of DUNDRUM-3 and DUNDRUM-4 for Māori in forensic mental health services in New Zealand: participatory action research. *BMC Psychiatry* 2020; 20 (1): 1–9.

175. Kennedy H. Limits of psychiatric evidence in criminal courts: morals and madness.

Medico-Legal Journal of Ireland 2005; 11: 1–17.

176. Kennedy H. Limits of psychiatric evidence in civil courts and tribunals: science and sensibility. *Irish Medical Journal* 2004; 10.

177. Rutledge E, Kennedy M, O'Neill H, Kennedy HG. Functional mental capacity is not independent of the severity of psychosis. *International Journal of Law and Psychiatry* 2008; 31 (1): 9–18.

178. Ganzini L, Volicer L, Nelson WA, Fox E, Derse AR. Ten myths about decision-making capacity. *Journal of the American Medical Directors Association* 2004; 5 (4): 263–7.

179. Marson DC, Hawkins L, McInturff B, Harrell LE. Cognitive models that predict physician judgments of capacity to consent in mild Alzheimer's disease. *Journal of the American Geriatrics Society* 1997; 45 (4): 458–64.

180. Marson DC, McInturff B, Hawkins L, Bartolucci A, Harrell LE. Consistency of physician judgments of capacity to consent in mild Alzheimer's disease. *Journal of the American Geriatrics Society* 1997; 45 (4): 453–7.

181. Moynihan G, O'Reilly K, O'Connor J, Kennedy HG. An evaluation of functional mental capacity in forensic mental health practice: the Dundrum capacity ladders validation study. *BMC Psychiatry* 2018; 18 (1): 78.

182. Appelbaum PS, Grisso T. Assessing patients' capacities to consent to treatment. *New England Journal of Medicine* 1988; 319 (25): 1635–8.

183. Grisso T. *Evaluating Competencies: Forensic Assessments and Instruments.* Cham: Springer Science & Business Media, 2006.

184. Grisso T, Appelbaum PS, Hill-Fotouhi C. The MacCAT-T: a clinical tool to assess patients' capacities to make treatment decisions. *Psychiatric Services* 1997; 48 (11): 1415–19.

185. Akinkunmi AA. The MacArthur Competence Assessment Tool – fitness to plead: a preliminary evaluation of a research instrument for assessing fitness to plead in England and Wales. *Journal of the American Academy of Psychiatry and the Law* 2002; 30 (4): 476–82.

186. Grisso T, Appelbaum PS. Comparison of standards for assessing patients' capacities to make treatment decisions. *American Journal of Psychiatry* 1995; 152 (7): 1033–7.

187. Grisso T, Appelbaum PS. *Assessing Competence to Consent to Treatment: A Guide for Physicians and Other Health Professionals.* New York, Oxford University Press, 1998.

188. Eastman N, Starling B. Mental disorder ethics: theory and empirical investigation. *Journal of medical ethics* 2006; 32 (2): 94–9.

189. Kenny A. *Freewill and Responsibility* (Routledge Revivals). London, Taylor & Francis, 2011.

190. Kenny A. *The Metaphysics of Mind.* Oxford, Oxford University Press, 1992.

191. Tan J, Hope T, Stewart A. Competence to refuse treatment in anorexia nervosa. *International Journal of Law and Psychiatry* 2003; 26 (6): 697–707.

192. Amador XF, David AS. *Insight and Psychosis: Awareness of Illness in Schizophrenia and Related Disorders.* Oxford, Oxford University Press, 2004.

193. David A, Buchanan A, Reed A, Almeida O. The assessment of insight in psychosis. *The British Journal of Psychiatry* 1992; 161 (5): 599–602.

194. Lewis A. The psychopathology of insight. *British Journal of Medical Psychology* 1934; 14 (4): 332–48.

195. Lysaker PH, Vohs J, Hasson-Ohayon I et al. Depression and insight in schizophrenia: comparisons of levels of deficits in social cognition and metacognition and internalized stigma across three profiles. *Schizophrenia Research* 2013; 148 (1–3): 18–23.

196. Owen GS, David AS, Richardson G et al. Mental capacity, diagnosis and insight in psychiatric in-patients: a cross-sectional

study. *Psychological Medicine* 2009; 39 (8): 1389.

197. Marson DC, Savage R, Phillips J. Financial capacity in persons with schizophrenia and serious mental illness: clinical and research ethics aspects. *Schizophrenia Bulletin* 2006; 32 (1): 81–91.

198. Fazel S, Hope T, Jacoby R. Assessment of competence to complete advance directives: validation of a patient centred approach. *BMJ* 1999; 318 (7182): 493–7.

199. Kennedy M, Dornan J, Rutledge E, O'Neill H, Kennedy HG. Extra information about treatment is too much for the patient with psychosis. *International Journal of Law and Psychiatry* 2009; 32 (6): 369–76.

200. Dornan J, Kennedy M, Garland J, Rutledge E, Kennedy HG. Functional mental capacity, treatment as usual and time: magnitude of change in secure hospital patients with major mental illness. *BMC Research Notes* 2015; 8: 566.

201. Re C (Adult: Refusal of Treatment). *Weekly Law Reports* 1993; 25 February: 290–6.

202. Cairns R, Maddock C, Buchanan A et al. Reliability of mental capacity assessments in psychiatric in-patients. *The British Journal of Psychiatry* 2005; 187 (4): 372–8.

203. Prat CS, Keller TA, Just MA. Individual differences in sentence comprehension: a functional magnetic resonance imaging investigation of syntactic and lexical processing demands. *Journal of Cognitive Neuroscience* 2007; 19 (12): 1950–63.

204. Calman KC, Royston G. Personal paper: risk language and dialects. *BMJ* 1997; 315 (7113): 939–42.

205. Knapp P, Berry DC, Raynor D. Testing two methods of presenting side effect risk information about common medicines. *International Journal of Pharmacy Practice* 2001, 9(S1) 6–6.

206. Edwards A, Elwyn G, Mulley A. Explaining risks: turning numerical data into meaningful pictures. *BMJ* 2002; 324 (7341): 827–30.

207. Mossman D, Noffsinger SG, Ash P et al. AAPL Practice Guideline for the forensic psychiatric evaluation of competence to stand trial. *Journal of the American Academy of Psychiatry and the Law* 2007; 35 (4 Suppl.): S3-72.

208. Hoge SK, Bonnie RJ, Poythress N et al. The MacArthur adjudicative competence study: development and validation of a research instrument. *Law and Human Behavior* 1997; 21 (2): 141–79.

209. Roesch R, Webster CD, Eaves D, Menzies RJ. *The Fitness Interview Test: A Method for Examining Fitness to Stand Trial.* Toronto, Centre of Criminology, University of Toronto, 1984.

210. Rogers R, Jordan MJ, Harrison KS. A critical review of published competency-to-confess measures. *Law and Human Behavior* 2004; 28 (6): 707–18; discussion 19–24.

211. Rogers R, Otal T, Drogin EY, Dean BM. Effectiveness of the Miranda acquiescence questionnaire for investigating impaired Miranda reasoning. *Journal of the American Academy of Psychiatry and the Law* 2020; 48 (2): 226–36.

212. Rogers R, Wasyliw OE, Cavanaugh JL. Evaluating insanity. *Law and Human Behavior* 1984; 8 (3–4): 293–303.

213. Dietz PE. Why the experts disagree: variations in the psychiatric evaluation of criminal insanity. *The Annals of the American Academy of Political and Social Science* 1985; 477 (1): 84–95.

214. Warren JI, Murrie DC, Chauhan P, Dietz PE, Morris J. Opinion formation in evaluating sanity at the time of the offense: an examination of 5175 pre-trial evaluations. *Behavioral Sciences & the Law* 2004; 22 (2): 171–86.

215. West DJ, Walk A (eds) *Daniel McNaughton: His Trial and the Aftermath.* London, Gaskell Books, 1977.

216. Parmigiani G, Mandarelli G, Meynen G, Carabellese F, Ferracuti S. Translating clinical findings to the legal norm: the Defendant's Insanity Assessment Support Scale (DIASS). *Translational Psychiatry* 2019; 9 (1): 278.

217. Mandarelli G, Carabellese F, Felthous AR et al. The factors associated with forensic psychiatrists' decisions in criminal responsibility and social dangerousness evaluations. *International Journal of Law and Psychiatry* 2019; 66: 101503.

218. Scarpazza C, Miolla A, Zampieri I et al. Translational application of a neuro-scientific multi-modal approach into forensic psychiatric evaluation: why and how? *Frontiers in Psychiatry* 2021; 12: 597918.

219. Giorgi-Guarnieri D, Janofsky J, Keram E et al. AAPL practice guideline for forensic psychiatric evaluation of defendants raising the insanity defense. *Journal of the American Academy of Psychiatry and the Law* 2002; 30 (2 Suppl.): S3-40.

220. Rogers R, Bender SD. *Clinical Assessment of Malingering and Deception*, 4th ed. New York, Guilford Publications, 2018.

221. Fenwick P. Automatism, medicine and the law. *Psychological Medicine Monograph Supplement* 1990; 17: 1–27.

Models of Care in Forensic Psychiatry

Harry Kennedy

Model of Care

Forensic psychiatry uniquely requires that its practitioners have expertise in the assessment of need for treatment of patients who represent a risk of violence to others, including not just their families and neighbours but also fellow patients and the clinicians who treat and care for them. Elsewhere in this volume, the assessment of risk and the available treatments are described. In this chapter the essential knowledge of therapeutic security is summarised as parts of a model of care that includes levels of therapeutic security so that violence itself can be treated.

The history of psychiatric hospitals is a cycle of idealism and enlightenment followed by growth. Growth leads to a decline in quality, eventually leading to dysfunctional decline, inquiries and reform before the cycle repeats. Secure forensic hospitals are bellwethers for this cycle [1] and need formal means of protecting against decline by ensuring not just quality standards but also excellence and the continuous improvement of outcomes for patients [2]. A model of care is a basis for preventing such entropic processes while ensuring that defined goals are reached and sustained over time [3].

Definition

A model of care broadly defines the way health services are delivered. It outlines best practice and services for a person, population group or patient cohort as they progress through the stages of the condition, injury or event. It aims to ensure that people get the right care, at the right time, by the right team and in the right place. A model of care often includes a logic model relating inputs (resources) to outputs (health gains). This definition is derived from the New South Wales Agency for Clinical Innovation [4]. A model of care is a document which is intended to be read by all new staff joining a service. The model of care bears the same relationship to policies that a constitution bears to laws. All policies, standard operating procedures and governance terms of reference should be implicit within it and compatible with it. A model of care should be written in plain English. However, it is not the same as a prospectus for patients or their families. Nor is it a contracting document. A model of care should be designed to last without major modification for about five years so that it can be evaluated properly. A model of care is typically written for the first time in consultation with commissioners, in order to instruct architects, software and clinical management system designers or as part of service reform. While a model of care cannot in itself cause a service to achieve its goals, it may be a precondition for success and it can contribute to a shared vision, mission and values.

A model of care can be written or compiled in many ways. Where no pre-existing model of care can be identified, a starting point is to map existing services, their estate, human resources and levels of activity, and pathways and processes. A common approach is to engage stakeholders in a process of participant action research. However, a model of care for a forensic psychiatry service cannot be written in a coherent way from grassroots up. A vision is necessary. Clinical science is consistent, methodical, cumulative and capable of being evaluated objectively. Human rights, medical ethics, legal structures and processes are 'given'. A final version of the model of care can only be valid if accepted by the clinicians who have clinical expertise and clinical responsibility. Contributory expertise, not inter-active expertise, is essential (see Chapter 6) [5].

Although the definition above is intended to be generic and applies to any health service or part of a service, the emphasis on relating needs to levels of service is so close in meaning to the risk-needs-responsive approach that the affinity for a forensic psychiatric/mental health service is clear.

Models of care can describe open systems, where there is no control or predictability over demand or outcomes, and closed systems in which there is total predictability over demand and outcomes. This overlaps with the problem of closed cultures in which dys-functional culture and practices can become normalised within an 'in-group'. In practice, a model of care for a healthcare organisation aims to bring both demand and outcomes into a predictable, manageable system that is resilient to those events that cannot be completely predictable and remains open to external scrutiny, national standards for quality and international standards for excellence.

Scientific Models and Systems

Forensic mental health services are integral parts of the larger mental health services for the population they serve, as a part of an interdependent system [6]. Any change in the delivery of care in one part of the overall mental health service will have effects on all the other parts [7, 8]. A whole-systems approach is always necessary when understanding the working of a model of care. General systems theory originates in the physiology of closed and open systems and their capacity to autoregulate to maintain homeostasis [9]. Systems theory has been reasserted as taking precedence over one directional deterministic theories and models, with a new emphasis on the emergence of systems at different levels that are interdependent. According to Noble [10], the (biological) ensemble behaves in a controlled way, the controls being those that maintain the constancy of the internal environment. Feedback mechanisms link the levels of a system. The 'insights obtained from higher-level analysis are needed in order to succeed even at the lower levels. The reason is that higher levels in biological systems impose boundary conditions on the lower levels. Without understanding those conditions and their effects, we will be seriously restricted in understanding the logic of living systems' (p. 16). Noble sets out rules for understanding biological systems, some of which are relevant here, including: (biological) functionality is multilevel; transmission of information is not one-way (a feedback mech-anism must operate and robustness is an essential feature of a (biological) system, with both bottom-up causal chains and top-down regulatory mechanisms to complete feedback loops); there is no privileged level of causality; there are no deterministic or purposeful 'programmes' at any level in a (biological) system; and more principles remain to be discovered since there is no 'genuine' theory of biology, though it is the goal of systems biology to find one. Higher-level control cannot be reduced to lower-level databases [10]. In services as distinct from biological systems, changes in, for example, mental health and criminal justice policy can be expected to have large effects on services [11, 12].

A 'model' in science is a bridge from a theory to hypotheses and experiments. A model is 'a simplified representation or description of a system or complex entity, especially one designed to facilitate calculations and predictions' [13]. A model is 'a representation of something else, designed for a special purpose . . . . All models have one characteristic in common, whatever their purpose. This characteristic is the mapping of elements in the system modelled onto the system' (p. 2). Beer quoted by McLaren [13] listed five steps in building a theoretical (mathematical) model: (i) the variables to be used in characterising and understanding the process must be specified; (ii) the forms of the relationships connecting these variables must be specified; (iii) ignorance and the need for simplicity will ensure that all relationships other than identities are subject to error and so, for purposes of efficient statistical estimation, these error terms must be specified; (iv) the parameters of the model must be estimated and the extent of its identification ascertained, after which, if this is inadequate, the model must be reformulated; and finally (v) the model must be kept up to date and used so that an impression can be formed of its robustness and reliability. Modelling in this scientific sense is reductive where being reductive is a virtue and a strength, a means of seeing the predictable processes underlying apparently complex phenomena.

Space has been given to explaining what a scientific model is because the term 'model' is often used inaccurately in psychiatry to refer to parts or fragments of a model of care or to aspirations for what a model might be [13]. The modelling of hospital activity, service demand, waiting list times, bed occupancy and length of stay are for the purposes of a model of care, considered in the same way as a scientific biological model. There is a useful literature on such modelling in other types of community and hospital service [14–16].

Elements of a Model of Care

There are four essential elements of a model of care:

- goals
- pathways and processes
- treatments
- evaluation and logic models.

Model of Care: Goals

Principles are typically derived from conventions on the rights of patients and from legislation. Lists of principles are seldom difficult to agree on, although the ordering and prioritising of principles can be very difficult. Good ideas are never good enough. Goals are therefore the most useful starting point for a model of care. Goals are derived from principles but goals are easier to prioritise or to order as a sequential process and to define in ways that are measurable and achievable. Goals also provide a protection against the introduction of 'good ideas' that cannot be related to outcomes or consequences. Falk set out basic goals for secure services: (a) sufficient physical security appropriate to the patients; (b) high staff ratios; and (c) a therapeutic policy which encompasses individual programmes [17]. Implicit in the last of these is the goal of achieving health gains for patients.

An emphasis should be placed on quality and excellence. Quality is static and ensures that a defined set of standards is treated as a floor below which the service will not fall. Excellence is dynamic and ensures continuously improving outcomes (health gains) for patients [2]. Because forensic mental health services are high risk, low volume and high cost, demonstrable excellence is a necessary part of ensuring a resilient service that can cope with adverse events.

Suggested goals for a model of care in forensic psychiatry:

- rights and recovery as defined in legal criteria
- zero target for violence by patients against patients and others
- managed culture of positive communication and constructive criticism
- prioritisation of effective treatments including physical health interventions over any other activity
- sustainable population-based levels of service
- active management of length of stay.

Pathways and Processes

Clinical Pathways

Criteria for a clinical pathway were defined following a systematic review [18, 19] as requiring that the intervention was a structured multidisciplinary plan of care, and any three of the following four: the intervention was used to channel the translation of guidelines or evidence into local structures; the intervention detailed the steps in a course of treatment or care in a plan, pathway, algorithm, guideline, protocol or other 'inventory of actions'; the intervention had time-frames or criteria-based progression (i.e. steps were taken if designated criteria were met); and the intervention aimed to standardise care for a specific clinical problem, procedure or episode of healthcare in a specific population. This works well for a forensic model of care.

The finished model of care document is the description of an organisation's system for using defined resources to perform a multidisciplinary plan of care to achieve planned health gains at the population level. Guidelines and evidence are channelled into local structures as described in the model of care under 'pathways and processes' and 'treatment'.

Steps in a course of care and treatment are set out in a plan of stratified therapeutic security, with inventory of actions concerning the elements of therapeutic security. The emphasis on active management of length of stay and criteria-based progression is set out in the description of structured professional judgements and judgement support frameworks for governance. Standardising the quality of healthcare for this patient group is defined within this model of care. The model of care should also ensure sufficient capacity to provide individualised care and treatment plans.

Mapping

Mapping is always necessary as a preliminary step. Static mapping should document the existing estate and human resources. Dynamic mapping then describes the referral, triage and admission processes, treatment and planned progression from high- to medium- to low-secure care and on to the community. There should also be a description of structured supports and patient pathways and processes. Forensic mental health services include a secure forensic hospital at their core. Secure forensic hospitals function as specialist tertiary referral centres. Typically, secure forensic hospitals and forensic mental health services sit at the centre of a complex intersection of pathways from the criminal justice system and from second-tier specialist psychiatric services, with complex pathways back to the community involving many agencies.

A population-based forensic mental health service must also include court liaison and diversion services [20–25], psychiatric in-reach clinics in remand [23, 26–28] and sentenced prisons [28–31], and community aftercare and supervision services [32–34], as well as consultation and liaison services for general adult mental health services and criminal justice agencies. Where these are not provided within one organisation, there should be clearly defined processes to ensure that pathways function quickly and responsively according to need [8, 35, 36].

Therapeutic Security

Risk management is the process of selecting and applying a range of intervention measures to prevent adverse outcomes including violence in therapeutic, custodial and community settings and in the post-release period or in the context of preventative supervision. The aim of risk management in forensic psychiatry services is to reduce the risk of very serious sexual or very serious violent crime against persons by patients under supervision. Secure forensic hospitals can always be described in terms of the elements of therapeutic security [37–39]: environmental or physical security; relational security (quantitative and qualitative); procedural security; and the specialist management and governance arrangements necessary to facilitate and sustain these. Therapeutic security is an essential pre-requisite for treatment since the prevention of violence is the means of ensuring that effective treatments can be delivered in an environment where the tension and anxiety caused by imminent violence is removed. This includes both overt acts of aggression, threats and violence [40] and more subtle bullying, intimidation and extortion [41].

Environmental Therapeutic Security

Physical or environmental therapeutic security includes the designed and built environment, maintenance of estate and fittings and the staff necessary to operate them. It includes perimeter security, secure entrances and exits, ligature-free environments, unobstructed sight lines and many other design essentials. The environment should be so robust that it can withstand attempts at destruction and cannot be used to produce weapons [42]. At medium- and high-secure levels the environment should be escape proof [43–46]. Although the concept of 'defensible space' relates to urban developments [47], a secure hospital campus should be designed for safety and reassurance on the same principles. The built environment should also be clean, constantly well maintained, with natural daylight and well-circulated air, and some control for patients over their own environment, for example heating and light [48]. It should be pleasing to the eye and uplifting in design and presentation. Although robust and secure, the built environment should not have obvious custodial, penal or non-therapeutic qualities. Access to gardens, vistas and variety (bedrooms, dayrooms, therapy areas, classrooms, workshops, gyms) should be built in to ensure preservation of skills for activities of daily living and social skills [49]. There should also be some form of engagement between the management of the secure hospital and the local community.

Relational Therapeutic Security

Relational therapeutic security can be divided into qualitative and quantitative relational therapeutic security. A common pattern in research literature is to concentrate on qualitative relational security while neglecting quantitative relational security. Staff-to-patient ratios are expensive and may even be considered commercially sensitive. However, this is the most important distinction between high, medium and low levels of therapeutic safety and security. Qualitative relational matters are much easier to discuss, although they are often coloured by intangible cultural and social matters properly studied by anthropologists.

Quantitative relational therapeutic security starts with the ratio of staff to patients at ward level and the amount of time spent in face-to-face contact [8]. This includes skills mix and the level and sophistication of training and experience. Qualitative relational therapeutic security is the balance between intrusiveness and openness; trust and safe boundaries between patients and professionals. Getting to know patients well includes the depth and breadth of knowledge of patients by the professionals. The ability to maintain a therapeutic relationship with a working alliance and interpersonal trust in forensic practice cannot be separated from systematically managing boundaries so that risk is recognised and managed. This balance represents one of the higher aspects of forensic psychiatric specialist training and expertise in each of the mental health professions [50, 51]. There are also systemic issues concerning the mix of patients on each ward and the ability to prevent bullying, exploitation and subversion of therapeutic security. Teams should be cohesive, communicative, consistent and have continuity over time, with a common purpose that is therapeutic and pro-social. Four key areas identified in the functioning of effective forensic hospital wards were: the 'whole care team', the 'other patients on the ward', the 'inside world experienced by patients' and the 'connections those patients have with the outside world' [52]. Another review identified eight areas of relational security 'boundaries', 'therapy', 'patient mix', 'patient dynamic', 'personal world', 'physical environment', 'visitors' and 'outward connections' [52, 53]. These aspects of qualitative relational security should be connected to risk management through the communicating of safety information reports to procedural security and governance structures.

Relational systems or process modes (sometimes incorrectly called models) are a sub-set of relational therapeutic security. These have origins in nursing processes [54]. All of these have in common an approach to structured communication, positive regard, the building of trust and a training element concerning how to achieve shared goal-setting in keeping with common factors for treatment [55] and generalised to day-to-day interactions on wards and in clinics. All have in common that they claim origins in either Delphi processes or qualitative research, though this does not explain the a priori assumptions that lead to such work. Most have an emphasis on modes of communication to demonstrate respect and to de-escalate or avert confrontations and frustrations. Safewards [56] and See-Think-Act [50, 52, 57, 58] are operationalised and are amenable to quantitative research (see Chapter 9). Dialog+ has also been subjected to some assessments of effectiveness with positive outcomes in community settings [59, 60]. A comparison of Safewards and Good Lives is reviewed in Chapter 15. The Recovery Model [61] is not a model but a relational system of laudable principles [62]. Like the biopsychosocial model [13], it is not actually a model, nor is it a care pathway. It has achieved an almost pre-eminent place in many state policies, without consistently defined goals or reliable evidence for effectiveness in achieving any specific goal or outcome.

The necessity and the possibility of developing a forensic recovery system has been discussed [63–68]. A co-produced set of self-rated outcome measures relevant to violence and measures of forensic recovery has been validated against real-world outcomes [69]. Concordance between staff-rated and self-rated outcomes proved to be the best predictor of objective outcomes relevant to forensic psychiatry patients. Some studies note that subjective outcomes such as satisfaction and perceived coercion are related to symptoms [70, 71]. In a forensic context, there is some evidence from observational studies that Safewards may reduce restrictive practices [72]. Trauma informed care is also currently popular. There is currently no obvious way to choose between these modes or processes and no information on whether any combination of two or more can be run at the same time.

Procedural therapeutic security serves the first two elements by ensuring that risk assessment and risk management are systematic, consistent across the service, tailored to individual need and dynamic. This includes policies and practices for controlling risk. At the patient level: systems and routines for the control and checking of patients' movements and communication generally. At the systems level: arrangements for professional governance, risk management, crisis and contingency planning, formalised reviews and transfer of responsibilities [38]. There should be a system to supplement individual risk assessments with a systemic collation of risk and security information reports, to prevent violence and bullying of patients by patients, to ensure that contraband (drugs, weapons, means of escape or illicit media) are not brought into the hospital or circulated within it [73, 74].

Management and governance structures and processes should be organised to maintain the elements of therapeutic security according to quality standards [75] and excellence [76], compliance with national and international standards, sustainability over time and resilience. This should include clarity regarding lines of responsibility: management of resources, lines of reporting and responsibility [38]. There should be processes for the weekly or monthly monitoring and benchmarking of admission, leave, transfer and discharge criteria. There should be processes for ensuring compliance with legal and policy requirements. There should be maintenance of inter-agency relationships and boundaries.

Structured Professional Judgement and Judgement Support Frameworks

A 'double-lock' structure should ensure that critical decisions regarding therapeutic risk-taking (triage decisions, giving or withholding accompanied and unaccompanied day leave, moves from more secure to less secure wards or settings, and conditional discharge, among others) should commence with the use of a structured professional judgement tool where a validated instrument exists, then is validated by a judgement support framework such as daily activity and hand-over reports, referrals and admissions panels [77, 78], leave panels with support frameworks of live activity reporting, peer review and audit, statutory review boards [79], and in some cases appeals mechanisms to ensure natural justice.

Resilience

Resilience in the face of serious adverse events (homicides [80], riots, hostage incidents [81], arson, absconding [82, 83] and coordinated escapes [84, 85], epidemic outbreaks [86, 87], surges in demand for services) requires comprehensive policies and standard operational procedures, but although these are necessary, they are not sufficient. Resilience also requires the ability to quickly respond to new and unanticipated challenges or errors by adopting practices from international experience, by innovation and improvisation requiring the highest levels of expertise, using continuous evaluation and design principles [88] and by working flexibly and responsively [89–91]. Expert clinical leadership [92, 93] is essential for such innovation and to motivate teams for such flexible working. Professional, non-clinical management is necessary to support expert clinical leadership.

Secure forensic hospitals can be organised according to principles of therapeutic security in a variety of ways. Very small services have relatively little choice in how they are organised; larger services can have more choice and a minimum size may be necessary for the critical mass to enable the delivery of specialist treatment programmes. The most common design is stratified therapeutic security in which distinctions are made between high security, medium security and low security as stages along a forensic recovery pathway. These may intersect with stratification from acute, subacute to medium-term and slow stream or long-term [8]. Special considerations arise concerning the provision of secure forensic services for women [27] (see Chapter 18), for adolescents (see Chapter 17) and for special needs groups.

Sustainable Levels of Service

Sustaining levels of service over time is an essential goal for a model of care. The process of understanding and quantifying admissions, lengths of stay and discharges and the factors that directly or indirectly affect these measures is 'modelling' in the scientific, quantitative sense. Any forensic hospital, service or system is liable to lose admission capacity if the numbers discharged in a given time period cannot keep pace with demand for admissions. This can be expressed in various ways. Bed occupancy should generally be managed at about 85% in order to cope with seasonal or other surges in demand [15, 16]. In practice many secure forensic hospitals run at 100% occupancy. Occupancy above 100% will reduce quantitative relational therapeutic security and is unsafe. The average length of stay in a ward or a hospital can be calculated in various ways. Operational research shows that length of stay is actually a mixed exponential function [14]. This can be approximated by thinking in terms of half-lives rather than mean length of stay [94]. The median length of stay is a rough but useful approximation [94]. For example, if length of stay has a half-life of 30 days, 50% of admissions would be discharged in 30 days, 75% discharged in 60 days and 87.5% in 90 days. In practice, however, there will always be some patients who require much longer lengths of stay [16, 95–98]. While the majority may be discharged back to the community or the criminal justice system, unless there is well-planned provision for those requiring much longer lengths of stay, admission capacity will quickly be lost [12, 14, 36, 97, 99].

In a stable hospital system in north London in 1999, of 1,054 beds ranging from high- and medium-secure forensic beds through acute and rehabilitation hospital beds and community high-support beds, 50% of beds were modelled as 'acute', with 93% of all admissions discharged with a half-life of 34 days; 6.2% of admissions became medium term, accounting for 28% of all beds and were discharged with a half-life of 273 days; and 0.8% of admissions became long term, accounting for 22% of all beds with a discharge half-life of 1,886 days (from [100] and [15]). In a stable secure forensic hospital with 89 beds, 36% of beds were modelled as 'acute' with 93% of admissions discharged with a half-life of 30 days; 6.9% of admissions were modelled as becoming medium term, occupying 34% of secure forensic beds with 5.4% discharged with a half-life of 474 days; and 1.1% of admissions became long term, occupying 40% of secure forensic beds and having a discharge half-life of 4,297 days (from [101] and [15]). These modelling exercises demonstrate that in a stable system, about 6% of all admissions will become medium term, occupying about 34% of secure forensic beds; and about 1% of all admissions will become long term, occupying about 40% of secure forensic beds. The great majority of admissions will be accommodated in about a third of available beds, characterised here as 'acute' or subacute. It is essential to plan for this.

Triage and Service Demands

Forensic psychiatrists typically act as gatekeepers for secure forensic hospitals to ensure that patients are detained in no greater or more restrictive a level of therapeutic security than is necessary and for no longer than is necessary. Structured professional judgement instruments based on validated criteria are increasingly used in decision support structures such as admissions panels and other governance structures for gatekeeping and goal-setting, including Mental Health Review Boards [26, 36, 77, 78, 102–107]. These guide but do not bind the clinician and the decision-maker.

In many jurisdictions the courts decide on committal to a forensic hospital or forensic psychiatry service based on expert evidence regarding mental disorder, then fitness to stand trial, then responsibility, and finally according to the need for treatment and the level of therapeutic security required. Forensic psychiatrists must have a role in relation to each of these steps. While the courts should be independent in the exercise of their powers, an effective secure forensic hospital service requires there to be some degree of consistency in decision-making by the courts and predictability in the numbers for admission from year to year [12]. A recent survey in the USA reported a median rate of forensic admissions of 9.5 per 100,000 per annum [108]. However, only a small proportion of these are likely to become psychiatric disposals by the courts, leading to long lengths of stay. A European survey showed widely varying incidence rates of new forensic hospital orders across Europe, ranging from 1 to 4 per 100,000 per annum [109]. In the UK, overall detention rates in all psychiatric in-patient units under the Mental Health Act were higher for males (83.2 per 100,000 population) than females (76.1 per 100,000 population). Known rates of use of Community Treatment Orders for males (11.4 per 100,000 population) were almost twice the rate for females (6.6 per 100,000 population), with wide variations for age groups and for black and ethnic minorities. A third of these (33%) are detained under forensic sections of the Act, though not all in secure forensic hospitals. For the four years 2013–16 admission orders under the forensic section of the Mental Health Act in England averaged 1,815 annually (3.2/100,000 per annum), with hospital orders with restrictions under section 37/41 (used in approximately the same way as not guilty by reason of insanity or not criminally responsible by reason of mental illness in other jurisdictions) averaging 446 annually (0.80/100,000 per annum) [110]. Of note, in England approximately 5,500 patients are subject to Community Treatment Orders at any one time. The low forensic admission rates may be in some dynamic relationship with Community Treatment Orders. About 4,500 patients are made subject to a Community Treatment Order per annum (8.1/100,000 per annum) and about 2,500 are fully discharged, usually by the treating psychiatrist; less than half of these civil Community Treatment Order patients are recalled, and two-thirds of recalls end in revocation [111].

International norms for secure forensic beds are variable. Northern European countries are fairly constant at 7 to 12 secure forensic beds (high and medium secure) per 100,000 population [112, 113]. Australian states and Canadian provinces often appear to have fewer beds and shorter lengths of stay. Need may be driven by differences in population deprivation scores [99, 114, 115], population density and deprivation [116], and in rural areas social cohesion [117]. Differences in case mix are probably most relevant [95, 118], though the increasing use of measures of need for therapeutic security (DUNDRUM-1 triage security scores) demonstrates consistent measures in most high-secure hospitals [78, 119], though not all [104], and consistency in medium-secure hospitals [77, 120] and at prison and court triage assessments for all levels [26, 27, 105].

It follows that when planning a model of care, the capacity to admit numbers of this order is essential, as is additional surge capacity. Modelling future needs should take account of annual admission rates and case mix (need for therapeutic security) and likely length of stay in half-lives.

Pathways Governance and Management

Modelling and prediction of secure bed need depends on reliable and consistent practice when triaging patients according to need for therapeutic security. The legal criteria for findings of unfitness to plead or stand trial and not criminally responsible by reason of mental illness are defined in law. However, clinical services increasingly use structured professional judgement instruments to assess need for therapeutic security in order to assist decision-makers regarding the appropriateness of detaining patients for treatment in high-, medium- or low-secure forensic hospitals [26, 77, 105, 121]. An admissions panel should act as gatekeeper and should then actively prioritise the waiting list for admission to the secure forensic hospital [77, 121].

This combination of structured professional judgement submitted to a decision support framework such as an admissions panel, leave panel or legal review board is designed to achieve this consistency, transparency and fairness. Similarly, the decision to move from high to medium to low security, from acute, to subacute, to medium or low security and the community, is heavily influenced by risk assessment using modern instruments to assist decision-making such as the Historical, Clinical and Risk Management (HCR)-20 [32, 79] and DUNDRUM toolkit [122–125]. A clinical audit of admissions using a validated instrument such as the DUNDRUM-1 triage security instrument [77, 78, 102, 104] would be an appropriate way of auditing this.

Progress along the pathway from admission and subacute to medium-secure and pre-discharge units is based on routine assessment of risk of violence [126–130] and suicide [128, 131] using structured professional judgement instruments in turn submitted to judgement support frameworks. In intensive care, acute and subacute settings, daily short-term assessments are used [132–134]. Equally important is the use of repeated measures of treatment programme completion (DUNDRUM-3) and forensic recovery (DUNDRUM-4) with measures of risk [64, 69, 122, 123, 135] to inform individual care planning and reports to Mental Health Review Boards.

Stratified Therapeutic Security and Active Management of Length of Stay

Acute Admission and Subacute Units

'Acute' here means requiring higher levels of care and more intensive or more complex treatments for a period of time which is taken to be dynamic. A 15-bed acute admission unit can accommodate 60 admissions per annum if the mean or median length of stay is approximately 90 days. Using the median as an estimate of half-life, 50% of admissions will be discharged in three months, 75% in six months and 87.5% in nine months. A 15-bed subacute admission unit can accommodate 15 admissions a year if the mean length of stay is limited to 12 months.

Intensive Care Unit

An intensive care unit with capacity of up to 10 patients should be supernumerary, with high staff-to-patient ratios and special skills in prevention and management of serious and frequent violence, in order to minimise use of restraint, seclusion and forced medication while aiming to achieve the goal of a 'zero' target for violence [136]. An intensive care unit for the most disruptive and challenging patients prevents loss of the therapeutic milieu in other units and is designed to minimise both injury and use of restrictive practices.

Medium-Term Medium-Secure Units

A governance structure should act as gatekeeper for passage between the subacute unit and the medium-term medium-secure units. Two 15-bed medium-term medium-secure wards can accommodate 10 admissions per annum if the mean or median length of stay is approximately three years. The emphasis here should be on intensive treatment to mitigate symptoms if this has not already been achieved, and on psychological and psychosocial interventions to reduce risk of future violence and the seriousness of violence.

A governance structure should act as gatekeeper and pathways manager between the medium-term medium-secure units and the pre-discharge unit which leads on to the community.

Slow-Stream Medium- and Low-Secure Units

Those who have treatment-resistant mental disorders or comorbidities including personality disorders or intellectual disabilities which impact on risk reduction, with persistent high levels of assaultiveness in hospital or risk of dangerous behaviour in the community, may need a slower-stream secure pathway [98, 119, 137–140]. Patients should be able to access slow-stream long-stay medium- or low-secure wards where the emphasis is on maintaining a safe therapeutic environment with quality-of-life activities for self actualisation and self-transcendence including education, occupation and creativity. If five patients move to this pathway each year, then a 20-bed slow-stream secure unit can remain accessible if the length of stay in that unit is four years; two 20-bed units can provide lengths of stay up to eight years; and three 20-bed units can remain accessible with lengths of stay in those units averaging 12 years.

Pre-Discharge Unit

A 20-bed pre-discharge unit can accommodate five admissions and discharges per annum if the mean or median length of stay is approximately four years, 10 admissions and discharges per annum with a mean or median length of stay of two years and 20 admissions and discharges per annum with a mean length of stay of one year. Most patients in such a unit should be capable of safely and reliably using unaccompanied leave in the community. Each patient is assessed each day for stability and short-term risk before accessing leave or other risk-tolerant programmes. There should be close attention to drug screening and searching for weapons and other contraband that might be brought back from leave. Typically this might include a two- or four-bed 'training apartment' where patients gain greater experience of independent living with occupational therapy and nursing support.

Specialist Pathways

Women generally make up 10–15% of patients in secure forensic hospitals, and for safety reasons require a single-sex ward [141], though many activities can be integrated with men patients. A minimum number is required to avoid mixing acutely unwell and high-risk patients with recovering and pre-discharge patients all in the one ward [142]. A 20-bed unit divided into a five-bed admission acute unit (20 acute admissions per annum with managed length of stay up to three months), a five-bed subacute unit (five of the 20 admissions could have a further 12 months of in-patient treatment) and a 10-bed medium-secure medium-term unit (divided into six treatment places and four rehabilitation and pre-discharge places) can accommodate two admissions a year with managed length of stay of five years before transitioning to supportive community places or to slow-stream secure units. A similar pathways design can be used for patients with intellectual or developmental disorders, acquired brain injury or other specialist needs.

Secure hospital provision for forensic child and adolescent patients may need further modification. A 10-bed unit can be organised in the same way, though with some difficulty.

Community Forensic Residences

Those who are on periods of trial leave in the community, or conditionally discharged for supervision in the community, may be placed in residential settings that also have a stratified system of therapeutic security, with minimal if any physical security but varying levels of relational and procedural therapeutic security. Staffing may vary from 24-hour nurse care to social care at varying levels, and frequent contact with the supervising community forensic mental health team. Patients may progress from higher to lower levels of support and supervision over time, until they settle in independent living or find the level of support necessary to remain stable and achieve their personal optimum recovery goals in a forensic context [143, 144]. Patients may be reintegrated into community mental health teams at the point of transition into the community (an integrated model), remain supervised by a forensic psychiatry service in the community (a parallel model) or reintegrate sometime after transition to the community [100, 145–147].

Higher ratios of staff to patients (high quantitative relational security) can be provided as specialist bespoke packages of care. These can safely accommodate even high-risk patients in the absence of locked secure environmental settings. These are increasingly common in longer-term provision for adolescents and in developmental and intellectual disability services. The level of risk and seriousness of risk that can be accommodated is limited by the tolerance for injury and adverse events to carers and in the local community, and by the expense of these highly resourced services.

Active Management of Length of Stay

This basic model supposes that a 90–100-bed male secure hospital pathway would, subject to the governance of a medically led admissions panel and subject to interactions with the courts, admit 60 patients per annum, of whom 45 would have a managed length of stay of approximately three months before returning to the criminal justice system or stepping down via the courts to community mental health teams; the remaining 15 would spend a further 12 months in a subacute unit. Five of these would then move to the criminal justice system or to community mental health teams. Ten of these would progress to medium-secure wards, having received a forensic mental health disposal from the courts.

An additional gatekeeping governance structure is required here. Two 15-bed medium-term medium-secure wards would admit and discharge 10 patients in a mean of three years. During that period, intensive psychological and psychosocial treatments should be delivered and outcomes assessed. Subject to evidence of progress and a further gatekeeping governance structure, 10 patients per annum could progress from the medium-secure wards to a 20-bed pre-discharge ward, with a view to two years' intensive rehabilitation and preparation for supervision and conditional discharge in supportive community places where further progression towards less structured, less highly staffed places would occur in accordance with the capacities of the patient. In the alternative, five of the 10 patients would progress to the pre-discharge ward each year, where four years would be available for rehabilitation and transition to the community. The other five patients, if assessed as unlikely to progress to the community in the medium term, would take a different pathway to a slow-stream secure ward or cluster of wards organised according to levels of need for therapeutic security and other specialist needs. Some alternative possible organisations of pathways and processes within secure forensic hospitals will be mentioned towards the end of this section.

Continuity of Care

Continuity of care is an essential aspect of qualitative relational security. A detailed knowledge of the history and the personality, dispositions and traits of each patient and of the milieu is central to the prevention of violence, the maintenance of therapeutic security and the provision of effective treatment and care. A number of systems for continuity of care can be compared. There may be one consultant psychiatrist-led team per ward. This is helpful for nurses who have to service only one ward round a week and can expect consistency. However, consultant forensic psychiatrists and other members of the multidisciplinary team will need to have wider horizons to maintain their expertise, including prison, community and court work. A more common solution is to operate wards in clusters – for example, acute and subacute, medium, pre-discharge and community. Two consultants will then follow their patients along a coherent part of the pathways, while also taking a role in the gatekeeping and transfer processes. With ward managers and senior allied health professionals, consistency can be expected in the planning of care and treatment according to individual and aggregated patient needs. For patients, changes of primary nurse, key workers and consultants represent a process of learning to develop and cultivate professional and supportive relationships [63, 148] with appropriate boundaries [50, 149] that avoid excessive personal dependence. This is essential for successful supervision in the community over periods of years.

A multidisciplinary team is not a transdisciplinary group or a committee. There are well-developed descriptions of how a medical team engages in dynamic decision-making, drawing on diverse skills but also drawing on first-hand knowledge based on work patterns and carefully observing levels of responsibility allocated according to experience and expertise [150]. The decision-making process in multidisciplinary teams is hierarchical, with the senior physician or psychiatrist defined as 'expert' while psychiatrists in training and nurses have related roles in gathering and collating information with specialist advice from other disciplines, and the final synthesis of information requires the overview, knowledge, experience and responsibility of the expert team leader [151, 152]. There is much evidence that each discipline contributes qualitatively different elements to the individual care and treatment plan, but there is little if any evidence that multidisciplinary teams as shared decision-makers achieve any measurable benefit in terms of improved risk assessment or management, shortened length of stay or improved patient satisfaction. Multidisciplinary teams impose administrative burdens on time [153] and reduce available face-to-face time for direct patient therapeutic contact. As a way of working, this can also lead to confusion regarding boundaries within the team and regarding clinical responsibility [154].

Model of Care: Treatments

Specialist Treatments

Treatment includes, but is not limited to, medical, psychological and/or social care for therapeutic purposes. It may serve to reduce the risk posed by the person and may include measures to improve the social dimension of the offender's life [155]. As a tertiary referral service, forensic mental health services should be able to provide specialist treatment programmes and interventions. The purpose of therapeutic security is to provide an environment where treatments can be delivered safely [8, 38] without fear of violence or aggression, including bullying and intimidation [41]. The primary goal of treatment may be aimed at the patient's specific mental illness, often in the context of treatment-resistant, life-shortening mental illnesses and complex comorbidities. In acute and intensive care settings there is a need for expert prescribing of bespoke medication and use of de-escalation and other skills, deployed as part of a highly skilled set of practices, in a proportionate way to prevent imminent violence or further violence [136]. There is also a need to deliver specialist treatments to reduce the risk of future violence and offending and to reduce the seriousness of any future risk of violence or adverse event [156].

Treatment Structures

Reviewing delinquency and violence, McGuire [157] concluded that the best evidence was for multimodal treatment programmes. For forensic patients with severe mental illnesses such as schizophrenia, the success of these treatments depends on successful pharmacological and biological treatments as a first step, and a safe, therapeutic milieu. A structuralist analysis suggests that secure forensic hospitals, like psychiatric services generally, deliver treatment programmes in seven domains or 'pillars'. These can be broadly classified as (i) physical health [158] which gained acute importance during the COVID-19 pandemic; (ii) mental health; (iii) substance misuse disorders; (iv) problem behaviours and criminogenic needs [159]; (v) self-care and activities of daily living; (vi) education occupation and creativity; and (vii) family relationships and intimacy [160, 161].

Treatment Frequency and Duration

McGuire [157] and Wampold [55] suggest that much greater attention should be paid to issues such as frequency and duration of each treatment programme, broadly understandable as 'dose'. In general each programme can be delivered in three phases: a short introductory phase that can be delivered in acute and subacute units, a substantive phase which may consist of multiple treatment programmes within each domain, and a maintenance, self-maintenance or 'recovery' phase, often commencing in the context of supervised or conditional discharge [162].

Tiered Skills and Individualised Treatment

While introductory phases of treatment can be delivered as Tier 1 or Tier 2 interventions, substantive programmes generally require Tier 3 or Tier 4 skills for the therapists or for the leaders of the programme. This enables the tailoring of treatments to the needs and neurocognitive learning style of the patient and an estimate of the likely dose–response relationship [163].

For example, within the pillar of mental health a patient with cognitive impairment arising from schizophrenia or a developmental disorder may commence interventions under the heading of mental health with anti-psychotic medication to achieve remission or minimise delusions, hallucinations, thought disorder and abnormal mood. This permits a cognitive remediation programme [164] to further optimise memory and concentration. This may be followed by a programme of metacognitive therapy [165, 166], addressing, for example, 'jumping to conclusions bias' or 'bias against disconfirmatory evidence'. Impaired capacity to generate alternative explanations may be more difficult to remedy. These are designed to enable the patient to benefit from further cognitive behaviour therapies or other forms of intervention. It should be possible to deliver talking therapies even while patients are at their most disturbed and most at risk of imminent violence, for example while in seclusion [136] or in an intensive care unit. This will present architectural challenges [49] as well as requirements for relational therapeutic security capacity.

Treatment Resources

The quality network for secure psychiatric services sets as a standard that every patient should have 25 hours a week of structured activities [167]. In the absence of better evidence regarding the relationship between 'dose' in terms of hours of face-to-face time with a therapist. and response or 'health gain' in terms of reduction in risk and the seriousness of risk and reduction in length of stay (the logic model), a reasonable goal is to deliver five hours a week of face-to-face interventions in four core therapy domains mental health, substance misuse, problem behaviours as criminogenic need and formal family therapy. The remaining 20 hours should be made up of activities of daily living and education, occupation and creativity focusing on quality of life [168], self-actualisation [68] and self-transcendence [125].

If each therapist can deliver 20 hours a week of face to face time with patients, then to deliver five hours a week of face-to-face core therapy time for 100 patients (500 hours) would require 25 whole-time equivalents of therapists with appropriate skills. The remainder of each therapist's time would be made up of supervision, training, treatment planning and related administrative burden. If face-to-face time is made up of three hours of one-to-one sessions and a two-hour group session consisting of eight patients and two therapists, this would require 17.5 whole-time equivalents. Further resource planning is required to ensure that therapists can deliver appropriately tiered therapies. Much attention is required to ensure that rooms in safe environments are available and scheduled to ensure access to treatment. Attention is also required to ensure that therapists are not diverted from face-to-face contact with patients by administrative and regulatory burden. Failure to deliver effective treatments at a frequency and duration that is effective is probably the single greatest failure of modern forensic mental health services [169–171]. Systems for measurement of input already exist [172].

Individual Care and Treatment Plans

Individual care and treatment plans are typically drafted very soon after admission and are revised in the light of reassessment and progress at least every six months, typically before a legal review of detention. These can be used at the individual level and at the aggregated level to assess need for general and specific treatment programmes. A governance system is required to ensure that needs are continuously aggregated in some meaningful way so that resources are systematically and flexibly brought to bear to meet these treatment needs. This is the first part of the 'logic model' of the model of care.

Model of Care: Evaluation

The logic model relates inputs (skilled resources and the therapeutic risks managed to deliver them) to outputs (health gains and recovery, specifically forensic recovery). The second essential part of the 'logic model' is a process of evaluation, relating the use of resources to the achievement of health gains. Evaluating outcomes is too important to be unresourced, unstructured and informal. An evaluation process is itself a marker of service quality and excellence.

The goals set by the model of care comprise outcomes that must be continuously evaluated. Three types of measure are typically taken as evaluations of the success of a model of care: key performance indicators, routine outcome measures and assessment of fidelity to the model.

Key Performance Indicators

Key performance indicators are of interest to public health programmes and to the commissioners of the service. Key performance indicators are usually expressed in terms of the population served. They may be designed for accountability concerning accessibility, equitably, effectiveness, efficiency and sustainability (see Table 7.1).

Further examples might include violent incidents/100 admissions per annum or per 100 beds per annum; self-harm incidents/100 admissions per annum and per 100 beds per annum; and escape incidents from within the secure campus per 100 patients per annum and absconding while on leave, per 1,000 episodes of day leave per annum.

Routine Outcome Measures

Routine outcome measures typically reflect clinician- and patient-focussed concerns for health gains and recovery. Routine outcome measures can be considered under four headings: personal recovery, symptomatic recovery, functional recovery and forensic / civil recovery [173] (see Table 7.2).

Forensic Recovery

Forensic or 'civil' recovery can be measured in milestones concerning increasing autonomy, responsibility and independence.

Symptomatic Recovery

Symptomatic recovery measures are important for alleviating suffering and distress as well as managing risk of violence and suicide.

Table 7.1 Performance measures

Item	Definition	Goals	Measures	Timescale
Accessibility	Ease of access	Admission criteria international guide 0.7/100,000/year	Admissions per 100,000 population per year	Annual
Equitability	Non-discrimination	Equality of access Equitability of access	Admissions per 100,000 by region, corrected for demographics and social variables	Annual
Effectiveness	Discharge rate	Objective return to functional autonomy and safety	Discharges per 100 beds and per 100 clinicians	Annual
	Moves to less secure places	Objective reduction in secure dependency needs	Positive moves per 100 beds and per 100 clinicians	Annual
Efficiency	Health gains per unit resource		Discharges per 100 beds per discharges per 100 clinicians	Annual
			Moves to less secure places per 100 beds per 100 clinicians	Annual
Sustainability	Year-on-year levels of service should not trend down	All of the above sustained over five-year periods		Five-year periods

Functional Recovery

Functional recovery is increasingly recognised as one of the most important goals of treatment in psychiatry. Forensic patients achieve functional recovery when they achieve their greatest potential for safe and independent living. This is typically measured in global occupational, social and symptomatic functioning, Functional capacity measures are described in Chapter 6.

Table 7.2 Four recoveries and routine outcome measures

Four Recoveries	Definition	Goals	Measures
Forensic / civil recovery	Ability to live safely with minimal secure care	Reduced need for therapeutic security	DASA; DRILL; HCR–20 dynamic; DUNDRUM–3; DUNDRUM–4
	Minimal substituted decision-making	Increasing autonomy	MacArthur Competence Assessment Tools Conditional discharge; absolute discharge
		Increasing responsibility	Concordance (minimal gap between staff-rated and patient-rated DUNDRUM–3 and DUNDRUM–4)
		Stability, insight, leave, working alliance, social integration	DUNDRUM–4
Symptomatic recovery	Subjective and objective signs and symptoms of illness or disorder	Reducing suffering	PANSS YMS HADS
		Reducing anger	Novaco B DASA
Functional recovery	Fulfilling roles in social, occupational and family life	Increasing independence	GAF/SOFAS AMPS-Process MCCB
		Resilience	Treatment completion, e.g. DUNDRUM–3
		Stress tolerance and coping skills	SAPROF
		Adjustment	CGI-C

Table 7.2 (cont.)

Four Recoveries	Definition	Goals	Measures
Personal recovery	Sense of personal control or agency	Working alliance and trust	Perceived coercion WAI/ITP
	Satisfaction with life and environment	–	EssenCES WHO-QOL
	Feeling safe		EssenCES
	Hope	Motivation	DUNDRUM–4 item 7

DASA: Dynamic Appraisal of Situational Aggression; DRILL: DUNDRUM Restrictions and Intrusions on Liberty Ladders; HCR-20: Historical, Clinical and Risk Management-20; PANSS: Positive and Negative Symptom Scale; YMS: Young Mania Scale; HADS: Hamilton Anxiety and Depression Scale; GAF: Global Assessment of Function; SOFAS: Social Occupational Function Assessment Scale; AMPS: Assessment of Motor and Process Skills; MCCB: Matrix Consensus Cognitive Battery; SAPROF: Structured Assessment of PROtective Factors for Violence; CGI-C: Clinical Global Impression-Corrections; WAI: Working Alliance Inventory; ITP: Interpersonal Trust in Physician; EssenCES: Essen Climate Evaluation Scale; WHO-QOL: World Health Organisation Quality of Life.

Personal Recovery

Personal recovery includes the generally recognised concept of subjective recovery measured by patient-reported outcome measures and patient-reported experience measures.

Assessment of Fidelity to the Model of Care

An assessment of fidelity to the model (so-called implementation science) is necessary for complex models of care such as a secure forensic hospital or a forensic mental health service. Implementation fidelity is 'the degree to which ... programs are implemented ... as intended by the program developers' (p. 1). This idea is sometimes also termed 'integrity' [174]. Implementation fidelity acts as a potential moderator of the relationship between interventions and their intended outcomes. This is also necessary so that 'mission drift' [175] is avoided, focus on the goals is maintained over the planned lifetime of the model of care and any future revision of the model of care will be informed by the evidence of the evaluations. Lack of fidelity to a model can lead to false pessimism about effectiveness of a treatment, intervention, programme or model of care [176, 177]; lack of fidelity can also lead to mistaken beliefs about untreatability or treatment resistance of the individual patient. In both instances, the most common reason for failure of a treatment that is otherwise known to be effective is failure to deliver, either systemically or through lack of adherence or compliance or through misdiagnosis. Barriers to implementation may include staff attitudes, difficulty engaging employers, and lack of performance indicators relevant to the model of care and facilitators, including the support of service managers and outside groups [178].

Measurement-Based Care

Measurement-based care is the practice of basing clinical care on patient data collected throughout treatment [179]. Although measurement in psychiatric treatment is not new, it is not yet standard clinical practice [180]; forensic psychiatry services are evidence driven and lend themselves to this excellent and progressive approach [181]. Measures of the four recoveries should be repeated at intervals of six months in a medium-term course of treatment in a secure forensic hospital. These should be reported to mental health review tribunals or boards as part of the treating consultant psychiatrist's report to the review board. This creates a virtuous cycle of transparency and goal-setting for the patient so that the review board hearing becomes a motivational engine for recovery. This also enables the active management of length of stay by focusing treatment resources on those most in need.

Variants of the Standard Model of Care

Much depends on the size of the population served.

Integrated Campus and Full Pathways Integration

In many jurisdictions, forensic mental health services are organised to serve population aggregates of 3 to 5 million. In the provinces of Canada and the states of Australia or the Länder of Germany, this allows a single integrated service to provide high, medium and low levels of therapeutic security on a single campus with seamless moves of patients between levels according to individual need. A critical mass can also be achieved to enable not only stratification according to levels of therapeutic security and risk but also specialised pathways in parallel groups such as women (typically 10–15% of forensic patients), patients with intellectual and developmental disorders, patients for whom complex needs arise mainly from personality disorders and other small specialist groups (elderly patients, patients with acquired brain injury, long-term/slow-stream patients).

Very Small Services or Small Populations

Very small services (20 to 30 beds) may not be able to stratify without architectural and staffing resources and improvisations. When patients are treated and discharged all in the same ward, this may be viable for very short-term crisis admissions but is disruptive for patients on the same wards engaged in medium-term treatments and rehabilitation.

Very Large Populations and Services

Very large populations (15 to 20 million) may opt to provide single highly specialised (Tier 4) high-security hospitals that are separate from multiple medium-secure and low-secure hospitals (serving 2 to 5 million). This requires strong central governance to ensure that patients do not suffer excessive delays when ready to move between levels of therapeutic security.

Long-Term Secure Care

There are predictable though small numbers of new long-stay patients who will continue to accumulate in forensic secure hospital services [101, 182] even when able to progress to less secure places [99] or to community high-support places [36, 96, 100, 183]. Those with lengths of stay over five years [138], or who have not progressed to safe discharge after three prolonged courses of treatment (in the Dutch TBS system of secure forensic clinics, three periods of treatment of three years each, usually in three different TBS clinics), may require a different approach. The characteristics of this group of patients may consist of those with very high levels of need for therapeutic security on admission [103], continuing high levels of need for therapeutic security and high levels of risk [119] or failure to progress in treatment programmes to reduce violence and risk [69, 122]. Appropriate services such as the model service in Zeeland are clear that providing for this group is their goal [184]. The model of care emphasises modified treatment goals such as quality of life [185], self-actualisation (self-expression through creativity) and self-transcendence (an appreciation of belonging, whether to a small group or to a society or culture) [119].

Prison In-Reach Services

A recent systematic review describes prison mental health services in terms of screening, triage, assessment, intervention and reintegration [186].

Prison In-Reach and Court Liaison Services

Prison in-reach services work best when closely integrated between court liaison and diversion services and remand prisons (jails) for those awaiting trial [23, 26, 29, 187, 188]. Systematic screening of all those received at such a prison works best as a two-stage process though unfortunately these seldom report their sensitivity or specificity. The disorders screened for typically include psychosis, major mood disorders, active suicidality or withdrawal from alcohol or other intoxicants [186]. A triage decision is then required regarding the appropriate level of care and treatment [26, 102]. This should lead seamlessly to court liaison, diversion to community mental health services or referral to a forensic hospital. This is an essential protection for the rights of the mentally ill, particularly when imprisonment can be related to mental health service strain at community and tier 2 level [6, 7].

Continuity and Monitoring in Sentenced Prisons

For prisoners in sentenced prisons, a system of psychiatric continuity of care and monitoring is necessary. This should also work best when closely integrated within the forensic mental health service and secure forensic hospital.

Integrated and Parallel Community Aftercare

Patients admitted to acute or subacute wards in a secure forensic hospital then diverted from the criminal justice system to community mental health services can best be thought of as following a pathway that is integrated between forensic and general adult mental health services. Patients conditionally discharged following a finding of not criminally responsible and medium- or longer-term treatment in a secure forensic hospital are most often placed in specialist community residences with high levels of community support. These patients are often followed both therapeutically and from the point of view of monitoring and supervision by community forensic mental health teams – a so-called parallel model. These may also be integrated with probation, parole and other voluntary sector agencies. This sort of forensic mental health pathway can be described as 'parallel' to general adult and community mental health services. It is in the interests of recovery and de-stigmatisation that reintegration into mainstream services should always remain as a medium- or longer-term goal [189].

Conclusions: Quality, Excellence and Dynamic Systems

Forensic psychiatry services may to some extent be a bellwether for both positive and problematic aspects of the larger model of care for mental health for a population, and may be the first places to see signs of service strain elsewhere [6, 7, 11, 190]. There are well-developed benchmark standards for quality of secure forensic services [75] described in this chapter. Where a service falls below any of these standards, it is not too difficult to correct this. Tertiary highly specialised services should also aim for excellence. This is particularly important in forensic services and low-volume, high-risk, high-cost services. Excellence is the process of leading continuous improvement of outcomes for patients through the virtuous cycle of research, development, teaching and training. Services that manage serious risks must ensure long-term sustainability and resilience. Investing in excellence and setting this as a key priority and value is essential [2].

References

1. Fallon PBR, Edwards B, Daniels G. *Report of the Committee of Inquiry into the Personality Disorder Unit, Ashworth Special Hospital.* London, The Stationery Office, 1999.

2. Kennedy HG, Simpson A, Haque Q. Perspective on excellence in forensic mental health services: what we can learn from oncology and other medical services. *Frontiers in Psychiatry* 2019; 10: 733.

3. Kennedy HG. Models of care in forensic psychiatry. *BJPsych Advances* 2021: 1–14.

4. Agency for Clinical Innovation. *Understanding the Process to Develop a Model of Care: An ACI Framework.*

Version 1.0, May. Chatsworth New South Wales Australia, NSW Agency for Clinical Innovation, 2013.

5. Collins H, Evans R. *Rethinking Expertise.* Chicago, IL, University of Chicago Press, 2008.

6. O'Grady J. The complementary roles of regional and local secure provision for psychiatric patients. *Health Trends* 1990; 22 (1): 14–16.

7. O'Reilly R, Allison S, Bastiampiallai T. Observed outcomes: an approach to calculate the optimum number of psychiatric beds. *Administration and Policy in Mental Health and Mental Health Services* 2019; 46 (4): 507–17.

8. Kennedy H. Therapeutic uses of security: mapping forensic mental health services by stratifying risk. *Advances in Psychiatric Treatment* 2002; 8 (6): 433–43.

9. Von Bertalanffy L. The meaning of general system theory. *General System Theory: Foundations, Development, Applications* 1973: 30–53.

10. Noble D. Claude Bernard, the first systems biologist, and the future of physiology. *Experimental Physiology* 2008; 93 (1): 16–26.

11. Yoon J, Domino ME, Norton EC, Cuddeback GS, Morrissey JP. The impact of changes in psychiatric bed supply on jail use by persons with severe mental illness. *The Journal of Mental Health Policy and Economics* 2013; 16 (2): 81–92.

12. Grove P, Macleod J, Godfrey D. Forecasting the prison population. *OR Insight* 1998; 11 (1): 3–9.

13. McLaren N. A critical review of the biopsychosocial model. *Australian & New Zealand Journal of Psychiatry* 1998; 32 (1): 86–92.

14. Harrison GW, Millard PH. Balancing acute and long-term care: the mathematics of throughput in departments of geriatric medicine. *Methods of Information in Medicine* 1991; 30 (3): 221–8.

15. McClean SI, Millard PH. Go *with the Flow: A Systems Approach to Healthcare Planning.* London, Royal Society of Medicine Press, 1996.

16. Millard PH, McClean SI. *Modelling Hospital Resource Use: A Different Approach to the Planning and Control of Health Care Systems.* London, Royal Society of Medicine Press, 1994.

17. Falk M. Secure facilities in local psychiatric hospitals. In Gostin L (ed.) *Secure Provision.* London, Tavistock, 1985.

18. Kinsman L, Rotter T, James E, Snow P, Willis J. What is a clinical pathway? Development of a definition to inform the debate. *BMC Medicine* 2010; 8 (1): 31.

19. Aspland E, Gartner D, Harper P. Clinical pathway modelling: a literature review. *Health Systems* 2021; 10 (1): 1–23.

20. James D. Court diversion at 10 years: can it work, does it work and has it a future? *The Journal of Forensic Psychiatry* 1999; 10 (3): 507–24.

21. Shaw J, Creed F, Price J, Huxley P, Tomenson B. Prevalence and detection of serious psychiatric disorder in defendants attending court. *The Lancet* 1999; 353 (9158): 1053–6.

22. Purchase ND, McCallum AK, Kennedy HG. Evaluation of a psychiatric court liaison scheme in north London. *BMJ* 1996; 313 (7056): 531–2.

23. Pierzchniak P, Purchase N, Kennedy H. Liaison between prison, court and psychiatric services. *Health Trends* 1997; 29 (1): 26–9.

24. Holloway J, Shaw J. Providing a forensic psychiatry service to a magistrates' court: a follow-up study. *The Journal of Forensic Psychiatry* 1993; 4 (3): 575–81.

25. Greenberg D, Nielsen B. Moving towards a statewide approach to court diversion services in NSW. *New South Wales Public Health Bulletin* 2003; 14 (12): 227–9.

26. O'Neill C, Smith D, Caddow M et al. STRESS-testing clinical activity and outcomes for a combined prison in-reach and court liaison service: a 3-year observational study of 6177 consecutive male remands. *International Journal of Mental Health Systems* 2016; 10: 67.

27. Jones RM, Patel K, Simpson AIF. Assessment of need for inpatient treatment

for mental disorder among female prisoners: a cross-sectional study of provincially detained women in Ontario. *BMC Psychiatry* 2019; 19 (1): 98.

28. Steel J, Thornicroft G, Birmingham L et al. Prison mental health inreach services. *British Journal of Psychiatry* 2007; 190 (5): 373–4.

29. Simpson AIF, Jones RM. Two challenges affecting access to care for inmates with serious mental illness: detecting illness and acceptable services. *The Canadian Journal of Psychiatry* 2018; 63 (10): 648–50.

30. Giblin Y, Kelly A, Kelly E, Kennedy HG, Mohan D. Reducing the use of seclusion for mental disorder in a prison: implementing a high support unit in a prison using participant action research. *International Journal of Mental Health Systems* 2012; 6 (1): 2.

31. Forrester A, Till A, Simpson A, Shaw J. Mental illness and the provision of mental health services in prisons. *British Medical Bulletin* 2018; 127 (1): 101–9.

32. Doyle M, Power LA, Coid J et al. Predicting post-discharge community violence in England and Wales using the HCR-20V3. *International Journal of Forensic Mental Health* 2014; 13 (2): 140–7.

33. Pratt D, Piper M, Appleby L, Webb R, Shaw J. Suicide in recently released prisoners: a population-based cohort study. *The Lancet* 2006; 368 (9530): 119–23.

34. Smith D, Harnett S, Flanagan A et al. Beyond the walls: an evaluation of a Pre-Release Planning (PReP) programme for sentenced mentally disordered offenders. *Frontiers in Psychiatry* 2018; 9: 549.

35. Cohen A, Eastman N. *Assessing Forensic Mental Health Need: Policy, Theory and Research*. London, RCPsych Publications, 2000.

36. Shaw J, Davies J, Morey H. An assessment of the security, dependency and treatment needs of all patients in secure services in a UK health region. *The Journal of Forensic Psychiatry* 2001; 12 (3): 610–37.

37. Kennedy HG. Therapeutic uses of security: mapping forensic mental health services by stratifying risk. *Advances in Psychiatric Treatment* 2002; 8 (6): 433–43.

38. Kaye C, Franey A. *Managing High Security Psychiatric Care*. London, Jessica Kingsley Publishers, 1998.

39. Crichton JHM. Defining high, medium, and low security in forensic mental healthcare: the development of the Matrix of Security in Scotland. *The Journal of Forensic Psychiatry & Psychology* 2009; 20 (3): 333–53.

40. Broderick C, Azizian A, Kornbluh R, Warburton K. Prevalence of physical violence in a forensic psychiatric hospital system during 2011–2013: patient assaults, staff assaults, and repeatedly violent patients. *CNS Spectrums* 2015; 20 (3): 319–30.

41. Sekol I, Farrington DP, Ireland JL. Bullying in secure settings. *Journal of Aggression, Conflict and Peace Research* 2016; 8 (2).

42. Department of Health. *Environmental Design Guide: Adult Medium Secure Services*. 15 April 2011.

43. Reed JL. *Report of the Working Group on High Security and Related Psychiatric Provision*. London, Department of Health, 1994.

44. Tilt RPB, Martin C, Maguire N, Preston M. *Report of the Review of Security at the High Security Hospitals*. London, Department of Health, 2000.

45. Hinton R, Kaye C, Franey A. The physical environment. *Managing High Security Psychiatric Care* 1998: 85–98.

46. Reed J. *Review of Health and Social Services for Mentally Disordered Offenders and Others Requiring Similar Services*. London, HM Stationery Office, 1992.

47. Newman O. *Defensible Space: People and Design in the Violent City*. London, Architectural Press, 1973.

48. Georgiou MNP, Jethwa J, Townsend K. *Physical Security in Secure Care*. London, Royal College of Psychiatrists Centre for Quality Improvement, 2020.

49. Seppanen A, Tormanen I, Shaw C, Kennedy H. Modern forensic psychiatric hospital design: clinical, legal and

structural aspects. *International Journal of Mental Health Systems* 2018; 12: 58.

50. Tighe J, Gudjonsson GH. See, Think, Act Scale: preliminary development and validation of a measure of relational security in medium- and low-secure units. *The Journal of Forensic Psychiatry & Psychology* 2012; 23 (2): 184–99.

51. James DV, Fineberg NA, Shah AK, Priest RG. An increase in violence on an acute psychiatric ward: a study of associated factors. *British Journal of Psychiatry* 1990; 156: 846–52.

52. Siu BW-M, Au-Yeung CC-Y, Chan AW-L et al. Measuring the profiles of the security needs of forensic psychiatric inpatients: validation of the See, Think, Act Scale. *Asia-Pacific Psychiatry* 2019; 11 (2): e12341.

53. Allen E. *See Think Act: Relational Security in Secure Mental Health Services*. London, Department of Health, 2010.

54. Doyle M, Jones P. Hodges' Health Career Model and its role and potential application in forensic mental health nursing. *Journal of Psychiatric and Mental Health Nursing* 2013; 20 (7): 631–40.

55. Wampold BE. How important are the common factors in psychotherapy? An update. *World Psychiatry: Official Journal of the World Psychiatric Association (WPA)* 2015; 14 (3): 270–7.

56. Bowers L, Alexander J, Bilgin H et al. Safewards: the empirical basis of the model and a critical appraisal. *Journal of Psychiatric and Mental Health Nursing* 2014; 21 (4): 354–64.

57. Allen E. *Your Guide to Relational Security: See Think Act*. London, Royal College of Psychiatrists Quality Network for Forensic Mental Health, 2016.

58. Chester V, Alexander RT, Morgan W. Measuring relational security in forensic mental health services. *BJPsych Bulletin* 2017; 41 (6): 358–63.

59. Priebe S, Kelley L, Omer S et al. The effectiveness of a patient-centred assessment with a solution-focused approach (DIALOG+) for patients with psychosis: a pragmatic cluster-randomised controlled trial in community care. *Psychotherapy and Psychosomatics* 2015; 84 (5): 304–13.

60. Omer S, Golden E, Priebe S. Exploring the mechanisms of a patient-centred assessment with a solution focused approach (DIALOG+) in the community treatment of patients with psychosis: a process evaluation within a cluster-randomised controlled trial. *PLoS One* 2016; 11 (2): e0148415.

61. Anthony WA. Recovery from mental illness: the guiding vision of the mental health service system in the 1990s. *Psychosocial Rehabilitation Journal* 1993; 16 (4): 11.

62. Warner R. Does the scientific evidence support the recovery model? *The Psychiatrist* 2010; 34 (1): 3–5.

63. Donnelly V, Lynch A, Devlin C et al. Therapeutic alliance in forensic mental health: coercion, consent and recovery. *Irish Journal of Psychological Medicine* 2011; 28 (1): 21–8.

64. McCullough S, Stanley C, Smith H et al. Outcome measures of risk and recovery in Broadmoor High Secure Forensic Hospital: stratification of care pathways and moves to medium secure hospitals. *BJPsych Open* 2020; 6 (4): e74.

65. Livingston JD, Nijdam-Jones A, Lapsley S, Calderwood C, Brink J. Supporting recovery by improving patient engagement in a forensic mental health hospital: Results from a demonstration project. *Journal of the American Psychiatric Nurses Association* 2013; 19 (3): 132–45.

66. Pouncey CL, Lukens JM. Madness versus badness: the ethical tension between the recovery movement and forensic psychiatry. *Theoretical Medicine and Bioethics* 2010; 31 (1): 93–105.

67. Simpson AI, Penney SR. The recovery paradigm in forensic mental health services. *Criminal Behaviour and Mental Health* 2011; 21 (5): 299–306.

68. Roychowdhury A. Bridging the gap between risk and recovery: a human needs approach. *The Psychiatrist* 2011; 35 (2): 68–73.

69. Davoren M, Hennessy S, Conway C et al. Recovery and concordance in a secure forensic psychiatry hospital: the self rated DUNDRUM-3 programme completion and DUNDRUM-4 recovery scales. *BMC Psychiatry* 2015; 15: 61.

70. Katsakou C, Bowers L, Amos T et al. Coercion and treatment satisfaction among involuntary patients. *Psychiatric Services* 2010; 61 (3): 286–92.

71. Hansson L, Björkman T, Priebe S. Are important patient-rated outcomes in community mental health care explained by only one factor? *Acta Psychiatrica Scandinavica* 2007; 116 (2): 113–18.

72. Stensgaard L, Andersen MK, Nordentoft M, Hjorthøj C. Implementation of the safewards model to reduce the use of coercive measures in adult psychiatric inpatient units: An interrupted time-series analysis. *Journal of Psychiatric Research* 2018; 105: 147–52.

73. Department of Health and Social Care. *Guidance on the High Security Psychiatric Services (Arrangements for Safety and Security) Directions 2019*. London, Community and Social Care/Mental Health, Disability and Dementia/Mental Health Policy, 2019.

74. Department for Health and Social Security. *High Security Psychiatric Services (Arrangements for Safety and Security) Directions 2019*. London, gov.uk, 2019.

75. Aimola L, Jasim S, Tripathi N et al. Impact of peer-led quality improvement networks on quality of inpatient mental health care: study protocol for a cluster randomized controlled trial. *BMC Psychiatry* 2016; 16 (1): 331.

76. Kennedy HG, Simpson A, Haque Q. Perspective on excellence in forensic mental health services: what we can learn from oncology and other medical services. *Frontiers in Psychiatry* 2019; 10.

77. Freestone M, Bull D, Brown R et al. Triage, decision-making and follow-up of patients referred to a UK forensic service: validation of the DUNDRUM toolkit. *BMC Psychiatry* 2015; 15: 239.

78. Williams HK, Senanayke M, Ross CC, Bates R, Davoren M. Security needs among patients referred for high secure care in Broadmoor Hospital England. *BJPsych Open* 2020; 6 (4): e55.

79. Crocker AG, Nicholls TL, Charette Y, Seto MC. Dynamic and static factors associated with discharge dispositions: the National Trajectory Project of Individuals Found Not Criminally Responsible on Account of Mental Disorder (NCRMD) in Canada. *Behavioral Sciences & the Law* 2014; 32 (5): 577–95.

80. Gordon H, Oyebode O, Minne C. Death by homicide in special hospitals. *Journal of Forensic Psychiatry* 1997; 8 (3): 602–19.

81. Völlm BA, Bickle A, Gibbon S. Incidents of hostage-taking in an English high-secure hospital. *The Journal of Forensic Psychiatry & Psychology* 2013; 24 (1): 16–30.

82. Wilkie T, Penney SR, Fernane S, Simpson AI. Characteristics and motivations of absconders from forensic mental health services: a case-control study. *BMC Psychiatry* 2014; 14 (1): 91.

83. Simpson AIF, Penney SR, Fernane S, Wilkie T. The impact of structured decision making on absconding by forensic psychiatric patients: results from an A-B design study. *BMC Psychiatry* 2015; 15 (1): 103.

84. Learmont J. *Review of Prison Service Security in England and Wales and the Escape from Parkhurst Prison on Tuesday 3rd January 1995*. London, HM Stationery Office, 1995.

85. Woodcock SJ. *Report of the Enquiry into the Escape of Six Prisoners from the Special Security Unit at Whitemoor Prison, Cambridgeshire, on Friday 9th September 1994*. London, HM Stationery Office, 1994.

86. Simpson AI, Chatterjee S, Darby P et al. Management of COVID-19 Response in a Secure Forensic Mental Health Setting: Réponse à la gestion de la COVID-19 dans un établissement sécurisé de santé mentale et de psychiatrie légale. *The Canadian Journal of Psychiatry* 2020; 65 (10): 695–700.

87. Kennedy HG, Mohan D, Davoren M. Forensic psychiatry and Covid-19: accelerating transformation in forensic psychiatry. *Irish Journal of Psychological Medicine* 2020: 1–26.

88. Horsky J, Schiff GD, Johnston D et al. Interface design principles for usable decision support: a targeted review of best practices for clinical prescribing interventions. *Journal of Biomedical Informatics* 2012; 45 (6): 1202–16.

89. Patel VL, Cohen TA, Murarka T et al. Recovery at the edge of error: debunking the myth of the infallible expert. *Journal of Biomedical Informatics* 2011; 44 (3): 413–24.

90. Patel VL, Cytryn KN, Shortliffe EH, Safran C. The collaborative health care team: the role of individual and group expertise. *Teaching and Learning in Medicine* 2000; 12: 117–32.

91. Patel VL, Groen GJ, Arocha JF. Medical expertise as a function of task difficulty. *Memory & Cognition* 1990; 18: 394–406.

92. Darzi A. *A High Quality Workforce: NHS Next Stage Review*. London, Department of Health, 2008.

93. Nicol E. Improving clinical leadership and management in the NHS. *Journal of Healthcare Leadership* 2012; 4: 59–69.

94. Priest RG, Fineberg N, Merson S, Kurian T. Length of stay of acute psychiatric inpatients: an exponential model. *Acta Psychiatrica Scandinavica* 1995; 92 (4): 315–17.

95. Sharma A, Dunn W, O'Toole C, Kennedy HG. The virtual institution: cross-sectional length of stay in general adult and forensic psychiatry beds. *International Journal of Mental Health Systems* 2015; 9 (1): 25.

96. Shah A, Waldron G, Boast N, Coid JW, Ullrich S. Factors associated with length of admission at a medium secure forensic psychiatric unit. *The Journal of Forensic Psychiatry & Psychology* 2011; 22 (4): 496–512.

97. Harty M-A, Shaw J, Thomas S et al. The security, clinical and social needs of patients in high security psychiatric hospitals in England. *The Journal of Forensic Psychiatry & Psychology* 2004; 15 (2): 208–21.

98. Völlm BA, Edworthy R, Huband N et al. Characteristics and pathways of long-stay patients in high and medium secure settings in England: a secondary publication from a large mixed-methods study. *Frontiers in Psychiatry* 2018; 9.

99. Pierzchniak P, Farnham F, Taranto N et al. Assessing the needs of patients in secure settings: a multi-disciplinary approach. The Journal of Forensic Psychiatry 1999; 10 (2): 343–54.

100. Sharma A, Dunn W, O'Toole C, Kennedy HG. The virtual institution: cross-sectional length of stay in general adult and forensic psychiatry beds. *International Journal of Mental Health Systems* 2015; 9: 25.

101. O'Neill C, Heffernan P, Goggins R et al. Long-stay forensic psychiatric inpatients in the Republic of Ireland: aggregated needs assessment. *Irish Journal of Psychological Medicine* 2003; 20 (4): 119–25.

102. Flynn G, O'Neill C, McInerney C, Kennedy HG. The DUNDRUM-1 structured professional judgment for triage to appropriate levels of therapeutic security: retrospective-cohort validation study. *BMC Psychiatry* 2011; 11: 43.

103. Davoren M, Byrne O, O'Connell P et al. Factors affecting length of stay in forensic hospital setting: need for therapeutic security and course of admission. *BMC Psychiatry* 2015; 15: 301.

104. Habets P, Jeandarme I, Kennedy HG. Applicability of the DUNDRUM-1 in a forensic Belgium setting. *Journal of Forensic Practice* 2019; 21 (1): 85–94.

105. Jeandarme I, Habets P, Kennedy H. Structured versus unstructured judgment: DUNDRUM-1 compared to court decisions. *International Journal of Law and Psychiatry* 2019; 64: 205–10.

106. Habets P, Jeandarme I, Kennedy HG. Determining security level in forensic psychiatry: a tug of war between the

DUNDRUM toolkit and the HoNOS-Secure. *Psychology, Crime & Law* 2020: 1–19.

107. Eastman N, Bellamy S. Admission Criteria for Secure Services Schedule (ACSeSS). London, St Georges Hospital Medical School, 1998.

108. Pinals DA FW, Warburton K, Wik A, Hollen V, Fisher WH. *Forensic Patients in State Psychiatric Hospitals: 1999–2016.* Alexandria, VA, National Association of State Mental Health Program Directors, Directors NAoSMHP, 2017. Report No. 9.

109. Salize HJ, Dressing H. Admission of mentally disordered offenders to specialized forensic care in fifteen European Union member states. *Social Psychiatry and Psychiatric Epidemiology* 2007; 42 (4): 336–42.

110. NHS Digital. *Mental Health Act Statistics, Annual Figures: 2016–17, Experimental Statistics.* London, NHS Digital, 2017.

111. Gupta S, Akyuz EU, Baldwin T, Curtis D. Community treatment orders in England: review of usage from national data. *BJPsych Bulletin* 2018; 42 (3): 119–22.

112. Chow WS, Priebe S. How has the extent of institutional mental healthcare changed in Western Europe? Analysis of data since 1990. *BMJ Open* 2016; 6 (4): e010188.

113. Tomlin J, Lega I, Braun P et al. Forensic mental health in Europe: some key figures. *Social Psychiatry and Psychiatric Epidemiology* 2020: 1–9.

114. DeTaranto N, Bester P, Pierczhniak P, Mccallum A, Kennedy H. Medium secure provision in NHS and private units. *The Journal of Forensic Psychiatry* 1998; 9 (2): 369–78.

115. Coid J, Kahtan N, Cook A, Gault S, Jarman B. Predicting admission rates to secure forensic psychiatry services. *Psychological Medicine* 2001; 31 (3): 531.

116. Kennedy HG, Iveson RC, Hill O. Violence, homicide and suicide: strong correlation and wide variation across districts. *British Journal of Psychiatry* 1999; 175: 462–6.

117. O'Neill C, Kelly A, Sinclair H, Kennedy H. Deprivation: different implications for forensic psychiatric need in urban and rural areas. *Social Psychiatry and Psychiatric Epidemiology* 2005; 40 (7): 551–6.

118. Davoren M, Byrne O, O'Connell P et al. Factors affecting length of stay in forensic hospital setting: need for therapeutic security and course of admission. *BMC Psychiatry* 2015; 15 (1): 301.

119. Eckert M, Schel SH, Kennedy HG, Bulten BH. Patient characteristics related to length of stay in Dutch forensic psychiatric care. *The Journal of Forensic Psychiatry & Psychology* 2017; 28 (6): 863–80.

120. Lawrence D, Davies TL, Bagshaw R et al. External validity and anchoring heuristics: application of DUNDRUM-1 to secure service gatekeeping in South Wales. *BJPsych Bulletin* 2018; 42 (1): 10–18.

121. Williams HK, Senanayke M, Ross CC, Bates R, Davoren M. Security needs among patients referred for high secure care in Broadmoor Hospital, England. *BJPsych Open* 2020; 6 (4).

122. Davoren M, Abidin Z, Naughton L et al. Prospective study of factors influencing conditional discharge from a forensic hospital: the DUNDRUM-3 programme completion and DUNDRUM-4 recovery structured professional judgement instruments and risk. *BMC Psychiatry* 2013; 13: 185.

123. Davoren M, O'Dwyer S, Abidin Z et al. Prospective in-patient cohort study of moves between levels of therapeutic security: the DUNDRUM-1 triage security, DUNDRUM-3 programme completion and DUNDRUM-4 recovery scales and the HCR-20. *BMC Psychiatry* 2012; 12: 80.

124. Adams J, Thomas SD, Mackinnon T, Eggleton D. The risks, needs and stages of recovery of a complete forensic patient cohort in an Australian state. *BMC Psychiatry* 2018; 18 (1): 35.

125. Wharewera-Mika J, Cooper E, Wiki N et al. The appropriateness of DUNDRUM-3 and DUNDRUM-4 for

Māori in forensic mental health services in New Zealand: participatory action research. *BMC Psychiatry* 2020; 20 (1): 1–9.

126. Müller-Isberner R, Webster CD, Gretenkord L. Measuring progress in hospital order treatment: relationship between levels of security and C and R scores of the HCR-20. *International Journal of Forensic Mental Health* 2007; 6 (2): 113–21.

127. Pillay SM, Oliver B, Butler L, Kennedy HG. Risk stratification and the care pathway. *Irish Journal of Psychological Medicine* 2008; 25 (4): 123–7.

128. Abidin Z, Davoren M, Naughton L et al. Susceptibility (risk and protective) factors for in-patient violence and self-harm: prospective study of structured professional judgement instruments START and SAPROF, DUNDRUM-3 and DUNDRUM-4 in forensic mental health services. *BMC Psychiatry* 2013; 13: 197.

129. Dolan M, Blattner R. The utility of the Historical Clinical Risk-20 Scale as a predictor of outcomes in decisions to transfer patients from high to lower levels of security: a UK perspective. *BMC Psychiatry* 2010; 10 (1): 76.

130. Dolan M, Khawaja A. The HCR–20 and post-discharge outcome in male patients discharged from medium security in the UK. *Aggressive Behavior: Official Journal of the International Society for Research on Aggression* 2004; 30 (6): 469–83.

131. SanSegundo MS, Ferrer-Cascales R, Bellido JH et al. Prediction of violence, suicide behaviors and suicide ideation in a sample of institutionalized offenders with schizophrenia and other psychosis. *Frontiers in Psychology* 2018; 9: 1385.

132. Ogloff JR, Daffern M. The dynamic appraisal of situational aggression: an instrument to assess risk for imminent aggression in psychiatric inpatients. *Behavioral Sciences & the Law* 2006; 24 (6): 799–813.

133. Hvidhjelm J, Sestoft D, Skovgaard LT et al. Aggression in psychiatric wards: effect of the use of a structured risk assessment. *Issues in Mental Health Nursing* 2016; 37 (12): 960–7.

134. Maguire T, Daffern M, Bowe SJ, McKenna B. Evaluating the impact of an electronic application of the Dynamic Appraisal of Situational Aggression with an embedded Aggression Prevention Protocol on aggression and restrictive interventions on a forensic mental health unit. *International Journal of Mental Health Nursing* 2019; 28 (5): 1186–97.

135. Kennedy HG, Davoren M, O'Flynn P, O'Sullivan OP. How to measure progress in forensic care. In Birgit Vollm PB (ed.) *Long-Term Forensic Psychiatric Care: Clinical, Ethical and Legal Challenges.* Cham, Switzerland Springer International Publishing, 2019, pp. 103–21.

136. Kennedy HG, Mullaney R, McKenna P et al. A tool to evaluate proportionality and necessity in the use of restrictive practices in forensic mental health settings: the DRILL tool (Dundrum restriction, intrusion and liberty ladders). *BMC Psychiatry* 2020; 20 (1): 515.

137. Reed J. The need for longer term psychiatric care in medium or low security. *Criminal Behaviour and Mental Health* 1997; 7 (3): 201–12.

138. Huband N, Furtado V, Schel S et al. Characteristics and needs of long-stay forensic psychiatric inpatients: a rapid review of the literature. *International Journal of Forensic Mental Health* 2018; 17 (1): 45–60.

139. Völlm B, Edworthy R, Holley J et al. A mixed-methods study exploring the characteristics and needs of long stay patients in high and medium secure settings in England: implications for service organisation. *Health Services and Delivery Research* 2017; 5 (11): 1–234.

140. O'Neill C, Heffernan P, Goggins R et al. Long-stay forensic psychiatric inpatients in the Republic of Ireland: aggregated needs assessment. *Irish Journal of Psychological Medicine* 2003; 20 (4): 119–25.

141. Mezey G, Hassell Y, Bartlett A. Safety of women in mixed-sex and single-sex

medium secure units: staff and patient perceptions. *British Journal of Psychiatry* 2005; 187: 579–82.

142. Harty M, Somers N, Bartlett A. Women's secure hospital services: national bed numbers and distribution. *The Journal of Forensic Psychiatry & Psychology* 2012; 23 (5–6): 590–600.

143. Davoren M, Hennessy S, Conway C et al. Recovery and concordance in a secure forensic psychiatry hospital: the self rated DUNDRUM-3 programme completion and DUNDRUM-4 recovery scales. *BMC Psychiatry* 2015; 15 (1): 61.

144. Adams J, Thomas SDM, Mackinnon T, Eggleton D. The risks, needs and stages of recovery of a complete forensic patient cohort in an Australian state. *BMC Psychiatry* 2018; 18 (1): 35.

145. Coid JW, Hickey N, Yang M. Comparison of outcomes following after-care from forensic and general adult psychiatric services. *British Journal of Psychiatry* 2007; 190: 509–14.

146. Leonard SJ, Webb RT, Shaw J. Service transitions, interventions and care pathways following remittal to prison from medium secure psychiatric services in England and Wales: national cohort study. *BJPsych Open* 2020; 6 (5): e80.

147. Snowden P, McKenna J, Jasper A. Management of conditionally discharged patients and others who present similar risks in the community: integrated or parallel? *The Journal of Forensic Psychiatry* 1999; 10 (3): 583–96.

148. Donnelly V, Lynch A, Mohan D, Kennedy HG. Working alliance, interpersonal trust and perceived coercion in mental health review hearings. *International Journal of Mental Health Systems* 2011; 5 (1): 29.

149. Allen E. *Your Guide to Relational Security: See, Think, Act*, 3rd ed. London, Royal College of Psychiatrists, 2023.

150. Patel VL, Kaufman DR, Magder SA. The acquisition of medical expertise in complex dynamic environments. In Ericsson A (ed.) *The Road to Excellence: The Acquisition of Expert Performance in the Arts and Sciences, Sports and Games.* Hillside, NJ, Lawrence Erlbaum Publishers, 1996, pp. 127–65.

151. Patel VL, Kaufman DR, Magder SA. The acquisition of medical expertise in complex dynamic environments. In Ericsson A (ed.) *The Road to Excellence: The Acquisition of Expert Performance in the Arts and Sciences, Sports and Games.* Hillside, NJ, Lawrence Erlbaum Publishers, 1996, pp. 127–65.

152. Galanter CA, Patel VL. Medical decision making: a selective review for child psychiatrists and psychologists. *Journal of Child Psychology and Psychiatry, and Allied Disciplines* 2005; 46 (7): 675–89.

153. Meehl PE. Why I do not attend case conferences. *Psychodiagnosis: Selected Papers* 1973: 225–302.

154. Haque Q, Webster CD. Staging the HCR-20: towards successful implementation of team-based structured professional judgement schemes. *Advances in Psychiatric Treatment* 2012; 18 (1): 59–66.

155. Council of Europe. *Dangerous Offenders: Recommendation CM/Rec(2014)3 and Explanatory Report.* Strasbourg, Council of Europe, 2014.

156. Richter MS, O'Reilly K, O'Sullivan D et al. Prospective observational cohort study of 'treatment as usual' over four years for patients with schizophrenia in a national forensic hospital. *BMC Psychiatry* 2018; 18 (1): 289.

157. McGuire J. A review of effective interventions for reducing aggression and violence. *Philosophical Transactions of the Royal Society of London Series B, Biological Sciences* 2008; 363 (1503): 2577–97.

158. Uhrskov Sørensen L, Bengtson S, Lund J, Ibsen M, Långström N. Mortality among male forensic and non-forensic psychiatric patients: matched cohort study of rates, predictors and causes-of-death. *Nordic Journal of Psychiatry* 2020: 1–8.

159. Clarke PDR, Gilchrist L, Johnstone L et al. Forensic mental health section. In NHS Education for Scotland (ed.) *The*

Matrix: A Guide to Delivering Evidence-Based Psychological Therapies in Scotland. Edinburgh, The Scottish Government, 2011, pp. 241–9.

160. Kennedy H. The DUNDRUM Toolkit V1.0.30. 2016.

161. Kennedy H, Castelletti L, O'Sullivan O. *Impact of Service Organisation on Teaching and Training*; a cross border study guide. In Goethals K (ed.) *Forensic Psychiatry and Psychology in Europe*. Cham, Springer, 2018, pp. 211–37.

162. Gunn J. Management of the mentally abnormal offender: integrated or parallel. *Journal of the Royal Society of Medicine* 1977; 70 (12): 877–80.

163. Campbell M. *The Matrix: A Guide to Delivering Evidence-Based Psychological Therapies in Scotland*. Edinburgh, The Scottish Government, 2011.

164. O'Reilly K, Donohoe G, O'Sullivan D et al. A randomized controlled trial of cognitive remediation for a national cohort of forensic patients with schizophrenia or schizoaffective disorder. *BMC Psychiatry* 2019; 19 (1): 27.

165. Moritz S, Kerstan A, Veckenstedt R et al. Further evidence for the efficacy of a metacognitive group training in schizophrenia. *Behaviour Research and Therapy* 2011; 49 (3): 151–7.

166. Naughton M, Nulty A, Abidin Z et al. Effects of group metacognitive training (MCT) on mental capacity and functioning in patients with psychosis in a secure forensic psychiatric hospital: a prospective-cohort waiting list controlled study. *BMC Research Notes* 2012; 5 (1): 302.

167. Worrall A. The service context for clinical guidelines: supporting guideline implementation by assuring and improving the quality of service in which clinicians work. *International Review of Psychiatry* 2011; 23 (4): 336–41.

168. O'Flynn P, O'Regan R, O'Reilly K, Kennedy HG. Predictors of quality of life among inpatients in forensic mental health: implications for occupational therapists. *BMC Psychiatry* 2018; 18 (1): 16.

169. Fortune Z, Rose D, Crawford M et al. An evaluation of new services for personality-disordered offenders: staff and service user perspectives. *International Journal of Social Psychiatry* 2010; 56 (2): 186–95.

170. Duggan C. Dangerous and severe personality disorder. *British Journal of Psychiatry* 2011; 198 (6): 431–3.

171. Tyrer P, Cooper S, Crawford M et al. The successes and failures of the DSPD experiment: the assessment and management of severe personality disorder. *Medicine, Science, and the Law* 2010; 50: 95–9.

172. Barrett B, Byford S. Collecting service use data for economic evaluation in DSPD populations Development of the Secure Facilities Service Use Schedule. The *British Journal of Psychiatry Supplement* 2007; 49: s75–8.

173. Kennedy HG, O'Reilly K, Davoren M, O'Flynn P, O'Sullivan OP. *How to Measure Progress in Forensic Care*. In Völm B, Braun P (eds) *Long-Term Forensic Psychiatric Care: Clinical, Ethical and Legal Challenges*. Cham, Springer, 2019, pp. 103–21.

174. Carroll C, Patterson M, Wood S et al. A conceptual framework for implementation fidelity. *Implementation Science* 2007; 2 (1): 40.

175. Bopp M, Saunders RP, Lattimore D. The tug-of-war: fidelity versus adaptation throughout the health promotion program life cycle. *The Journal of Primary Prevention* 2013; 34 (3): 193–207.

176. Vincent GM, Guy LS, Gershenson BG, McCabe P. Does risk assessment make a difference? Results of implementing the SAVRY in juvenile probation. *Behavioral Sciences & the Law* 2012; 30 (4): 384–405.

177. Vincent GM, Guy LS, Perrault RT, Gershenson B. Risk assessment matters, but only when implemented well: a multisite study in juvenile probation. *Law and Human Behavior* 2016; 40 (6): 683–96.

178. Talbot E, Bird Y, Russell J et al. Implementation of individual placement and support (IPS) into community

forensic mental health settings: lessons learned. *British Journal of Occupational Therapy* 2018; 81 (6): 338–47.

179. Scott K, Lewis CC. Using measurement-based care to enhance any treatment. *Cognitive and Behavioral Practice* 2015; 22 (1): 49–59.

180. Harding KJK, Rush AJ, Arbuckle M, Trivedi MH, Pincus HA. Measurement-based care in psychiatric practice: a policy framework for implementation. *The Journal of Clinical Psychiatry* 2011; 72 (8): 1136–43.

181. Glancy G, Choptiany M, Jones R, Chatterjee S. Measurement-based care in forensic psychiatry. *International Journal of Law and Psychiatry* 2021; 74: 101650.

182. Bulten E, Verkes RJ. Long stay in Europe: a systems-oriented approach. In Völlm B, Braun P (eds) *Long-Term Forensic Psychiatric Care: Clinical, Ethical and Legal Challenges*. Cham, Springer International Publishing, 2019, pp. 27–45.

183. Taylor PJ, Maden A, Jones D. Long-term medium-security hospital units: a service gap of the 1990s? *Criminal Behaviour and Mental Health* 1996; 6 (3): 213–29.

184. Smeekens MV, Braun P. Long-term forensic psychiatric care: the Dutch perspective. In Völlm B, Braun P (eds) *Long-Term Forensic Psychiatric Care: Clinical, Ethical and Legal Challenges*. Cham, Springer International Publishing, 2019, pp. 235–50.

185. Vorstenbosch ECW, Escuder-Romeva G. Quality of life in long-term clinical forensic psychiatry. In Völlm B, Braun P (eds) *Long-Term Forensic Psychiatric Care: Clinical, Ethical and Legal Challenges*. Cham, Springer International Publishing, 2019, pp. 139–59.

186. Simpson AIF, Gerritsen C, Maheandiran M et al. A systematic review of reviews of correctional mental health services using the STAIR framework. *Frontiers in Psychiatry* 2022; 12.

187. McInerney C, Davoren M, Flynn G et al. Implementing a court diversion and liaison scheme in a remand prison by systematic screening of new receptions: a 6 year participatory action research study of 20,084 consecutive male remands. *International Journal of Mental Health Systems* 2013; 7: 18.

188. Greenberg D, Nielsen B. Court diversion in NSW for people with mental health problems and disorders. *New South Wales Public Health Bulletin* 2002; 13 (7): 158–60.

189. Gunn J. *Management of the Mentally Abnormal Offender: Integrated or Parallel. Proceedings of the Royal Society of Medicine* 1977; 70 (12): 877–80.

190. Khosla V, Davison P, Gordon H, Joseph V. The interface between general and forensic psychiatry: the present day. *Advances in Psychiatric Treatment* 2014; 20 (5): 359–65.

Psychopharmacology of Chronic Aggression and Violence in Forensic Settings

Michael A. Cummings, Ai-Li W. Arias, George J. Proctor and Stephen M. Stahl

Introduction

Before the 1990s there had been considerable debate as to whether those individuals suffering with chronic severe mental illness exhibited elevated rates of aggression and violence compared to the general population. In 1990, Swanson et al. analysed data from the National Institute of Mental Health (NIMH) Epidemiological Catchment Area Surveys and concluded that although the mentally ill accounted for only around 5% of violent offences, they did exhibit elevated rates of aggressive and violent behaviour compared to the general population [1]. More recent observations have confirmed the conclusion of Swanson's analysis, finding that mentally ill individuals with a single prior offence were 3.97 times as likely to have further violent offences, while those with multiple prior violent offences were 6.18 times as likely as the general population to engage in further aggression and violence. Moreover, ratio comparisons to the general population were similar for men and women, as well as for psychotic and non-psychotic disorders among forensic mentally disordered samples [2]. Moreover, a 38-year total population study in Sweden found that persons suffering from chronic schizophrenia, the most represented group in forensic settings, showed elevated levels of violent offending, suicide and mortality compared to the general population. Men in this study had an elevated hazard ratio of 7.5 for violence, suicide and early mortality, while women exhibited a hazard ratio of 11.1 for the same variables [3]. These hazard ratios were significant at $P < 0.05$. Taken together, these and numerous smaller studies have confirmed that violent offending is a substantial problem in forensic psychiatric populations.

To effectively address persisting violence and aggression, it is vital that clinicians differentiate the source or sources of aggression and violence in a given case [4]. Note that in this context, aggression refers to a broad range of threats or acts that may psychologically or physically harm others or oneself. Violence is then defined as a subcategory of aggression characterised by physical acts that may lead to property damage or the injury or death of others. Considered broadly, persisting violent behaviour can be divided into three categories: psychotically driven violence based on persecutory thoughts and perceptions coupled with anger, impulsive violence related to affective arousal coupled with inadequate top-down inhibition of impulsive behaviour, and instrumental or predatory violence and aggression related to antisocial personality features. Substance use appears to add to violence risk for all three categories [4, 5]. Moreover, in forensic settings, impulsive violence appears to be most common, predatory violence next most common and psychotically driven violence least common [6]. It was noted that psychotically driven aggression and violence may be the least prevalent because this category has the largest and most effective array of pharmacological tools available to treat the underlying psychosis. In contrast, predatory or instrumental aggression and violence interventions are largely limited to custodial and psychosocial approaches, while impulsive aggression and violence involves a pleomorphic array of causes and a limited number of effective pharmacological interventions [7, 8, 4, 5]. Moreover, the majority of cases of persisting impulsive aggression and violence in forensic settings occur most frequently among individuals suffering from schizophrenia, traumatic brain injury (TBI) and neurocognitive disorders [4, 5].

The goal of this chapter is to give the reader a systematic approach to the assessment and treatment of aggression and violence arising from psychosis and a review of evidence-based pharmacological interventions for aggression and violence arising from impulsivity in the context of TBI or neurocognitive disorder. In turn, we will consider an algorithmic approach to the assessment and treatment of psychotically driven aggression and violence, the approach to treatment resistance in schizophrenia-spectrum disorders, data-supported treatment of aggression and violence related to TBI, and, finally, data-supported pharmacological treatment of aggression and violence in the context of major neurocognitive disorder.

Psychotically Driven Aggression and Violence

In community settings, the most common barriers to independent living, employment and stable interpersonal relationships for patients suffering from schizophrenia-spectrum disorders or other psychotic disorders are negative symptoms and cognitive deficits [9]. In contrast, severely mentally ill psychotic patients, often incarcerated or chronically institutionalised, more frequently experience substantial barriers related to positive psychotic symptoms leading to aggression or violence [10]. This is not to say that among the chronically institutionalised severely mentally ill population positive psychotic symptoms are the only or even majority source of aggressive and violent behaviours. As briefly referenced at the start of the chapter, a survey conducted within the California Department of State Hospitals, an approximately 7,000-bed system dedicated to the treatment of conserved and forensically committed patients, reviewed 839 episodes of aggression or violence by 88 persistently aggressive in-patients and found that 54% of such episodes were impulsive, 39% were predatory or instrumental, and 17% were psychotically driven [6]. Nevertheless, amelioration or control of positive psychotic symptoms commonly forms the initial treatment focus among the severely mentally ill [4].

Elevated dopamine signal transduction in the meso-limbic dopamine pathway (ventral tegmentum to temporal lobe) and/or inadequate top-down glutamate modulation of dopamine signalling in the meso-limbic dopamine circuit by frontal lobe structures is thought to underlie the expression of such positive psychotic signs and symptoms such as illusions, hallucinations, delusions and psychomotor agitation. Respectively, these views of the roles of dopamine and glutamate have been termed the dopamine and glutamate hypotheses of psychosis [11, 12].

As in all of medicine, the initial step in treatment is evaluation. Table 8.1 outlines the initial evaluation of patients in whom preliminary data points to positive psychotic signs and symptoms as a principal source of problematic behaviours and impairment of psychosocial functioning.

Table 8.1 Initial review and treatment of severely ill psychotic patients [39–43]

Decisions	Assessments	Brief Comments

Aggressive/violent behaviours arise from psychosis
• Yes, continue
• No, alternate treatment approaches
	Review prior history and assessments
	• Frequency of problem behaviours
	• Severity of problem behaviours
	• Patient factors associated with problem behaviours
	• Environmental factors associated with problem behaviours
	• Cause of latest decompensation
	• Comorbid violence factor
	  – Substance abuse
	  – Impulse dyscontrol
	  – Predatory violence	

Patient poses an immediate risk • Yes, then decide level of control • No, then repeat risk assessment as clinically indicated	Evaluate need for segregation or restraint • Clinical observation • Clinical interview • Use of rating scale, e.g. Dynamic Appraisal of Situational Aggression (DASA)	Be familiar with relevant regulations/procedures governing seclusion or use of physical restraints
Physical conditions contribute to behaviour risk • No, continue • Yes, treat physical condition	Physical evaluations • Psychomotor agitation • Evaluate for akathisia • Evaluate for pain or physical discomfort • Evaluate for delirium • Evaluate for intoxication or withdrawal • Evaluate for complex partial seizures • Evaluate sleep	

Abnormal labs contribute to problem behaviours

- Yes, correct underlying abnormality
- No, continue

Evaluation of laboratory data

- Plasma glucose
- Plasma calcium
- White blood cell count to rule out sepsis
- Infectious disease screens as clinically indicated
- Plasma sodium to rule out hyponatremia or hypernatremia
- Oxygen saturation if suspect
- Serum ammonia if suspect
- Thyroid status
- Sedimentation rate and C-reactive protein if history of inflammatory disease

Serum ammonia useful only if elements of delirium clinically present

A second important element in approaching the treatment of positive psychotic symptoms is evaluation of past treatment responses and of elements that may affect medication responses such as non-adherence to oral medications, altered medication kinetics or past pharmacodynamic issues. A systematic approach is described in Table 8.2.

After evaluation of the patient and of the patient's pharmacotherapy, the next step is to design the primary pharmacological approach to the patient's illness. In this context, it should be remembered that all medication trials have one of three end points: (1) the patient's illness improves; (2) intolerable adverse effects occur which cannot be adequately addressed to permit continuation of the medication trial; or (3) a point of futility is reached. An example of reaching a point of futility would be a patient whose olanzapine plasma concentration has reached approximately 150 ng/ml without improvement over four to six weeks. By a plasma concentration of approximately 150 ng/ml, olanzapine's receptor occupancy curve for dopamine D2 receptors has become very flat, such that doubling the drug's plasma concentration would increase receptor occupancy by only an additional 2–3%. More broadly, the point of futility is often described as the point at which further medication titration carries a < 5% chance of producing substantial clinical improvement [5]. An approach to a choice of a principal medication trial is outlined in Table 8.3.

In many cases of severe psychotic illness, even optimal anti-psychotic treatment may not adequately address all the patient's target symptoms. In this context, while the effect sizes of adjunctive treatments are typically modest, they may exert important effects on specific illness domains [13]. An outline of the approach to the use of adjunctive medications is given in Table 8.4.

While a patient's routine treatment regimen is expected to be the mainstay of pharmacological treatment, fluctuations in symptom severity or behaviour may require as needed or *pro re nata* (PRN) medications. This is especially true early in treatment prior to achieving an optimal response from the patient's routine psychopharmacological treatment. Principles and practice in using PRN or stat medications are described in Table 8.5.

An important issue among individuals suffering from psychotic severe mental illness is that a substantial portion of such patients are treatment resistant [14]. John Kane et al. defined treatment-resistant schizophrenia according to very stringent criteria. These included failures of three anti-psychotic trials of at least six weeks' duration at doses of at least 1000 mg chlorpromazine equivalents, absence of any period of good functioning during the prior five years and failure of a prospective high-dose (haloperidol 60 mg per day or greater) trial to produce a significant reduction in psychotic signs and symptoms [15]. Because the criteria created by Kane et al. are difficult to complete outside a research setting, treatment resistance has more recently been redefined as failure of two six-week trials of anti-psychotic medications from two different classes at doses of at least 600 mg chlorpromazine equivalents per day. If one of the anti-psychotics was a long-acting injectable formulation, then the trial duration should have been four months. One check of plasma concentration, as well as two other measures of medication adherence, was defined as a minimal requirement. Optimal assurance of medication adherence was held to include two measurements of plasma concentration separated by at least two weeks without informing the patient prior to laboratory sampling [12].

The development of treatment resistance is critically important because the vast majority of anti-psychotic medications become largely ineffective in this context. That

Table 8.2 Evaluation of psychopharmacology for severe psychosis [44, 45, 4]

Decisions	Assessments	Brief Comments
Inadequate treatment contributes • Yes, adjust treatment • No, observe treatment response	Evaluate adequacy of current treatment • Duration (4–6 weeks) • Dose (at least standard) • Dosing (e.g. with food if needed) • Adherence • Plasma concentrations • Hepatic inducers, e.g. carbamazepine or phenytoin	

Adverse medication effects present
 	
• Yes, adjust treatment or treat adverse effect
• No, continue
	Presence of adverse anti-psychotic effects
	• Neurological
	  – Akathisia
	  – Dystonia
	  – Parkinsonism
	• Sedation
	• Orthostasis
	
	Presence of adverse anticonvulsant effects
	• Ataxia
	• Tremor
	• Cognitive impairment
	
	Presence of adverse lithium effects
	• Polyuria
	• Nausea, vomiting, diarrhoea
	• Tremor
	• Cognitive impairment
		• Many adverse effects respond to time or gradual dose reduction

Table 8.2 (cont.)

Decisions	Assessments	Brief Comments
	Presence of adverse beta-blocker effects • Hypotension • Bronchospasm • Bradycardia	
Patient is responding to treatment • Yes, optimise and continue • No, alter treatment approach	Evaluate response to current treatment • Partial response • No response	• A partial response (< 20% to 30% improvement on the Positive and Negative Symptom Score (PANSS) or Brief Psychiatric Rating Scale (BPRS) with minimal or no adverse effects argues for a higher-dose trial of the present anti-psychotic • Failure of ≥ 2 adequate trials with at least one being a second-generation anti-psychotic argues for a clozapine trial • A partial response (small decline in BIS–11) with adequate anticonvulsant plasma concentrations argues for the addition of an anticonvulsant or other medication with distinct mechanism of action

Table 8.3 Principal medication choice (excluding elderly demented) [4, 5, 46]

Decisions	Assessments	Brief Comments
Patient responding to optimal treatment • Yes, continue • No, adjust treatment	Patient's frequency and severity of problem behaviours are improving with adequate dose and plasma concentration, then continue present treatment	Note that although no response by weeks 4 to 6 of adequate to high-dose treatment portends a poor outcome, many patients show ongoing improvement for many weeks to months following a favourable, albeit partial, response to early treatment
Patient response absent • Yes, check adherence • No, consider alternative treatment	Patient has demonstrated an inadequate response in problem behaviours frequency or severity to present anti-psychotic treatment • Adherent to oral medications • Not adherent to oral medications	• Preferred oral agents: amisulpride; olanzapine; fluphenazine; haloperidol • Preferred long-acting injectable agents: fluphenazine; haloperidol; paliperidone
Plasma concentrations are adequate • Yes, continue • No, adjust dosing or switch to long-acting injectable	Dosing and plasma concentrations (oral medications)	• Olanzapine: 40–60 mg/d with plasma concentration 120–150 ng/mL • Fluphenazine: 20–60 mg/d with plasma concentration 0.8–2.0 ng/mL • Haloperidol: 20–80 mg/d with plasma concentration 5–18 ng/mL
Plasma concentrations are adequate • Yes, continue • No, adjust dosing	Dosing and plasma concentrations (depot medications)	• Fluphenazine: 25–100 mg/14d with plasma concentration 0.8–2.0 ng/mL • Haloperidol: 200–300 mg/28d after loading with 200–300 mg weekly times 3 with steady state plasma concentrations 5–18 ng/mL • Paliperidone: 234 mg followed 1 week by 156 mg then continuing at 117–234 mg every 28d

Table 8.4 Adjunctive medications [47, 5]

Decisions	Assessments	Brief Comments
Mood stabilisers	• Irritability • Mood lability • Bipolar diathesis • Suicidality (lithium)	• Valproate (VPA) can be loaded at 20–30 mg/Kg, reaching steady state at circa 3 days • Lithium can be initiated at 600 mg once per day and titrated by 300 mg every other day to 900–1200 mg once per day. Lithium also can be loaded at 30 mg/Kg up to 3000 mg by giving 3 emergency room doses at 1600, 1800 and 2000 hours on day 1 and then measuring a plasma concentration the following morning. If the plasma concentration is < 1.0 mMol/L, then give 1200 mg immediate release (IR) q (once daily) at bedtime. If the plasma concentration is > 1.0 mMol/L, then give 900 mg IR q at bedtime. Once per day dosing spares renal function. Plasma concentrations should be 0.6–1.0 mMol/L • Lamotrigine may be helpful for dysphoric or negative symptoms but may promote hypomania or mania
Clonazepam	• Agitation or anxiety incompletely responsive to primary treatment	Dose at 0.5–2.0 mg TID and then taper as the patient stabilises. Avoid use in major neurocognitive disorders
SSRI antidepressants	• Residual negative symptoms • Impulsive behaviour or suicidality	Avoid use in patients in whom bipolarity may be present. May increase irritability in brain-injured or autism patients. Avoid use of fluvoxamine with clozapine or olanzapine, as fluvoxamine may increase clozapine or olanzapine plasma concentrations 5- to 10-fold
Sedatives	• Insomnia worsens irritability, dysphoria, agitation and mood lability in many patients	Note that antihistamines may cause idiosyncratic excitation and agitation and that diphenhydramine, but not hydroxyzine, will add to anticholinergic burden

	• Consider trials of zolpidem 5–10 mg at bedtime, eszopiclone 1–8 mg at bedtime, hydroxyzine 100 mg at bedtime, diphenhydramine 25–50 mg at bedtime or trazodone 25–100 mg at bedtime until the patient stabilises
Beta blockers	• Propranolol has excellent CNS penetration and the most evidence for response	Propranolol contraindicated in those with asthma. Monitor blood pressure to avoid hypotension
	• ECT	If adjunctive medications fail, then ECT should be considered. This is especially true if the patient is taking clozapine and continues to have inadequate response

Table 8.5 PRN and stat medications [48]

Decisions	Assessments	Brief Comments
Patient unstable · No, continue · Yes, provide frequent PRN or stat treatment	Estimate severity of agitation · Mild · Moderate · Severe	· For mild agitation, give lorazepam 1–2 mg or hydroxyzine 25–50 mg PO or IM every 2 hours not to exceed 4 doses per 24 hours. Titrate against agitation based on observation, not patient complaint · For moderate to severe agitation, give anti-psychotic ± lorazepam 2 mg ± diphenhydramine 25–50 mg or hydroxyzine 25–50 mg PO or IM not to exceed 4 doses per 24 hours (see caveats in text)
Stability improved · No, continue frequent PRN or stat medications and adjust primary treatment · Yes, simplify PRN and stat treatment and eventually discontinue	Estimate frequency of breakthrough agitation · Seldom · Moderately frequent · Very frequent	As determined by frequency and severity of breakthrough psychomotor agitation, gradually increase PRN dose interval and reduce the number of medications or doses prescribed. Once agitation is controlled, discontinue PRN orders for agitation

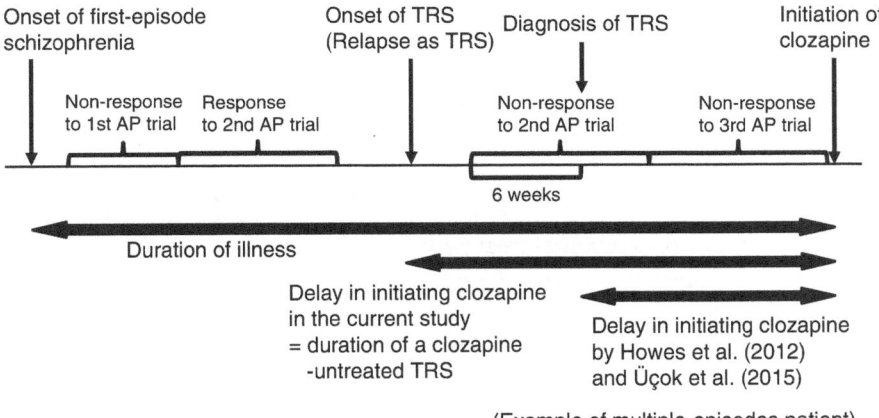

Figure 8.1 Delaying the time to starting clozapine reduces the likelihood of response in resistant schizophrenia.

is, response rates to almost all anti-psychotic medications are 0–5% in treatment-resistant psychosis. High-plasma-concentration olanzapine (120 ng/ml to 150 ng/ml) does slightly better at 7%. Fortunately, in treatment-resistant psychotic patients clozapine at plasma concentrations of 350 ng/ml to approximately 1000 ng/ml produces a decrease in psychotic signs and symptoms of at least 20–30% in up to 60% of such patients [15, 16]. Even clozapine, however, begins to show a decline in efficacy after resistant psychosis has been ongoing for > 2.8 years, arguing strongly for not delaying clozapine treatment among patients determined to be treatment resistant [17]. The decline in clozapine response is illustrated in Figure 8.1.

Clozapine has also been found to be effective in decreasing impulsive violence among schizophrenic individuals. In the New York State Hospital system, a 12-week-long, randomised, double-blind, parallel-group study of chronically physically assaultive non-treatment-resistant male in-patients with schizophrenia or schizoaffective disorder were prescribed either clozapine, olanzapine or haloperidol with no significant differences in change in PANSS scores across all three groups. However, the total aggression scores (Modified Objective Aggression Scale, MOAS) showed that clozapine significantly reduced verbal and physical aggression compared to haloperidol or olanzapine presumably due to related improvements in executive functions stemming from glutamate modulation in the prefrontal cortex. Because of its anti-aggressive property independent of its effect on psychosis, clozapine is the preferred agent for schizophrenia patients treated with optimal non-clozapine anti-psychotics who continue to have impulsive aggression [18].

One case series even suggested that clozapine may reduce violence among severely antisocial (psychopathic) individuals. A retrospective review of case notes and recorded violent or aggressive incidents for patients with a primary diagnosis of antisocial personality disorder (ASPD) and high psychopathy scores treated with clozapine was conducted. The researchers concluded that clozapine was beneficial in that it decreased impulsive behavioural dyscontrol and anger at lower plasma concentration levels of < 350 ng/mL (mean plasma concentration = 171 ng/ml) [19].

Take-Home Points

- Positive psychotic symptoms are frequently the cause of institutionalisation or incarceration for chronically severely mentally ill psychotic patients. Delusions associated with anger are a common pathway to aggressive and violent behaviour.
- Positive psychotic symptoms are driven by dopaminergic overactivity in the meso-limbic circuit, making dopamine antagonist anti-psychotics the first step in treatment.
- Failure to respond to two adequate dopamine antagonist anti-psychotic trials should strongly prompt consideration of treatment with clozapine.
- Even clozapine's superior anti-psychotic efficacy begins to fade after about 2.8 years of treatment-resistant status, indicating that use of clozapine should not be delayed in such cases.
- Clozapine reduces impulsive as well as psychotically driven aggression and violence, likely by improving executive cognitive functions.

Treatment of Aggression and Violence in TBI and Neurocognitive Disorders

Of the many behavioural disturbances associated with severe mental and neurocognitive disorders, impulsive behaviours, including agitation and aggression, present unique challenges. Frontal inhibition, cognitive impairments and executive dysfunction commonly combine to promote behavioural disturbances in severe mental and neurocognitive disorders, and this interplay between brain structures and circuits may explain a mechanism for the impulsive behaviours, agitation and aggression. A circuit of periaqueductal grey matter, hippocampus, amygdala and hypothalamus mediates threat response, a bottom-up impulse to be aggressive or violent. Prefrontal cortex (PFC) serves a top-down role to inhibit those bottom-up impulses, and PFC dysfunction impairs a person's ability to recognise social cues and increases the risk of impulsive aggressive responses by a person failing to make appropriate risk/reward assessments for inhibiting responses. Added sensory deficits in hearing, vision or pain together with sensory processing and appraisal deficits in cognition combine to foster behavioural disturbances of agitation, aggression and impulsive acts [20]. Of the PFC, specifically the ventromedial PFC and its connections to lower structures, such as the amygdala, serve this top-down inhibitory function [20, 5]. PFC–amygdala circuit connectivity is disrupted by dysfunction in associated serotonin and dopamine systems in several mental conditions. Enhancing serotonergic and dopaminergic signalling in and around this circuit provides a theoretical approach to pharmacologic agent selection for many of these behavioural disturbances. Severe mental and neurocognitive disorders, including TBI, often show pathology in the brain regions associated with top-down and bottom-up structures, as described earlier [21].

TBI occurs in 50 million persons globally [22]. Behavioural disturbances of concern in post-acute TBI include agitation, irritability, impulsive violence and aggression [5, 22]. There are few studies providing strong support for particular pharmacologic interventions in TBI. Systematic reviews reveal limited evidence of efficacy for individual agents. Nevertheless, there is data to suggest that certain medications can be used in a manner consistent with good clinical practice [5, 23].

Systematic reviews highlight trials of amantadine, propranolol and valproic acid as most supported for efficacy in TBI behavioural disturbances. Support from systematic reviews also exists for methylphenidate and carbamazepine, though the evidence for methylphenidate is not as strong as for the weak dopamine agonist amantadine, and use of carbamazepine has many disadvantages, including the need for slow titration to minimise ataxia, risk of hyponatremia and potent induction of both CYP 450 3A4 and the efflux transporter P-glycoprotein. Asian patients should be screened for the HLA-B*1502 allele due to its association with carbamazepine-induced Stevens-Johnson syndrome [24–26, 5, 27]. Antidepressants, in particular SSRIs, do show efficacy for depressive symptoms in TBI patients but not for aggression and agitation [28, 5]. Medication classes associated with only negative outcomes or side effects across multiple publications include benzodiazepines, phenytoin and opiates [22].

Importantly, while anti-psychotics have frequently been used to target agitation in TBI patients, a 2019 systematic review found that 'while the class may reduce agitation, it is advisable to consider if other classes, such as beta-blockers or anti-epileptics, might provide a similar effect' (p. 146) with greater literature support and lesser risks of cognitive decrements [22].

Major neurocognitive disorders (dementias) consist of a heterogeneous group of disorders, but the majority of studies have focussed on the most common type, Alzheimer's disease (AD), and to a lesser extent on vascular dementia.

Behavioural disturbances of most concern are similar to those found in TBI patients, though psychosocial interventions for dementias have the greatest literature support and are more likely to show effect in dementia patients, and, therefore, they should be considered before the addition of pharmacologic interventions.

Psychosocial interventions including correcting visual and hearing impairments, ensuring adequate lighting, alleviation of pain, empiric routine use of nonopioid analgesics when patients' verbal abilities are limited, bright light therapy and orientating strategies have modest efficacy data [5].

Acetylcholinesterase inhibitors (AChEIs) have the strongest evidence of the pharmacologic options supporting their use for behavioural disturbances associated with mild to moderate AD by delaying the progression of the underlying illness [29, 5]. Memantine has also shown low- to moderate-quality evidence of efficacy in AD both as monotherapy and combined with AChEIs [30, 5].

SSRI antidepressants have a significant efficacy for aggressive dementia patients such that a 2011 Cochrane review concluded SSRIs and trazadone seemed to be reasonably well tolerated compared to placebo and anti-psychotics. Of the SSRIs, citalopram and escitalopram are most studied but have QTc warnings, whereas sertraline does not and may be considered desirable from a drug–drug interaction risk standpoint as well [31, 5].

A large, naturalistic study from the US Veterans Health Administration (VHA) provided mortality risk estimates for various agents in a population of 46,008 veterans with dementia 65 years of age or older. The study clarified the risk–benefit landscape when treating behavioural disturbances in patients with dementia. The number needed to harm (NNH), with harm defined as mortality over six months, ranged for anti-psychotics from 8 for haloperidol to 31 for quetiapine. Antidepressant use, on the other hand, was associated with a decreased risk of mortality. Takeaways from this study include that anti-psychotics should not be considered as first-line agents in patients with dementia, and, if used, low doses of atypical anti-psychotics, such as risperidone 0.25 mg/d or quetiapine 25 mg bid, should be considered [32, 5]. Nevertheless, anti-psychotics may be considered in certain situations, such as continued agitation despite nonpharmacologic interventions, or when behavioural agitation or aggression are dangerous to the patient or others [33]. Atypical anti-psychotics, including aripiprazole, should be considered due to greater tolerability. Once used for four months, anti-psychotics may be tapered and discontinued often without worsening of behavioural disturbances [34, 33], with the possible exception of patients with significant psychosis [35, 33].

Evidence for use of anticonvulsants in dementia patients with behavioural disturbances is largely negative. In the VHA study, valproate was found to have a NNH of 20. Data with carbamazepine use is conflicting, and both tolerability and kinetic concerns limit its use. Low-dose lamotrigine (mean dose at study endpoint 46.3 ± 24.2 mg/d, range 25–100 mg/d) showed modest benefit in a 16-week trial with 40 in-patients to the extent that the doses of concomitant anti-psychotics could be lowered [36, 32, 37].

Finally, although benzodiazepines are occasionally used on an emergency basis for acute agitation, there is no evidence to support their efficacy for persistent aggression, with significant concerns about tolerability [38]. Relevant medications are summarised in Table 8.6.

Take-Home Points

- Aggressive and violent behavioural disturbances cause increased risk of physical harm for both patients and caregivers.
- For dementia, psychosocial treatments have stronger evidence supporting efficacy than pharmacological interventions.
- For patients with behavioural disturbance, few pharmacological interventions have strong evidence to support their use.
- All pharmacological interventions with evidence of efficacy for behavioural disturbance have adverse associated risks that must be taken into account when considering a patient's risk–benefit analysis for a particular medication. In particular, anti-psychotics worsen cognitive performance in TBI patients and increase mortality risk among elderly patients with major neurocognitive disorders.
- Note that some patients may require higher than cited anti-psychotic plasma concentrations to achieve stabilisation, such as haloperidol up to > 20 ng/mL or fluphenazine up to 4.0 ng/mL. In general, however, receptor saturation for haloperidol and fluphenazine occur at about 4.0 and 18.0 ng/ml, respectively. Note that in converting from oral haloperidol to haloperidol decanoate, haloperidol decanoate should be loaded at 10 times the daily oral dose, while maintenance dosing is 20 times the daily oral dose. If injections > 300 mg are needed, then increase dose frequency to twice per month.
- Caveats: whenever possible, choose an anti-psychotic that is also being used as part of the primary treatment. Available dose forms may limit this option.
- The most commonly prescribed PRN and stat anti-psychotics are haloperidol, fluphenazine, chlorpromazine, olanzapine and risperidone. Of these, haloperidol, fluphenazine, chlorpromazine, olanzapine and ziprasidone are available in oral and injectable formulations.
- Haloperidol and fluphenazine carry the highest risks of acute neurological adverse effects, especially given parenterally. Chlorpromazine carries a risk of orthostasis. Olanzapine is not effective orally due to an absorption time to peak plasma concentration of 6–9 hours. Olanzapine, especially at higher parenteral doses, is prone to cause severe orthostasis if combined with a benzodiazepine, usually lorazepam.

Table 8.6 Medications for behavioural disturbances [32, 5, 49, 33, 23, 50, 22]

Medication	Indications	Comments
AChEIs	Mild to moderate AD Dz No TBI indication	• Differential response among agents, so try another if first one fails • Not for acute agitation
Amantadine	No dementia indication Behavioural disturbance in TBI	
Anticonvulsants	Behavioural disturbance in dementia	• Scarce support of efficacy • Increased mortality risk with dementia • If used, consider: Valproate 40–60 mcg/mL Lamotrigine 25–100 mg/d
	Behavioural disturbance in TBI	• Positive findings supporting use • Carbamazepine has pharmacokinetic risks, ataxia, sedation, Stevens-Johnson risk in Asians make it less desirable • Phenytoin also has pharmacokinetic risks, side effects make it less desirable • Valproate has the most evidence support • Valproate 1000–1800 mg/d
Antidepressants	Behavioural disturbance in dementia	• Modest efficacy • SSRIs are the most studied for behavioural disturbance in dementia • Not effective for affective symptoms • Citalopram and escitalopram QT risks • Citalopram/escitalopram 10–20 mg/d
	Behavioural disturbance in TBI	Sertraline 25–100 mg/d Trazodone 12.5–200 mg/d (multiple daily dosing)

Table 8.6 (cont.)

Medication	Indications	Comments
		• Positive findings of weak quality
		• Have been helpful for depressive symptoms in TBI
Atypical anti-psychotics	Behavioural disturbance in dementia	• Increased mortality risk with dementia
		• Modest benefit for behavioural disturbances
		• More effective if psychosis present
		• Less effective if severe dementia
		• Try to taper after 4 months of use
		• Aripiprazole 2–10 mg/d
		• Olanzapine 5–10 mg/d
		• Risperidone 0.5–2.0 mg/d
		• Quetiapine 25–300 mg/d
	Behavioural disturbance in TBI	• No evidence of efficacy for routine use for behavioural disturbance in TBI
		• If used, only consider quick treatment of a few doses for severe agitation
		• Consider second line to amantadine, propranolol, valproate
(Typical) anti-psychotics	Avoid in either dementia or TBI	• Risks too high with dementia
		• No supporting evidence for TBI
Benzodiazepines	Behavioural disturbance in dementia	• Known risks, no substantial benefits – avoid
	Behavioural disturbance in TBI	• Mostly negative findings for efficacy
		• May use only short term for acute agitation
Buspirone	Behavioural disturbance in dementia	• No supporting evidence
	Behavioural disturbance in TBI	• Low level of evidence, may be considered second line

Dopamine agonists	Behavioural disturbance in dementia	• No supporting evidence
	Behavioural disturbance in TBI	• Amantadine has strongest evidence of efficacy of possible agents for behavioural disturbance in TBI
		• Initiate > 4 weeks post-TBI
		• Amantadine 100–300 mg/d
		• Methylphenidate only mixed efficacy data for anger, inferior to amantadine
Lithium	Behavioural disturbance in dementia	• No supporting evidence
	Behavioural disturbance in TBI	• Insufficient evidence to recommend
Propranolol	Behavioural disturbance in dementia	• No supporting evidence
	Behavioural disturbance in TBI	• Positive findings support for behavioural disturbance in TBI
		• Titrate to 40–80 mg/d

Intramuscular ziprasidone should be limited to two doses of 20 mg per 24 hours, especially if given in addition to oral ziprasidone.

- Diphenhydramine, but not hydroxyzine, adds to anticholinergic burden.
- Limit doses of potent dopamine antagonists in Parkinson's disease and major cognitive disorder with Lewy bodies. Pimavanserin and lumateperone may be better choices in these contexts. Limit benzodiazepine and anticholinergic use in all major neurocognitive disorders.

References

1. Swanson JW, Holzer CE, Ganju VK et al. Violence and psychiatric disorder in the community: evidence from the epidemiologic catchment area surveys [erratum appears in *Hospital & Community Psychiatry* 1991; 42 (9): 954–5]. *Hospital & Community Psychiatry* 1990; 41: 761–70.

2. Stevens H, Agerbo E, Dean K et al. Offending prior to first psychiatric contact: a population-based register study. *Psychological Medicine* 2012; 42: 2673–84.

3. Fazel S, Wolf A, Palm C et al. Violent crime, suicide, and premature mortality in patients with schizophrenia and related disorders: a 38-year total population study in Sweden. *Lancet Psychiatry* 2014; 1: 44–54.

4. Stahl SM, Morrissette DA, Cummings M et al. California State Hospital Violence Assessment and Treatment (Cal-VAT) guidelines. *CNS Spectrums* 2014; 19: 449–65.

5. Meyer JM, Cummings MA, Proctor G et al. Psychopharmacology of persistent violence and aggression. *Psychiatric Clinics of North America* 2016; 39: 541–56.

6. Quanbeck CD, McDermott BE, Lam J et al. Categorization of aggressive acts committed by chronically assaultive state hospital patients. *Psychiatric Services* 2007; 58: 521–8.

7. Kennedy HG. Therapeutic uses of security: mapping forensic mental health services by stratifying risk. *Advances in Psychiatric Treatment* 2002; 8: 433–43.

8. Bonta J, Andrews DA. *Risk-Need-Responsivity Model for Offender Assessment and Rehabilitation*. Ottawa, Her Majesty the Queen in Right of Canada, 2007.

9. Kaneko K. Negative symptoms and cognitive impairments in schizophrenia: two key symptoms negatively influencing social functioning. *Yonago Acta Medica* 2018; 61: 91–102.

10. Dack C, Ross J, Papadopoulos C et al. A review and meta-analysis of the patient factors associated with psychiatric in-patient aggression. *Acta Psychiatrica Scandinavica* 2013; 127: 255–68.

11. Merritt K, McGuire P, Egerton A. Relationship between glutamate dysfunction and symptoms and cognitive function in psychosis. *Frontiers in Psychiatry* 2013; 4: 151.

12. Howes OD, McCutcheon R, Agid O et al. Treatment-resistant schizophrenia: Treatment Response and Resistance in Psychosis (TRRIP) working group consensus guidelines on diagnosis and terminology. *The American Journal of Psychiatry* 2017; 174: 216–29.

13. Galling B, Roldan A, Hagi K et al. Antipsychotic augmentation vs. monotherapy in schizophrenia: systematic review, meta-analysis and meta-regression analysis. *World Psychiatry* 2017; 16: 77–89.

14. Nucifora FC Jr, Woznica E, Lee BJ et al. Treatment resistant schizophrenia: clinical, biological, and therapeutic perspectives. *Neurobiology of Disease* 2019; 131: 104257.

15. Kane J, Honigfeld G, Singer J et al. Clozapine for the treatment-resistant schizophrenic: a double-blind comparison with chlorpromazine. *Archives of General Psychiatry* 1988; 45: 789–96.

16. Stroup TS, Gerhard T, Crystal S et al. Comparative effectiveness of clozapine and standard antipsychotic treatment in adults with schizophrenia. *The American Journal of Psychiatry* 2016; 173: 166–73.

17. Yoshimura B, Yada Y, So R et al. The critical treatment window of clozapine in treatment-resistant schizophrenia: secondary analysis of an observational study. *Psychiatry Research* 2017; 250: 65–70.

18. Krakowski MI, Czobor P, Citrome L et al. Atypical antipsychotic agents in the treatment of violent patients with schizophrenia and schizoaffective disorder. *Archives of General Psychiatry* 2006; 63: 622–9.

19. Brown D, Larkin F, Sengupta S et al. Clozapine: an effective treatment for seriously violent and psychopathic men with antisocial personality disorder in a UK high-security hospital. *CNS Spectrums* 2014; 19: 391–402.

20. Siever LJ. Neurobiology of aggression and violence. *The American Journal of Psychiatry* 2008; 165: 429–42.

21. Rosenbloom MH, Schmahmann JD, Price BH. The functional neuroanatomy of decision-making. *The Journal of Neuropsychiatry and Clinical Neurosciences* 2012; 24: 266–77.

22. Nash RP, Weinberg MS, Laughon SL et al. Acute pharmacological management of behavioral and emotional dysregulation following a traumatic brain injury: a systematic review of the literature. *Psychosomatics* 2019; 60: 139–52.

23. Hicks AJ, Clay FJ, Hopwood M et al. The efficacy and harms of pharmacological interventions for aggression after traumatic brain injury-systematic review. *Frontiers in Neurology* 2019; 10: 1169.

24. Tangamornsuksan W, Chaiyakunapruk N, Somkrua R et al. Relationship between the HLA-B*1502 allele and carbamazepine-induced Stevens-Johnson syndrome and toxic epidermal necrolysis: a systematic review and meta-analysis. *JAMA Dermatology* 2013; 149: 1025–32.

25. Hammond FM, Bickett AK, Norton JH et al. Effectiveness of amantadine hydrochloride in the reduction of chronic traumatic brain injury irritability and aggression. *The Journal of Head Trauma Rehabilitation* 2014; 29: 391–9.

26. Sami MB, Faruqui R. The effectiveness of dopamine agonists for treatment of neuropsychiatric symptoms post brain injury and stroke. *Acta Neuropsychiatrica* 2015; 27: 317–26.

27. Hammond FM, Malec JF, Zafonte RD et al. Potential impact of amantadine on aggression in chronic traumatic brain injury. *The Journal of Head Trauma Rehabilitation* 2017; 32: 308–18.

28. Hammond FM, Sherer M, Malec JF et al. Amantadine effect on perceptions of irritability after traumatic brain injury: results of the amantadine irritability multisite study. *Journal of Neurotrauma* 2015; 32: 1230–8.

29. Cummings J, Lai TJ, Hemrungrojn S et al. Role of donepezil in the management of neuropsychiatric symptoms in Alzheimer's Disease and dementia with Lewy bodies. *CNS Neuroscience & Therapeutics* 2016; 22: 159–66.

30. Gareri P, Putignano D, Castagna A et al. Retrospective study on the benefits of combined memantine and cholinesterase inhibitor treatment in aged patients affected with Alzheimer's disease: the MEMAGE study. *Journal of Alzheimer's Disease* 2014; 41: 633–40.

31. Seitz DP, Adunuri N, Gill SS et al. Antidepressants for agitation and psychosis in dementia. *Cochrane Database of Systematic Reviews* 2011; CD008191.

32. Maust DT, Kim HM, Seyfried LS et al. Antipsychotics, other psychotropics, and the risk of death in patients with dementia: number needed to harm. *JAMA Psychiatry* 2015; 72: 438–45.

33. Deardorff WJ, Grossberg GT. Behavioral and psychological symptoms in Alzheimer's dementia and vascular dementia. *Handbook of Clinical Neurology* 2019; 165: 5–32.

34. Reus VI, Fochtmann LJ, Eyler AE et al. The American Psychiatric Association practice guideline on the use of antipsychotics to treat agitation or psychosis in patients with dementia. *The American Journal of Psychiatry* 2016; 173: 543–6.

35. Devanand DP, Mintzer J, Schultz S et al. The antipsychotic discontinuation in Alzheimer disease trial: clinical rationale and study design. *The American Journal of Geriatric Psychiatry* 2012; 20: 362–73.

36. Gallagher D, Herrmann N. Antiepileptic drugs for the treatment of agitation and aggression in dementia: do they have a place in therapy? *Drugs* 2014; 74: 1747–55.

37. Suzuki H, Gen K. Clinical efficacy of lamotrigine and changes in the dosages of concomitantly used psychotropic drugs in Alzheimer's disease with behavioural and psychological symptoms of dementia: a preliminary open-label trial. *Psychogeriatrics* 2015; 15: 32–7.

38. Tampi RR, Tampi DJ. Efficacy and tolerability of benzodiazepines for the treatment of behavioral and psychological symptoms of dementia: a systematic review of randomized controlled trials. *American Journal of Alzheimer's Disease & Other Dementias* 2014; 29: 565–74.

39. Ogloff JR, Daffern M. The dynamic appraisal of situational aggression: an instrument to assess risk for imminent aggression in psychiatric inpatients. *Behavioral Sciences & the Law* 2006; 24: 799–813.

40. Hankin CS, Bronstone A, Koran LM. Agitation in the inpatient psychiatric setting: a review of clinical presentation, burden, and treatment. *Journal of Psychiatric Practice* 2011; 17: 170–85.

41. Vaaler AE, Iversen VC, Morken G et al. Short-term prediction of threatening and violent behaviour in an Acute Psychiatric Intensive Care Unit based on patient and environment characteristics. *BMC Psychiatry* 2011; 11: 44.

42. Volavka J, Citrome L. Pathways to aggression in schizophrenia affect results of treatment. *Schizophrenia Bulletin* 2011; 37: 921–9.

43. Joshi A, Krishnamurthy VB, Purichia H et al. 'What's in a name?' Delirium by any other name would be as deadly: a review of the nature of delirium consultations. *Journal of Psychiatric Practice* 2012; 18: 413–18.

44. Ruberg SJ, Chen L, Stauffer V et al. Identification of early changes in specific symptoms that predict longer-term response to atypical antipsychotics in the treatment of patients with schizophrenia. *BMC Psychiatry* 2011; 11: 23.

45. Lopez LV, Kane JM. Plasma levels of second-generation antipsychotics and clinical response in acute psychosis: a review of the literature. *Schizophrenia Research* 2013; 147: 368–74.

46. Siskind D, Siskind V, Kisely S. Clozapine response rates among people with treatment-resistant schizophrenia: data from a systematic review and meta-analysis. *The Canadian Journal of Psychiatry* 2017; 62: 772–7.

47. Lally J, Tully J, Robertson D et al. Augmentation of clozapine with electroconvulsive therapy in treatment resistant schizophrenia: a systematic review and meta-analysis. *Schizophrenia Research* 2016; 171: 215–24.

48. Stein-Parbury J, Reid K, Smith N et al. Use of pro re nata medications in acute inpatient care. *Australian and New Zealand Journal of Psychiatry* 2008; 42: 283–92.

49. Plantier D, Luaute J. Drugs for behavior disorders after traumatic brain injury: systematic review and expert consensus leading to French recommendations for good practice. *Annals of Physical and Rehabilitation Medicine* 2016; 59: 42–57.

50. Keszycki RM, Fisher DW, Dong H. The hyperactivity-impulsivity-irritiability-disinhibition-aggression-agitation domain in Alzheimer's disease: current management and future directions. *Frontiers in Pharmacology* 2019; 10: 1109.

Ward Milieu and the Management of In-Patient Violence
Use of Seclusion and Other Restrictive Practices

Mary Davoren and Peter Turner

Introduction

Secure forensic mental health services provide care and treatment to mentally disordered offenders with a history of serious violence [1]. While most violence in the community is not linked to mental disorder, it is important for all clinicians in mental health services to acknowledge that there is a small but significant association between major mental illness and violence [2]. This is independent of the risk related to substance misuse; however, it is well established that substance misuse raises this risk even further. There are high rates of trauma among those who attend mental health services, including forensic mental health services. Many have witnessed significant levels of violence from a young age, and in forensic services these patients have moved on to use violence themselves. It is therefore vital that any secure forensic mental health service works to break the cycle of violence and to absolutely minimise any violence on in-patient wards, due to the effect these incidents have on both the victims and perpetrators of that violence as well as on other patients and clinical staff who may witness such violence. The effects on the victims are often both physical and emotional, but the effect on the perpetrator includes the renewing of the cycle of violence that brought them to secure services in the beginning. This should not be underestimated. Violence must be seen as an unmet treatment need, something to be addressed in an appropriate and supportive manner during the course of the admission to the forensic service.

Increasingly, secure forensic mental health services must balance reducing restrictive practices on one hand with keeping a therapeutically safe and violence-free environment on the other. Nursing staff and other hospital clinicians have the right to work in a safe environment. They should not be subject to intimidation and assaults in the work setting. Patients have the right to care in a safe environment and they need to have confidence that staff members can keep them safe during their in-patient stay. Minimising in-patient violence and minimising past violence for forensic patients undermines the accurate assessment of an area of significant treatment need which may, in turn, seriously limit the patient's chance of a future successful discharge in the community. We posit in this chapter that active and careful management of ward milieu and dynamics, and active treatment of psychotic and other symptoms, together with proportionate use only of restrictive practices and good evaluation of any and all restrictive practices, is the most effective way of managing a forensic in-patient setting to reduce and prevent incidents of violence.

Therapeutic Security

The purpose of security in prisons is to provide safe custody. Therapeutic security such as exists in secure forensic hospitals, in contrast to custodial settings such as prisons, aims to offer a safe space for patients to be therapeutically challenged. Challenge is inherent in all effective therapy, and patients in forensic and secure settings have a history of using violence when challenged, uncomfortable or distressed. When working with patients who have a history of significant violence, therapeutic security is required to allow the therapist to challenge the patient appropriately, without fear of violence, such as when having discussions about their past violence, drug use or other issues. It also places the patient in a position whereby they cannot respond with violence to the feelings of challenge in their therapeutic encounters, such that they need to develop different more pro-social coping skills. These can include taking some time out, speaking to a primary nurse or doctor, or learning self-soothing skills. This breaks the cycle of violence and allows the patient to develop the skills needed to minimise future violent behaviour, thus allowing progress to less secure settings and eventually the to the community. This is the purpose of therapeutic security in forensic settings.

Therapeutic security in forensic mental health settings consists of three component parts: physical security, procedural security and relational security [3]. Physical security consists of the physical infrastructure of the ward and hospital designed to provide safe and secure care, for example the perimeter fence and walls and secure doors and locks. These are built to national specifications; for example, in NHS England, a medium-secure unit must have a single perimeter fence a minimum of 5 metres high, while a high-secure unit in England must have a double fence or fence and wall each measuring a minimum of 5 metres high. Procedural security consists of the procedures, protocols and policies a hospital puts in place to manage therapeutic security. It is largely focussed on preventing prohibited items entering the hospital space such as searches for weapons or drugs. These procedural security policies and practices also vary depending on the level of therapeutic security the hospital is placed at. They should have a statutory basis in law for the individual jurisdiction concerned.

Relational security is somewhat more difficult to define. It is based on the knowledge clinicians have of the individual patient, including their usual presentation, their signature signs of relapse and their individual risks and needs. In 1974 Scott stated that forensic psychiatric hospitals needed to be 'high in quality and quantity of staff' [4]. It has also been shown that units with higher levels of bank staff on wards have higher rates of incidents of violence. Clinicians are the most expensive resource input in any healthcare setting, and keeping a mix of senior nursing staff on wards is a challenge both from a recruitment perspective and an economic perspective. The nursing-staff-to-patient ratio is a very important consideration in management of any in-patient forensic setting, and we would argue in the safe and effective running of any mental health setting. Objectively, better staff skill mixes with higher numbers of more senior nursing staff regularly present on wards may be one of the most vital resources a hospital has to limit in-patient violence and therefore to limit associated need for restrictive practice. In modern practice many hospitals have diluted the nursing skills mix (proportion of nursing staff who are trained and registered) on forensic wards and are therefore increasingly dependent on the physical and procedural aspects of security to manage risk. This is a concern. Any service that is truly focussed on improving quality of care for patients and reducing in-patient violence and the associated need for restrictive practice must address the nursing skills mix on wards. This cannot be overlooked in the quest to make financial savings. It is also essential that services recognise and utilise the existing expertise within the wider staff groups, such as specialised trainers, practitioners and advisors in the prevention and management of aggression and violence. Such expertise is often restricted to the training environment and only used after an incident to provide their views on whether the taught procedures were applied correctly. A proactive approach should exploit all opportunities to embed this level of expertise into the multidisciplinary approach to bridge the gap between the training arena and operational settings. Training, feedback and guidance within this complex area of practice should continue within the ward settings, to provide timely leadership, advice, support and opportunities to learn from events and to maximise their abilities to act as positive role models to drive and create a positive and proactive culture.

Relational Security and Working Alliance

Implementing good relational security starts with the clinician getting to know the patient to develop a good rapport and working alliance. Multiple assessments and reviews over the short and longer term will be required to effectively achieve this. The clinician must read all supporting background documents, including the Historical Clinical and Risk Management-20 (HCR-20) for violence risk assessments [5], individual care plans, and medical pre-admission reports, court reports and books of evidence in relation to the index offence to ascertain a longitudinal history of the patients presentations.

The findings from the inquiry into the care and treatment of A.R. (the Falling Shadow Inquiry report) [6] are particularly relevant here. Every clinician should understand the importance of reading objective accounts of the index offence and past offending behaviour rather than simply relying on one account alone, whether that is from the patient or another staff member. This is further discussed in Chapter 2. There is evidence that approaches to better communication and boundary-setting can reduce both violence and the use of restrictive practices. Safewards [7, 8] is one example, as is the use of the See Think Act process [9, 10].

Making Promises You Cannot Keep

Care should be taken not to make promises one cannot keep, for obvious reasons. Promises, for example agreeing to advocate at ward rounds for community leave or reductions in medication or early discharge, can be tempting to make, but honesty and an upfront approach are vital in forensic settings. If these care plans would not be appropriate for the patient, then they cannot safely proceed. Many patients have come from challenging home or early life environments with failures in care during childhood, and this may result in patients feeling highly sensitive to perceived rejection, betrayal or broken commitments and trust. It is vital that staff members do not fall into a habit or custom where they are unknowingly or absent-mindedly repeating these patterns. To do so risks seriously undermining the therapeutic working alliance with a vulnerable patient.

Splitting and Ward Dynamics

All clinicians working in secure forensic mental health settings should have a good knowledge of splitting dynamics, as these are common in groups with a significant history of trauma and high rates of emotionally unstable personality traits or emotionally unstable personality disorder (EUPD). Clinicians in secure forensic settings will at times need to deliver news that is not welcome from the patient perspective, for example if the relevant Department of Justice or Ministry of Justice declines community leave or if a mental health tribunal does not agree to discharge. It is vital to resist the temptation to engage in splitting behaviours at those times. Statements such as 'I would have given you this leave but the department said no or the clinical director said no' are rarely helpful and can seriously disempower a patient.

The correct approach is to advise the patient of the reasons why the request was declined in a manner that engages the patient to work on that area with their therapist's and their team's support; for example, advising the patient that the relevant department or manager will accept a new referral once the patient is incident-free for a period of time, or once they have successfully completed a piece of individual or group work in the relevant area. The patient can move forward with that advice and work towards their self-identified goal in a positive manner. All patients have individual risks and needs, and it is important to develop a good working alliance with a patient as soon as possible. Without a good working alliance when things are going well, it will be almost impossible to intervene and verbally de-escalate a patient at a future time of distress.

Ward Milieu and Atmosphere

Ward milieu or ward 'temperature' is very important in forensic settings, and arguably in all mental health services. Managing the ward atmosphere is a core responsibility of the consultant forensic psychiatrist and nurse managers. It is important for consultant forensic psychiatrists to be able to reflect on ward atmosphere and have a good under-standing of when the atmosphere is positive or more challenging, as well as understanding changes in the atmosphere. The Essen-Climate Evaluation Scale (Essen-CES) can be used to ask patients and staff about their views in relation to ward atmosphere and how safe they feel in the setting [11]. It is important to note that even one new patient or staff member transferred into a ward can significantly alter a ward dynamic. Senior clinicians should visit their in-patient ward frequently and regularly, predictably and unpredictably to monitor the atmosphere. A weekly community meeting is often a very good starting point for this; for example, reflecting on the attendance of patients and staff – do all patients and staff speak up or is the conversation dominated by one or two group members?

It is important to note that it may be only after an individual is moved from a ward that others will speak up about how intimidated they felt around that person. Reassurances while the individual remains on the ward may not always be genuine. Ward atmosphere tempera-ture charts are easily utilised on forensic wards on a day-to-day basis. These simply consist of a traffic-light-style scale with a list of patient names and each patient being coded 'green', 'amber' or 'red' to demonstrate an at-a-glance view of the level of symptomatology or distress each patient is presenting with on that day (see Figure 9.1). The board can quickly and clearly identify which patients need additional staff input and staff support on a day in question, and also give an indication of the overall ward atmosphere on a given day. It can support staff in ensuring that patients who might have additional needs on a given day are identified, as well as ensuring that staff new to the ward or visiting the ward for short periods understand the group dynamic on the day in question.

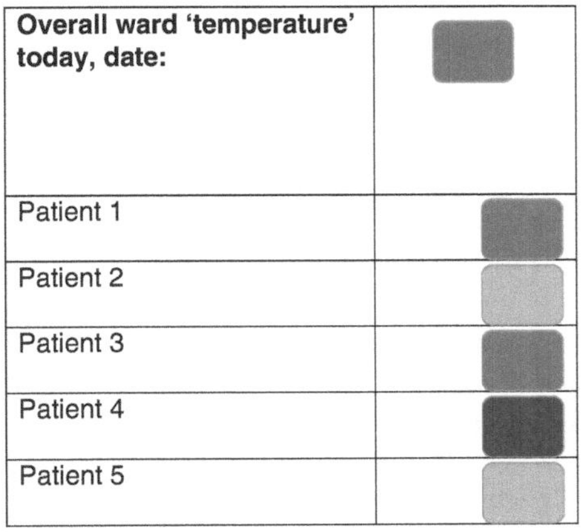

Overall ward 'temperature' today, date:	
Patient 1	
Patient 2	
Patient 3	
Patient 4	
Patient 5	

Figure 9.1 Ward atmosphere 'temperature' chart. Light grey: this patient is doing well; usual observations are sufficient. Medium grey: please be mindful of this patient; they might need some extra support today. Dark grey: please have extra awareness of this patient's needs today; their presentation is not as stable as is usual for them.

Substance Misuse on the Ward

Substance misuse is significantly associated with violence and will increase impulsivity and therefore also increase risk of self-harm. There must therefore be zero tolerance to alcohol or illicit drugs in an in-patient setting, be that general psychiatry or forensic psychiatry. Keeping illicit drugs out of forensic hospital settings can pose a serious challenge. The most common methods of illicit drugs coming into units include visitors or staff members bringing them in or patients bringing them back from unescorted community leave. It is important to have a clear policy in place for random urinary drug screening and searching on entering the secure premises to protect vulnerable patients from being offered illicit drugs. Contraband drugs will cause relapse of mental illness, relapse of addiction symptoms, violence and self-harm. It is important for clinicians to have an awareness of novel psychoactive substances, such as synthetic cannabis and synthetic cocaine. These have major effects on mental state but will not show up on conventional drug screens. Because of the widespread availability of these substances, unfortunately a clear urinary drug screen can no longer reassure a clinician of the absence of illicit drugs.

Clinicians should have an awareness of the risk of addiction issues comorbid with major mental disorders in forensic settings. This is a key vulnerability for many patients. While in the hospital setting, home brewing of alcohol can take place; staff should have an awareness of this if items such as bottles of juice are found in dark areas or bottles of juice with bread (or other yeast-containing foods) are found. Items such as alcohol hand sanitisers, aftershave and perfume may be consumed, indicating serious alcohol dependence. Dependence on prescription medications such as benzodiazepines and their congeners is another key concern. Benzodiazepines are cross-tolerant with alcohol and may also have a disinhibiting effect post-ingestion. Interviews and assessments with the aim of accessing prescriptions for benzodiazepines are rarely of genuine therapeutic benefit. Nicotine replacement therapy is in place in many secure settings as health services implement smoke-free environments. The introduction of smoke-free campuses in forensic settings is not associated with an increase in violent or other incidents, but nicotine replacement therapy, especially lozenges, can act as a currency in forensic settings and can be traded. E-cigarettes can be utilised as delivery devices for novel psychoactive substances and care must be taken in relation to these items given the rates of substance misuse noted in forensic patient groups who are often highly vulnerable in this area.

Therapeutic Boundary Issues on the Ward

All patients admitted to secure forensic hospitals have a serious history of violence. Those admitted to medium-secure units are deemed to pose a high risk to the public, while those in high security pose a 'grave and immediate risk' to the public. Therefore, all these patients have by definition broken major societal boundaries. Boundary-breaching behaviour including violence is a significant target for treatment in secure forensic settings. Patients in these settings benefit from clear and consistent boundary-setting from staff, so that they develop an awareness of their behaviour and what is acceptable. There is an association between units that manage boundaries well and higher-quality forensic services. Clinicians should have a clear understanding of their role and the role of others on their team, and senior clinicians in forensic settings should tutor more junior staff in this area. It is vitally important that all staff, but particularly less experienced staff members, are taught the difference between being 'friendly and professional' and being 'friends'. Patients already have friends and family; they are attending a health service for the purpose of seeing mental health professionals. Blurring of role boundaries can lead to significant confusion and adverse outcomes for patients and can seriously undermine therapy.

Consistency of approach from senior clinicians is vital in secure forensic mental health settings. Patients in secure forensic settings have high rates of comorbid personality disorder.

A Structured Approach to Short-Term Assessments of Violence Risk in In-Patient Settings

The best predictor of future behaviour is past behaviour. The use of structured professional judgement instruments such as the HCR-20 is almost universal in forensic psychiatric hospitals [12]. These are important documents and should be completed in a highly detailed manner and updated regularly. However, these instruments provide a high-level overview of past violence and support the development of overall management, treatment and care plans for patients to target risk factors for violence. Short-term violence risk, on a day-to-day basis, requires a different type of instrument. Structured instruments such as the Brøset scale or Dynamic Assessment of Situational Aggression (DASA) scale meet this need [13, 14]. These instruments allow the rating of short-term violence risk and short-term risk of incidents on mental health wards. They are internationally validated and the aim is that each patient is rated against their own usual baseline. Any escalation above a patient's usual baseline, which is different for each individual, is noted and scored. If a patient scores above a certain level, staff are prompted to consider an intervention, such as a review of mental state, the offer of an 'as required' medication or some time out, depending on the level of escalation. The use of these scales prompts ward staff to intervene quickly when a patient is escalating in behaviour, with the intervention aimed at reducing the risk of the situation progressing to an incident. In this way these instruments are used with the aim of reducing the overall rate of incidents on the ward and consequently reducing the associated need for restrictive practices such as seclusion [15, 16].

De-escalation

The root causes of incidents of aggression and acts of violence are extremely complex in nature. As discussed previously, and supported by current thinking and research, there are a plethora of variables to consider during the prediction, prevention and management of conflict resolution. Wide ranging and varied, often the primary cause of aggression and violence is related to an unmet need, an action or inaction that can often be observed within the system, environment and people. Such observations within these domains may independently or interactively play a key role in positively de-escalating and/or negatively escalating the behaviour of self and others. Therefore, if such themes are unnoticed or not addressed in a timely way, they will lead to a cycle of events and responses that misses the opportunity to predict and prevent. Instead, there may be a cycle of staff responding and managing the initial aggressive or violent act through more habitual restrictive means (physical restraint, seclusion, extra medication, etc.).

Over-reliance on the use of reactive measures can negatively shape the organisation's culture, resilience and tolerance to violence, with less early responses to behavioural changes. Such cultures can inadvertently develop negative grassroots adjustments by staff to their daily routines, practices and procedures to keep themselves and others safe, such as implementing blanket restrictions, zero tolerance for patients actively expressing themselves (non-violently), restricting liberty (de facto seclusion) and so on, thus continuing the cycle of conflict and confirming the need to apply restrictive procedures or unregulated coercive responses to maintain their status, safety and order.

A ward is a small community within itself. Therefore, an initiative-taking whole-systems approach must be continually applied to strive to understand, achieve and maintain the complexities of a state of 'equilibrium' among the people, community and populations. All this must be accomplished while maintaining a realistic understanding that complete 'unanimity' and 'adaptation' between people and the environment may not always or even often happen within this rapidly changing and evolving setting. Healthcare staff and clinical teams must strive tirelessly to establish concord between these warring challenges to reach a desirable state of 'harmony' that preserves human rights for all, remains within the boundaries of legal and ethical frameworks, and creates safe physical and social spaces within which to disperse such operational duties with empathy, care, compassion and kindness.

Understanding these complexities when designing and delivering 'training' and while practising as a clinician in a secure hospital setting cannot be overemphasised. Training in the prediction and prevention of aggression and violence must consider the 'vulnerabilities' and 'conflicts' within people, the system and environment in order to strive for a culture that becomes solution-focussed, has the confidence to recognise when change is necessary and has the courage to change direction, no matter how difficult and challenging this may be.

De-escalation (prevention) is rightly placed as a key priority within national guidance, codes of practices, organisational violence reduction strategies and local policies of mental health services in the UK, Ireland, Canada, Australia and other jurisdictions. Staff training in de-escalation within forensic mental health settings sits as the core foundation of a hierarchical response that promotes the least restrictive response to reducing aggression and violence. However, it should be noted that verbal de-escalation is not a singular approach. Often it may be necessary to intervene physically to contain the risk and to safely support the patient through their episode of acute behavioural disturbance.

Kaplan and Wheeler identified the following five phases of pending violence: the triggering event(s), escalation, crisis point, recovery and post-crisis depression [17]. Therefore, it is essential that staff are aware of these various stages so that they understand the complexities of each, and how to safely respond or disengage if necessary.

Verbal de-escalation at the point of conflict is complex and often frightening, as it is likely that both the victim's and perpetrator's baseline behaviour has been triggered and may be following a similar path along the stages of the assault cycle as described by Kaplan and Wheeler. Therefore, during this stressful process, staff must be aware of the impact of their own behaviour and responses in order to avoid escalation. Resolving conflict is an exceedingly difficult and challenging task, especially considering the innate physiological fight, flight or freeze responses that occur in such circumstances. Although de-escalation training puts a great deal of emphasis on verbal de-escalation skills and will in turn develop the clinician's confidence in applying these in practice, there is no defined gold standard of de-escalation training, and there are no magic words or actions that will immediately resolve human conflict.

During verbal de-escalation it is vital for clinicians to determine their own safety, and where possible maintain a safe distance with an awareness of the adjacent spaces, exits and other staff. Has an alarm been sounded to summon support? The clinician on site should strive to exhibit behaviours such as positive and open body language, remaining calm throughout, using a clear tone of voice and adjusting communication and conflict resolution styles to respond to the risks and to understand the patient. The successful clinician on the spot will have a positive and initiative-taking attitude, being open and honest, remaining collaborative and focussed on problem solving. The clinician engaged in de-escalation will maintain a person-centred approach that is trauma-informed, and, when safe to do so, will take positive risks. In simple terms de-escalation is about humanising the process, showing empathy, and being compassionate, kind and keeping one another safe while avenues are being explored to collaboratively reach a state of equilibrium.

Seclusion, Restraint and Other Restrictive Practices

All clinicians working in secure forensic mental health settings acknowledge that violence can and does happen in these settings, as in any mental health setting. Allowing in-patient violence to go unchecked is counter-therapeutic and dangerous. At times, to ensure safety and to even preserve life, restrictive practices such as seclusion and restraint are required. Patients admitted to psychiatric units, regardless of the level of security, are entitled to be in a safe and therapeutic ward environment, free from the risk of assault and intimidation from others, where they can progress towards their own recovery. Staff members also have a right to a safe place of work. Increasingly there is significant pressure on mental health services to eliminate all restrictive practices, including seclusion and restraint, but at the same time these services are pressurised to have a zero rate of in-patient violence. The appropriate aim is for care in the least restrictive manner that is safely possible and to ensure that each and every incident of restrictive practice is absolutely necessary and proportionate to the risk of violence posed at that given time for that individual patient. It is also important to note that the Committee for Prevention of Torture and Inhuman or

Degrading Treatment (CPT) from the Council of Europe does not advocate a ban on seclusion and other restrictive practices. Rather, they recognise:

> the restraint of violent psychiatric patients who represent a danger to themselves or others may exceptionally be necessary. The means of restraint should always be applied with the principles of legality, necessity, proportionality and accountability. All types of restraint, and the criteria for their use should be regulated by law. Patients should only be restrained as a measure of last resort to prevent imminent harm to themselves or others and restraints should always be used for the shortest and safest time possible. [18]

It is vital for all consultant forensic psychiatrists to be aware that it is never appropriate to utilise seclusion or other restrictive practices due to staffing shortages, inadequate staffing experience levels or other service-based considerations, or to use any such measure that is not in accordance with the law.

The Medical Seclusion Review

The role of the duty doctor or duty consultant when called to a violent incident, for example in response to an alarm, is not to get directly involved in the management of the response to the incident unless it is very prolonged. Most incidents are safely brought to a peaceful conclusion by highly skilled, ward-based nursing staff within a minute or two. The doctor responding to an alarm should proceed to the site knowing they will not be the first responder and that a trained team will already be managing the situation. Before contributing further, the doctor must first fully inform themselves of the identity of the patient and their medical and psychiatric background. Reading the care plan and any special care plan for managing violence, plus the medication chart and any cautions recorded there, is essential, as is speaking to the ward staff who are not directly involved in the incident. A psychiatrist in training is always wise to consult the duty consultant or treating consultant. There may then be a need for the doctor to retrospectively authorise any legally regulated restraint that has been used, to consider the use of extra 'as required' medication that may be needed, including the option of forced medication by injection (by far the highest risk of the possible interventions given that it involves the injection of a medication with potentially cardiac-irritant side effects at a time of arousal and agitation), and to review an episode of seclusion.

The role of the doctor is to be an objective medical professional making decisions in consultation with the nurses and team and, where possible, in consultation with the patient. It is always necessary to examine and interview the patient, even if this is only possible while the patient is restrained or secluded. The safety, dignity and engagement of the patient is always the first priority for the doctor. It is the role of the doctor to observe whether approved safe techniques are being used or have been used in a way that is medically necessary and proportionate to prevent violence. The doctor will be required to decide whether to authorise by signing legal forms, and must support this with a detailed clinical note, signed with date, time and registration number.

In keeping with the stages of the assault cycle, in particular the recovery phase, it is likely that until the patient has returned to their baseline behaviour and the risks have reduced to a safe level, any interaction within the unlocked environment will remain volatile and unpredictable. In an ideal world, all reviews of a patient who is in seclusion following an imminent or actual violent incident should take place through an open-door process. If the risk of violence remains high, keeping the door locked will reduce the likelihood of physical assaults. However, this approach must be continually reviewed by the multidisciplinary team to ensure that this remains necessary and proportionate to the risks presented and the patient's liberty is not restricted for any longer than is lawfully necessary. Once the risks have reduced and before considering unlocking the door and entering the patient's personal space, it may be prudent to conduct a series of open-door reviews. On each occasion the nurse or doctor leading the review should inform and reassure the patient of the planned process and procedures.

The clinicians should reiterate to the patient that they will not enter unless invited, that by request they will exit and the door will be closed, and if any sudden movements are observed, the staff will close and contain the door. Staff training for this procedure should include open-door procedures whereby the appropriate number of trained staff are present, positioned in a safe place away from the aperture of the door, but within proximity and in readiness to respond to a sudden escalation of risk such as attempts to breach the door. It is important to reduce the number of staff positioned within the aperture of the door since this can appear threatening, negatively impact on the patient's beliefs and mental state, and potentially activate past traumas and repeat the cycle of violence, which may influence the use of seclusion being believed to be the safest option. Only the nominated person should be safely positioned at the door to aid a single route of communication. Unless it is necessary to enter the seclusion room, preserving the patient's personal space should always be respected to promote autonomy, feeling safe, collaboration and trust and to develop a rapport. Slowing down the interaction will reduce foreseeable incidents to enable safer environmental desensitisation and to enable all avenues of de-escalation. This approach is of vital importance during both short-term and long-term uses of seclusion. Too often, the locked door is only opened when there is a need to do something to the patient, rather than taking frequent opportunities to safely open the door just to have a conversation, humanising the restricted process.

In the event of a patient being secluded, it is essential for the nursing team to develop a care plan to support and meet the needs of the patient while contained. In addition to this there should be an operational plan to safely manage any other foreseeable risks such as medical emergencies, fire evacuations, barricaded incidents, hostage-taking, and risk to self and others (ligatures/weapons/violence, etc.). Staff and the system should be prepared for the intended interventions required to manage these foreseeable risks, and the appropriately trained staff and equipment should be available onsite to aid a safe, timely and informed response. Failure to prepare will create confusion and unnecessary delays, lead to poor decision-making, and may place the patient and staff at greater risk of harm.

The purpose of the medical review of seclusion is to review the patient's continued need for care in seclusion and to ascertain if that is the least restrictive option possible to safely manage the risk to others posed by the patient at that point in time. Seclusion can only be legally used to manage risk to others; it is not to be used for the management of self-harm. Other aims during a medical seclusion review include a brief assessment of mental state and an assessment of any physical health issues or injuries.

Prior to commencing the medical seclusion review, the doctor and nursing team who plan to complete the review should meet in a ward meeting room or the nurses' station, but always away from the secluded patient. Too often, this discussion takes place outside of the patient's door and prior to entry, where the patient can hear but not clearly understand what is happening. A clear handover should take place to discuss the patient's presentation and reason for seclusion, which is generally led by the ward nurse in charge. This discussion should ascertain if the patient is eating and drinking normally, how their mental state is at the time of the review, any recent incidents in the seclusion room and if the nursing staff have any concerns about the patient's physical health – whether or not nursing staff have been able to take vital signs and if they are stable. Any potential for illicit drug misuse should be considered with the staff, bearing in mind that novel psychoactive substances will likely not show up on a urinary drug screen. It is important to ascertain whether or not the patient may have been injured during a physical encounter prior to seclusion or whether or not the patient was restrained, as this is likely to increase the potential of a restraint-related injury and/or activation or reactivation of trauma.

Once the pre-seclusion briefing discussion has been completed, the ward nurse in charge will allocate individual roles and responsibilities to each member of the nursing team. The number of clinicians and resources required will depend on the intended task and presented risks. The trained clinicians who have been identified to physically intervene if needed should not be allocated other roles such as carrying equipment or food. In the event of a sudden escalation of behaviour, clinicians who have been allocated to respond should be free from hazards (objects they are carrying or restrictions on movement) to manage the situation in a timely manner. Nurses carrying out other functions should only enter the environment with items such as blood pressure and pulse monitors, food, and so on when instructed to do so. All clinicians, medical and nursing, should clearly understand their role and the importance of exiting the room with all items accounted for after the review or especially after an incident. The person managing the door is best placed to coordinate the flow and number of staff and items entering and exiting the room. It is vital that there is no confusion regarding roles in the event of an urgent situation as this can lead to injuries to patients and staff or the need for a restraint being applied longer than might be necessary. (See later section on 'Incidents during Seclusion Reviews' which explores a decision-making tool to aid staff in risk assessment and planning.) It is only once each team member is clear on their role that the team will approach the seclusion room door. A team member who has a good relationship with the patient should then speak to the patient via the door panel to attempt to gain cooperation and will ask the patient to sit on the mattress at the far end of the room with their legs facing the door. If cooperation is not achievable at this stage, an informed decision will be made by the nurse in charge to ascertain if it is necessary to enter and if the risks presented to all during entry are proportionate to the intended task and current needs of the patient. If it is not safe to enter, and there is no urgent need, time should be taken to seek cooperation so as to minimise the risk of an incident.

If cooperation is possible, and the patient is willing to let the nurses open the door and enter the room, the nurse in charge will direct the nurse managing the door to open it. The nurses will speak to the patient and enter the room and position themselves safely to enable the nominated clinicians to safely enter and complete the agreed tasks and assessments. Once nurses have finished these tasks, items such as empty cups and plates and vitals monitors should be moved out of the room immediately, and trained clinicians nominated to respond physically should remain in position until all risk items have been removed by the exiting clinicians. Only then should these trained staff, whose role was to complete vital observations and offer food items, exit the room, and maintain eye contact with the patient until they have safely exited the room.

The medical review can then commence either within the room or utilising the open-door review process if the risks suggest this is a safer option at this stage of the patient's recovery. The psychiatrist should speak to the patient and inquire about their views of the incident leading to the seclusion and about any overt symptoms, including any risk issues to both self and others. The doctor should ascertain if the patient continues to present a high and immediate risk of violence to others such that seclusion needs to continue. The patient's level of cooperation with any possible care plans to support seclusion ending should be assessed. It is vital the doctor observes the patient carefully to ascertain if there are any overt physical health issues. It is also of paramount importance that a doctor does not make promises that cannot be safely kept, such as offering the patient time out of seclusion or additional personal items in the seclusion room that have not been considered in advance by the team at the pre-seclusion briefing. To make a promise that might subsequently not be possible to keep risks damaging the working alliance with the patient when they are in a difficult situation. Requests should be listened to carefully and the patient advised it will be discussed with the team and feedback given after the review separately. In summer it is particularly important for the patient to be provided with adequate fluids and in winter the team should have an awareness of the temperature of the seclusion room as they can be cold at times. Once the doctor has completed the brief review, the doctor should exit the room and the nursing staff will then work together as a team to safely exit and close the door. It is vital at this point that the doctor has an awareness of not standing in the swinging arc of the door or not standing in the way of nursing staff such as to prevent additional staff entering urgently in the event of an emergency.

While the review is underway, the doctor and all staff must have an awareness of the signs that a patient may be becoming irritable or angry. This includes non-verbal cues such as fist-clenching and intense staring eye contact. This can escalate to verbal cues such as the patient's speech becoming louder or angrier in tone. If this occurs, thank the patient for their time and end the review promptly and safely. Prolonging the review at that stage is rarely effective. Often this presentation means the patient is not yet ready to have a conversation about safety issues relevant to future violence; the patient may experience the team being in the seclusion room or remaining outside as intrusive and hostile. If a patient is escalating in demeanour after an incident brought them to seclusion, it is clearly not the correct time to end seclusion. The chances of the termination being successful at that stage are very poor and that is tantamount to setting the patient up for a failed re-integration with the ward. End the review politely, offer the patient space and quiet in the seclusion room, and review again at the next medical review time to see if things have improved.

Once the seclusion review has ended, the team should return to the ward office and discuss how the review went (repeat the National Decision Model (NDM) cycle). Mention and record any positives or evidence of progress and evidence of good practice. Areas for improvement of the team performance should also be highlighted. For example, were all the staff members and the doctor happy with the information provided within the initial brief; positions they stood in; did anyone block the door; did team members go too close to the patient, making the patient feel uncomfortable during the review or placing themselves at risk? The patient's presentation and level of cooperation is then discussed. Does the patient still need to remain in seclusion? What care plan could be considered to support the patient re-entering the ward area? Does the patient require refractory clothing and blankets due to risk to self, or could they be safely managed in their own clothing? The patient's own clothing will be best, if possible, from a risk perspective. Any requests made by the patient should be discussed carefully and feedback on these given to the patient later. Any incidents or emergency situations that took place during the review are discussed – did these go well, were they managed appropriately and what might have been done differently to ensure the best possible outcome?

At the end of the post-seclusion briefing, the decision is taken whether to continue or discontinue seclusion. Any statutory forms required such as seclusion registers and restraint registers are carefully completed and signed as prescribed by law or regulations. The doctor will write a detailed note in the patient's medical record, as will the nurse in charge, and the doctor will then exit the ward.

It is important to note that ultimate clinical responsibility for the care and treatment of the patient lies with the responsible clinician (in most cases the treating consultant psychiatrist); however, great care must be taken to consider the nursing view very carefully in this area, as it will be the nursing staff members on the ward who manage the risk posed once the patient returns to the ward area. A general agreement from all parties is the best outcome to aim for. A registrar or senior registrar in forensic psychiatry who disagrees with a decision regarding the need for seclusion must escalate that matter to the consultant forensic psychiatrist, as this is a very significant decision that balances the rights of the patient with the risk to other patients and staff on the ward.

Incidents during Seclusion Reviews

Incidents within a seclusion environment are common and often predictable. By the very nature of caring for a patient within a seclusion environment, it is inevitable that personal space to provide care and treatment may be compromised, therefore elevating the risk of close-contact physical violence.

During the planning phase for a seclusion review, staff should consider following a structured decision-making model to introduce a structured rationale of what they did during an intervention and why. For example, we consider here the National Decision

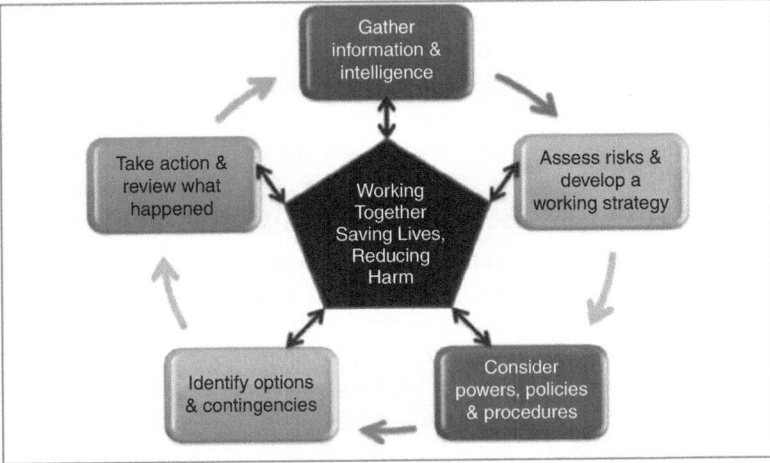

Figure 9.2 National Decision Model, College of Policing, UK.

Model (NDM) of the College of Policing in the UK (see Figure 9.2). This model has been successfully adopted into staff Professional Management of Violence and Aggression (PMVA) training within the high-secure mental health services in England and can provide a tool for both planned and unplanned dynamic responses to managing risk.

The NDM has six key elements:

1. Code of ethics (central to the process).
2. Gather information and intelligence.
3. Assess threat and risk and develop a working strategy.
4. Consider powers and policy.
5. Identify options and contingences.
6. Take action and review what happened.

Too often, during planned interventions within a seclusion environment or responses to incidents on wards, such informed processes are not utilised and this is a missed opportunity to safely reduce and manage foreseeable risks. Furthermore, planning high-risk interventions without a visual structure can lead to inconsistencies within the team's decision-making culture for the management of aggression and violence. Poor preparation by staff may lead to responses to sudden violence that are less than ideal, and this may in turn lead to further need for restrictive practices as the situation is escalating rather than de-escalating.

Planned Interventions in the Seclusion Area

The levels of risk within a seclusion environment can rapidly escalate to a level that poses a significant risk to those who enter the locked environment. Such incidents may consist of severe damage to property, fashioned weapons, barricades, trip, slip and biohazards, and hostage-taking. Each forensic mental health service must identify, plan and develop safe systems of work to contain, manage and resolve such distressing and potentially life-threatening events at a management level. The situations where restrictive responses such as the use of personal protective equipment (PPE), including body armour, helmets and shields, are required should be carefully considered in advance and only used by specifically trained members of staff. A system of escalated responsibility should be in place so that only senior clinician managers can authorise such escalation. This should only be in the context of the management of severe levels of violence risk. If needed, the support of other agencies such as the police can be considered who will have legal authority to deploy a higher level of tactics outside a clinical context within policing powers, should the situation be significantly threatening to merit that level of response to maintain safety.

Reducing Restrictive Practice Interventions

Reducing restrictive practices including seclusion, restraint and all other restrictive practices should be a key goal for all forensic mental health services. However, it is important to note that the aim should not be zero restrictive practices; rather, the aim should be zero in-patient violence. The key aim for these interventions should be to ensure that any restrictive practice used should be both medically necessary and proportionate. Even one episode of seclusion that was not proportionate or the least restrictive option that would have managed that patient's risk at that time is not acceptable. However, several episodes of seclusion, if they were all the absolutely least restrictive method of preventing violence and were proportionate to the need at the time, is acceptable. Many mental health settings including forensic units in NHS hospitals in England are incentivised to minimise their use of restrictive practices. This is an important goal for services.

Having adequate numbers of highly specialised, highly trained nurses with an appropriate level of seniority on the ward is one of the most effective ways of reducing restrictive practice. Forensic wards that are struggling to maintain nursing staff numbers or struggling to maintain appropriate levels of skills mix among nursing staff will always be at higher risk of violent incidents. It is the violent incidents that lead to restrictive practices. It is vital that in the quest to reduce restrictive practices, clinicians do not permit wards to become unsafe places and normalise violence in forensic settings. This is not in the best interests of this vulnerable patient group and it results in an unsafe place for nurses and other clinicians. It is important to note that entirely prohibiting seclusion and restrictive practices to manage acute violence in in-patient settings would likely lead to patients who pose a risk of violence when unwell being refused admission to hospitals, and instead remaining in prisons, leading to exclusion of a vulnerable, unwell patient group from healthcare services.

Demonstrating Proportionality in the Use of Restrictive Practice in Forensic Hospitals

There is a small but significant association between mental illness and violence, and violence does happen on psychiatric wards and hospitals [19]. Hospitals are mandated to provide a safe space for patients and staff have the right to a safe place of work. Therefore at times, to manage acute risk of violence towards others, seclusion and other restrictive practices are used. This must be used only when absolutely necessary to prevent imminent violence; it must be proportionate to the risk and seriousness of the risk posed and can be used only in accordance with the law [18].

When seclusion or restrictive practices are used in in-patient settings, it can often be challenging for consultants, nurse managers, hospitals or services to demonstrate that the incident of restrictive practice was both necessary and proportionate. The Dundrum Restriction and Intrusion on Liberty Ladders (DRILL) tool is a structured professional judgement instrument designed to assess incidents of violence and the response of the team or service to ascertain if the response was proportionate to the incident [20]. The DRILL tool may be of assistance to the doctor or nurse in charge as a means of structured understanding of how incidents arise and are managed. This sets out a series of scales or 'ladders' that quantify a range of disruptive and violent behaviours including violence, self-harm, risk to others, absconding and non-compliance. Typically several of these may occur together and may escalate over time. Interventions are similarly deployed by the ward team and doctors in a highly trained and professionally skilled way, deploying a selected number of options, each ranging from low grade to more restrictive and drawn from de-escalation, enhanced observations, ad hoc personal searches, extra medication, situational control, manual restraint, seclusion and mechanical restraint. Low-grade incidents should elicit low-grade interventions while in theory more serious incidents may require a more restrictive intervention such as seclusion.

The DRILL tool allows a team or a service to review the incident, quantify its severity and quantify the level of the response and intervention. It does not bind the clinician; rather, it guides, and highlights episodes where there appears to be a mismatch in the level of incident and level of the corresponding intervention. This does not mean the intervention was incorrect but rather that it should be reviewed and reflected upon. Video recording is increasingly available for an objective review of the antecedents, behaviours, interventions and consequences of a violent incident – or a prevented incident – and the DRILL tool can be used as a means of measuring proportionality. The DRILL tool allows a service to demonstrate proportionality of interventions and restrictive practice to commissioners, managers, patients and others in an evidence-based way. It can also be used for teaching, reflective practice and ongoing learning among the clinical team.

In conclusion, the management of the therapeutic milieu in in-patient settings and providing patients and clinicians with a safe hospital space are vital to treating mental illness and treating violence. Providing safe care and treatment and managing risk in such settings requires sufficient numbers of highly trained clinicians and good planning, combined with effective training and a positive approach. The use of proactive approaches such as Safewards and the DASA scale to prompt interventions has been shown to be effective in reducing violent incidents. Restrictive practices should only be used to prevent imminent violence to others, only when absolutely necessary and proportionate to the risk posed, and always compliant with the law in the relevant jurisdiction.

References

1. Williams HK, Senanayke M, Ross CC, Bates R, Davoren M. Security needs among patients referred for high secure care in Broadmoor Hospital England. *BJPsych Open* 2020; 6 (4): e55.

2. Coid JW, Ullrich S, Kallis C et al. The relationship between delusions and violence: findings from the East London first episode psychosis study. *JAMA Psychiatry* 2013; 70 (5): 465–71.

3. Kennedy HG. Therapeutic uses of security: mapping forensic mental health services by stratifying risk. *Advances in Psychiatric Treatment* 2002; 8 (6): 433–43.

4. Scott PD. Solutions to the problem of the dangerous offender. *The BMJ* 1974; 4 (5945): 640–1.

5. Douglas KS, Hart SD, Webster CD et al. Historical-clinical-risk management-20, version 3 (HCR-20V3): development and overview. *International Journal of Forensic Mental Health* 2014; 13 (2): 93–108.

6. Blom-Cooper LJ, Hally H. *The Falling Shadow: One Patient's Mental Health Care, 1978–1993*. Report of the Committee of Inquiry into the Events Leading Up to and Surrounding the Fatal Incident at the Edith Morgan Centre, Torbay, on 1 September 1993. London, Duckworth, 1995.

7. Bowers L, Alexander J, Bilgin H et al. Safewards: the empirical basis of the model and a critical appraisal. *Journal of Psychiatric and Mental Health Nursing* 2014; 21 (4): 354–64.

8. Stensgaard L, Andersen MK, Nordentoft M, Hjorthøj C. Implementation of the safewards model to reduce the use of coercive measures in adult psychiatric inpatient units: an interrupted time-series analysis. *Journal of Psychiatric Research* 2018; 105: 147–52.

9. Allen E. *Your Guide to Relational Security: See, Think, Act*, 3rd ed. London, Royal College of Psychiatrists, 2023.

10. Tighe J, Gudjonsson GH. See, Think, Act Scale: preliminary development and validation of a measure of relational security in medium- and low-secure units. *The Journal of Forensic Psychiatry & Psychology* 2012; 23 (2): 184–99.

11. Schalast N, Redies M, Collins M, Stacey J, Howells K. EssenCES, a short questionnaire for assessing the social

climate of forensic psychiatric wards. *Criminal Behaviour and Mental Health* 2008; 18 (1): 49–58.

12. Douglas KS, Webster CD, Hart SD, Belfrage H. *HCR-20v3: Assessing Risk for Violence: User Guide.* 3rd ed. Burnaby, Mental Health, Law, and Policy Institute, Simon Fraser University, 2013.

13. Almvik R, Woods P, Rasmussen K. The Brøset Violence Checklist: sensitivity, specificity, and interrater reliability. *Journal of Interpersonal Violence* 2000; 15 (12): 1284–96.

14. Ogloff JR, Daffern M. The dynamic appraisal of situational aggression: an instrument to assess risk for imminent aggression in psychiatric inpatients. *Behavioral Sciences & the Law* 2006; 24 (6): 799–813.

15. Hvidhjelm J, Sestoft D, Skovgaard LT et al. Aggression in psychiatric wards: effect of the use of a structured risk assessment. *Issues in Mental Health Nursing* 2016; 37 (12): 960–7.

16. Griffith JJ, Meyer D, Maguire T, Ogloff JRP, Daffern M. A clinical decision support system to prevent aggression and reduce restrictive practices in a forensic mental health service. *Psychiatric Services* 2021; 72 (8): 885–90.

17. Kaplan SG, Wheeler EG. Survival skills for working with potentially violent clients. *Social Casework* 1983; 64 (6): 339–46.

18. European Committee for the Prevention of Torture and Inhuman or Degrading Treatment or Punishment (CPT). *Means of Restraint in Psychiatric Establishments for Adults (Revised CPT Standards).* Strasbourg, 21 March 2017, CPT/Inf(2017) 6, p. 2. https://rm.coe.int/16807001c.

19. Broderick C, Azizian A, Kornbluh R, Warburton K. Prevalence of physical violence in a forensic psychiatric hospital system during 2011–2013: Patient assaults, staff assaults, and repeatedly violent patients. *CNS Spectrums* 2015; 20 (3): 319–30.

20. Kennedy HG, Mullaney R, McKenna P et al. A tool to evaluate proportionality and necessity in the use of restrictive practices in forensic mental health settings: the DRILL tool (Dundrum restriction, intrusion and liberty ladders). *BMC Psychiatry* 2020; 20 (1): 1–20.

10

Community Forensic Psychiatry Including Liaison with Health, Criminal Justice and Public Protection Agencies

Lindsay Thomson

Introduction

Within forensic mental health services, we assess, care for, treat and manage people with major mental disorders who at times present a high risk to the safety of others. Undoubtedly, the practice setting that manages the highest risk is the community. It is there that the constant application of relational security between patient and staff is no longer present, and continuous monitoring and supervision are no longer possible. Increased patient stability in terms of their mental health and additional risks such as substance misuse and better compliance with medication and care plans will be expected as factors that allowed the individual to reach the community, but may of course change. All decisions around risk and care should be taken within the framework of human rights legislation.

Community forensic psychiatry includes the work of community forensic mental health teams, specialist services to the criminal justice system (police, courts, prison and probation) and liaison with general adult and public protection agencies.

Community Forensic Mental Health Services

Development of Forensic Community Care

The area of psychiatric practice that moved most slowly towards community provision was forensic. Traditionally, it was seen as in-patient dominant with those who reached the community returning largely to general adult psychiatric or intellectual disability services. In some areas, there were specialist forensic out-patient services, for example the Douglas Inch Clinic in Glasgow or the Portman Clinic in London, but these were rare and seldom dealt with patients with psychosis. The literature shows some development of thinking in the 1990s and some service descriptions and outcome studies in the following decade. Initially care of mentally disordered offenders (MDOs) in the community was carried out by general Community Mental Health Teams (CMHTs). One study demonstrated that 7% of a CMHT caseload consisted of MDOs [1]. Reluctance by CMHTs to accept such patients was linked to lack of training in offending and substance misuse. Secure forensic services were seen as remote with little access to their expertise.

Assertive community treatment (ACT) was developed within general adult psychiatry in the 1970s. Its essential components are home-delivered treatment, 24-hour service delivery, integrated substance misuse treatment with involvement of specialists, access to rehabilitative therapies, and from a service perspective a small case load and involvement of a psychiatrist. This model has been successfully evaluated in terms of reducing the number and length of hospital admissions, and improving quality of life, compliance, clinical outcomes and patient satisfaction [2]. The UK700 randomised controlled study, however, found no change in incidents of physical assault (22.7% vs. 21.9%) in those who received intensive case management (defined by case manager load of 10–15 patients) compared to standardised case management (case load of 30–35) over a two-year period [1]). A study in the USA found that violence was reduced with Out Patient Commitment and this was attributed to supervised compliance with medication and abstinence from intoxicants [3].

ACT did not impact on forensic outcome measures such as recidivism, so adapted forensic ACT (FACT) models were developed. These included recognition of forensic rehabilitation models such as Risk Needs Responsivity or the Good Lives Models; detailed risk assessment and management; and control by legal sanction in conjunction with improved communication, for example with probation officers, alongside care and treatment including, where appropriate, specialist input such as trauma-informed care. A systematic review of FACT found that there were significant methodological problems in comparing studies but overall arrest rates were low, although admissions increased, suggesting that this was being used as a major risk management tool [4]. A randomised controlled trial (RCT) found a reduction in hospital admissions as well, but this was a court diversion model with input and sanctions for non-compliance by a judge and would not be relevant to all jurisdictions [5]. A similar model was used in an RCT in Belgium involving internees diverted to the forensic mental health system and it found reduced arrests but increased hospital admissions [6]. The latter should not be interpreted as a poor outcome but as a functioning, responsive service.

Models of Forensic Community Care

Three models for the delivery of care to MDOs in the community are in existence: integrated, parallel and combined. In the integrated model patients are moved from forensic in-patient care to the out-patient care of GAP or intellectual disability services. In the parallel model, patients remain within forensic services. The former benefited from access to community mental health services such as day hospital and the latter benefited from good links with the criminal justice system, specialist line management and supervision, access to specialist services such as forensic psychology, capped caseloads and separate referral processes [7]. A third combined model has been used whereby patients move to general adult services who hold clinical responsibility for these individuals but have access to specialist forensic advice or treatments. Now with the development of multiple specialist teams in GAP, it is perhaps inevitable that the parallel model will be more prominent where population density permits. It would probably be more helpful to see the two models as a continuum, with patients moving between services depending on their needs rather than two discrete services, but in general this has not happened.

The crucial aspects of forensic practice that differentiate it from other areas of psychiatry are set out in Box 10.1.

Box 10.1 Aspects of Forensic Psychiatric Practice

(i) Willingness to say 'no' when patients ask to reduce or stop medicine, to revert to 'controlled drinking' or 'less harmful drugs'
(ii) Willingness to use structures of control such as conditional discharge or community treatment orders and probation orders, and willingness to breach
(iii) Ability to be consistent, reliable and 'wise' or a source of wisdom for the patient in respect of these recurrent lapses of judgement by patients
(iv) Willingness to work across agencies while managing dual mandate and duty to breach confidentiality at critical times
(v) Ability to manage and prevent splitting
(vi) Ability to manage boundaries appropriately
(vii) Willingness to maintain a long-term therapeutic relationship.

Community Forensic Mental Health Team Components

Community Forensic Mental Health Teams (CFMHTs) were established to deliver care and treatment to MDOs in the community, and to provide ongoing assessment and management of their risk. Components of a successful functioning CFMHT include: a community location, team mobility, team accessibility out of hours, formation of an effective therapeutic alliance with the patient, high frequency of contacts, ease of access to services such as housing and welfare, family and friend engagement, access to specialist treatments for mental health and criminogenic needs, return to hospital if required with bed availability, use of legal proceedings to promote engagement, and joint mental health and criminal justice working to ensure effective problem-solving. In addition, the team should be culturally informed and demonstrate flexible thinking, for example in considering daily prescribing if an individual has serious side effects from a depot. The team's work should be underpinned by an understanding of the Recovery Model [8, 9] and firmly based on risk assessment and risk management informed care plans. Safe forensic practice will inevitably place limitations on the autonomy supported by the Recovery Model but the aim of the latter remains important. In an ideal world, the move from in-patient to community care should be seamless and the legal controls to which many of our patients are subject make this more likely with, for example, leave of absence or suspension of detention and conditional discharge. Undoubtedly, the more the relationship between the patient and the professionals is viewed as a contract rather than a coercive mechanism, the more likely it is to succeed [10].

CFMHT Patients

A typical cohort of CFMHT patients will be male (86.6%), white (80%), single (never married, 47.7%), aged in their early 30s (32, SD 11.2) and commonly with drug (28.7%) or alcohol (25.8%) dependence, and a history of a serious index offence (homicide 17.1%, violence 52.9%, sexual offending 7.8%) and of previous offending (70.8%). Over a third will be on a restriction order (38.3%) [11]. Most will have schizophrenia as their primary diagnosis, although comorbid personality disorder and substance misuse will be common.

CFMHT Assessment and Management of Risk

A key component to the work of CFMHTs is the assessment and management of risk of harm to others. Chapter 6 covers this in detail. Risk assessment and management plans are used in the direct care of forensic patients but also to assist other services, chiefly criminal justice, in ensuring the correct placement and care package for an individual. In summary, a detailed structured professional judgement risk assessment should be carried out and a formulation developed outlining a patient's predisposing, precipitating, perpetuating, protective and presenting (warning signs) factors for their mental disorder and offending behaviours. This forms the basis for scenario planning which speculates about future situations and should encompass repeat, escalation, twist and improvement scenarios, and a risk management plan. The risk management plan consists of four components: monitoring such as surveillance or drug testing; supervision, for example of prohibited contacts or areas; treatment of mental disorder and criminogenic needs using medication and psychological therapies as indicated; and victim safety planning with the use, for example, of exclusion zones, home security and crisis plans.

Even from this brief summary, the reader will gather that the final document is likely to be complex and long. The major risk in a community setting is that this document is not available to staff or not used due to these factors. No amount of brilliant work is of any help if it is not utilised in practice. To get around these problems, simplified risk management systems have been put in place such as the traffic lights system [12]. This is a simple table that sets out each early warning sign or relapse indicator and the contingency actions to be taken under green, amber or red. This will cover areas such as mental illness, substance misuse, therapeutic engagement, violence or absconsion risk. For example, alcohol use may be an early warning sign: green would state no sign of alcohol use and complying with random breathalyser tests – continue with current management plan; amber: missed tests or signs of use such as an empty bottle or can – inform responsible medical officer and counsel patient; red: clear use of alcohol – immediate recall to hospital. Such plans are completely individualised. In some cases an empty can of beer may be an indicator for recall.

Understanding of this system comes to life with the example of a patient found by a nursing assistant mopping the stairs in his block of flats. On discussion, he said he had been sick the night before because he had drunk too much alcohol and asked her not to tell anyone as he was embarrassed. While the social embarrassment is understandable and possibly recognised by many a reader, the member of staff was completely familiar with the patient's traffic light indicators and this was a red. This incident was reported immediately and the patient was recalled.

Recent research concerning patients' understanding of risk shows that compliance is seen as their primary aim in moving on through the forensic system rather than internalisation and understanding of their risks that would assist with self-management. As the controls reduce on movement from an in-patient or custodial setting to the community, so compliance controls are reduced, increasing the risks. To address this, efforts have been made at shared decision-making. One randomised controlled study compared this approach to risk against treatment as usual and found no difference [13]. However, there was a clear dose effect in that most participants only had one session of shared risk decision-making.

Housing

Undoubtedly, a major component in the successful management of a mentally disordered offender in the community is suitable housing. Homelessness, temporary accommodation or housing in the setting of an antisocial peer group are unlikely to lead to successful rehabilitation. Many patients benefit from transitional housing such as hostels or supported accommodation where skills training, safety, company, integration and promotion of independence are present [14]. The downside of transitional housing is that it can be temporary. Careful thought should be given if proposing to move an individual from a successful setting to another. The care package around the individual may need to be increased, not decreased. Ideally, any transitional arrangement will have longer-term options nearby to allow the development of community links. It is essential to capture an individual's needs, provide information and support in applications, plan additional support, and consider the service user's views [15]. Some countries such as Canada have formalised programmes to transition from hospital with supported housing to the community [16].

Outcomes of Forensic Patients

The outcomes for forensic patients vary depending on the factor considered. Overall, they are reasonably good in terms of progression through the mental health system to the community, recidivism and symptom alleviation; but they are very poor for premature morbidity and social integration. For example, one study of 169 patients with schizophrenia drawn from high security and followed up for 10 years found that by the end of the study, 46 (27.2%) patients were in high security, 43 (25.5%) in medium- or low-secure units, 35 (20.7%) in an open ward, 3 (1.8%) in prison and 40 (23.7%) in the community. Violence occurred in 75% of patients over the 10-year follow-up period, and this was serious in 25%, although further convictions were rare and most violence occurred in the first two years. Continuous positive symptoms of psychosis were present in over one third. One third had self-harmed during this period but there was only one known suicide and 11 (6.5%) deaths in total. At the end of the study there was only one person in voluntary employment; 18 (12.7%) were living independently and 10 (7.1%) were in a relationship [17]. A study of morbidity and mortality in forensic patients over a 21-year average period found that 36% of the cohort had died at an average age of 56, losing 15 years of their expected potential lives. Death was caused largely by respiratory and cardiac problems rather than suicide [18].

The debate over parallel versus integrated systems of out-patient care continues. With the expansion of CFMHT services in England and Wales, a study was carried out to see which was better [11]. All patients were discharged from medium security and 409 were followed up by forensic services and 652 by general adult services on the outcome measures of mortality, hospital readmission and recidivism over an average of 6.2 years. No differences were found in terms of readmission and recidivism rates, with around one quarter of patients reoffending or being readmitted; 5% committed a violent offence and 4.9% died, 2.4% by suicide. The general adult psychiatry group had an increased risk of natural death (not by suicide) and the forensic group of earlier violent recidivism. However, the groups were not the same, with those with a more serious offending history, more primary or comorbid personality disorder being placed in the forensic cohort and those with a label of treatment-resistant schizophrenia in the general adult psychiatry group.

Specialist CFMHT Groups

Community Forensic Intellectual Disability Service

The components of CFMHTs equally well apply to services for MDOs with intellectual disability. Community forensic intellectual disability (ID) teams (CFIDTs) support least restrictive care; reduce need for in-patient beds and decrease costs; provide a pathway for support in and out of prison and hospital; and deliver specialist ID-adapted interventions. The multidisciplinary make-up of the team should be as a CFMHT but also include speech and language therapists. A study of a CFIDT followed 70 service users over an average of 123 weeks (range 1–443): 94.3% were male with an average age of 37.1 years (SD 12, range 18–58), 74.3% had mild learning disability and comorbidity was common, 38.6% with autism, 32.9% physical health problems, 28.6% drug and alcohol misuse, 21.4% personality disorder, 20% psychosis, 20% depression and 14.3% ADHD. Almost half had been the victim of physical or sexual abuse or neglect. Offences leading to service referral included sexual (52.9%), assaults (20%) and fire-setting (14.3%). These reduced on follow-up respectively to 14.3%, 17.2% and 1.4%; and over half (51.4%) had no further offending [19].

Similar positive outcomes were found in a study of 309 referrals to a local CFIDT service between 1985 and 2008 [20]. The cohort consisted of 156 sex offenders, 126 other offenders, chiefly assaults, and 27 women. One person was lost to follow-up. Seventy-six of 272 (27.9%) men reoffended over a 1–20-year period: 24 (15.4%) of the sex offender group, 52 (42.6%) of the other offences group and 6 (23%) women. A comparison of offending rates 2 years before and up to 20 years after involvement with the service showed a significant reduction. While the outcome chosen was recidivism, the description of the service components was comprehensive with detailed assessment and care planning, access to a day centre and day treatment, back-up of a 10-bedded open unit, and treatment availability including medication, anger management, social problem-solving, anxiety management, alcohol education, sexual offending group treatment, individual psychological treatment, and daily and community living skills training adapted for a population with ID.

Personality Disorder

Personality disorder (PD) is known to be a common diagnosis among offenders. Health engagement in the management of these offenders has grown. In the UK the concept of dangerous and severe PD developed in the late 1990s. Huge investment was made in this public safety initiative, largely in the high-secure hospital and prison setting. One benefit of this was the development of some community-based initiatives for people with PD. For example, specialist hostels (probation/bail) were opened for high-risk PD offenders and managed by the probation service with significant mental health input [21]. One study showed that 50 of 80 men left the hostel for positive and agreed reasons and one fifth were rearrested during their stay, which was lower than expected. Failure in the hostel setting was associated with higher psychopathy scores and previous offending. This was seen as a successful example of justice and health joint working.

Women

As in all aspects of life, equality should be promoted. The fundamental problem for female MDOs is that they are a small group, 10–20% at most, of the total MDOs. Most of the research and measures in use are based on male populations. No one would wish to advocate an increase in female offending to address this problem, but it does mean that this offender group is often an add-on to a predominantly male service. It is recognised that the offending patterns, precipitants and needs of female offenders are different to many of their male counterparts, so obtaining equality in service provision is important but difficult [22]. There may be population-dense areas where the provision of a female CFMHT is feasible, but for most services the individually tailored approach to care will be the best option.

Neurodevelopmental Disorders and Acquired Brain Injuries

Severe brain injury can result in cognitive and emotional deficits, and in changes in personality. Impairments in problem-solving, memory, empathy, tolerance, impulse and aggression control make keeping to societal norms more difficult and involvement with criminal justice services more likely. The cause of these difficulties may not be obvious and require routine enquiry about brain injuries. Interventions include advice on management, psychological interventions or neurorehabilitation. In reality, brain injury services are limited and CFMHTs may be called upon to manage these individuals [23]. The independent sector may provide intensive individualised packages of care combining disability-adapted residential accommodation, 24-hour care and the support of a CFMHT. These can be expensive and may require funding from disability, criminal justice and health sources.

Autism spectrum disorders (ASDs) including autism, Asperger's syndrome and pervasive development disorder are manifested by difficulties with social interaction and communication and restricted, repetitive stereotyped behaviours. Unlike acquired brain injuries (ABIs), people with ASD are more likely to be rule keepers and involvement with the criminal justice system is less likely. It can occur when behavioural patterns are disturbed, the rules of social engagement are misunderstood or there is resentment caused by rejection or bullying, over-sensitivity to sound or an intense interest in weapons or death. A study of ASD in the prison population found no evidence of higher rates than in the community [24].

Liaison with Health, Criminal Justice and Public Protection Agencies

Liaison within Health Services

The interface between forensic psychiatry and GAP, ID, child and adolescent or old age psychiatric services is essential to describe in local services, for example whether the parallel or continuous models of forensic service delivery discussed earlier are in use. Referral criteria and defined patient pathways assist clarity on both sides.

Continuity of care is a major factor in successful outcomes of forensic patients in the community. For reasons of imprisonment or hospitalisation, the move to the community may not be from a local facility. This is particularly true when patients are moved to independent providers of forensic mental healthcare and geographically dislocated from the home, family and local services.

Liaison with Criminal Justice Services

The work of CFMHTs will include liaison with the different components of criminal justice services, including police, courts, prisons and probation services.

Police

The primary purpose of any police force is to keep the peace, prevent offending and apprehend offenders. However, in reality the police do a great deal of social care in their interactions with the young, elderly and those with mental disorders. Training in mental disorders and systems to support officers in their work are therefore important. In the UK, the different jurisdictions have place of safety orders which allow the police to take an individual to an identified place of safety if they think the person may have a mental disorder or be in immediate need of care or treatment, and that it is in their interests or necessary for the protection of others. Places of safety are usually hospitals so the involvement of CFMHT staff in this setting is unlikely.

CFMHT staff may become involved in providing psychiatric services to police stations. This will be dependent on local agreements. In some areas, such services are provided by a wider psychiatric rota and in others there will be no provision but forensic medical examiners who are usually general practitioners with training in forensic procedures will refer on to psychiatric services as required. Decisions to be taken in a police station setting include: fitness to remain in custody; assessment and management of identified health needs; and fitness to be interviewed.

Courts

Involvement with courts can be pre-trial and psychiatric recommendations may include informal treatment, compulsory treatment under civil mental health legislation, assessment or treatment as a bail requirement, or remand to hospital for assessment or treatment. Psychiatric issues to be considered at the time of trial include fitness for trial and responsibility for any alleged act on grounds of mental disorder. Post-conviction, consideration may be required of assessment and treatment insofar as these are relevant to sentencing considerations by the court or final disposal. Court disposals may include community options with psychiatric or psychological treatment requirements, hospital care and treatment, or guardianship or intervention orders for those with capacity issues.

Services to courts are often provided by CFMHTs. Many will have a system to respond to and allocate requests for psychiatric reports. Others will have formal systems to attend the court on a daily or on-call basis and will assess individuals at the request of the prosecution service or following concerns raised by police or custody staff. Such services often use nurse screening followed by psychiatric assessment and recommendations under mental health legislation as required. These services may vary in name, being known as diversion or liaison services. In reality, most will do both.

Diversion and Liaison Services

Two main services have developed around the criminal justice service and both are aimed at ensuring individuals with mental disorder get the required care and treatment. In reality these services only exist in urban areas where there is sufficient population density and court throughput to make them worthwhile, and they are difficult to sustain [25].

Diversion concerns the transfer of responsibility for an individual from criminal justice to health services with a discontinuation of prosecution or criminal justice involvement. There are five main steps involved in the diversion process: screening, formal assessment, liaison with prosecutors and mental health services, disposal and monitoring. In some countries this will involve Mental Health Courts which may require a guilty plea and violent offenders may be excluded. The court may have the option of an alternative sentence if the participant fails to adhere to the conditions set for treatment. In the UK, diversion from prosecution only occurs in more minor cases where the individual is willing to accept treatment. No conditions are set.

Much more common is the liaison system with joint working between mental health and criminal justice. Under this pathway the individual will go through the criminal justice system but will have access to assessment and treatment, in hospital if necessary, pre-trial and pre-sentencing, and may ultimately be fully diverted to the mental health system under a final disposal but the prosecution will have proceeded. Prosecution may go ahead at the same time as the assessment and treatment or at a later stage. Hybrid options also exist whereby the individual can be given a suspended sentence dependent on the outcome of treatment or compliance with treatment, made subject to a community justice or probation order with a condition of psychiatric or psychological treatment, or given a sentence but sent to psychiatric hospital under a hospital direction.

Prisons: Throughcare

Linking prisoners with mental disorders into treatment services following release is critical to prevent their deterioration and possible recidivism, but is often poorly done. Indeed, meeting their wider needs of accommodation and support is also required. Standard throughcare operated by many prisons endeavours to do this with social work and health colleagues making strenuous efforts, but in reality many prisoners leave with a bed in temporary accommodation but otherwise homeless, unregistered with a primary care or general practice service, with a short supply of any medication required and with a letter in their pocket to be handed to health professionals outlining their needs. For longer-term and more serious prisoners who are released on licence conditions, such supports are easier to put in place because of the need to have a fixed address. Depending on local arrangements, CFMHTs may be involved in this work, providing in-reach into local prisons or liaison with prison mental health services over transfer of care [26].

Two models have been developed to endeavour to improve through care: adapted Forensic Assertive Community Treatment (FACT) and Critical Time Intervention (CTI) [27]. What matters in both models is engagement with the prisoner and a holistic approach addressing mental health, housing, welfare, and vocational and social needs. The adapted FACT model is focussed on prisoners with mental disorder and their return to the community. The aim is to prevent further imprisonment and there is often ongoing criminal justice involvement which can be used to promote compliance. It is described as a 'long-term wrap-around approach' to optimise continuity of care by placing all services within an interdisciplinary team. It is ongoing as long as the need is there. CTI promotes contacts with external services through engagement between a CTI case manager and the prisoner in the latter stages of their custody and into the community setting. It is time limited and usually lasts three to nine months. It promotes self-reliance and aims to assist the prisoner in building community connections. A qualitative comparison of the two models found that both promoted engagement but had basic differences in philosophy and available resources.

Probation Services

Probation services exist to supervise individuals who have offended in the community. They have either been given a community sentence or have been released from prison on parole or licence. Conditions will be set for any period of probation and include regular meetings with a probation officer, unpaid work, attendance at education or training courses, and treatment programmes, for example for sex offending or substance misuse. CFMHTs are likely to work closely with probation officers managing specific individuals in the community or in a bail or parole hostel (approved premises) setting. In England there are a small number of approved premises specifically for MDOs [28]. Terminology varies in this field and probation officers in one jurisdiction can be offender managers or criminal justice social workers elsewhere. Regardless of this, most jurisdictions will have an option for psychiatric or psychological treatment as part of their probation orders or community payback orders. Such treatment does not have to be with a forensic specialist.

Specialist Community-Based Offender Services

Some specialist clinics focus on management of problem behaviours and high-risk offenders, often in conjunction with criminal justice services, rather than on specific psychopathological symptoms or diagnoses as the primary reason for referral. Such behaviours include sexual offending, stalking, arson, threatening or violence (Forensicare Problem Behaviour Clinic – Melbourne). Others offer a joint working model between health and criminal justice services to improve public safety and offender outcomes, and to reduce risk and recidivism (Serious Offender Liaison Service, Edinburgh). This is based on consultation, assessment and advice on psychologically informed interventions to criminal justice staff involved in the management of complex cases. Direct treatment is rare. Other specialist services such as the Fixated Threat Assessment Centre (London) or PREVENT mental health hubs (England) focus on one issue such as threats to politicians or royalty, or prevention of terrorism, and provide a national or regional service with liaison with local services [30–34]. There is a great deal to learn from these approaches for CFMHTs.

Public Safety Systems

A major change in the management of MDOs in the community in recent years has been the development of formal multi-agency working arrangements. This reflects the complexity in managing some high-risk offenders and MDOs. This multi-agency working is defined as 'the coming together of people from different professional backgrounds, organisations and services, sometimes with varying primary purposes, but with the common aim of improving public safety and decreasing an individual's risk of harm to others' [29] (p. 154). Such multi-agency working may improve risk management by formal case review with a broader perspective, engagement with individuals who may otherwise be rejected by mental health services, sharing of and clarity on responsibilities, continuity of care, information sharing on a proportionate basis, opportunities to develop cross-agency relationships and for informal working, and wider training opportunities.

Ultimately, the aim of multi-agency working is to reduce reoffending. Potential disadvantages to multi-agency working should be acknowledged and include breach of confidentiality, intrusion into an individual's private life, and potential financial and opportunity costs for the agencies involved. Examples of multi-agency working are in place in Germany, the UK, the Netherlands and Denmark [29].

Germany: The Round Table

The round table in Germany is a process of formal meetings of police, probation officers and out-patient mental health services to review a proposed package of care, and to consider additional requirements to further the integration of the patient into the community and to improve public safety. Other parties such as social work, housing or the legal profession may be invited as relevant to an individual case. An evaluation of the round-table approach found improved outcomes with recidivism rates for violence reducing from 15% to 6% after the introduction of forensic out-patient care and to 1.8% following the development of round tables. In addition, this development has led to joint educational seminars, improved discharge planning and a greater clinical focus on prevention of violence.

United Kingdom: Multi-Agency Public Protection Arrangements

Multi-Agency Public Protection Arrangements (MAPPAs) exist in all four countries of the UK, although there may be some variation in name and practice. They were introduced in 2003 to manage the risk of harm to others and are enshrined in law: Criminal Justice Act 2003 (sections 325–327) in England and Wales; Criminal Justice (NI) Order 2008 in Northern Ireland; and the Management of Offenders etc. (Scotland) Act 2005.

MAPPA mandates the police, prison and probation services to collaborate to manage the risks presented in the community by dangerous offenders. Other services such as health, social care, education, housing, welfare, employment, electronic monitoring, youth offending and the UK Border Agency have a statutory duty to participate. MAPPA is divided into three response levels dependent on an individual's level of risk, press interest and management complexity, usually judged by the number of agencies involved in coordinating care. Cases in level one will usually involve only one agency and level two will have more than one agency involved due to the complexity of an individual's needs. There are a small number of cases with complex requirements with or without a high media interest which merit level three MAPPA. Level one and two cases involve a careful check of the plan in place and advice, whereas a multi-agency public protection panel is called to review in detail arrangements for level three cases.

In 2019, there were 82,921 offenders under MAPPA in England and Wales: 73% were registered sex offenders, 27% chiefly violent offenders and less than 1% other dangerous offenders; 98% of cases were managed at level one and 140 cases (0.2%) at level three; 179 MAPPA offenders were charged with serious further offences.

Public Protection Arrangements are in place in Northern Ireland (PPANI). Initially voluntary from 2001 under Multi-Agency Sex Offender Risk Assessment and Management (MASRAM), it became statutory in 2008. PPANI has many similarities to MAPPA but has Local Area Public Protection Panels (LAPPPs) and two lay members of the public on its senior management boards. In 2018–19, there were 440 LAPPPs; 151 were category 2 (clear and identifiable evidence that they could cause serious harm through carrying out a contact sexual or violent offence) and 32 were category 3 (highly likely) offender reviews.

MAPPA was established in Scotland in 2007 and is very similar to the model in England and Wales. Initially the focus was on registered sex offenders but this extended to restricted patients in 2008 and to other risk of serious harm offenders in 2016. Key agencies or responsible authorities include Police Scotland, Local Authorities, Scottish Prison Services and the health boards for restricted patients. Developments have included an information-sharing concordat between the NHS and MAPPA partners, a Forensic Network MAPPA Health Group and training through the School of Forensic Mental Health.

On 31 March 2019 there were 4,218 registered sex offenders being managed in the community, with 97% of these being managed on MAPPA level one and 114 at level two or three [12]. Of these, 1.9% were convicted of a violent or further sexual offence and 6% were reported for failing to comply with notification requirements. Figures on violent offenders or restricted patients managed under MAPPA were not provided.

Netherlands: Safety Houses

There are 25 safety houses in the Netherlands involving local authorities, the criminal justice and mental health services. It is a collaborative concept, not a building. Their remit is wider than those multi-agency developments in Germany and the UK and includes reduction of nuisance, as well as domestic violence and criminality, but the cases will be complex and meet the following criteria:

> multiple problems in one or more areas of living that will result in criminal behaviour and / or nuisance, or further social decline; cooperation between partners in multiple areas is required to achieve an effective approach; the problem is influenced by and has an impact on the family and social system and / or the immediate social environment (or is expected to have an influence on it); and there are severe local or area-specific safety problems, which require a multiple service response approach.

Safety houses function under a national framework developed by the Ministry of Safety and Justice of the Netherlands. This sets out four main aspects to their work: firstly, it should be person-orientated and based on an individual plan; secondly, it is territorial with each local authority area able to join; thirdly, it examines systems in which the individual is based such as family or peer group, and targets interventions accordingly; and lastly, it is victim-orientated and will provide information to victims, mediation and support in completing a victim impact statement.

Denmark: Police, Social Services and Psychiatry Cooperation

The Police, Social Services and Psychiatry (PSP) Cooperation began in Denmark in 2004 but became a national system in 2009. It involves multi-agency working between the police, social services and psychiatry to manage vulnerable individuals aged 18 or over with mental disorder, substance misuse and/or social problems in the community. It is divided into managerial and operational functions: the former has responsibility for strategy and train-ing, and the latter for specific cases and coordination. This system applies currently only to individuals over the age of 18. The PSP gathers information on each individual regarding their background and needs, and meeting these is assigned to a lead body. Concerns about the sharing of information and confidentiality were addressed by amendments to the Danish Judicial Code and to the Administration of Justice Act and Processing of Personal Data Act in 2009. A qualitative evaluation of the PSP model found that it improved service coordination, feedback and sharing of experiences.

There will be other multi-agency systems in operation elsewhere in the world but many countries lack these. The advantages and disadvantages of such systems are set out above. As multidisciplinary working was once considered challenging and is now the norm, so it is likely that we will see a similar pattern in the development of multi-agency working. To be successful it requires joint educational initiatives, resources, peer review, clarity on roles and procedures, evaluation and development of outcome measures, and data-sharing protocols to address concerns around confidentiality.

Cohesion Systems: Forensic Network

Cohesion and mechanisms for debate and development are essential for any system to grow and function well. This can be seen above in the development of multi-agency systems but it is equally true for disparate systems that may sit under one body such as health. Managed care networks have been introduced across health to address these issues. One example is the Forensic Mental Health Service Managed Care Network which was established by Scottish Government in 2003 to provide a pan-Scotland approach to the planning of services, address fragmentation across the forensic mental health estate, determine the most effective care for MDOs, consider wider issues surrounding patient pathways, align strategic planning across Scotland, and address teaching, training and research needs. The Forensic Network's multi-agency approach facilitates information sharing across the estate, criminal justice services, the voluntary sector and social services, and encourages the development of strong working relationships which assist with the planning of services and the patient journey through the forensic mental health estate.

Governance of the Forensic Network is via a multi-agency board which deals with national oversight and matters of strategic direction. The Network's structure is shown in Figure 10.1. The Network Inter-Regional Group manages operational issues and consists of regional and clinical leads. In addition, there are Network professional groups for lead nurses, allied health professionals, psychology, pharmacy, carer coordinators and social work, as well as a Carer Forum. The clinical fora were created to develop educational and networking opportunities, alongside the identification of any policy or operational issues, and have been developed in the areas of ID, risk, services for women, sexual harm, prisoner mental health, addictions, PD and problem behaviours, victims and trauma, and MAPPAs. The Network commissions short-life working groups, for example on electronic monitoring.

Managerial control of services sits with each of the geographical health boards or the national high-security State Hospitals Health Board for Scotland. The Forensic Network

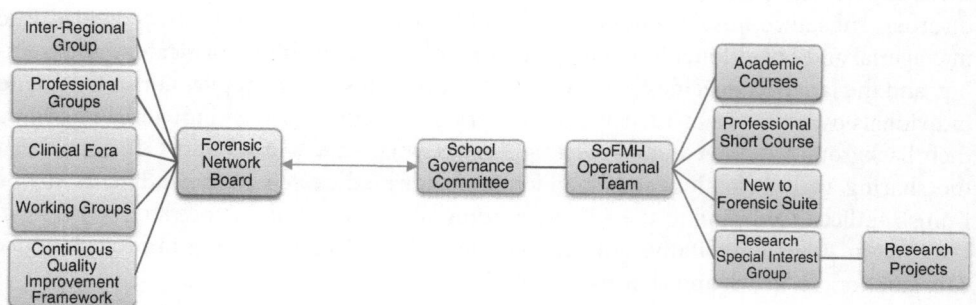

Figure 10.1 Structure of the Forensic Network and School of Forensic Mental Health.

provides a forum to discuss and agree strategic and operational issues such as the configuration of the forensic estate, patient pathways, services for women, ID services, and high- and medium-secure referral criteria, and to plan the annual Forensic Network census, which provides data for research and planning.

The Network has developed a mechanism for conflict resolution and has a continuous quality improvement framework whereby within each cycle there is agreement on new standards, self-assessment, peer review visits with a report and recommendations, and a locally developed action plan. The current over-arching themes are on assessment, care planning and treatment; physical health; risk; management of violence; physical environment; and teams, skills and staffing.

The Forensic Network established the School of Forensic Mental Health (SoFMH) in 2007. The School delivers a range of short courses, has established an online MSc in Forensic Mental Health and has introduced the 'New to Forensic' suite of programmes. This initial course involves all staff, clinical and non-clinical, new to the forensic field and takes them through a mentored programme with chapters covering different aspects of the patient's journey and professional, user and carer issues. Versions of this programme have been adapted for other countries and the third sector. 'New to the Essentials of Psychological Care in Forensic Practice' and 'New to Forensic Medicine' complete this suite of courses.

References

1. Walsh E, Gilvarry C, Samele C et al. Reducing violence in severe mental illness: randomised controlled trial of intensive case management compared with standard care. *BMJ* (Clinical research ed.) 2001; 323 (7321): 1093–6.

2. Lamberti JS, Weisman RL, Cerulli C et al. A randomized controlled trial of the Rochester forensic assertive community treatment model. *Psychiatric Services* 2017; 68 (10): 1016–24.

3. Swanson JW, Swartz MS, Wagner HR et al. Involuntary out-patient commitment and reduction of violent behaviour in persons with severe mental illness. *The British Journal of Psychiatry* 2000; 176 (4): 324–31.

4. Marquant T, Sabbe B, Van Nuffel M, Goethals K. Forensic assertive community treatment: a review of the literature. *Community Mental Health Journal* 2016; 52 (8): 873–81.

5. Cusack KJ, Morrissey JP, Cuddeback GS, Prins A, Williams DM. Criminal justice involvement, behavioral health service use, and costs of forensic assertive community

treatment: a randomized trial. *Community Mental Health Journal* 2010; 46 (4): 356–63.

6. Marquant T, Sabbe B, Van Nuffel M, Verelst R, Goethals K. Forensic assertive community treatment in a continuum of care for male internees in Belgium: results after 33 months. *Community Mental Health Journal* 2018; 54: 58–65.

7. Mohan R, Slade M, Fahy TA. Clinical characteristics of community forensic mental health services. *Psychiatric Services* 2004; 55 (11): 1294–8.

8. Jacobson N, Greenley D. What is recovery? A conceptual model and explication. *Psychiatric Services* 2001; 52 (4): 482–5.

9. Clarke C, Lumbard D, Sambrook S, Kerr K. What does recovery mean to a forensic mental health patient? A systematic review and narrative synthesis of the qualitative literature. *The Journal of Forensic Psychiatry & Psychology* 2016; 27 (1): 38–54.

10. Bonnie RJ, Monahan J. From coercion to contract: reframing the debate on mandated community treatment for people

with mental disorders. *Law and Human Behavior* 2005; 29: 485–503.

11. Coid JW, Hickey N, Yang M. Comparison of outcomes following after-care from forensic and general adult psychiatric services. *British Journal of Psychiatry* 2007; 190: 509–14.

12. Scottish Government. *Memorandum of Procedure on Restricted Patients. ANNEX H – Risk Management Traffic Lights for All Levels of Security*. Edinburgh, Scottish Government, 2010.

13. Troquete NA, van den Brink RH, Beintema H et al. Risk assessment and shared care planning in out-patient forensic psychiatry: cluster randomised controlled trial. *British Journal of Psychiatry* 2013; 202 (5): 365–71.

14. Kelly BL, Barrenger SL, Watson AC, Angell B. Forensic assertive community treatment: recidivism, hospitalization, and the role of housing and support. *Social Work in Mental Health* 2017; 15 (5): 567–87.

15. Heard CP, Scott J, Tetzlaff A, Lumley H. Transitional housing in forensic mental health: considering consumer lived experience. *Health & Justice* 2019; 7 (1): 1–9.

16. Leclair MC, Deveaux F, Roy L et al. The impact of Housing First on criminal justice outcomes among homeless people with mental illness: a systematic review. *The Canadian Journal of Psychiatry* 2019; 64 (8): 525–30.

17. Darjee R, Øfstegaard M, Thomson L. Schizophrenia in a high-security hospital: long-term forensic, clinical, administrative and social outcomes. *The Journal of Forensic Psychiatry & Psychology* 2017; 28 (4): 525–47.

18. Rees C, Thomson L. Exploration of morbidity, suicide and all-cause mortality in a Scottish forensic cohort over 20 years. *BJPsych Open* 2020; 6 (4): e62.

19. Browning M, Gray R, Tomlins R. A community forensic team for people with intellectual disabilities. *Journal of Forensic Practice* 2016; 18 (4): 274–82.

20. Lindsay WR, Steptoe L, Wallace L, Haut F, Brewster E. An evaluation and 20-year follow-up of a community forensic intellectual disability service. *Criminal Behaviour and Mental Health* 2013; 23 (2): 138–49.

21. Blumenthal S, Craissati J, Minchin L. The development of a specialist hostel for the community management of personality disordered offenders. *Criminal Behaviour and Mental Health* 2009; 19 (1): 43–53.

22. Thomson LD, Bogue JP, Humphreys MS, Johnstone EC. A survey of female patients in high security psychiatric care in Scotland. *Criminal Behaviour and Mental Health* 2001; 11 (2): 86–93.

23. Network NPH. *Brain Injury and Offending: Report to National Prisoner Network Committee*. Edinburgh, Scottish Government, 2016, p. 57.

24. Robinson L, Spencer MD, Thomson LD et al. Evaluation of a screening instrument for autism spectrum disorders in prisoners. *PLoS One* 2012; 7 (5): e36078.

25. James DV. Court diversion in perspective. *Australian & New Zealand Journal of Psychiatry* 2006; 40 (6–7): 529–38.

26. Smith D, Harnett S, Flanagan A et al. Beyond the walls: an evaluation of a Pre-Release Planning (PReP) programme for sentenced mentally disordered offenders. *Frontiers in Psychiatry* 2018; 9: 549.

27. Shaw J, Conover S, Herman D et al. *Critical Time Intervention for Severely Mentally Ill Prisoners (CrISP): A Randomised Controlled Trial*. Southampton, NIHR Journals Library, 2017. www.ncbi.nlm.nih .gov/books/NBK424457. doi: 10.3310/ hsdr05080.

28. Bourne R, Rajput R, Field R. Working with probation services and mentally disordered offenders. *BJPsych Advances* 2015; 21 (4): 273–80.

29. Thomson L, Goethals K, Nedopil N. Multi agency working in forensic psychiatry: theory and practice in Europe. *Criminal Behaviour and Mental Health* 2016; 26 (3): 153–60.

30. Barry-Walsh J, James DV, Mullen PE. Fixated Threat Assessment Centers: preventing harm and facilitating care in public figure threat cases and those thought to be at risk of lone-actor grievance-fueled violence. *CNS Spectr.* 2020; 25 (5): 630–7.

31. Gill P, Corner E, Farnham F et al. Predictors of varying levels of risks posed by fixated individuals to British public figures. *Journal of Forensic Sciences* 2021; 66 (4): 1364–6.

32. Sydes M, Wine L, Higginson A et al. Criminal justice interventions for preventing radicalisation, violent extremism and terrorism: an evidence and gap map. *Campbell Systematic Reviews* 2023; 19 (4): e1366.

33. Wilson S, Farnham F, Taylor A, Taylor R. Reflections on working in public-figure threat management. *Medicine, Science and the Law* 2019; 59 (4): 275–81.

34. Pathé MT, Lowry TJ, Haworth DJ, Winterbourne P, Day L. Public figure fixation: cautionary findings for mental health practitioners. *Behavioral Sciences & the Law* 2016; 34 (5): 681–92.

Assessment of Personality Disorder, Psychopathy and Associated Offending Behaviour

Jeremy W. Coid

The assessment of personality disorder (PD) and of associated violent and other criminal behaviour are among the most complex tasks for a forensic psychiatrist. Assessment is complicated by high levels of comorbidity with clinical mental disorders, the high hetero-geneity of violent and criminal behaviour, and differing and sometimes conflicting views on how PD should be conceptualised and diagnosed. It therefore requires a high level of diagnostic competence and ability to think flexibly regarding different models of mental disorder and diagnostic approaches.

Some knowledge of psychodynamics can be very helpful in the assessment of offenders with PD and their management, together with awareness of the strong feelings these patients arouse in those who work with them, and why. People with PD can be difficult to manage, treat and interact with, and they can be disliked by mental health professionals. It is therefore important to gain experience and competency of working with PD patients, together with a good training. This is thought to improve staff competency, reduce staff turnover in units with PD patients and improve service and treatment outcomes [1]. At consultant level, it is important to be aware of how PD patients can result in over-involvement, staff-burnout, manipulation of staff and 'splitting' of staff teams. This can impact heavily on nursing staff who spend longest periods in face-to-face contact and at consultant level it is important to be aware of the pressures on nurses, but also on less experienced medical staff. However, it can also adversely influence the decision-making of experienced clinicians. Awareness of counter-transference is therefore essential in working with and assessing PD patients. A psychodynamic understanding can also be helpful in assessments, where the primitive symbolism and underlying meaning of offending behav-iour, which can sometimes have a dream-like quality, can become clearer during an assessment.

This chapter is not helped by being written at a time when traditional diagnostic categories in the International Classification of Diseases, 10th edition (ICD-10) [67] are about to be abandoned and replaced by broad severity dimensions of personality function-ing within a new framework. There is no available evidence to suggest how forensic psychiatrists will use this new framework in future clinical practice or when presenting evidence as an expert witness. Inevitably, this chapter must rely on evidence from research and personal clinical practice using traditional categories. Because, in the past, standardised instruments based on ICD-10 were slow in being developed and have poor reliability, much of this chapter is based on successive versions of the US *Diagnostic and Statistical Manual* (DSM) diagnostic system [2]. That does not mean that the chapter is automatically outdated and that a new, more appropriate era of PD measurement is about to begin. Because the new system is untested in the forensic clinical sphere, its utility will need to be demonstrated and proved over time. Clinical services may mandate that the new system is entered into clinical case notes in a centrally controlled National Health Service. But if it cannot be used to reliably explain the association between PD and offending behaviour to a court or convey helpful information to other disciplines in tribunals and for parole board assessments of future risk of reoffending, together with deciding on clinical management and treatment interventions, it will ultimately fail. It is recommended at this stage that trainees develop expertise in a tested categorical system such as DSM and additionally train in the forthcoming dimensional system to develop their own style of assessment, based on new research, their increasing clinical experience over time and observation of other clinicians.

Clinical experience with the severe personality pathology encountered in forensic clinical practice can be very confusing at first if a rigid approach is taken to the underlying theoretical basis of PDs. It is important to be aware that the notion of a PD as something that is best measured using psychological trait theory is a relatively recent claim. It does not always fit the clinical reality. For example, schizoid PD as defined by DSM, and originally derived from psychodynamic principles, is likely to show features of 'detachment' in the forthcoming ICD-11 [3]. However, in prisons and secure settings, schizoid PD often shows remarkable similarities to Asperger's syndrome or high-functioning autism. It is more likely to receive these latter diagnoses now that better training has been developed for the developmental disorders. It is, of course, highly questionable whether a patient should be given a primary diagnosis of PD when they have autism. Similarly, borderline (or emotionally unstable) PD, as typically encountered in secure settings, often shows such severe affective disturbance that 'negative affectivity' in the new ICD-11 system is unlikely to do the observed psychopathology of intense rapid cycling mood swings adequate justice.

Key issues to remember when encountering patients with PD in forensic practice are firstly that they show high levels of comorbidity with other PDs as well as other clinical syndromes. Research using standardised diagnostic instruments typically produces multiple diagnostic categories and it will initially be difficult to ascertain which is the primary condition. Although the new ICD-11 system is expected to overcome this problem, it cannot and will inevitably show multiple, high dimensional scores for many forensic patients. Secondly, the PDs encountered (however measured) are typically severe, resulting in multiple forms of dysfunction in the patient's daily living. It is sobering to reflect that severe cases of borderline PD, which often do not respond to conventional treatments such as psychotherapy [4], or are too disturbed to cooperate in talking treatments, may require long periods in security and are often prescribed long-term medication. Some psychopaths remain as socially disabled as any patient with schizophrenia and, by default, become institutionalised for long periods, usually in prison, often for the protection of others.

So how to advise the trainee forensic psychiatrist when assessing PD and offending behaviour? Firstly, there have been few studies investigating the associations and those that have usually used the DSM glossary. It is possible that ICD-11 will present a framework to rely on, but in the absence of any empirical support for this at present, trainees should primarily adhere to the DSM framework, despite its shortcomings. ICD-10 has multiple shortcomings and dissocial PD is not fit for purpose due to a lack of diagnostic validity and should always be replaced with DSM antisocial personality disorder in the forensic assessment. Psychopathy will not be dealt with adequately by the new ICD system and is not included in successive versions of the DSM. This means that trainees should obtain a full training in making the diagnosis of psychopathy using the Psychopathy Checklist – Revised (PCL-R) [5] from an expert trainer. Do not rely on short courses and opt for the full training of at least two days. Do not rely on other disciplines to make the diagnosis of PD for you. Ensure you can confidently achieve this yourself because it will be essential in your clinical practice and you may need to justify your diagnosis and its individual criteria in a court. Beware of self-report instruments sometimes used by clinical psychologists, such as the *Millon Clinical Multiaxial Inventory Manual* (MCMI) [6]. They often cannot distinguish between a severe mental illness and PD and have a low threshold for a PD diagnosis, although they can be useful in research. For PD, it will be necessary to have a training in diagnosing DSM categories pending the development of ICD-11 methods in forensic samples and in settings such as security, and for its applicability to courts. In the UK, different instruments are used but tend to achieve similar results. But these can be time-consuming until the trainee becomes skilled in administering them. It is best to take copies of research instruments with you to assessments. An instrument such as the Structured Clinical Interview for DSM-IV Axis II Personality Disorders (SCID-II) [7] is more useful for a psychiatrist despite complaints of the 'halo' effect when making diagnoses. However, this is likely a problem in research settings rather than for experienced clinicians.

A further key issue is being able to differentiate between PD and clinical syndromes. For some PDs – for example, schizotypal – it is impossible to do so. It should be remembered that there is no diagnosis of schizotypal PD in the ICD system and that schizotypal is a category among the schizophrenias in ICD-10. Avoidant PD (often comorbid with borderline PD) is remarkably similar to social phobia and in many cases is indistinguishable [8]. Similarly, paranoid PD can be indistinguishable from delusional disorder, if sufficiently severe. Trainees should be careful not to miss a diagnosis of delusional disorder and should opt for the latter diagnosis if necessary. Both may respond favourably to anti-psychotic medication. It is also important to remember that in forensic settings, paranoid PD is often comorbid with antisocial PD (ASPD). Irrespective of these issues, it is best to conduct a full clinical assessment of the patient or client for lifetime history of clinical syndromes first before progressing to assessing presence of PD. In some centres, the lifetime approach is not always emphasised but should be a cornerstone of forensic clinical assessment. There are research diagnostic instruments that help and experience with these will soon demonstrate that mental illness can fluctuate and at times will not be present. It will also show that great caution should be used regarding fluctuating and relapsing conditions such as psychosis before a diagnosis of PD can confidently be made. In general, it is best to take a hierarchical approach where the clinical syndrome takes priority over the diagnosis of PD as the primary condition, with extreme caution over attributing a PD diagnosis in the presence of severe mental disorder. What will become clear with experience is that in the forensic setting, patients and clients are more likely to receive multiple PD diagnoses together with multiple clinical syndromes over the lifetime.

Epidemiology of Personality Disorder and Violence

DSM Personality Disorders

PD in the household population of the UK showed an overall weighted prevalence of 'any' PD of 4.4% (95%CI 2.9–6.7), using DSM Axis II categories in a survey carried out in 2000 [9]. The survey involved screening the population using a self-report instrument in a first phase, followed by clinical diagnostic instruments administered by trained clinicians in a second phase. However, if PD 'unspecified' was used (participants with a cut-off number of traits/symptoms but not meeting any defined DSM category), the prevalence nearly doubled, indicating that many people have abnormal personality features which do not necessarily fit with the diagnostic categories in current glossaries. Rates of PD were higher among men than women and people who were separated or divorced, unemployed, and residing in urban locations. These individuals had a high use of healthcare, but this was confounded by their high levels of comorbid clinical syndromes and substance misuse. A vulnerable group were identified with Cluster B disorders (antisocial, borderline, narcissistic) who are often in care during childhood and enter the criminal justice system when young, suggesting the need for preventative interventions at the public health level. Although borderline PD is thought to be commoner among women and is the commonest category among in-patients, the 2000 survey was important in showing this was not the case.

Table 11.1 compares the prevalence of PD in the national population of the UK in 2000 [9] and among prisoners in 1995 [10]. These studies are the most comprehensive available for the UK and prevalence of PD using sound survey methods and representative sample have not been completed since. The surveys used the same instruments to diagnose PD and are derived from face-to-face interviews. The prevalences are presented in a deliberately simplistic manner to show the differences in prevalence of different PDs between men and women, and between prison settings and the general population. Table 11.1 shows that PD is considerably more prevalent among prisoners and among men. Borderline PD was more prevalent among men in contrast to many studies of borderline PD where it is assumed incorrectly that the reverse is the case. This is because women with borderline PD are more likely to be accepted as referrals for psychiatric treatment than men and particularly to be hospitalised more than men. Obsessive-compulsive was the most prevalent PD in the community and ASPD was the most prevalent among prisoners. ASPD showed a marked difference in prevalence between men and women, although this was less marked among prisoners. Although there is no evidence within Table 11.1, the findings would suggest that in addition to ASPD, diagnoses of borderline PD and paranoid PD are likely to have a direct bearing on becoming a prisoner.

Data from the first phase of the British National Household Survey of Psychiatric Morbidity was also used to measure associations between PD categories and self-reported violence [11]. DSM categories were created using a self-report instrument in this study. Although self-report instruments tend to have a lower threshold and over-diagnose categories of personality disorder, this method was used because it measured statistical *associations* between violence and PD, was the best available for this purpose and was applied to a large population sample. One aim was to measure independent associations by adjusting for comorbid PDs and clinical syndromes. The study then found that men who reported violence in the past five years showed independent associations with a limited number of categories of paranoid, antisocial and borderline PDs, and women only with ASPD. However, the odds of association with violent behaviour together with ASPD were twice as high among women, even though ASPD was less prevalent among women.

ASPD was independently associated with severity of the violence measured according to victim injury, repetitive violence and violence when intoxicated, and more likely to occur in pubs and bars. There were fewer associations with other categories: paranoid was associated with repetitive violence and violence when intoxicated; obsessive-compulsive, although not independently associated with violence, was associated with more serious violence which

Table 11.1 Comparison of prevalence of different categories of personality disorder in the general population of Britain in 2000 and prisons in England and Wales in 1995

General population				Prisons					
Men		Women		Men (remand)		Men (sentenced)		Women	
diagnosis	%	diagnosis	%	diagnosis	%	diagnosis	%	diagnosis	%
Obsessive-compulsive	2.6	Obsessive-compulsive	1.3	Antisocial	63	Antisocial	49	Antisocial	31
Paranoid	1.2	Schizoid	0.8	Paranoid	29	Paranoid	20	Borderline	20
Antisocial	1.0	Avoidant	0.7	Borderline	23	Borderline	14	Paranoid	16
Borderline	1.0	Borderline	0.4	Avoidant	14	Obsessive-compulsive	10	Avoidant	11
Avoidant	1.0	Paranoid	0.3	Schizoid	8	Narcissistic	7	Obsessive-compulsive	10
Schizoid	0.9	Antisocial	0.2	Narcissistic	8	Avoidant	7	Narcissistic	6
Dependent	0.2	Schizotypal	0.1	Obsessive-compulsive	7	Schizoid	6	Dependent	5
Schizotypal	0.9	Dependent	–	Dependent	4	Schizotypal	2	Schizoid	4
Narcissistic	–	Narcissistic	–	Schizotypal	2	Histrionic	2	Histrionic	4
Histrionic	–	Histrionic	–	Histrionic	1	Dependent	1	Schizotypal	4
Any	5.4		3.4		78		64		50

resulted in victim injury. Avoidant PD showed a specific, *negative* association with repetitive violence. ASPD was associated with multiple victim types, including intimate partners, family members, strangers and the police, and was more likely to occur in pubs/bars, outside/in the street and in the workplace. Paranoid PD was associated with violence towards friends, persons known to the perpetrator as well as intimate partners, and incidents were more likely to occur in the street, outdoors, and pubs and bars. Histrionic PD was associated with violence towards the police and incidents occurring in the home; narcissistic PD was associated with violence towards intimate partners and in the home. Reports of violence increased linearly with increasing numbers of comorbid PDs, and there was a general trend of increasing violence with increasing numbers of comorbid clinical syndromes.

ASPD was the most important PD for violence at the population level. Using self-report data, this condition showed a prevalence of about 4% (usually around 1–2% in most population studies when using standardised interviews) but accounted for 22% of all violent incidents in the population, representing a significant public health problem of violence and burden of care, including physical injuries inflicted by the perpetrator and received from others, together with the psychological impact on victims and witnesses, including children in households. ASPD was relatively uncommon in women, but when it did occur it posed an even greater risk of violence than among men. It is thought that ASPD and comorbid anxiety disorder constitute a distinct subcategory of ASPD with different aetiology, requiring different treatment interventions [12]. This was confirmed in another epidemiological study of the British household population which showed a different pattern of adult antisocial behaviour compared to participants with ASPD alone [13]. This subcategory was also associated with more symptoms of psychosis, contrasting with participants with anxiety disorder alone and where the symptoms of the subtype were strongly associated with comorbid anxiety disorder. The subtype appeared to be more unstable in different areas of daily living and these individuals more likely to seek help from mental health services.

Causality in Personality Disorder and Offending

The finding of a diagnosis of PD in an offender does not necessarily mean a causal connection with criminal behaviour. Howard [14] has argued that to establish causality, three criteria have to be met, including: (1) the PD must occur before the offending. This would at first seem straightforward in that PDs are supposed to be lifelong and first appear in childhood or adolescence. However, experience shows that some PDs such as borderline PD show considerable fluctuation of intensity and appearance of associated symptoms, with features at times more similar to a clinical mental illness. This means that however the PD diagnosis is made, it will be necessary to demonstrate a direct impact of symptoms (or traits) on the offending behaviour and not simply by making a categorical diagnosis of PD (or attributing a score on a dimensional scale), then saying that these explain the offending behaviour; (2) alternative explanations for the relationship should be excluded, such as alcohol abuse; and (3) a causal mechanism linking PD with the offending needs to be specified in order to address the question of how PD causes violence. The latter is perhaps the most difficult component of the assessment because there has been little research to identify theoretical causal mechanisms. However, a potential framework for future research involves the role of PD in offender decision-making and motivation [15]. Social cognition researchers regard decision-making as a continuous mental process that precedes behaviour, based on an individual's interaction with the environment. In this context, researchers are concerned with the manner in which individual decisions are guided by logic and rationality. Decision-making is a problem-solving pursuit that ends when an acceptable or suitable solution is reached. Breaking the law (i.e. criminality) is a social behaviour that requires the decision-making process to be engaged in, just as with other social behaviours.

To guide assessment, a research framework was developed relying on temporal analysis strategy to understand the nature of offender decision-making influenced by the offender's background, with interviews focussing on four areas: motivation (where the notion to commit an offence first came to the offender's mind and why); planning (the process of offence preparation just prior to the decision to commit an offence); enactment (those decisions and actions taken during the commission of a crime); and aftermath (those decisions, perceptions and actions which take place immediately following the offence, and which may have consequences for future offences). This has been used in studies of burglary [16, 17] and robbery [18, 19], but with less application to offences more likely to be assessed by a forensic psychiatrist, such as serious violent and sexual offences.

The four components of motivation, planning, enactment and aftermath should be routinely included in a forensic assessment of offending behaviour. Each of these may be influenced by PD or may even have a direct causal association. In clinical practice, mental health evaluations of offenders typically involve the deconstruction of the criminal act, examining the various identified components in relation to identified psychopathology. However, criminal behaviour is determined by law and motivation does not necessarily affect legal liability of the ultimate finding of guilt in some jurisdictions. Nevertheless, it is highly important for a forensic psychiatrist to attempt to establish motivation and whether psychopathology such as PD influenced this. Criminal behaviour can be broken down into characteristics that explain the act itself, including the four components above, characteristics of the victim and offender, and their relationship. In addition, there may be motivating factors that induced the offender to act in a certain way, with additional shaping factors such as disinhibition through intoxication, encouragement by others and so on. Several of these factors may show a dynamic relationship in a single act that needs to be understood by the psychiatrist. It is also important to establish the time frame for these interactions together with their relationship to any key external factors in the lives of offenders [20]. This process is similar to all forensic assessments, including those of psychotic individuals, which include reading depositions and statements regarding the offence in depth, obtaining previous criminal records and going through the details with the offender. Taking a full family history and ascertaining the relationship between the offender and family members to understand their development and whether this influenced their criminal career is essential, as well as establishing a developmental timeline leading up to the offending behaviour, including development of other clinical syndromes and substance misuse. However, it is also essential to make a sound diagnosis following training in PD and psychopathy assessment. This means understanding some of the theoretical bases for the aetiology of the different PDs as well as getting a 'feel' for each condition. With experience, it will be seen that PD categories usually contain considerably more psychopathology than are considered 'personality traits'. The question then is how to link these with the offending behaviour.

One further consideration in the assessment of PD and offending behaviour is that two aspects of the effects on the behaviour need to be considered: firstly, where there is a direct effect and the PD directly drives the pathway, for example motivation in the following discussion; secondly, where PD acts as a vulnerability or predisposing factor to offending, but where other factors will be necessary, such as intoxication or provocation (which might be minimal compared to a normal person, or specific and symbolic for the PD individual based on previous experience such as childhood maltreatment), shaping the behaviour of the offence itself and associated behaviour such as efforts to conceal evidence, pretending to help the police in searching for the victim and so on. There is no 'either/or' and more than one of these can be observed in a single case.

Cognitive Theory of Motivation

Using a cognitive model, it was hypothesised that individuals with PD demonstrate a predisposition, operating in the form of pre-existing PD, which leads to the development of 'schemas' that integrate and attach meaning to events in the environment. These schemas lead to attributions and motivations, which in turn result in action in the form of violence or criminal behaviour [21].

Cognitive theory proposes that dysfunctional feelings are largely due to functions of 'schemas' [22–24] that tend to produce consistently biased judgements and corresponding tendency to make cognitive errors in certain types of situation [25]. This theory considers cognitive structures as organising experience and behaviour. Beliefs and rules represent the content of these schemas and consequently determine the content of an individual's thinking, affect and behaviour. However, the basic tenet of this model is that attributional bias, rather than motivational or response bias, is the main source of dysfunctional affect and conduct [26–29].

The term 'motivational' in cognitive theory can be potentially confusing when applied to criminal behaviour as it differs from establishing motivation for crime. In cognitive theory, motivational theories of personality are constructed as basic drives and differentiated from attributions which are considered more important in the development of abnormal cognitive processing. In PDs, schemas are considered to operate on a continuous basis in processing information and regulating cognition, affect, motivation and tendency to action, inhibition of behaviour, and directing an individual's actions. Some schemas are concerned with evaluations of other persons and oneself and are thought to operate in a logical and linear progression from perception through to behaviour, as shown in Figure 11.1. In Figure 11.1, exposure to a stimulus may activate the relevant schema, such as perceiving a situation or another person as posing a risk (cognitive schema). For example, an individual with paranoid PD might think that other persons are talking about them, followed by anxiety that they might be plotting to attack them, together with increasing anger (affective schema). This is then followed by an urge to retaliate violently by carrying out a pre-emptive strike (motivational schema) and next becoming mobilised for the attack by obtaining a suitable weapon (action or instrumental schema). But, as Figure 11.1 shows, if the individual judges that attacking the person is counter-productive, for example if there is a good chance of being apprehended by the police or suffering injury, then they may inhibit the impulse (control schema). Importantly, comorbid personality pathology together with paranoid PD, for example psychopathy or borderline PD, can have major effects on whether the individuals is able to inhibit the impulse [21].

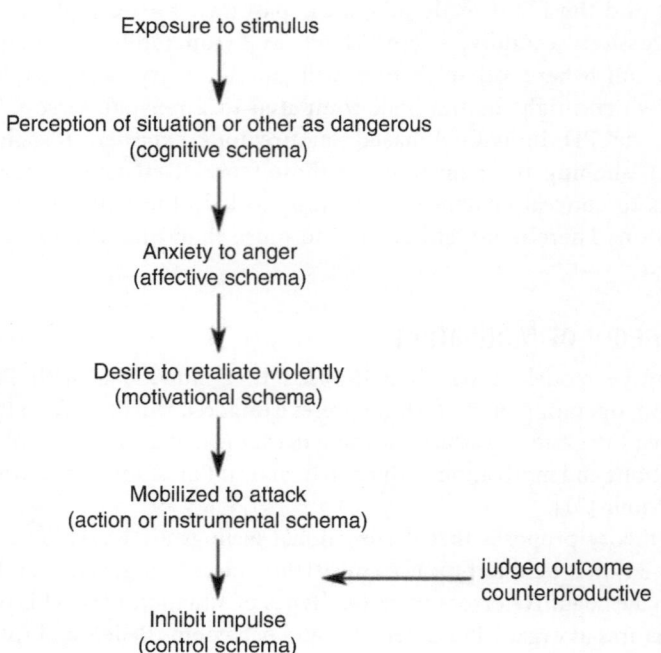

Exposure to stimulus

↓

Perception of situation or other as dangerous
(cognitive schema)

↓

Anxiety to anger
(affective schema)

↓

Desire to retaliate violently
(motivational schema)

↓

Mobilized to attack
(action or instrumental schema)

↓ ← judged outcome
counterproductive

Inhibit impulse
(control schema)

Figure 11.1 Logical and linear progression from perception to behaviour. Coid JW. Personality disorders in prisoners and their motivation for dangerous and disruptive behaviour. *Criminal Behaviour and Mental Health* 2002; 12: 209–26. Reproduced with permission from John Wiley and Sons.

Motivation and Dispositional Factors in the Offence

A descriptive model was developed and evaluated on the basis of motivations and dispositions at the time of offending in a descriptive study of serious violent, sexual and arson offenders with PD [20]. A new typology was created, based on motivational factors that had led to the behaviour and the key situational variables, and by establishing these and certain relevant antecedents with the offender at interview. However, it was essential to have available documented evidence from witness statements as PD patients may diverge from official and witness accounts of what took place. Certain categories were included which were derived from previous research, for example a motivational typology of rape [30]. Although the intention was to concentrate primarily on motivating factors, it also included shaping or dispositional factors, such as intoxication with substances, whether carried out in a gang or group and so on. The typology is shown in Appendix 11.1. Independent associations, controlling for other PD categories and clinical syndromes, were first established with categories of offending. There was a moderate degree of association between offences of robbery, firearms offences and theft with a PD. This was as expected, corresponding to criteria for ASPD. However, associations of narcissistic with homicide offences, paranoid with attempted murder, and wounding and kidnap with schizoid PD may have reflected the sample being both extreme and unusual, detained in high-security hospitals and special prison units for difficult and dangerous offenders. Among the sample, a small number of offenders were found to have had episodes of severe psychosis. Closer examination revealed they had been suffering from schizophrenia or delusional disorder at the time of the offence.

The motivation had been psychotic and on the basis of psychotic symptoms. This was despite the fact they had been managed and treated for PD, and where the psychosis had never been diagnosed previously in certain cases. This is important because differentiating and excluding a diagnosis of psychosis is an essential part of the forensic assessment of PD patients. The findings of this research study mirror what many forensic trainees will experience in their future clinical practice. Trainees need to gain sound clinical competence in making and excluding a diagnosis of psychosis, with an ability to resist labelling a psychotic patient as having a PD merely because they are difficult to manage, and with the result they are excluded from conventional mental health services. Furthermore, it is important to remember that patients with psychosis sometimes do not respond well to certain treatments for PD, such as challenging group therapy, and their symptoms can be exacerbated by these interventions.

Taxonomy. Categories of PDs can be associated with motivations and dispositions criminal behaviour. After statistical adjustments for confounding from other comorbid PDs and clinical syndromes, the following axis II and motivations for serious criminal behaviour emerged. ASPD can be related to offending for financial gain, offending due to irritability or as part of gang or group activity. Borderline PD may be related to motivations including relief of tension and dysphoria, a desire to resolve problems, irritability, revenge, displaced aggression, exhilaration and excitement, pyromania, and homicidal urges. Histrionic PD may motivate offending for financial gain and to avoid arrest. Narcissistic PD may lead to offending through a motivation to dominate, control, gain or maintain control, or in reaction to a blow to self-esteem. Paranoid PD may motivate for revenge or under-controlled aggression. Schizoid PD may be related to expressive aggression and sometimes to offending through excitement or exhilaration. Obsessive-compulsive PD may be related to irritability, displaced aggression and as a reaction to loss [20].

Antisocial Personality Disorder

Antisocial Personality Disorder DSM 301.7

A. A pervasive pattern of disregard for and violation of the rights of others, occurring since age 15 years, as indicated by three or more of the following:

1. Failure to conform to social norms with respect to lawful behaviours, as indicated by repeatedly performing acts that are grounds for arrest.
2. Deceitfulness, as indicated by repeated lying, use of aliases, or conning others for personal profit or pleasure.
3. Impulsivity or failure to plan ahead.
4. Irritability and aggressiveness, as indicated by repeated physical fights or assaults.
5. Reckless disregard for safety of self and others.
6. Consistent irresponsibility, as indicated by repeated failure to sustain consistent work behaviour or honour financial obligations.
7. Lack of remorse, as indicated by being indifferent to or rationalizing having hurt, mistreated, or stolen from another.

B. The individual is at least age 18 years.
C. There is evidence of conduct disorder before age 15 years.

D. The occurrence of antisocial behaviour is not exclusively during the course of schizophrenia or bipolar disorder.

This should be assessed together with conduct disorder. This will be investigated retrospectively in adults.

Conduct Disorder

A repetitive and persistent pattern of behaviour in which the rights of others or major age-appropriate social norms or rules are violated, as manifested by the presence of at least 3 of the following 15 criteria in the past 12 months from any of the categories below, with at least one criterion present in the past 6 months.

Aggression to People and Animals

1. Often bullies, threatens, or intimidates others.
2. Often initiates physical fights.
3. Has used a weapon that can cause serious physical harm to others (e.g. a bat, brick, broken bottle, knife gun).
4. Has been physically cruel to people.
5. Has been physically cruel to animals.
6. Has stolen while confronting a victim (e.g. mugging, purse snatching, extortion, armed robbery).
7. Has forced someone into sexual activity.

Destruction of Property

8. Has deliberately engaged in fire-setting with the intention of causing serious damage.
9. Has deliberately destroyed others' property (other than by fire-setting).

Deceitfulness or Theft

10. Has broken into someone else's house, building, or car.
11. Often lies to obtain goods or favours or to avoid obligations (i.e. cons others).
12. Has stolen items of non-trivial value without confronting a victim (e.g. shoplifting, but without breaking or entering; forgery).

Serious Violations of Rules

13. Often stays out at night despite parental prohibitions, beginning before age 13 years.
14. Has run away from home overnight at least twice while living in the parental home, or once without returning for a lengthy period.
15. Is often truant from school, beginning before age 13 years.

The disturbance in behaviour causes clinically significant impairment in social, academic, or occupational functioning.

The concept of a psychiatric 'syndrome' of persistent antisocial behaviour from childhood to adulthood is embodied in the diagnostic construct of ASPD. The diagnosis differs strikingly from other DSM categories (and the forthcoming ICD-11 approach) by being composed almost entirely of behaviours rather than personality traits. It is one of the most reliable diagnoses in psychiatry and the only PD category in any glossary derived from empirical longitudinal research. In her seminal study, *Deviant Children Grown Up* (1966), Lee Robins [31] followed up children referred and assessed at a child guidance clinic 30 years later, including those referred for antisocial behaviour, those referred for other reasons and a control group from local schools. The original conduct-disordered sample had parents of low social status and only a third were with both parents when referred, with a third spending at least six months in a foster home. Many fathers had deserted their families and/or drank heavily; mothers tended to be unable to keep house or neglected their children. A large proportion had siblings with behavioural disorders, most were behind at school, and half the boys and a third of girls had juvenile convictions. Girls had more disrupted lives than boys.

When followed up, the antisocial children were more likely to have left their area of origin, with 75% of men and 40% of women arrested for non-traffic offences, and with half the men arrested for at least one major crime. Women were more likely to have been married more than once and tended to choose men who were unfaithful and failed to support them. There was a higher rate of childlessness in the antisocial group and those with children had children who also had behavioural problems. Participants were thought to show remission in their fourth and fifth decades, but only in 12%. Improvement took place over each decade in terms of their reduction in antisocial behaviour rather than suddenly. Most importantly, 60% showed little or no improvement. It was thought that special life circumstances, such as threat of further punishments following arrest, were a decisive factor among those who improved. However, Robins believed that neither hospitalisation nor the experience of psychotherapy had any positive association with improvement. In contrast, there was less consistency over time among children who were referred for other conditions, mainly psychoneurotic conditions of childhood, although this group were more likely to show diagnoses of depression and anxiety at follow-up.

Using these findings, Robins derived the criteria for 'sociopathic personality disorder' in an early DSM glossary, which was later changed and termed ASPD. Because the original cohort was entirely white, the study was later replicated in different parts of the USA among young black males and later Vietnam veterans [32, 33]. The study also showed many similarities to other longitudinal studies of delinquency. Robins concluded that her findings indicated that adult and childhood antisocial behaviour formed two syndromes and that both were closely connected. She also concluded that adult antisocial behaviour is a pervasive syndrome requiring a preceding pattern of childhood antisocial behaviour, although the majority of children with conduct disorder would not go on to become adults with ASPD. It was observed that the variety of childhood behaviour was a better predictor of future ASPD than any individual behaviour, and also that the childhood behaviour was a better predictor than family background or social class. Earlier age of onset led to greater persistence into adulthood. Correspondingly, Moffitt [34] later proposed a theoretical framework with predictions about which risk and protective factors should be related to early onset conduct disorder. Life-course persistent (or early onset) was proposed as having its earliest origins in both neurological deficits and exposure to environmental risk, such as poor parenting and parental antisocial behaviour. Neurological deficits were thought to give rise to difficult temperament, leading to the child being vulnerable to poor parenting from caretakers. Adolescent-limited individuals were proposed as beginning their antisocial behaviour during the adolescent period and desisting after reaching adulthood.

ASPD is more common among first-degree relatives of those with ASPD than the general population, with the risk greater among biological relatives of females with the disorder than males with the disorder. Biological relatives are also more likely to have somatic disorder and substance misuse disorder. Adoption studies suggest that both genetic and environmental factors contribute to risk of ASPD. Earlier study of aetiological risk factors showed that in forensic settings, patients with ASPD were more likely to be male, younger and of low social class, with family members with PD, having low full-scale IQ, more likely to have lost a parent in childhood by divorce or desertion and to have been in local authority care, brought up in poverty, experienced parental discord in the family home or cruelty in childhood, and more likely to have been sexually assaulted and to have delinquent siblings and criminal parents [35].

Table 11.2 shows that ASPD was independently associated with offences committed for financial gain, such as thefts, robberies and firearm offences. ASPD is a pervasive pattern of disregard for and violation of the rights of others and shows considerable overlap with the criminological construct of the career criminal. Individuals with ASPD have more extensive histories of acquisitive offending than other PDs and more are involved in criminal organisations, corresponding to group and gang activity, as in Table 11.1. A subgroup are involved in crimes of violence and violence was often involved in the commission of acquisitive offences. In some cases, offences had been preceded by intense irritability, sometimes precipitated by minimal provocation, and corresponding to criterion 4 of irritability and aggressiveness, as indicated by repeated physical fights or assaults.

Case 1. Antisocial, narcissistic PD: A 30-year-old man had a history of offending from the age of 11 years, starting with thefts and progressing to burglaries by his mid-teens, resulting in sentences to youth offender institutions. He was often in fights during childhood, had run away from home on numerous occasions and regularly truanted from school. He had regularly offended with his younger brother who was convicted of murder in his late teens. The subject had initially also been arrested for the offence, but the prosecution was dropped due to lack of evidence. He was from a large criminal family which was well known locally in a poor part of an industrial town. His mother had been convicted for shoplifting offences, had been in a psychiatric hospital following self-harm and was known to have lived off prostitution during his childhood, when he would be taken into care on occasions, together with his siblings. His paternity was uncertain, but he claimed his father was a professional criminal who had served prison sentences for repeated violence. He was known to social services for violence towards his female partners and children. He abused alcohol heavily and would get into fights in clubs and bars. He claimed to dislike drugs. In his early 20s, he had become involved with professional criminals and had served sentences for robbery (mugging), then armed robbery and possession of a firearm, resulting in a long period of imprisonment. He was in fights in prison and made weapons to use on other prisoners, resulting in periods in solitary confinement. He was involved in selling drugs to other prisoners, although he claimed not to abuse drugs himself. Prison officers perceived him as an arrogant bully who would exploit weaker and vulnerable prisoners. He expressed little convincing concern about his future or alternatives to a life involving crime. He would typically begin crime reduction courses with prison psychologists but would not complete these.

It is recommended that trainees become well acquainted with the diagnostic criteria for ASPD and apply this routinely in all forensic assessments. Unlike other PD categories, the criteria can be reliably applied to patients with psychosis and experience will show that in many patients treated in secure settings, the difficult behaviour of in patients with diagnoses of schizophrenia can be due to these underlying features rather than their psychotic

Table 11.2 Motivations/dispositions and categories of DSM personality disorder: independent associations between motivations and dispositions and criminal behaviour after statistical adjustments for confounding from other comorbid personality disorders and clinical syndromes

Motivation for offending	DSM personality disorder category						
	antisocial	borderline	histrionic	narcissistic	paranoid	schizoid	compulsive
Financial gain	✓		✓				
Hyer-irritability	✓						✓
Gang/group activity	✓						
Relief of tension/dysphoria		✓					
Homicidal urge		✓					
Revenge		✓			✓		✓
Displaced aggression		✓					
Excitement/exhilaration		✓				✓	
Resolve problems		✓					
Pyromania		✓					
Avoid arrest			✓				
Power, dominate, control				✓			
Blow to self-esteem				✓	✓		
Under-controlled aggression						✓	
Expressive aggression						✓	
Loss							✓

Coid JW. Axis II disorders and motivation for serious criminal behaviour. In AE Skodol (ed.) *Psychopathology and Violent Crime*. Washington, DC, American Psychiatric Association, 1998, pp. 53–94 [20]

symptoms – although this must be carefully excluded because this observation is not uniform. In childhood, conduct disorder is often accompanied by comorbid ADHD and in adulthood by substance misuse. Among forensic populations, ASPD is frequently comorbid with paranoid and borderline PDs, rendering these patients difficult to manage, with some suggestion of interactive effects between the personality pathology which multiply the difficult and challenging behaviour. As shown in the epidemiological studies described earlier, ASPD is associated with multiple types of potential victim (among those who are violent), including intimate partners as well as strangers, and in multiple locations. ASPD is the most prevalent diagnosis found among prisoners. DSM recommends that because deceit and manipulation are central themes of ASPD, it is important to integrate information from systematic clinical assessment with information from collateral sources.

Borderline (Emotionally Unstable) Personality Disorder

F 60.3 emotionally unstable personality disorder (ICD-10) will be referred to as borderline PD in this chapter, according to personal preference. This is largely because diagnostic research instruments which can be used routinely in clinical settings were originally developed in the USA using the DSM system. ICD-10 also refers to two subtypes: F60.30 impulsive type and F60.31 borderline type. It is concerning but important for trainees to learn that diagnoses in all glossaries are finally decided by committees rather than on the basis of intensive research or general consensus. In the original discussions for ICD-10 PDs, a committee member forcefully argued that there were two subtypes based on his genetic research. Sadly, the research was not replicated by others and ICD-10 was left subsequently with subtypes F60.30 and F60.31. In contrast, the US DSM committees saw no reason to make this division and promoted a single diagnosis of borderline PD.

Table 11.2 shows that individuals with borderline PD are most likely to commit serious offences motived by multiple factors including relief of tension/dysphoria as part of a syndrome of mood disturbance associated with the condition, compulsive homicidal urges, a severe mood state of hyper-irritability which can result in violence, revenge, displaced aggression, deliberately carried out for excitement/exhilaration, and to resolve problems, and is seen in cases of fire-setting where pyromania is present.

Borderline Personality Disorder 301.83

Borderline PD is defined as a pervasive pattern of instability in personal relationships, self-image and affects, and marked impulsivity, beginning in young adulthood and present in a variety of contexts as indicated by five or more of:

1. Frantic efforts to avoid real or imagined abandonment.
2. A pattern of unstable and intense interpersonal relationships characterised by alternating between extremes of idealisation and devaluation.
3. Identity disturbance: markedly and persistently unstable self-image or sense of self.
4. Impulsivity in at least two areas that are potentially self-damaging (e.g. spending, sex, substance abuse, reckless driving, binge eating).
5. Recurrent suicidal behaviour, gestures or threats, or self-mutilating behaviour.
6. Affective instability due to masked reactivity of mood (e.g. intense episodic dysphoria).
7. Chronic feelings of emptiness.

8. Inappropriate, intense anger or difficulty controlling anger (e.g. frequent displays of temper, constant anger, recurrent physical fights).
9. Transient, stress-related paranoid ideation or severe dissociative symptoms.

Apart from suicidal behaviour and chronic feelings of emptiness, each of these criteria can be observed to potentially influence criminal behaviour by individuals with borderline PD, sometimes having a peripheral or shaping effect on the events, sometimes impacting directly and possibly causally by driving the behaviour. For example, clinical assessment will sometimes reveal that individuals with borderline PD can be driven to behave irresponsibly and manipulatively to prevent abandonment by others or to force others to intervene to protect or care for them. Alternating extremes of idealisation and devaluation can typically lead to violence in close relationships and this feature typically leads to break-ups of relationships, followed by behaviour related to their fear of the inevitable abandonment by their partner. In forensic settings, identity disturbance can sometimes be extreme and fluctuating; for example, sexual identity linked with serious, serial sexual crimes, with a small group of male offenders carrying out rapes they claim to have been a 'lesbian' rape, with insistence they should be sent to a women's prison because they wish to transition and become a woman. These cases typically show no convincing history of true transsexualism in childhood. The fluctuating feelings of being like a woman, possibly or actually 'being' a woman, and with a 'true' female identity, typically start during adolescence rather than childhood. It is sometimes observed that when these feelings of 'other' identity become particularly intense, the individual is particularly dangerous and likely to offend or seek out victims to offend against.

Forensic psychiatrists should be very clear about such cases after a full investigation and not support applications for transfers to locations such as women's prisons, where they can find more victims, or sanction extreme medical measures such as gender reassignment in unstable cases of identity disturbance relating to borderline PD. This is typically fluctuating over time and unlikely to be successful despite the patient's insistence that they will recover if reassignment is carried out. Additional forms of identity disturbance are seen, for example so-called multiple identity disorder, where the offender claims they have multiple personalities, some good, some bad, and where it is the 'bad' or 'evil' one who has carried out the offence and not the others. These cases are now rare but were not uncommon two decades ago, particularly in the USA, where defences to murder were run on the basis of multiple personality and where there was commonly a strong iatrogenic effect. These cases became less common as courts became more acquainted with them and where 'experts' in multiple identity sometimes had their evidence discredited in court.

Impulsivity, although potentially self-damaging, can also result in behaviours which are damaging to others. Impulsive behaviours which damage the self can also be substituted for by impulsive behaviours aimed to harm others or put others at risk. Among forensic patients with borderline PD, impulsivity can take on features of compulsivity. An affective state of intense or recurrent anger can clearly result in violence and harms to other persons, particularly if combined with stress-related paranoid ideation. However, a feature of borderline PD which is strongly related to offending behaviour among forensic populations is criterion 6, 'Affective instability due to marked reactivity of mood'. This is worth considering carefully because some cases encountered in prisons and secure hospitals are so severe that it has to be questioned whether the individual is suffering from personality pathology.

If the nine criteria of borderline PD are reflected upon, these are clearly an uneasy mix of behaviours with underlying interpersonal dynamics (1 and 2), unexplained self-harming or self-destructive behaviours (4 and 5), an unrelated single item of identity disturbance (3), severe transient symptoms of paranoia and anxiety (9), and three items of abnormal affect (6, 7 and 8). None of the criteria conveniently fit personality traits, although borderline PD is often associated with a particular personality style, behaviour that draws attention and help-seeking behaviour.

Secure hospitals and prisons can give trainees a misleading impression of the sex ratio for borderline PD. The national household survey of the UK [9] showed that borderline PD was somewhat more prevalent among men than women (see Table 11.1). Patients with borderline PD are particularly help-seeking and because men sometimes show aggressive behaviour, women are thought more manageable in a hospital setting. However, a key issue is that borderline PD has multiple symptoms and behaviours that are associated with mental disorder and with experience so that many trainees will question whether patients with borderline PD are really presenting with a PD. Among prisoners, borderline PD is the most prevalent category among women, whereas ASPD is most prevalent among men. Borderline PD is often associated with younger age in many samples. This may be because the condition ameliorates with age in most individuals, although there is a wide range of outcomes as shown in longitudinal studies. There is usually a negative association between borderline PD and having children and many individuals remain single throughout their life. In the serious offenders sample, borderline PD was associated with lower full-scale IQ. Early childhood environment is often characterised by different forms of adversity and difficulties between parents. Borderline PD is highly comorbid with other PDs and clinical syndromes, although it is important to control for confounding. Studies that adjust for other diagnostic categories find less comorbidity. In a study of serious offenders, borderline PD tended to show comorbidity more with clinical symptoms than other PDs. These included independent associations with depression, dysthymia, brief unspecified psychotic episodes, phobias, somatisation and transsexualism [36]. The risk of suicide among borderline PD patients should not be underestimated or minimised as 'attention-seeking', with follow-up studies suggesting around 9%.

Case 2. Borderline PD: A 30-year-old woman was assessed in a high-secure hospital where she had been sent under a compulsory order of the Mental Health Act following a conviction for arson with intent. Although diagnosed with borderline PD, her childhood was relatively normal. She was from a large working-class family and had been described as supportive to her mother in caring for her siblings during their upbringing. She worked as a waitress after leaving school and married, having two children. Her behaviour rapidly deteriorated at some stage after her first child and she began to be increasingly argumentative and violent towards her husband. She had episodes of depression and was treated by her primary care physician with antidepressants, but her deterioration continued with frequent episodes of self-harm and increasingly heavy drinking. She would disappear for periods from the family home with men she met in bars and failed to care for her children who had become increasingly afraid of her rages. She was excluded from the family home by her husband who took out an injunction against her and went to live with her mother. Their relationship deteriorated and she was at times violent towards her mother. She was locked out one evening after an argument. She obtained paper and lighter fuel and pushed burning materials through the letterbox. Her mother had to be rescued by the fire brigade from a serious blaze in the hallway. She had locked the back door to prevent her mother from escaping. On remand, she was violent and frequently cut her wrists and made ligatures.

The diagnosis was at first uncertain and it was questioned whether she suffered from bipolar disorder, but a consensus of opinions concluded that she had borderline PD. Following transfer to the secure hospital, her condition continued to deteriorate and she intermittently required transfer to the most secure ward with the highest levels of observation, where she was frequently secluded after assaults on staff and patients, a pattern that continued over the next five years. When interviewed, she was a small woman who was polite, pleasant and cooperative, the interviewer spending most of an afternoon with the patient. The intention was to see her on a second occasion two weeks later, but interview was impossible. She was secluded after assaulting the senior ward nurse and could be heard screaming abuse at ward staff. She was spoken to through the door hatch and appeared in a state of hyper-irritability. Nurses would only unlock the door if three were present.

An Affective Syndrome?

Prior to borderline PD being included in DSM, these patients often confused clinicians. Research prior to DSM III suggested that patients with these features were found in families of persons with affective disorders and that the patients themselves had features of abnormal affect and were highly prone to affective disorders. They were thought on the 'border' or within the diagnostic 'borderland' with affective disorder – hence the unfortunate decision to use 'borderline' to classify them. What also persisted was the insistence that the primary psychopathology was one of PD and that this was not a clinical syndrome, with the criteria being altered in DSM over time so that the affective criterion appeared more like a personality trait than a symptom. Trainees will be taught that the condition is a PD but may also question why these patients are the most common PD admitted to hospital, why they are commonly treated with antidepressants and anti-psychotic medication, particularly in secure settings, why psychotherapy and talking treatments do not improve them, or why they are too unwell to cooperate in these treatments for long periods, despite National Institute for Health and Care Excellence (NICE) guidelines [4], and why they receive different diagnoses at different times over the lifespan, with disagreements common among professionals. A further interesting observation is the wide range of severity and persistence over time of the condition, with some of the most severe cases being found in secure settings and prisons. Epidemiological study has found that the majority of patients with borderline PD are not managed by mental health professionals or in prison but are managed by their primary care physician [37].

Figure 11.2 shows a model of the association between affective symptoms and behavioural disorder observed in a hospitalised group of female patients in maximum security. All women with borderline PD showed rapid cycling episodes of a mixture of symptoms classified into four subgroups of anxiety, anger, depression and tension. The women could go for long periods without showing cycling when their behaviour and demeanour was normal except for those with additional ASPD or psychopathic personalities. Typically, the mood swings would appear with increasing intensification of the symptoms and a growing sense of compulsion to act out in various ways that the patient had found would relieve the symptoms. Self-mutilation was the most common. Acting out would be followed by symptom relief, followed by a resolution phase, and in these chronic cases this would then be followed by a further bout of symptom intensification. External stress factors would bring on the symptoms but in many cases the

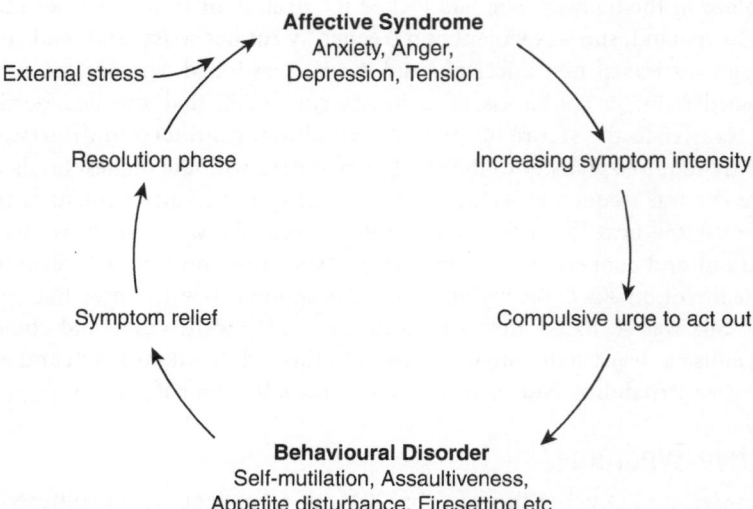

Figure 11.2 Association between affective syndrome and behavioural disorder. Coid JW. An affective syndrome in psychopaths with borderline personality disorder? *British Journal of Psychiatry* 1993; 162: 641–50 [38].

episodes would be brought on by no apparent external stressor. In this unusual sample, behaviours included fire-setting with features of pyromania and compulsive urges to kill which excited the patient but which also appeared to give them relief by acting out the behaviour.

Narcissistic Personality Disorder

Narcissistic PD was not formally included in ICD-10 and was listed among 'other' PDs, but ICD-11 will include a number of narcissistic traits. The committee to determine narcissistic PD for the DSM glossary was largely made up of psychiatrists with a psychodynamic approach. Narcissistic PD in the DSM is actually a poor representation of a complex psychodynamic construct which does not fit well with a criterion-based system used to define the DSM PDs. Trainees are recommended to read Akhtar and Thomson [39] for a lucid review of the construct using a psychodynamic approach. Trainees will find that a deeper understanding of the dynamics of narcissistic PD (as well as becoming well acquainted with the DSM criteria) will repay the effort because narcissistic PD is one of the most important concepts in forensic psychiatric practice, particularly in the assessment of extreme violence and also in cases of intimate partner violence.

Table 11.1 shows that serious offenders with narcissistic PD are likely to be motivated by need for power, domination and control and/or a blow to their self-esteem.

Narcissistic Personality Disorder 301.81

Narcissistic PD is defined as a pervasive pattern of grandiosity (in fantasy or behaviour), need for admiration and lack of empathy, beginning by early adulthood and present in a variety of contexts, as indicated by five or more of the following:

1. Has a grandiose sense of self-importance (e.g. exaggerates achievements and talents, expects to be recognized as superior without commensurate achievements).

2. Is preoccupied with fantasies of unlimited success, power, brilliance, beauty, or ideal love.
3. Believes that he or she is 'special' and unique and can only be understood by, or should associate with, other special or high-status people (or institutions).
4. Requires excessive admiration.
5. Has a sense of entitlement (i.e. unreasonable expectations of especially favourable treatment or automatic compliance with his or her expectations).
6. Is interpersonally exploitative (i.e. takes advantage of others to achieve his or her own ends).
7. Lacks empathy, is unwilling to recognize or identify with the feelings and needs of others.
8. Is often envious of others or believes that others are envious of him or her.
9. Shows arrogant, haughty behaviours or attitudes.

The key descriptions of narcissistic PD were developed on the basis of psychodynamic theory and typically these individuals would be in therapy before the features (that were later refined into DSM criteria) would become apparent. In the national survey in the UK (see Table 11.1), no cases were found at the second stage when a representative sample of the population were interviewed – either because the condition is rarer than other PDs or because there was not sufficient supporting background information to make the diagnosis by trained interviewers interviewing people in households on a one-off basis. However, cases were diagnosed using a self-report instrument in a larger sample in the first phase. The implications of these epidemiological findings are that clinicians will need to have available considerable information. However, with experience, a forensic psychiatrist should be able to observe certain aspects in the manner and behaviour of narcissistic individuals at interview, such as attitudes towards crimes and victims in relation to themselves and in the nature of the offending.

Kernberg [40] described individuals with 'narcissistic personality' as having excessive admiration, intense ambition, grandiose fantasies, overdependence on acclaim and an unremitting need to search for brilliance and power. However, behind this, Kernberg described them as having a pathological inner world despite their superficially adaptive behaviour manifested as an inability to love, lack of empathy, chronic feelings of boredom, emptiness, uncertainty about their identity and exploitation of others. In addition, they would have chronic envy and defences against this in the form of devaluation, omnipotent control and narcissistic withdrawal. This would appear in contempt and attachment to or avoidance of others they secretly admired. These individuals often had a tendency towards promiscuity, sexual paraphilia, substance abuse, a readiness to shift values quickly to gain power and a peculiarly corruptible conscience. To further understand these dynamic components, Akhtar and Thomson [39] described both overt and covert features of narcissistic PD. In terms of their self-concept, they would appear to have an inflated self-regard, show haughty grandiosity, have fantasies of wealth and power and have a sense of entitlement. But behind this they would have inordinate sensitivity and feelings of inferiority and worthlessness, with a continuous search for glory. Their relations with others would appear superficial, with contempt and devaluation, but behind this would be intense envy and enormous hunger for acclaim. Their social adaptation would include social success and intense ambition, behind which would be chronic boredom and dissatisfaction with social identity. Their ethical standards and ideals would show zeal and enthusiasm, behind which was a lack of genuine commitment and a corruptible conscience. In love and sex they were often seductive, promiscuous and lacked inhibitions, with frequent infatuations, behind which was an inability to love and a propensity to use others as an extension of themselves, sometimes with perverse fantasies [41]. Their cognitive style included an egocentric perception of reality; they would be articulate and rhetorical but circumstantial, behind which could be observed inattention to objective aspects of events and subtle gaps in memory, sometimes with autocratic use of language.

Case 3. Narcissistic PD: Brian Blackwell lived at home with his parents, an accountant and an antiques dealer, in an affluent village in northern England. It is believed his parents were over-indulgent, over-protective and controlling of minor aspects of his life in his childhood. He was an under-18 tennis champion at a local club and a good student, obtaining a scholarship to college and intending to study medicine. He regularly told innocuous lies, such as embellishing his academic achievements, but his lying escalated in the two months leading up to killing his parents in 2004, age 18 years. He applied for 13 credit cards in his father's name and attempted to obtain a cash advance from a bank by falsely claiming to be a professional tennis player who needed money to pay to play in the French Open tournament. His girlfriend believed he was a professional tennis player with a sponsorship from Nike and that he had a Mercedes and an apartment in the same building as a famous football player. With savings his parents had intended for his university education, he bought expensive gifts for his girlfriend and 'hired' her as his manager, writing her a cheque that bounced. When his mother found out, she contacted his bank manager. He killed his parents soon after in their home, bludgeoning them with a hammer and stabbing them repeatedly with a carving knife. He then took his unaware girlfriend on a lavish holiday to the USA, returning home to live at his girlfriend's address. The decomposed bodies of his parents were then found at their home and he was arrested the next day. He initially denied the offence, then said he acted in self-defence – although blows to the top of his father's head suggested the latter had been sitting down when attacked.

He finally admitted at trial that he had become enraged when his parents expressed concern about extravagant spending and tried to stop him travelling to the USA with his girlfriend. He pleaded guilty to the lesser charge of manslaughter due to diminished responsibility after being diagnosed with narcissistic PD by psychiatrists, which was accepted by the court. However, he was sentenced to life imprisonment after recommendations of being sent to a hospital under the Mental Health Act were rejected by the judge because he could be released by a tribunal from hospital and because the judge doubted he would be safe for release in the future.

Kernberg's patients, on whom narcissistic PD theory was developed, were seen in private psychodynamic practice in the USA and tended to be wealthy, middle- and upper-class individuals, differing considerably from those typically seen in forensic clinical practice, although the case of Brian Blackwood shows considerable overlap. Many of the features described above can be observed in the histories of and interactions with individuals encountered in prisons and sometimes secure hospitals. The question then arises why persons with features of narcissistic PD can become successful heads of business corporations or of academic departments of universities (while having considerable personal problems), whereas others can be found in prison. Wilson [42] suggested two levels of adaptation among those with narcissistic pathology, where Level 1 constitutes a more severe and dysfunctional subgroup, prone to episodes of paranoia, sometimes progressing to temporary paranoid psychotic symptoms, and with features of comorbid borderline PD. In addition, they are thought prone to depressive episodes characterised by an 'empty' depression and contrast with Type 2 where the depression has features of guilt. Type 2 pathology is considered less severe and dysfunctional and would predispose the individual to high-flying and superficially successful adaptation in which the individual can competently navigate the occupational and social demands of an external world despite the presence of severe object-relational impairments and where they can be driven by their psychopathology to succeed.

Wilson's division is helpful but is based on psychodynamic thinking which some readers may find difficult to understand. Alternative ways of conceptualising a division whereby narcissism manifests as superficially successful and highly unsuccessful variants can include a dimensional approach: firstly, that the unsuccessful type has additional comorbid psychopathology such as additional ASPD, borderline PD or paranoid PD: secondly, that the psychopathology of individuals encountered in forensic practice is more likely to include psychopathic traits whereby the narcissistic features are particularly severe and dysfunctional along a spectrum of severity with psychopathy at the most severe end. Narcissistic PD is found to characterise many individuals with psychopathy and is statistically associated with the interpersonal facet [1] using a four-facet model of psychopathy.

Narcissistic Rage

An alternative psychodynamic perspective on narcissistic PD to that of Kernberg is given by Kohut. However, this is somewhat complex. For forensic psychiatrists, an important paper for understanding violence in the context of triggering factors is Kohut's 'Thoughts on Narcissism and Narcissistic Rage' [43]. Kohut's theory and the paper may be difficult for those without psychodynamic training, but his description of narcissistic rage should be understandable for most clinicians. Narcissistic rage is part of a continuum from fleeting annoyance to unbridled rage seen during homicide. Kohut described five important components that trainees will sometimes experience in their assessments, typically in homicides and in cases of intimate partner violence:

1. Need for revenge.
2. Undoing of a hurt or righting of a wrong.
3. Relentless pursuit by whatever means.
4. Utter disregard for reasonable limitations or consequences of their actions, with total lack of empathy for the victim or person who triggers the particular rage response.
5. A vengeful attitude in which reasoning is not only intact but sharpened, despite its irrationality, leading to ruthless completion of the act.

Rosen [44] has described the importance of childhood rearing experiences and the individual's perception of their own worth in the eyes of parents or parental figures in a process known as 'mirroring'. Everyone attempts to maintain their self-esteem within a given range. But some individuals will resort to any means to redress the balance and counteract feelings of devaluation. This includes physical action and aggression, sexual stimulation, alcohol, drugs or risk-taking. Regulation of self-esteem is considered a key component of narcissistic rage. Should self-esteem suddenly fall or be threatened, trigger mechanisms operate in susceptible persons and violence may be triggered by a narcissistically wounding experience.

A further dynamic phenomenon typically seen in cases of intimate partner violence involving narcissistic PD is the 'core complex' [45], originally described in cases of sexual perversion but fitting the oscillation backwards and forwards within dysfunctional close relationships due to narcissistic psychopathology. Typically these individuals long for deep closeness in their relationships, containment by their partner and close bonding to the extent of 'merging' with them. However, this threatens them with a permanent loss of their sense of self and separateness to the extent of extreme, unbearable anxiety. This then leads to strategies to distance themselves from their partner (flight to a safe distance or 'narcissistic withdrawal') such as infidelity, substance misuse, infidelity or temporarily leaving the home, which reassures them and reduces the anxiety. However, this then leads to painful affects and feelings of anxiety from isolation, sometimes accompanied by feelings of humiliation and anger due to rejection. This circular process can result in these individuals becoming at high risk of violence to partners when accompanied by severe narcissistic pathology.

Case 4. Narcissistic PD: A 22-year-old man was referred for a forensic assessment by his psychiatrist, concerned about his risk to future female partners. He had served a prison sentence for manslaughter of the new boyfriend of his former girlfriend. Since his release, he had formed another relationship and had seriously attacked his new girlfriend. She refused to press charges against him because he had agreed to accept psychiatric treatment. Closer assessment of the assault showed it would have had more serious consequences had the weapon he had grabbed in a rage and beaten her with not broken, allowing her to escape. He would typically form relationships with women who had had multiple former sexual partners, claiming unconvincingly that he was not a jealous person. He would usually cohabit with them but would then find himself other partners, leaving them for periods of time, whereupon they would form a relationship with another man. This pattern would then result in him becoming extremely jealous and violent towards his partners. The repeated pattern suggested that he could tolerate neither emotional closeness from his partners or separation. He would typically idealise his partners at the beginning of the relationship then become disinterested in them after unreasonable behaviour and demands on his part, followed by going absent from their home, sometimes staying with friends or a temporary new girlfriend.

The original homicide had occurred after he had separated from a former girlfriend and become increasingly desperate and subjectively depressed, contemplating suicide. She had become afraid, refused to see him and her mother had moved in with her at her request. He had repeatedly phoned her, attempting to persuade her to let him return. On the day of the offence, he had telephoned and had argued with her. He had left some clothing at her home and had angrily insisted during the argument that she should give the coat she had given him as a birthday present to her new boyfriend. Her mother who had been listening on the extension suddenly interrupted and said there was no point in giving it to the new boyfriend as the coat would be too small for him. The man then slammed the phone down, left his accommodation and took a bus, followed by a train, to his ex-girlfriend's address, stopping at a hardware shop to buy a carving knife with the deliberate intention of killing her and possibly her mother. He was confronted by the new boyfriend on arrival, who was physically larger and stronger, and stabbed him to death in a struggle after he had forcibly entered the house. He was subsequently convicted of manslaughter due to provocation and served a short prison sentence.

Writers on narcissistic rage have drawn attention to its relationship to extreme, unusual and often transient mental states, usually affective states that can be diminished by the explosion of rage. Kohut believed there could be cases of chronic narcissistic rage. Although this chapter deals with violence, narcissistic rage is thought to be able to result in self-harm, particularly suicide attempts and completed suicide. The behaviour can be repetitive and patients with these conditions are difficult to treat and often treatment resistant. They typically cause strong personal feelings in clinicians (counter-transference). DSM describes a fragile self-esteem in individuals with narcissistic PD leading to social withdrawal as well as rage and repetitive impaired interpersonal relationships. In addition, narcissistic PD is described as comorbid with anorexia nervosa, substance use disorders (particularly cocaine), hypomanic mood, and dysthymia and depressive disorder. Careful examination of cases after extreme violence will sometimes reveal a complex dynamic relationship with the violence, sometimes with relief of apparent severe symptoms of depression following achieving violent revenge. It is not uncommon for cases to be treated for depression and referred for transfer to hospital after being remanded into prison custody following serious violence against a close person in a state of narcissistic rage. Cases may also be referred for assessment of possible defences such as diminished responsibility to a charge of murder when appearing in court.

Case 5. Narcissistic, paranoid PD, depressive disorder: A 28-year-old man was admitted to a secure hospital unit from prison due to concerns about his mental state. He was charged with murder of his girlfriend and an offence under the Animal Welfare Act 2006 after killing her dog. He had appeared depressed on occasions while on remand, but insisted with near-delusional intensity that he had done nothing wrong and that his girlfriend and her parents should be in his place, not himself. He had cohabited for some months with his girlfriend and she had become pregnant, after which he developed an obsessive concern about her weight, health and the development of the baby. This resulted in a progressive deterioration of their relationship and episodes of violence. He had meanwhile begun maltreating his girlfriend's dog and she had left their home to stay with her parents. He was arrested after causing a disturbance outside their home. He then became severely depressed and was prescribed antidepressants. He deteriorated, could not eat or sleep and would spend time lying on the floor of his apartment, crying, with his mobile phone, waiting for his girlfriend to phone him after leaving her multiple messages.

Eventually he waited for her outside her place of work shortly after his phone messages had become increasingly threatening. He seriously assaulted her, leaving her on the pavement and subsequently requiring neurosurgery for head injuries, from which she later died. He then went to her parents' home from where he took her dog, taking it on a long walk and drowning it in a pond, returning with the dog lead and leaving it on her parents' doorstep. He described his symptoms of severe depression lifting after the killing of the dog and a sense of inner peace that he, she and the dog were now 'at peace' but her parents were not at peace. He continued to insist he bore no responsibility and his mood in hospital was characterised by simmering anger and resentment. He had a grandiose sense of his own importance and looked down on the other patients on his ward who had severe mental illness. Information was obtained that he had become obsessed with a previous girlfriend after she became pregnant and had been convicted of assaulting her and a police officer who had attempted to intervene. Interviews during the assessment destabilised him by challenging his defences. He was prescribed antidepressants after becoming depressed, but then required transfer to a high-security hospital after threatening female nurses, then assaulting one. He was convicted of manslaughter due to diminished responsibility but served a prison sentence because he was thought to be untreatable under the conditions of mental health legislation.

Histrionic Personality Disorder

Histrionic PD in a forensic context is rarely if ever seen as a standalone diagnosis and is commonly comorbid with narcissistic and borderline PD and ASPD. The category has been criticised as being applied frequently to women, although this was not found in the British national survey. In the Dangerous Offenders study, the diagnosis was most commonly observed among a group of difficult prisoners posing major problems of control and was one aspect of the multiple PD pathology of certain professional career criminals, often with records of armed robbery with high status in the prison setting among other prisoners.

Careful examination of the criteria showed a degree of overlap with facet 1 of psychopathy and these individuals, largely men, had high PCL-R scores, usually near but below the cut-off for a full diagnosis. They posed severe problems for prison officers in their general interactions on a day-to-day basis, attracting attention to themselves by constant challenging of rules and regulations openly to gain status. They were highly volatile, bullied other prisoners and were generally highly demanding. Features of over-dramatic, reactive and intensely expressed behaviour, with characteristic disturbances in interpersonal relationships due to shallowness, egocentricity, and vain and demanding behaviour in histrionic individuals typically appeared as a need to advertise their toughness but with minimal ability to tolerate stress. They had typically used excessive force in the course of crimes for financial gain, such as robbery. They enjoyed the status their crimes gave them and were boastful about their prowess in violence and the enjoyment of the proceeds of crime in terms of cars and women. They would be highly flirtatious with female visitors and staff and boasted of their violence. Similar features were apparent among the smaller subgroup of women with histrionic PD, although few had been involved in professional crime and involvement in prostitution was not uncommon.

Histrionic Personality Disorder 301.50

A pervasive pattern of excessive emotionality and attention-seeking, beginning in early adulthood and present in a variety of contexts, as indicated by five or more of the following:

1. Is uncomfortable in situations in which he or she is not the center of attention.
2. Interaction with others is often characterized by inappropriate sexually seductive or provocative behavior.
3. Displays rapidly shifting and shallow expression of emotions.
4. Consistently uses physical appearance to draw attention to self.
5. Has a style of speech that is excessively impressionistic and lacking in detail.
6. Shows self-dramatization, theatricality, and exaggerated expression of emotion.
7. Is suggestible (i.e. easily influenced by others and circumstances).
8. Considers relationships to be more intimate than they really are.

Case 6. ASPD, narcissistic and histrionic PD (score 28 PCL-R): A 30-year-old man was serving a sentence of 25 years for armed robbery with additional extensions of his sentence due to attempts to escape from prison custody. He was a lifelong offender with his first conviction at the age of eight years. He had not spent longer than 12 months out of custody since age 18 years and his offences had become increasingly serious and the sentences longer as he had got older. He was well acquainted with other high-ranking offenders in organised crime who he had met in the prison system and had carried out crimes that had been devised by others. He had a reputation for being able to use controlled but, if necessary, extreme violence to intimidate building society staff to hand over cash, usually at gunpoint. He had been involved in serious fights and injured others in prison, and had spent all his sentences in maximum-security institutions.

His last conviction had been for escape from custody and possession of a firearm. He had seduced a female prison officer and had been having sexual relations with her, eventually persuading her to bring him a disguise and let him out of prison, to where a car was waiting, and with a loaded revolver. She was now also serving a prison sentence for aiding his escape. At interview, he was an imposing man with a heavily tattooed, muscular body he delighted in showing, with his shirt off, even though it was winter. He spoke disparagingly about the prison officer and her unhappy marriage, which had now broken up, and said she was ugly and that he had to shut his eyes to have sex with her. This was at the top of his voice for the benefit of other prisoners who might be listening, although an attempt was made to keep the interview confidential. He said he was now the 'minder' of a notorious gangster in the prison. The interview had to be handled carefully because doubts regarding details of his history would antagonise him, and also because he seemed to have considerable sensitivity and problems with self-esteem, despite his arrogance and boasting. He said that he intermittently suffered from panic attacks.

Paranoid Personality Disorder

Unlike community samples, paranoid PD is highly prevalent in prison populations and is often a feature of cases with personality disorder that will be assessed in forensic settings. Paranoid PD is typically comorbid with ASPD and the paranoid sensitive and vengeful traits add an extra dimension of potential risk to their pre-existing criminal disposition operating through ASPD, often with a tendency to become involved in fights with minimal provocation. Chronic vigilance for signs of malicious intent by others and the view that they cannot be trusted will sometimes result in their behaviour being perceived as intentional and malicious and therefore deserving of retaliation. For the most severe examples, protests that the behaviour was unintentional or accidental can be perceived as further evidence of deception and proof. Clinical experience will sometimes include expression of distress at what they perceive as orchestrated mistreatment and malevolent intent, sometimes resulting in additional feelings of humiliation (particularly when comorbid with narcissistic PD) and planning a revenge attack with meticulous care [21]. Table 11.1 shows these individuals were most likely to commit violent offences in a state of under-controlled aggression and/or for revenge.

Paranoid Personality Disorder 301.0

A pervasive distrust and suspiciousness of others such that their motives are interpreted as malevolent, beginning by early childhood and present in a variety of contexts, as indicated by four or more of the following:

1. Suspects, without sufficient basis, that others are exploiting, harming, or are deceiving him or her.
2. Is preoccupied by unjustified doubts about the loyalty or trustworthiness of friends or associates.
3. Is reluctant to confide in other because of unwarranted fear that the information will be used maliciously against him or her.
4. Reads hidden demeaning or threatening meanings into benign remarks or events.
5. Persistently bears grudges (i.e. is unforgiving of insults, injuries, or slights).
6. Perceives attacks on his or her character or reputation that are not apparent to others and is quick to react angrily or counterattack.
7. Has recurrent suspicions, without justification, regarding fidelity of spouse or sexual partner.

Case 7. Paranoid PD: A 26-year-old man who had worked in a bank but had lost his job due to conflict with other staff was convicted of two counts of murder, one of attempted murder and one of animal cruelty. He claimed to have been in a close relationship with a 23-year-old woman who had agreed to marry him but who had decided to finish the relationship. She gave the history of him always being difficult and irritable, highly jealous of her friends and family, that she had never agreed to marry him, and that his behaviour had progressively deteriorated over time. She would attempt to avoid him, but he would appear wherever she went and she had been considering an injunction on the grounds of harassment. She eventually told him the relationship was over on the telephone, having been encouraged by her father. He travelled next day to the family home where he shot her father dead in the hallway with a shotgun he had bought from local criminals in the town where he lived. When he found she was not at home he put her kitten in the microwave and texted her a photo. Still in a rage, he continued to search for the girlfriend and shot dead an unknown male stranger who encountered him and asked what he was doing. He fired shots at a second man he encountered who ran off and notified the police.

He was eventually arrested by armed police following a 'siege' at his mother's home. While on remand, he expressed no remorse and blamed the entire series of events on her. Following his conviction and life sentence, he posed numerous problems of control in the prison system and although not a career criminal, he was quite prepared to fight with anyone who he perceived as disrespecting or criticising him. He tended to be avoided by other violent offenders in prison. He made two serious assaults on other prisoners by pouring boiling water over them containing dissolved sugar. He threatened revenge on prison officers who tried to contain his behaviour and spent long periods in solitary confinement. His degree of denial of responsibility caused visiting psychiatrists to sometimes question whether the correct diagnosis was delusional disorder.

Schizoid Personality Disorder

Most commentaries on schizoid PD note that it is rarely found in clinical settings and rarely comes to the attention of psychiatrists. However, this is not entirely the case; offenders and cases meeting the criteria are sometimes found in high-secure hospitals and prisons. The three main features of the condition are a tendency to social isolation, lack of emotion and a tendency to withdraw into internal fantasy. Commentaries usually describe their lack of sexuality in terms of their lack of interest in sexual acts or romance. However, from an anecdotal perspective, these cases are most likely to appear among sex offenders and individuals with sadistic pre-occupations and fantasies, sometime with non-sexualised compulsions to kill and harm others.

The Dangerous Offenders study showed that expressive aggression and excitement/exhilaration were most likely to characterise their offending behaviour. However, this included an extreme group of unusual violent and sexual offenders in high security. The key feature was that although their motivation may have been pleasure from the harm inflicted on others and accompanying excitement, this was not an overt feature, these offenders spending long periods in their fantasies, often with meticulous planning and researching. During interviews, it was often not difficult to elicit the underlying fantasies and compulsions that had driven or shaped their offending behaviour (although this was not always the case).

For example, one patient assessed following his arrival in a high-secure hospital, having carried out a killing where he had dissected the blood supply to the victim's head with a scalpel, complained bitterly that his collection of books on anatomy and vampires had been removed from his possession, asking if the author could use his 'influence' to restore them. Lack of social-emotional reciprocity, lack of facial expression and unusual body language, and narrow, fixed interests, with deficits of developing, maintaining and understanding relationships, were often present at interview and in the clinical history in schizoid PD established using a structured diagnostic instrument.

Schizoid Personality Disorder 301.20

A pervasive pattern of detachment from social relationships and a restricted range of expression of emotions in interpersonal settings, beginning by early adulthood and present in a variety of contexts, as indicated by four (or more) of the following:

1. Neither desires or enjoys close relationships, including being part of a family.
2. Almost always chooses solitary activities.
3. Has little, if any, interest in having sexual experiences with another person.
4. Takes pleasure in few, if any, activities.
5. Lacks close friends and confidants other than first degree relatives.
6. Appears indifferent to the praise and criticism of others.
7. Shows emotional coldness, detachment, or flattened affectivity.

Schizoid PD does not occur exclusively during the course of schizophrenia, a bipolar disorder or depressive disorder with psychotic features, another psychotic disorder, or autism spectrum disorder and is not attributable to the physiological effects of another medical condition.

DSM describes the condition as sometimes being premorbid to schizophrenia and delusional disorder. It also describes 'great difficulty' differentiating schizoid PD from those with milder forms of autism spectrum disorder which it says may be differentiated by more severely impaired social interaction and stereotyped behaviours and interests. In the Dangerous Offenders study, most cases were subsequently reviewed and considered to be indistinguishable from Asperger's syndrome or autism spectrum disorder and this should be considered if using a diagnostic instrument or these criteria when carrying out a PD assessment. Furthermore, a subgroup of these individuals were subsequently found to develop schizophrenia following their conviction, usually several years into prison sentences or in secure hospitals. From a diagnostic perspective, trainees who assess these cases should bear in mind that these criteria may represent an intermediate phase of a psychotic illness or constitute autistic spectrum disorder, rather than constituting a true PD. They should therefore receive a diagnostic assessment for the latter and screen for psychotic experiences and symptoms.

Case 8. Graham Young was only 14 years old when admitted to Broadmoor maximum-security hospital. His mother died when he was an infant and he was placed in the care of his aunt and uncle. He was thought to show distress if separated from his aunt, but was described as later becoming a peculiar child, solitary in his habits, and made no efforts to socialise with others his age. By the time he could read, he was noticed to be interested in notorious poisoners and developed a fascination with Adolf Hitler, wearing swastikas. He was known to sacrifice cats in occult ceremonies. He developed a detailed knowledge of chemistry and began to build up a quantity of poisons, including thallium. His first victim was a fellow science pupil who became ill but was thought to have survived because he could not closely monitor the effects. He therefore turned to his own family.

His eldest sister was found to have been poisoned by belladonna and recovered. His stepmother was later found writhing in agony in the back garden, with Young watching in fascination. He had been slowly poisoning her with antimony but sped up the process with thallium and she died. Her body was cremated, as he had suggested to his father. After her death, he moved on to his father, who he poisoned with antimony. His school chemistry master then contacted the police after discovering poisons and materials about poisoners in his school desk. He was convicted of poisoning his family but not his stepmother who had been cremated. Soon after admission to Broadmoor hospital, another patient died who he claimed he had poisoned with laurel leaves from which he had extracted cyanide, but his confession was not taken seriously. He is thought to have poisoned a tea urn and continued reading about his obsession, but tended to keep this hidden so he could gain his release. He informed a nurse he would kill someone for every year he was detained in the hospital, but was nevertheless released age 23 years.

He continued to stock up on his poisons in London and another hostel resident, where he had been placed, soon exhibited stomach cramps. He found work in photo laboratories which gave him access to poison supplies. His fellow workers began to exhibit debilitating ailments associated with thallium poisoning, two dying. He described his frustration at the time the second victim took to die in his diary. By this time, many of his fellow workers had experienced symptoms. When the visiting doctor reassured them at a meeting, Young challenged him in front of his colleagues and asked if he had ever considered thallium poisoning. The doctor then informed police of his concerns and Young's poisons were uncovered, together with his meticulous diaries recording dosages administered and his victims' reactions over time.

He was sentenced to life imprisonment and formed an association with Ian Brady, a notorious serial killer, playing chess and bonding over their mutual fascination with Nazi Germany. Young would sometimes grow a Hitler moustache in prison. In his diary, Brady described Young as genuinely asexual, excited only by power, clinical experimentation, observation and death. Young was later thrilled that a waxwork of himself was added to Madame Tussauds Chamber of Horrors in London next to his childhood hero, another poisoner.

Obsessive-Compulsive Personality Disorder

Obsessive-compulsive personality disorder (OCPD) is often considered the most high-functioning of the PDs and obsessive traits are often helpful in ensuring that tasks get completed. However, persons with OCPD are often highly rigid and can become angry and explosive when their demands for order are not met. In the Dangerous Offenders study, most cases of OCPD were comorbid with other PDs such as borderline PD, and in a small number of cases ASPD, although the latter was an unusual combination and unlikely to be encountered in community samples. Motivating factors appeared to be displaced aggression and loss, and the offences were carried out in a state of hyper-irritability. Loss or threatened loss was often difficult to cope with in a personality characterised by rigid and inflexible traits. In some cases when combined with borderline PD, the obsessive characteristics appeared to combine to make the reaction more explosive when the individual had felt abandoned in the course of the break-up of a relationship. Where there had been an unstable and intense interpersonal relationship, this was more likely to result in extremes of idealisation and devaluation due to the OCPD features observed in behaviour in the relationship over time. In some cases the anger had been displaced onto inanimate objects or other persons less highly valued than the original provoking person until the final violent outburst. Typically, the outburst had occurred when the other person had failed to submit to their way of doing things or carrying out what was expected of them.

However, in a subgroup of cases OCPD as a single category was combined with paraphilias to impact on their sex offending. The crime scenes in these latter cases showed particular features of orderliness and the behaviour had been rehearsed over a prolonged period in fantasy and carefully planned. Most importantly, however, OCPD was not the primary psychopathology leading to offending in any of the clinical cases on which this section of the chapter is based and was generally a feature which intensified behaviour together with the effects of other PD psychopathology or shaped features of the behaviour.

Obsessive-Compulsive Personality Disorder 301.4

A pervasive pattern of preoccupation with orderliness, perfectionism and mental and interpersonal control, at the expense of flexibility, openness and efficiency, beginning by early adulthood and present in a variety of contexts, as indicated by four of the following:

1. Is preoccupied with details, rules, lists, order, organization, or schedules to the extent that the major point of the activity is lost.
2. Shows perfectionism that interferes with task completion (e.g. is unable to complete a project because his or her own overly strict standards are not met).
3. Is excessively devoted to work and productivity to the exclusion of leisure activities and friendships (not accounted for by obvious economic necessity).
4. Is over conscientious, scrupulous, and inflexible about matters of morality, ethics, or values (not accounted for by cultural or religious identification).
5. Is unable to discard worn-out or worthless objects even when they have no sentimental value.
6. Is reluctant to delegate tasks or to work with others unless they submit to exactly his or her way of doing things.
7. Adopts a miserly spending style towards both self and others; money is viewed as something to be hoarded for future catastrophes.
8. Shows rigidity and stubbornness.

Case 9. Sexual sadism, paedophilia and OCPD: A 59-year-old man was assessed in prison for a parole hearing after receiving a life sentence for murder and rape of a 7-year-old girl when he was age 27 years. His previous criminal history showed he had no previous convictions for acquisitive offences but multiple convictions for sexual assaults on children starting from the age of 15 years. There had been an escalation in the level of violence inflicted on his victims, culminating in the murder. Previous assessment had revealed that he had had a long-standing sexual fantasy of asphyxiation of male and female child victims, which had escalated in intensity and intrusiveness into his thinking, coming to dominate his daily living. He had been sexually assaulted himself in childhood but had made what appeared to be a successful adjustment in adulthood, doing well at work and being able to buy his own apartment. He had no friends and spent his spare time on the internet, playing computer games remotely with opponents. He sometimes dated adult men for brief sexual encounters which involved mutual strangulation, but these were generally unsatisfactory. He kept a collection of leather belts which he used to facilitate masturbation and asphyxiation of partners, one of which was used on his victim.

Following his arrest, police noticed the extreme orderliness of his apartment and that he had carefully folded his victim's clothing and placed her shoes neatly side by side. At interview, he described masturbatory sadistic fantasies of strangling children during the act of rape, which he varied over time, and which had become impossible to push out of his mind in the weeks leading up to the murder. These were perceived as intrusive and compulsive, but at the same time exciting and sexually gratifying. He claimed they had not been present for many years. However, he had engaged in sexual activities with other prisoners and one had complained that he had tried to strangle him five years earlier. During the interview the offender was polite but at times showed barely concealed rage if the interviewer deviated from his description of what had occurred in terms of fine detail. He would repeatedly go over the details with the interviewer to ensure that he fully understood and wrote it down correctly, in a highly controlling manner.

Psychopathic Disorder

Psychopathy Criteria

The syndrome of psychopathy was originally described by Cleckley [46] who observed a series of specific features among these individuals, including superficial charm and good intelligence; absence of delusions and other signs of irrational thinking; absence of nervousness or psychoneurotic manifestations; unreliability; untruthfulness or insincerity; lack of remorse or shame; inadequately motivated antisocial behaviour; poor judgement and failure to learn from experience; pathologic egocentricity and incapacity for love; general poverty in major affective relations; specific loss of insight; unresponsiveness in general interpersonal relations; fantastic and uninviting behaviour with drink and sometimes without; suicide rarely carried out; sex life impersonal, trivial and poorly integrated; and failure to follow any life plan. These criteria from Cleckley's textbook were based on clinical observations of a subgroup of patients admitted to psychiatric hospitals in the mid-twentieth century and formed the basis of the PCL-R which was later refined and developed by Hare.

As described earlier, psychopathy is best measured using the Revised Psychopathy Checklist which requires full training to gain competence to complete. There are 20 items which score 0, 1 or 2, with a maximum score of 40, and at a cut-off of 30 or more an individual is rated as a psychopath.

Items in the Revised Psychopathy Checklist (5)

1. Glibness/superficial charm.
2. Grandiose sense of self-worth.
3. Need for stimulation/proneness to boredom.
4. Pathological lying.
5. Conning/manipulative.
6. Lack of remorse or guilt.
7. Shallow affect.
8. Callous/lack of empathy.
9. Parasitic lifestyle.
10. Poor behavioural controls.
11. Promiscuous sexual behaviour.
12. Early behavioural problems.
13. Lack of realistic long-term goals.
14. Impulsivity.
15. Irresponsibility.
16. Failure to accept responsibility for own actions.
17. Many short-term marital relationships.
18. Juvenile delinquency.
19. Revocation of conditional release.
20. Criminal versatility.

Psychopathy has an early onset and the items in the checklist are characteristic of the individual's social functioning or disability. Features are first evident by middle to late childhood, can be reliably assessed in adolescence and are chronic, persisting into adulthood, although there may be some changes in symptom pattern after 45 years. The condition is associated with unstable interpersonal relations, poor occupational functioning and increased risk of involvement in criminal activity. Hare has described the condition as

> differentiated from other personality disorders on the basis of its pattern of interpersonal, affective, and behavioural symptoms. Interpersonally, psychopaths are grandiose, egocentric, manipulative, dominant, forceful, and cold-hearted. Affectively, they display shallow and labile emotions, are unable to form long-lasting bonds to people, principles, or goals, and are lacking in empathy, anxiety, and genuine guilt and remorse. Behaviourally, they are impulsive and sensation-seeking, and they readily violate social norms. [47, p. 5]

Epidemiology

Psychopathy is a rare condition in the general population. Using the same British household survey described earlier, it was estimated that the prevalence of the population scoring 11 or more on the PCL:SV (screening version of the PCL-R) was 1.8%, for 13 or more 0.6% (possible psychopathy), and only 1 subject (0.16%) above the recommended cut-off for probable psychopathy of 18, who scored 20. Psychopathy showed a quasi-continuous population distribution, accounted for by a small subgroup, and 70.8% of the population had no psychopathic traits. Scores were higher among men than women and correlated with lower intelligence. There were independent associations between total scores and antisocial, borderline and histrionic traits, meaning that there was overlap in the symptoms of the conditions in the two diagnostic systems. When the scores were divided into the four-facet model of psychopathy, facet 1 (interpersonal) was associated with narcissistic PD; facet 2 (affective) with schizoid and antisocial PDs; facet 3 (lifestyle) with histrionic, borderline and antisocial PDs; and facet 4 (antisocial) with conduct disorder and adult ASPD.

Psychopathy was also associated with drug misuse, criminal convictions, prison sentences, violence in the past five years, homelessness, psychiatric hospital admission and suicide attempts. It was of interest that there were no associations with either psychoneurotic or psychotic symptoms, corresponding to Cleckley's original 1941 description of the syndrome of psychopathy [46]. In general, the findings indicated that psychopathy among non-incarcerated and non-psychiatric individuals in the general population is rare but represents a disabling condition with various negative outcomes, similar to those found in forensic and psychiatric samples. As it is a rare condition, it might at first be thought that psychopathy would not have a high impact on violence at the population level. However, despite individuals with scores of 11 or above in the general population demonstrating a prevalence of 2.1%, they still accounted for 18.7% of violent incidents, a population-attributable risk of 16.6%, indicating a significant public health impact. Psychopathic traits correlated with victim injury, multiple victim subtypes and multiple locations for violence [48, 49].

Psychopathy was also measured in the second stage of a two-stage survey of prisoners in England and Wales in 1997 [50], using the Revised Psychopathy Checklist (PCL-R). The prevalence of categorically diagnosed psychopathy at the standard cut-off of 30 was 7.7% (95% CI 5.2–10.9) in men and 1.9% (95% CI 0.2–6.9) in women. Psychopathy correlated with younger age among prisoners, no educational qualifications, repeated imprisonment, detention in a higher level of security, disciplinary infractions, antisocial, narcissistic, histrionic and schizoid PDs, and substance misuse (including alcohol), but not neurotic disorders or schizophrenia. Using the four-facet model, associations with DSM PD categories were similar to those observed in the British household survey. The findings indicated that psychopathic prisoners were more likely to have extreme features along a spectrum of multiple social and behavioural problems among prisoners. Despite notions of psychopathy being associated with extremes of violence, the most common conviction was for theft, reflecting the multiple forms of offending associated with the condition (criminal versatility).

Four-Facet Model

Hare later carried out further development of assessment using the PCL-R, firstly using factor analysis to show a correlated two-factor model (equivalent to combining factors 1 and 2 and factors 3 and 4) and later a four-facet model [52].

The four facets are interpersonal, affective, lifestyle and antisocial. Factor 1, 'interpersonal', includes item 1: glibness, superficial charm; item 2: grandiose sense of self-worth; item 4: pathological lying; and item 5: conning, manipulative. Factor 2, 'affective', includes item 6: lack of remorse or guilt; item 7: shallow affect; item 8: callous, lack of empathy; and item 16: failure to accept responsibility for own actions. Factor 3, 'lifestyle', includes item 3: need for stimulation, proneness to boredom; item 9: parasitic lifestyle; item 13: lack of realistic long-term goals; item 14: impulsivity; and item 15: irresponsibility. Factor 4, 'antisocial', includes item 10: poor behavioural controls; item 12: early behavioural problems; item 18: juvenile delinquency; item 19: revocation of conditional release; and item 20: criminal versatility [52].

The four-facet model is recommended and courses will teach how to score this. Offending behaviours often tend to associate with these facets somewhat differently, although all tend to be correlated. Some have suggested that facet 2 contains the 'core' features of the psychopathic personality, although it might be argued that all must be present. Facet 4 shows a major problem in the study of criminal behaviour and psychopathy because features of the individual's criminal history constitute the facet, meaning that arguments for the association are circular based on facet 4.

Two issues should be considered, however. Many studies have used the preceding two-factor model when testing theories and correlates with psychopathy. This is unfortunate because it is probable that the underlying aetiological factors will differ, particularly for facets 1 and 2. Secondly, it is important when considering previous research into psychopathy to look carefully at the cut-off used to consider that a participant is a psychopath. Many have lowered that cut-off to 25 and above to increase sample size. Clinical experience will show in forensic settings that 30 should be the minimum before making the diagnosis. There are arguments that facet 4 does not fit the clinical picture and that some psychopaths manage to avoid an intensive criminal history. These arguments are beyond the scope of this chapter. However, research that has used prison and secure hospital samples and included scores of 25–29 in their studies should be discounted. These individuals are largely non-psychopaths and likely to be career criminals with some psychopathic traits. Psychopathy was developed as a continuous scale. However, there are arguments that it should be considered as a categorical entity which are also beyond the scope of this chapter.

Clinical experience of cases with high scores, 33 and above, often show very unusual features in terms of their interactions with others, for example at interview, and in their criminal behaviour which are not all covered by the PCL-R. Each of the four facets are apparent, but certain symptoms become more striking or are more likely to be present at high overall score levels, for example pathological lying; grandiosity which is totally at odds with the life history and current situation of the individual. Similarly, lifetime parasitic use of others and a meaningless quality to their behaviour and existence in the community become clearer. All symptoms of the affective facet are likely to be present but the disconnect between what the individual says in terms of their reasoning and motivations for their criminal behaviour and their description of their affect, as they say they experienced it, becomes more apparent.

Although psychopathy is presented as personality psychopathology, spending time with very high PCL-R scorers often suggests to the careful clinical observer that they are in the presence of an individual suffering from severe mental illness or a not entirely defined cognitive deficit state rather than someone whose condition is a mere disorder of personality. There is a repeated disconnect between the logic behind their behaviour, as they describe it, the affect associated with the behaviour, as they describe it, and their general demeanour in the context of their current situation. In cases of pathological lying it is difficult to be sure both whether they believe the lies themselves and whether they truly believe that they are likely to be believed by the clinician [51].

Case 10. Psychopathy: A 49-year-old who had spent most of his adolescence and adult life in prison was serving a life sentence for the murder of a homeless man when he was age 26 years. Prior to that he had been convicted of crimes such as burglary and theft which had started before the age of 10 years, when he was first convicted. These offences had been continuous throughout his life and he would steal food or alcohol when he felt hungry or needed to drink, never having worked at any time in his life. The offences were impulsive and unplanned, solely to meet his immediate needs. He never lasted for more than weeks outside of prison since his teenage years, often only lasting for days. When in prison, he was often in trouble for fighting with other prisoners and prison officers and would become enraged easily if told to do anything he did not want to. Long periods of solitary confinement had no impact. There was no evidence that he had changed in any way during his sentence or that he was safe for release. He had encountered the victim sleeping in a derelict house where he had joined him and had consumed his alcohol, not having any of his own. It appeared that the deceased had shared his food with him. In the middle of the night, he had torn a door off its hinges in the house, thrown it on top of the man and proceeded to stamp up and down on the door until he was crushed to death beneath it.

He had never given a satisfactory explanation for this behaviour. His explanations that the man had made sexual advances towards him, and later that he had feared for his life due to the man's threats, which were given before his trial, were not pushed with any degree of conviction by the man to help his case and were totally unconvincing. At interview, many years later, he was again asked to explain his behaviour. His manner was generally cheerful and forthright. He began an unconvincing monologue about how the deceased had done something to annoy him, without being clear what it actually was, and seemed to be addressing the interviewer when he started to say things like, 'Right, we are going to teach you a good lesson for that!' 'Now you are going to see what happens to people who do these things!' 'I am going to show you now!' He stood up to give a dramatic demonstration of how he stamped on top of the door, reassuring the interviewer he was talking about the deceased and not him.

He scored 32 on the PCL-R and might have scored higher except for scoring low on superficial charm, conning/manipulative and criminal versatility. Otherwise, he fulfilled the criteria of each of the facets of the four-facet model. His affect was markedly abnormal and inappropriate in the interview, with abnormality of his cognition, to the extent that the interviewer considered whether he might be suffering from a chronic psychotic illness or even brain damage. However, no symptoms could be elicited over the life-course and previous psychological testing did not suggest overt cognitive dysfunction, although his intelligence was at the bottom of the normal range.

Psychopathy and Offending Behaviour

Studies show that psychopaths account for a large amount of criminal and violent behaviour, as would be expected from their personality structure and cognitions about the world around them. However, their offending behaviour often lacks purpose and long-range planning. In many cases, their violence is often callous and cold-blooded or part of an aggressive or macho display, without the affective colouring or understandable motives seen in non-psychopathic offenders [47]. When comparing criminal histories of psychopathic with non-psychopathic offenders, psychopathic offenders tend to be charged with violent crimes twice as often [53], although these earlier studies often included male samples from a single prison. Looking at larger samples, robbery appeared a more common primary offence in a large UK sample [21].

Psychopaths' offences tend to be both predatory, with premeditation and instrumentality, and reactive where they are unable to reliably control their behaviour. Because of skilled use of deception through verbal and non-verbal communication, their potential for uninhibited aggression and violence can be disguised by charm, gregariousness and an outward appearance of being normal [54]. Overall, however, some authors observe that psychopaths commit more instrumental violent offences than reactive. However, some have also observed an impulsive component to their violent instrumental behaviour, including considerably more violence than necessary to obtain what they want, for example drugs, money or sex. In addition, and despite these observations of impulsivity, psychopathic violent offenders are more likely to self-report low emotional arousal at the time they offended.

Deception is a major issue in psychopathy and there have been concerns in the press and among professionals that psychopaths are adept at fooling even professionals. What is clear is that a subgroup appear to derive pleasure from lying, although clinical experience shows that the process is complex. Occasionally, psychopaths will be more inclined to lie when under stress. Meloy has referred to psychopaths' use of deception as 'endogenous' [55], compulsively fuelled to protect the narcissistic self. It has also been observed that some psychopaths pile untruths one upon the other. However, Cooper and Yuile argued that pathological lying in the psychopath is not synonymous with being a good liar, but refer to 'duping delight' to describe the feelings they experience when 'putting one over' other people [56]. Cooper and Yuile argued that psychopaths do not necessarily have a superior ability to fool others or overcome a polygraph test if the person administering it is skilled. However, they are good at identifying when others are less experienced or do not have information at hand, and are skilled at manipulating others who are not prepared.

An important component of psychopathic disorder is lack of empathy and the relationship to the propensity for repeated criminal and violent behaviour without conscience or remorse. This needs to be qualified because on certain levels, some psychopaths are remarkably empathic in understanding what others want and how to manipulate them. Empathy has been described as on three levels, including (i) an affective component, sharing the emotion of the target individual (e.g. feeling another's distress), (ii) a cognitive component, involving the capacity to take the perspective of another person, and (iii) a regulatory component, in which one is able to monitor the origins of the feelings. It is thought that only the affective component is deficient in psychopathy while the cognitive functioning remains relatively normal [57]. Psychopaths are also thought to be less sensitive to fear than others and less responsive to fear conditioning, resulting in a fear response [58]. The fearlessness model of psychopathy posits that deficiency in the capacity to experience anxiety and/or fear gives rise to other aspects such as lack of remorse, superficial charm, callousness and impulsivity.

Another theory is that psychopaths' brains are strongly drawn to reward to the extent it overwhelms the sense of risk or concern about punishment, possibly due to dysfunction dopamine responses. It is thought that psychopaths have an impaired sense of potential threat but that their anticipation of reward overwhelms those concerns. This has been thought to relate to strong associations observed between psychopathy and substance abuse [59]. Early research concentrated on excessive slow wave activity in the EEG among psychopaths, particularly in the temporal or parietal regions. Because these patterns were similar to immature brains of children, this gave rise to the theory of 'cortical immaturity' [60]. A particularly interesting early theory was that the slow waves indicated a low level of brain excitement and that offending behaviour might represent a mechanism whereby the psychopath tried to alter their brain functioning in order to redress this unpleasant state.

More recently, decrease of alpha frequency indicating disrupted communication between different brain regions has been postulated, with attenuation of alpha activity linked to shallow affect and failure to accept responsibility [61]. A study by Herpertz et al.

[62] supported the theory that psychopaths are characterised by a pronounced lack of fear in response to aversive events. Furthermore, the results suggested a general deficit in processing affective information with emotional hypo-responsiveness, regardless of whether stimuli were negative or positive. Hypo-emotionality in psychopaths was thought to predispose them to violence because it prevents them from experiencing emotions that naturally inhibit the execution of violent impulses.

These studies, while interesting and raising possibilities of underlying causes for the features of psychopathy, all tend to show inconsistencies with difficulties in replication. Few studies have established a link between motivation and crime for psychopathy. Most rely on deficit theories to explain the behaviour and drive to commit offences. These are helpful and indeed plausible explanations of mechanisms that facilitate offending by psychopaths but few provide examples of driving factors. Considering the four-facet model, this approach would suggest that the psychopath commits crimes of fraud and deception because, for example, their personality structure as captured by facet 1 is to be conning and manipulative with a tendency to lying. However, scoring these same PD characteristics is itself dependent on behaviours such as conning others in the course of a fraud.

The facet structure does not satisfactorily describe what drives the psychopath to commit these crimes. Facet 2 would appear to be a more powerful potential explanation as a deficit model in normal affective functioning. However, it has been argued that theories of psychopathy that focus solely on deficit theories fail to explain why psychopaths carry out criminal and other high-risk behaviour. In the Dangerous Offenders study, psychopaths committed offences that seemed to result in a sense of exhilaration and achievement, with violence committed at times when they appeared to be hyper-irritable, resulting from minimal provocation. Several seemed to commit offences deliberately to experience excitement, which seemed ultimately pointless, with short-term planning, and highly likely to be detected or observed by others. In a prisoners study, robbery appeared to fulfil many of the characteristics of psychopaths' offending, the majority being unplanned and driven by the immediate need for money which would be largely spent on drugs or alcohol. These offences could involve not only robberies in premises such as shops but also individuals ('mugging') who would be subdued with violence. Among cases involving psychopaths, an element of excitement was often thought present but usually denied at interview.

In a detailed review of contemporary research some decades ago, Hare [63] suggested that much of the behaviour of psychopaths serves to increase sensory input and arousal to more optimal levels because of their low cortical arousal. Situations that would be frightening to most persons would be merely exciting to psychopaths and actively sought out. Similarly, drugs such as stimulants would be preferable and an early study suggested that psychopaths' behaviour could be temporarily improved by prescription of amphetamines [64]. It was also thought that psychopaths may have abnormal sleep patterns and disturbances in REM sleep so that it was necessary to obtain inordinate sensory input during waking hours to make up for low levels of REM sleep [63]. These theories have declined in their importance over time but still provide the most interesting theoretical base for further study into what could underlie and drive psychopaths' criminal behaviour, coupled with the important deficit of being unaware of or inattentive to the many subtle cues required for the guidance of behaviour and necessary for effective social functioning.

The elements of thrill-seeking, searching for exhilaration and excitement, sometimes associated with conning and manipulative behaviour and pathological lying, have not been adequately studied but can be seen from anecdotal accounts of offending behaviours. These can sometimes be seen to include behaviour that draws attention to the individual and their guilt, as if the excitement from the behaviour overcomes common sense or the understanding that it is ultimately self-defeating. Examples include: a man who had raped and murdered a neighbour's teenage daughter and hidden her body and soon after led the search by local villagers to find her; a man appearing on TV and tearfully pleading with the public to give information on a missing family victim he had murdered then concealed; a man who persuaded a friend to help him murder an older man for excitement and who told his girlfriend what he had done, but then decided that he would poison her because she worked in a shop and would probably tell someone, resulting in her informing the police when she realised a sandwich he made her contained rat poison; a man who had murdered his brother for no understandable motive as a juvenile and who had come close to being paroled several years later, but had then started threatening the life of another weaker prisoner he had previously been friendly with (no reason for the behaviour could be identified except that with less supervision he had more opportunity and was thought to be enjoying frightening him); a convicted sex offender trying to bring legal action against a prison for not actively treating him, but where it subsequently emerged that he had been organising an exchange between prisoners in group therapy of the depositions and statements of each group member's sex crimes against women and children; and a psychiatrist approached by a lawyer to carry out an assessment of a man on remand, but only if he could fulfil his client's stipulation that he must be a fully believing 'Christian' psychiatrist (the defendant was charged with raping a female priest).

Future research needs to investigate the disconnect between the psychopath's cognitive functioning and understanding of the likely outcome of their behaviour and the motivating drives for the behaviour. Trainees will need to have all the information available for these assessments. Psychopaths, like many offenders, will often say they cannot remember or were intoxicated at the time. Occasionally, they will give a fantastic story to account for the offence or simply dismiss the offending as not worth deeper consideration. A long story consisting of multiple lies is worth recording but should not become the focus of an assessment. With experience, trainees will learn when to challenge the account or move on to another issue in the history. It is important to go through each element of the offence to form a professional opinion of what occurred and what motivated the behaviour and compare this to the individual's account both of the facts and their accompanying affect and explanation.

Case studies in this chapter are based on clinical cases seen by the author but details have been deliberately changed for confidentiality purposes. Each case study was constructed as an amalgam of elements observed in different cases which matched the diagnosis described. The case of Brian Blackwell was widely reported and diagnosed by a forensic psychiatrist but was not assessed by the author.

Appendix 11.1 Taxonomy of Motivation

This taxonomy is a shortened version of that previously published as a chapter in an American Psychiatric Association publication [20]. It evolved inductively from clinical practice and research interviews with offenders with severe personality disorder in secure settings. The categories are not mutually exclusive and different motivations can exist simultaneously. Additional modifying factors can occur while the offence is carried out. In the original publication, clinical examples are given of more difficult motivations to classify and understand.

1. Expressive aggression

High levels of expressive aggression are observed during the offence, often in excess of force necessary to gain victim compliance, such as anger rape [30, 65]. Offences predominantly impulse-driven and can involve displaced aggression which compensates for an accumulation of real or imagined insults or humiliations from others.

2. Power, domination, control

Involves need to achieve dominance and control over victim. Typically in 'power-assurance rape' [65] where the assault is an expression of rape fantasies. Offender often compensates for acutely felt inadequacies.

3. Sexual gratification

Offence involves gratification of sexual desire, including sexual deviations.

4. Sadistic sexual fantasy

Offence is enactment of a sadistic sexual fantasy with previous rehearsal in imagination, reinforced by masturbation, and may be a 'try-out' or follow previous try-outs [66].

5. Paraphilia

Offence involves acting upon one or more paraphilias.

6. Sexual conflict

Offences are precipitated rather than motivated by unresolved conscious or subconscious conflicts resulting from earlier experiences, such as sexual abuse.

7. Hyper-irritability

State of intense anger or irritability prior to the offence, but which has not been provoked by the victim. Victim may have been provocative or there may have been some minimal stress, but the anger or irritability is independent of the circumstances and has no clear cause or focus for the offender.

8. Relief of tension/dysphoria

Offence preceded by intense feelings of anxiety, tension, anger and/or dysphoria. Symptoms often relieved by the offending behaviour and may be carried out deliberately for this purpose.

9. Excitement/exhilaration

Deliberately carried out for pleasurable (non-sexual) excitement and/or exhilaration.

10. Compulsive urge to harm/kill

Offending explained by compulsive urges to harm others which are not provoked or for revenge. May take form of obsessive and intrusive thoughts and may attempt to resist urges.

11. Blow to self-esteem

Precipitated by words or actions of victim, resulting in blow to self-esteem and accompanying feelings of humiliation, devaluation and consequent rage [44].

12. Threatened or actual loss

Offence precipitated by loss or threatened loss of another person, object or supportive situation such as accommodation, resulting in extreme anxiety, distress and anger.

13. Under-controlled aggression

History of low threshold for violence following minimal provocation, 'short fuse'.

14. Victim precipitation

Undisputed evidence that victim provoked the behaviour of the offender.

15. Revenge

Retaliation for a perceived wrong. Real, imagined or delusional.

16. Jealousy

Can be coded when offender discovers true infidelity or jealousy is 'morbid'.

17. Displaced aggression

Offence committed on another person or object in place of the individual who originally provoked reaction of anger in the offender.

18. Problem resolution/attention-seeking

Committed to draw attention to situation, persuade others to resolve problems, or gain attention or care.

19. Financial gain

Intention and expectation of financial gain.

20. Escape arrest

Designed to avoid detection or escape arrest.

21. Pyromania

Fire-setting in context of clearly defined pyromania.

22. Gang/group activity

Carried out as part of a group or organised gang.

23. Psychotic

Offence directly motivated by symptoms of psychotic illness or where symptoms demonstrated substantial influence on motivation.

24. To be a hero

Offence committed so that others are blamed and in which they take credit for subsequent events, such as alerting authorities, rescue.

25. Intoxication

Intoxicated with alcohol/drugs at time of offence (not a 'motivation' but key modifier of offence-related behaviour).

26. Impulsivity

Impulsivity is not a motivation but a modifying factor and is a predisposition to react rapidly and without planning to internal and external stimuli with lack of regard for short- and long-term consequences. Often thought to be a feature of abnormal personality, it can be a characteristic of several mental disorders. It is also highly complex and can involve emotional impulsivity which differs from cognitive impulsivity [14].

References

1. Freestone MC, Wilson K, Jones R et al. The impact on staff of working with personality disordered offenders: a systematic review. *PLoS One* 2015; 10 (8): e0136378.

2. American Psychiatric Association. *Diagnostic and Statistical Manual of Mental Disorders, fifth edition text revision: DSM-5-TR.* Arlington, VA, American Psychiatric Association, 2022.

3. Reed GM, First MB, Kogan CS et al. Innovations and changes in the ICD-11 classification of mental, behavioural and neurodevelopmental disorders. *World Psychiatry* 2019; 18 (1): 3–19.

4. National Collaborating Centre for Mental Health. *National Institute for Health and Care Excellence: Guidelines. Borderline Personality Disorder: Treatment and Management.* Leicester, The British Psychological Society and The Royal College of Psychiatrists, 2009.

5. Hare RD. *The Hare Psychopathy Checklist: Revised* [PCL-R; manual]. North Tonawanda, NY, Multi-Health Systems, 1991.

6. Millon T, Grossman S. *MCMI-IV: Millon Clinical Multiaxial Inventory Manual.* Bloomington, IN, NCS Pearson, 2015.

7. First M, Gibbon M, Spitzer R, Williams J, Benjamin L. Structured Clinical Interview for DSM-IV Axis II Personality Disorders (SCID-II). Washington, DC, American Psychiatric Press, 1997.

8. Reich J. Avoidant personality disorder and its relationship to social phobia. *Social Anxiety* 2010: 207–22.

9. Coid JW, Yang M, Tyrer P, Roberts A, Ullrich S. Prevalence and correlates of personality disorder in Great Britain. *British Journal of Psychiatry* 2006; 188: 423–31.

10. Singleton N, Gatward R, Meltzer H. *Psychiatric Morbidity among Prisoners in England and Wales.* London, Stationery Office, 1998.

11. Coid JW, Gonzalez R, Igoumenou A et al. Personality disorder and violence in the national household population of Britain. *The Journal of Forensic Psychiatry & Psychology* 2017; 28 (5): 620–38.

12. Hodgins S. Persistent violent offending: what do we know? *The British Journal of Psychiatry* 2007; 190 (S49): s12–s14.

13. Coid JW, Ullrich S. Antisocial personality disorder is on a continuum with psychopathy. *Comprehensive Psychiatry* 2010; 51 (4): 426–33.

14. Howard R. Personality disorders and violence: what is the link? *Borderline Personality Disorder and Emotion Dysregulation* 2015; 2 (1): 1–11.

15. Topalli V. *Offender Decision-Making and Motivation.* Oxford, Oxford University Press, 2011.

16. Bennett T, Wright R. *Burglars on Burglary: Prevention and the Offender.* Farnham, Gower, 1984.

17. Wright R, Decker S. *Burglars on the Job: Streetlife and Residential Break-Ins.* Boston, MA, Northeastern University Press, 1996.

18. Wright R, Decker S. *Armed Robbers in Action: Stickups and Street Culture.* Boston, MA, Northeastern University Press, 1997.

19. Jacobs BA, Topalli V, Wright R. Managing retaliation: drug robbery and informal sanction threats. *Criminology* 2000; 38: 171–98.

20. Coid JW. Axis II disorders and motivation for serious criminal behavior. In Skodol AE (ed.) *Psychopathology and Violent Crime.* Washington, DC; American Psychiatric Press Inc., 1998, pp. 53–97.

21. Coid JW. Personality disorders in prisoners and their motivation for dangerous and disruptive behaviour. *Criminal Behaviour and Mental Health* 2002; 12 (3): 209–26.

22. Beck AT. Thinking and depression: II. Theory and therapy. *Archives of General Psychiatry* 1964; 10 (6): 561–71.

23. Beck A. Depression: Clinical, Experimental, and Theoretical Aspects. New York, Harper & Row, 1972.

24. Freeman A, Pretzer J, Fleming B, Simon KM. *Clinical Applications of Cognitive Therapy.* New York, Springer, 1990.

25. Beck AT, Davis DD, Freeman A. *Cognitive Therapy of Personality Disorders.* London, Guilford Publications, 2015.

26. Hollon SD, Kendall PC, Lumry A. Specificity of depressotypic cognitions in clinical depression. *Journal of Abnormal Psychology* 1986; 95 (1): 52.

27. MacLeod C, Mathews A, Tata P. Attentional bias in emotional disorders. *Journal of Abnormal Psychology* 1986; 95 (1): 15.

28. Mathews A, MacLeod C. Discrimination of threat cues without awareness in anxiety states. *Journal of Abnormal Psychology* 1986; 95 (2): 131.

29. Zwemer WA, Deffenbacher JL. Irrational beliefs, anger, and anxiety. *Journal of Counseling Psychology* 1984; 31 (3): 391.

30. Groth A. with Birnbaum HJ. *Men Who Rape*. New York, Plenum Press, 1979.

31. Robins LN. *Deviant Children Grown Up: A Sociological and Psychiatric Study of Sociopathic Personality*. Baltimore, MD, Williams and Wilkins, 1966.

32. Hare EH, Wing JK. *Psychiatric Epidemiology: Proceedings of the International Symposium Held at Aberdeen University 22–25 July, 1969*. New York, Oxford University Press, 1970.

33. Robins LN. Sturdy childhood predictors of adult antisocial behaviour: replications from longitudinal studies. *Psychological Medicine* 1978; 8 (4): 611–22.

34. Moffitt TE. Life-course-persistent and adolescence-limited antisocial behavior: a developmental taxonomy. *Psychological Review* 1993; 100 (4): 674–701.

35. Coid JW. Formulating strategies for the primary prevention of adult antisocial behaviour: 'high risk' or 'population' strategies. *Early Prevention of Adult Antisocial Behaviour* 2003: 32–78.

36. Coid J. The co-morbidity of personality disorder and lifetime clinical syndromes in dangerous offenders. *Journal of Forensic Psychiatry & Psychology* 2003; 14 (2): 341–66.

37. Coid J, Yang M, Bebbington P et al. Borderline personality disorder: health service use and social functioning among a national household population. *Psychological Medicine* 2009; 39 (10): 1721–31.

38. Coid JW. An affective syndrome in psychopaths with borderline personality disorder? *The British Journal of Psychiatry: The Journal of Mental Science* 1993; 162: 641–50.

39. Salman Akhtar M, Thomson Jr JA. Overview: Narcissistic personality disorder. *The American Journal of Psychiatry* 1982; 139 (1): 12–20.

40. Kernberg OF. *Borderline Conditions and Pathological Narcissism*. New York, Jason Aronson, 1975.

41. Katz J. *Seductions of Crime: Moral and Sensual Attractions in Doing Evil*. New York, Basic Books, 1988.

42. Wilson A. Levels of adaptation and narcissistic psychopathology. *Psychiatry* 1989; 52 (2): 218–36.

43. Kohut H. Thoughts on narcissism and narcissistic rage. *The Psychoanalytic Study of the Child* 1972; 27 (1): 360–400.

44. Rosen I. Self-esteem as a factor in social and domestic violence. *The British Journal of Psychiatry* 1991; 158 (1): 18–23.

45. Glasser M. Aggression and sadism in the perversions. In Rosen I (ed.) *Sexual Deviation* (3rd ed.). Oxford, Oxford University Press, 1996, pp. 279–99.

46. Cleckley HM. *The Mask of Sanity: An Attempt to Clarify Some Issues about the So-Called Psychopathic Personality*. St Louis, MO, Mosby, 1941.

47. Hare RD. *Hare Psychopathy Checklist: Revised*. Toronto, Multi-Health Systems, 1991.

48. Coid J, Yang M. The impact of psychopathy on violence among the household population of Great Britain. *Social Psychiatry and Psychiatric Epidemiology* 2011; 46: 473–80.

49. Coid J, Yang M, Ullrich S, Roberts A, Hare RD. Prevalence and correlates of psychopathic traits in the household population of Great Britain. *International Journal of Law and Psychiatry* 2009; 32 (2): 65–73.

50. Coid J, Yang M, Ullrich S et al. Psychopathy among prisoners in England and Wales. *International Journal of Law and Psychiatry* 2009; 32 (3): 134–41.

51. Shover N. *Great Pretenders: Pursuits and Careers of Persistent Thieves*. Boulder, CO, Westview, 1996.

52. Hare RD. *Manual for the Revised Psychopathy Checklist*. Toronto, ON, Multi-Health Systems, 2003.

53. Hare RD, Jutai JW. Psychopathy and cerebral asymmetry in semantic

processing. *Personality and Individual Differences* 1988; 9 (2): 329–37.

54. Porter S, Woodworth M, Black PJ. Psychopathy and aggression. In Patrick CJ (ed.) *Handbook of Psychopathy*, 2nd ed. New York, Guilford Press, 2019, pp. 481–94.

55. Meloy JR. *The Psychopathic Mind: Origins, Dynamics, and Treatment*. Lanham, MD, Rowman & Littlefield, 1988.

56. Cooper BS, Yuille JC. *Psychopathy and Deception: The Psychopath*. London, Routledge, 2017, pp. 487–503.

57. Blair RJR. Responding to the emotions of others: dissociating forms of empathy through the study of typical and psychiatric populations. *Consciousness and Cognition* 2005; 14 (4): 698–718.

58. Blair RJR. The amygdala and ventromedial prefrontal cortex in morality and psychopathy. *Trends in Cognitive Sciences* 2007; 11 (9): 387–92.

59. Buckholtz JW, Treadway MT, Cowan RL et al. Mesolimbic dopamine reward system hypersensitivity in individuals with psychopathic traits. *Nature Neuroscience* 2010; 13 (4): 419–21.

60. Schirmann F. 'The wondrous eyes of a new technology': a history of the early electroencephalography (EEG) of psychopathy, delinquency, and immorality. *Frontiers in Human Neuroscience* 2014; 8: 232.

61. Konicar L, Radev S, Silvoni S et al. Balancing the brain of offenders with psychopathy? Resting state EEG and electrodermal activity after a pilot study of brain self-regulation training. *Plos One* 2021; 16 (1): e0242830.

62. Herpertz SC, Werth U, Lukas G et al. Emotion in criminal offenders with psychopathy and borderline personality disorder. *Archives of General Psychiatry* 2001; 58 (8): 737–45.

63. Hare RD. *Psychopathy: Theory and Research*. New York, Wiley, 1970.

64. Hill D. Amphetamine in psychopathic states. *British Journal of Addiction to Alcohol & Other Drugs* 1947; 44 (2): 50–4.

65. Douglas JE, Burgess AW, Burgess AG, Ressler RK. *Crime Classification Manual: A Standard System for Investigating and Classifying Violent Crime*. New York, John Wiley & Sons, 2013.

66. MacCulloch MJ, Snowden PR, Wood PJ, Mills HE. Sadistic fantasy, sadistic behaviour and offending. *British Journal of Psychiatry* 1983; 143: 20–9.

67. World Health Organization. *The ICD-10 Classification of Mental and Behavioural Disorders: Diagnostic Criteria for Research*. Geneva, World Health Organization, 1993.

Stalking and Threats to Harm and Kill

Paul E. Mullen

Stalking

Stalking is a problem behaviour which involves a course of conduct in which one individual imposes repeated unwanted contacts and/or communications on another in a manner which creates distress and/or fear [1]. Stalking as a criminal offence is defined in different ways in different jurisdictions as their legislators struggle with a victim-defined crime (the subjective report of distress and/or fear) and, above all, with the criminalisation of a series of acts, each of which may be legal when considered in isolation.

The contacts may involve loitering nearby, following, maintaining surveillance and approaches. Unwanted communications cover the whole gamut of the oral and written, delivered in diverse ways, among the commonest being emails. The stalking can progress to behaviours which are in themselves criminal acts, such as assaults (from touching through to violent assaults) and communications involving threats or slanderous utterances intended to damage the target's reputation or disrupt their lawful functioning [2]. Another form of harassment involves ordering or cancelling goods and services in the victim's name [3].

Widely varying estimates of the frequency of stalking are generated by using different definitions and different ascertainment methods in different cultures and socioeconomic groups. In the English-speaking world, somewhere between 25% and 40% of people will experience some form of stalking. In about half of cases this will involve a series of intrusions lasting days to a couple of weeks. Those that persist beyond two weeks can continue for months or years. Women are more frequently the victims; men are almost always the perpetrators. The evidence suggests stalking rates have escalated over recent decades. A number of contemporary social and cultural factors probably contribute to this increase. If stalking continues beyond a few days, or reoccurs, serious psychological and social damage (including reputational and financial) may be inflicted [1]. The primary sufferer is the victim but in most cases of longer-term pursuit the stalker is also adversely affected. Victims may suffer physical and/or sexual assault, as in some cases may stalkers [9]. In one of my cases [1] the victim killed their stalker, and in several others the victim, or their supporters, inflicted serious injuries on the stalker. As a topic, this subject has passed into popular culture and general knowledge [10, 11], which may complicate assessment.

Risk Assessment and Management

Almost all medical practice is based on applying probabilities derived from research to direct the management of the consenting patient for their benefit. For better or for worse, forensic mental health professionals have been drawn into offering probability-based assessments of risk on individuals to a range of authorities which can be used to legitimise inflicting punishment or other actions not in the interests of their patient. In most clinical situations the fact that estimates of probability apply only to groups, not to individuals, is a reason for caution about their application, particularly about the relevance of the research data to the risk–benefit analysis in a particular case. In forensic practice neither consent nor the patient's likely benefit can be assumed. If this does not stop you entirely, it should motivate an even more careful and sceptical examination of any database on which you rely in estimating risk.

Most of the databases used in forensic practice, both in actuarial and research-based risk estimates, are problematic. Estimates of reoffending based on populations which come from different jurisdictions and cultural contexts can be misleading. For example, the offender population in US studies contains a high proportion of African-American and Hispanic people, which makes any studies on reoffending of dubious relevance to offenders in, say, Bristol or Dublin. Even more concerning is the use of studies of reoffending, which almost always use figures from a wide range of offences from the relatively minor to the serious, with the preponderance being minor, and apply them to questions about the risk of serious violence or the more extreme forms of sexual offending.

Risk management is on far firmer ground for the forensic clinician; after all, that is our job (though not that of that chimera, the American forensicist). I may not be able to give the court a reliable estimate of reoffending, but whatever that risk may be, I can usually provide clear guidance on what will reduce it. Personally, I regard those I assess as patients (from the Latin: ones who suffer), not clients (from the Latin: supplicants to patricians), who have offended. Part of our responsibility to our patients is to reduce the chances of them harming themselves by continuing to harm others.

In the real world, courts and tribunals have become used to obtaining assessments of risk and dangerousness and will not always accept the scientifically and ethically sound response that a reliable estimate in this individual is not possible, though you can express an opinion on what will reduce that risk. One way around this is to be clear and precise in your responses to questions of risk. An individual may fall into a high-risk group for reoffending on the assessment tools you are using.

In almost all research, whatever the rate of future offending may be, in the high-risk group (say, 70%) the 95% confidence limits are likely to span 50% (e.g. 70% plus or minus 25%). This indicates that you cannot say whether the individual is more likely than not to reoffend. Even if the 95% confidence limits do not span 50% (e.g. 80% with 95% confidence, 93% to 67%), it is essential to alert those intending to use the risk estimate of the range covered by that estimate. If whatever approach you employ does not have data on 95% confidence limits available, then assume that high risk indicates a range of possibilities, including a less than 50% chance. Also make clear you are relying on data based on a range of offences from populations which may differ in important ways from your own community. Do all this and nothing more; then your opinion may never be asked again.

Assessing and Managing Stalkers

Forensic mental health professionals confront the problems being created by stalking in situations involving:

- assessing and managing the stalker
- assessing and managing victims of stalking

- advising criminal and civil courts about stalking
- advising organisations (including health services) how to respond to best protect staff and the organisation from stalkers
- advising forensic mental health professionals as victims of stalking.

This section will focus on assessing and managing stalkers who target members of the general community.

The Stalker

Stalking can involve different types of people and occur in different types of relational and social contexts. Stalkers can have different types of motivations and different types of psychopathology. Victims respond in different ways, some of which, however well intentioned, can aggravate the problem. The duration and intensity of stalking is highly variable. It is a reasonable assumption that such differences may all affect the likely damage suffered both by the victim and the perpetrator, as well as impacting on assessment and management.

There were early attempts to use the stalker's psychopathology as defined in the *Diagnostic and Statistical Manual of Mental Disorders* (DSM) as a guide to their assessment. This approach created more problems than solutions, in large part because most stalkers do not have easily classifiable mental disorders directly related to their behaviour. Attempts employing attachment style also fell by the wayside, as did the use of multidimensional models using the stalking behaviours such as following, phoning, gifts and property damage.

Stalkers can be divided on the basis of the type of victim, such as strangers, ex-partners, acquaintances, celebrities, royalty and heads of state. Separation on the basis of victim type can inform risk assessment and management, being particularly useful when, for example, considering royalty, who attract those with a different spectrum of motivations and who are far more likely to have major mental disorders. Such approaches usually also take account of threats, overt violence and escalation of intensity. In practice there are considerable overlaps between the relational and motivational typologies.

The approach to be described here has a motivational typology as its starting point but can also encompass relational and victim variables [1]. This approach has had some validation from research on outcomes. Equally important, it encourages treating both perpetrator and victim as human beings trapped in a situation created by the perpetrator to which the victim attempts to respond. What follows is not a classification but a typology of stalkers which implies some overlap between the groupings and an occasional case which will fit ill wherever placed.

The Rejected

The stalking emerges in the context of separation from someone with whom they have had a close relationship, usually sexual and emotional. The initial motivation is often a varying mixture of the desire for reconciliation and the desire to punish the perceived desertion. The stalking is often sustained either because it becomes a twisted substitute which fills the void left by the lost relationship or because of an ongoing desire to exact revenge for the rejection. The vast majority of rejected stalkers are male. They rarely have major mental disorders, though a variety of social and psychological vulnerabilities are found.

The increasing rates of stalking in Western societies are, in no small part, because of the escalating numbers of breakdowns in sexual and emotional relationships in what at least one of the partners considered to be established and permanent. A century ago, most people married young and stayed together for a lifetime, with or without the occasional extra-marital indulgence. Today, not only do a large number of marriages end in separation but also a pattern of what could be called serial monogamy is common before even attempting to 'settle down'. The end of every relationship is a potential cause of stalking by a partner who regards themselves as wronged by the 'abandonment'. Sexual jealousy of an actual or imagined rival can complicate the Rejected's response, though less commonly than might be thought. The Rejected Stalker usually constructs themselves as a victim, not of sexual infidelity but of injustice, and of error based on the partner's failure to credit their many positive features. The type of infidelity most commonly complained of is to vows, commitments and God's laws.

On the positive side, the changed nature of intimate relationships reflects the slow progress in women's social position, including increased financial security, which offers the capacity to discontinue relationships which were abusive or just failed to meet their needs. Once men deserted; now women depart. Men need to come to terms with the new reality.

The Rejected Type encompasses a wide range of dysfunctional traits and beliefs. Some of the Rejected are simply acting on the basis of religious tenets and social attitudes about women and marriage which were common 50 years ago but are no longer acceptable to their ex-partners, or the vast majority of their fellow citizens. Some are overly dependent and incapable of envisioning, let alone accepting, an end to the relationship. Some are so self-absorbed and self-centred that they cannot accept their partner's right to end a relationship; as one such stalker said: 'I leave women, women don't leave me.' Some Rejected stalkers, to be fair, are genuinely confused about their partner's intentions – a confusion sometimes fostered by the departing partner's best intentions. Kindness, consideration and the wish to transition from a sexual/emotional partnership to a friendship are laudable aims as long as the intention to end the relationship is made clear. The exiting partner's own guilt can be the source of words and actions which foster the erroneous expectation that the relationship is not over or can be revived with a touch of persistent pursuit.

The Incompetent Suitor

The context in which the stalking of the Incompetent Suitor emerges is usually one of loneliness and/or sexual frustration. The victims are selected from casual contacts or complete strangers. The stalker is not seeking love but is motivated by the desire for friendship, a date or simply sex. They are almost all males. Their problem is their incapacity or unwillingness to negotiate the social interactions which might bring success in establishing a relationship. They persist despite their advances being repelled because they fail to recognise, or are indifferent to, the negative and often fearful responses produced by their inept approaches. In most cases they stop after the failure of repeated attempts, with few persisting beyond a week or so. Those who do persist for longer usually have some connection to the victim through, for example, their workplace, educational establishment or living in the same neighbourhood. Unsurprisingly, autism spectrum disorders occasionally turn up in this group.

The modern world has lost many of the informal mechanisms by which the less socially able and less attractive males were paired off with women susceptible, for one reason or another, to family and social pressures. More importantly, marriage is no longer the only option for women, who are increasingly able to choose between potential partners and reject the lot if they so desire. At the same time, a culture of sexualisation, where sexual acts are projected unencumbered by emotional or social contingencies, encourages the notion of a sexual free-for-all from which the Incompetent Suitor feels excluded. As one such stalker said, 'You're getting it, they're all getting it, why aren't I getting it, it's not fair.'

Intimacy Seekers

Intimacy Seekers are not seeking to 'get it' through some brief encounter but are pursuing true love, or at least an intimate long-term relationship. Unlike the Incompetent Suitors, they are almost all females. The context is usually that of loneliness and a lack of someone to love or even to feel close to. Not all Intimacy Seekers are solitary as a painful loneliness can coexist both with marriage and extensive though superficial social networks. The intimacy-seeking type are pursuing a loving relationship which they believe, against all evidence, either already exists or which their efforts will eventually create. They may use a range of approaches and communications. Some are insistent and intrusive, whereas others are satisfied to wait in expectation with only the occasional reminder to their beau of their continuing love. These are the most persistent type of all stalkers. In some of our cases the pursuit had continued for decades, albeit in some only with a quiet insistence rather than the more dramatic forms of harassment.

Psychiatry has a long history of engagement with Intimacy Seekers and their stalking behaviours through the notion of erotomania. Originally the concept covered a wide range of pathologies of love from exaggerated forms of infatuation to delusions. Over time, the concept of erotomania was whittled away to leave just a rare condition involving delusions of being loved by another. One effect of the adoption of anti-stalking legislation was to bring to clinical attention numerous examples of Intimacy Seekers, not all of whom fitted into the current delusional disorder erotomanic type concept.

Intimacy Seekers all share an intense preoccupation with an individual with whom they thought they are, or would be, romantically involved. Some believed the love was mutual, some that they were responding to the other's romantic advances, and some knew no relationship yet existed but were convinced that eventually their love would be reciprocated. Whether the stalking of the Intimacy Seekers has become more common is, unlike other forms of stalking, uncertain, as is what (if any) cultural and social influences are at play. Health professionals are one of the more common targets.

Clinically, three broad types are found.

(1) Those with pre-existing psychotic disorders, usually of a schizophrenic type, though occasionally manic or organic, in the context of which the erotomania emerged.
(2) Those who could be regarded as having a delusional disorder.
(3) Those who have pathological infatuations.

Resentful Stalkers

Resentful Stalkers can be subdivided first into those who try to remain anonymous while conducting covert harassment, and second into those who make no secret of who they are and how they are attempting to exact revenge. Both types are motivated by the desire for vengeance directed at an individual, an organisation or a representative of a group by whom they believe they have been injured. The supposed injury has usually been in the form of injustice or humiliation.

Both the overt and covert Resentful Types have failed to express their anger at the time to the perceived injustice or humiliation in the form of acts of disagreement or retaliation. Instead, they become preoccupied long term with the hurt and by their need to strike back [12]. Typically, they ruminate for long periods about the supposed insult or injury before initiating their campaign of harassment. Typical behaviours found in the Resentful Stalker involve indirect and implied threats rather than direct threats, malicious complaints, false accusations, internet trolling and sometimes property damage. Resentful Stalkers with the requisite skills may hack into computers to create distress and disruption. One of our cases started rumours of the malfeasance and imminent bankruptcy of a company backed up by forged documents. Another, claiming to be a whistleblower, cast doubt on his employer's safe handling of toxic waste. Both produced the disruption and disquiet they desired, at least for a time.

The Resentful Stalkers probably persist because of the unaccustomed sense of power and control they derive from the success of their campaign. They conceive of themselves as victims fighting back against the powerful and privileged when, for the most part, they target the more vulnerable members among their supposed oppressors. This group may have personality traits disposing them to suspiciousness and oversensitivity, though a few have obvious mental disorders. Identifying those who act anonymously is a problem. Bringing any Resentful Stalker into treatment is difficult, rarely occurring without conviction and a court order.

Health professionals are one of the groups who attract stalking from those who become resentful about aspects of their treatment. Professionals of all types are vulnerable to malicious complaints made to registration bodies and agencies of accountability whose starting point is to assume the complaint, however outlandish, is justified. Such complaints organisations all too often turn justice on its head, demanding proof of innocence rather than evidence of guilt. As those trained in science know, it is difficult, if not impossible, to prove a negative.

Predatory Type

The Predatory Type are fortunately rarely encountered. They are men who follow and watch a victim while planning a sexual attack. They differ from most perpetrators of serial sexual attacks in how much of their satisfaction comes from the extended periods, lasting weeks or months, of surveillance, during which they indulge in fantasies of the coming attack. One of our cases was eventually caught and convicted of five rapes over a period of 10 years. Subsequently he described multiple instances in which he followed and spied on women for weeks on end, fantasising about the coming rape, even though in many cases he did not progress to an attack.

Another case was of a man who had been following and spying on a woman while he planned and fantasised about raping and strangling her. He then intended to hang himself. He hired a van, rented a secluded holiday cabin, purchased ropes and ties, and even acquired a supply of ether. At that point, for some reason the horror of what he was about to undertake dawned. He sought help from a local primary care physician, who arranged an immediate assessment at our community clinic. To my surprise, the long-term outcome was favourable. This man was never charged and had no prior convictions. Managing a patient on a voluntary basis you know has come close to committing a dreadful act, whom you have not informed the police about, in part because no crime was committed, is one of the challenges of forensic practice, and provides one of the rewards if all goes well.

Assessing and Managing Risk in Stalking

The risks for the victim of stalking are:

(1) That the stalking will persist.

(2) That the stalking, if it has ceased, will reoccur.

(3) That the stalking will inflict serious psychological and social damage.

(4) That levels of depression and anxiety will escalate, leading to a risk of suicide.

(5) That the stalker may launch a physical or sexual assault.

The risks for the stalker are:

(1) That their stalking will continue and become an all-consuming preoccupation which erodes their social and financial situation.

(2) That their actions will attract condemnation from their peers and eventually criminal sanctions.

(3) That their psychological functioning will be undermined and they will suffer significant ongoing impairment.

(4) That they may become depressed, despairing and potentially suicidal.

In a significant minority, stalking is a self-limiting problem. The Incompetent Type rarely persists beyond a week or two, and only the repeat offenders of this type are likely to be seen clinically. Rejected and Resentful Types may desist when their behaviour is exposed and an active police intervention, even if only a caution, ensues (civil proceedings leading to restraining orders are far less effective). A joint police and mental health professional response group is the gold standard for the initial approach to the management of all types of stalking.

The general management of the different types of stalker who do persist long enough to reach a forensic clinic will now be considered. The issue of threats and violence will be considered separately.

The *Intimacy Seekers* are the most persistent type, though not usually the most intrusive. The very length of the pursuit places considerable psychological and social stress on both victim and stalker. The stalker does have the compensation of the fantasy of love and the hope of future joy, whereas the victim has no such comforts. This type always requires primarily a mental health solution.

The Intimacy Seeker type includes pursuit by those with schizophrenic or manic disorders who have developed a delusional attachment to the target. The stalking usually, but not always, ceases with effective treatment of the active symptoms of the psychosis, though it may return with a relapse, either focussing on a new victim or returning to the original target.

Delusional disorders with a fixed belief that a loving relationship exists with their target are found frequently among the Intimacy Seekers. Contrary to some writings on erotomania, the belief that they are the unwilling recipient of the love of the target is uncommon. In most cases they believe a mutual affection exists. The management of delusional disorders is often time-consuming and of uncertain outcome. Our practice is to focus initially on reducing the intrusive behaviours using the patient's convictions that their love will last and eventually be victorious. So why risk upsetting or alienating their supposed lover? The force of the pursuit comes in part from the loneliness and emptiness of so many of the lives of this group. Part of the solution can be encouraging and facilitating various forms of social interactions. This can, however, have unexpected consequences. One of my patients ceased her decade-long pursuit, though not her hopes for love, when she joined a women's social club. All might have been well but for the weekly jaunts to play the 'pockies' (slot machines), which set off an enthusiastic and financially ruinous gambling behaviour. The management of delusional disorders in general remains a contested area with the role of medication, of the psychotherapies and of social interventions unresolved.

Among the intimacy-seeking type are individuals who have been conceptualised as cases of morbid infatuation, who fit ill with both the current nosology and notions about delusion. They will accept their target does not yet return their affection. They will often agree that the pursuit of the beloved has to date not advanced their courtship. But they insist that their love will triumph. One of our cases had a rhinoplasty and a hair transplant, in addition to dedicated bodybuilding, in case his failure to obtain a date with his beloved had been due to some defect in his appearance. In our experience the morbid infatuations are the most intrusive of the Intimacy Seekers and the subgroup most likely to become violent. Our only homicide among our Intimacy Seeker group was a man with a morbid infatuation who killed his hoped-for wife-to-be when her engagement to another was announced in the newspaper.

The *Rejected Type* form the majority of referrals to our clinic from the courts. In most cases they had persisted despite police cautions, prior conviction or civil restraining orders. In some, threats and assaults had precipitated the referral. Most of these *men* regarded themselves as the victim in the situation, either of an unjust system or of their ex-partner. It was their rights which were being infringed – rights which variously included to intrude, to pursue, to threaten and even to assault in pursuit of a notion of justice which often included a curious mix of restoration of the relationship and punishment of the deserter. The vehemence of their self-justifications was often increased where there were children from the relationship. Religion was not infrequently invoked as a justification. This type is almost always intrusive both in person and via communications.

There is no pill for misplaced enthusiasms, or denials of the obvious, let alone fundamentalist religiosity. To stop the intrusions, short of locking them up and throwing away the key, you have to change those attitudes, desires and contexts which sustain the behaviours. This requires establishing the patient's acceptance, however reluctant, that they will attempt to cease the stalking. Without that, there is little a mental health service can offer beyond becoming part of the problem.

In managing this group, as with so many problem behaviours, an appeal to self-interest is a good place to start. In those focussed on reconciliation, the price they are paying, and will pay, can be contrasted with the lack of benefits and with suggestions it may be time to give up the unequal struggle. This can be placed in a manner flattering to their ego (such dedication is rare) and emphasising the dire consequences of persistence. Those seeking vengeance may be less evoking of sympathy but more likely to respond to appeals to self-interest. The stalker can experience an increased temptation to attempt contacting the ex-partner at certain times, such as late at night or Sunday morning; in certain states, notably intoxications; during certain activities like reviewing old photos; and when visiting certain places which recall the lost relationship.

The stalker can be helped to manage triggers by avoiding them where possible or preparing strategies to control the urges to contact the lost love. Developing new interests, not just amorous, is worth encouraging, though many of the Rejected tend to be obsessive, which can be problematic (think gambling, dieting, collecting, etc.). Managing this group sometimes amounts to throwing lifeline after lifeline in the hope they finally grab a way out. Attitudes in all of us are difficult to change, but particularly in the aggrieved obsessive who make up so many of the Rejected Type. Pointing out why their partner may have departed, however tempting, does not help. Equally unhelpful is mediating any contact between stalker and victim. The time for marriage guidance is past. The key is time, persuasion and persistence in an ongoing contact with a consistent therapist or therapists (sadly a big ask in most mental health services). The Rejected are the stalker type most likely to threaten and attack and many of those who reach our services have already acted in these ways.

The *Resentful Type*, in my experience, is usually encountered when consulting for organisations plagued by such a stalker the identity of whom is uncertain. The Resentful Type are the master of the indirect threat and the anonymous spiteful communication. In practice, once a Resentful Stalker is identified and faced with the consequences of their actions, they often desist. The exceptions are those who have convinced themselves they are on a quest for justice, not just for themselves but also for the wider community. This subtype overlaps with the abnormally persistent complainers and litigants who are notoriously difficult to manage.

The *Incompetent Suitor* only comes our way if they are repeat offenders or have committed an assault (usually minor). The problem is managing either social ineptitude, or gross interpersonal insensitivity, or poor impulse control, or social isolation, or all of the above. Those who can be squeezed into the autism spectrum have, potentially, services available if they, and the service, can be persuaded to accept the referral. A significant minority have low levels of intellectual function but few qualify for intellectual disability services. Clinical psychologists may assist with social skills training, and social workers can sometimes slot these patients into groups tolerant of, and often made up of similarly, vulnerable people. A degree of community support combined with occasional sessions to reinforce the message of avoiding stalking behaviours can sometimes work and at least shows the service tried.

Threats and Violence

One of our patients, who had suffered long-term stalking at the hands of an ex-partner, described how when he finally struck her, after recovering from the initial shock, she experienced a sense of relief at the thought that now the police might act to protect her from this man who was destroying her life. I tell this story to emphasise that in most cases much of the victim's suffering results not from uttered threats or actual violence but from the stress inflicted by the stalking itself. Threats and potential violence are complicating factors which need to be managed as part of the stalking but should rarely be the prime focus.

All the stalking types described can on occasion make threats and launch attacks. The Rejected are the type most likely to behave in this way and the Intimacy Seekers the least, but it is a potential complication which needs to be considered in all stalkers. The violence of stalking occurs in the community. Our role is to assess threats and the risk of violence and do what we can to manage the stalker in a manner which reduces the chances of an assault.

Working with the police opens up the possibility of more direct interventions. The assessment and management of threats is considered later in this chapter.

We know something about what increases the risk of violence in a stalker – first and foremost, threats which reflect some commitment to action. The Rejected resort to violence more often than other types. The usual risk factors for violence apply to some extent but many of the stalkers who launch attacks are sober, previously law-abiding citizens, with rigid rather than impulsive traits, who are not usually assertive, let alone aggressive. A pattern of escalating intrusiveness particularly combined with threats is concerning.

It is essential to make clear to the stalker the dire consequences for them of the resort to violence. Prudence only inhibits violence in those able to both calculate their own advantage and envision a future worth protecting. Prudential wisdom is curtailed in the despairing, the depressed, those of limited intellect, those totally dedicated to their own desires and the suicidal. As clinicians, we should recognise and manage depression and the suicidal and at least attempt to alleviate despair. There are situations when the stalker patient is directly or indirectly threatening violence with few protective factors obvious. In those already subject to court orders, the responsible probation/community corrections officer should be informed, though in the absence of direct police mental health stalking prevention units, this is often of limited value. The question of informing the potential victim, and ideally their support professionals if they exist, needs careful consideration.

When You Are the Target of Stalking

Health professionals have a greater than usual chance of being stalked. In most instances it is an Intimacy Seeker or Resentful Stalker. Interestingly, those referred for stalking rarely stalk those treating them; after all, they have already found their target. Professionals are stalked because of the patients they see, not because of some failing in them. The research is clear: experienced professionals are just as likely to be stalked by patients as more junior staff. When a colleague is stalked, we owe them full support, not veiled criticism or retrospective 'wisdom'.

An awareness of possible early signs is useful. The potential Intimacy Seekers may give warning signs. A gift, of flowers, sweets, a book or the like, can be an appropriate expression of gratitude. Repeated gifts or strange offerings should raise concerns. Similarly, a thank you card is one thing; multiple notes and billet doux another. Requesting more appointments, waiting around to speak to you after the clinic or 'chance' encounters in shops or the street may all occur quite innocently on occasion but not repeatedly. If there are warning signs, it is important to make clear you are finding the repeated contacts disturbing and they must stop. Even at this stage, serious consideration should be given to transferring the patient to another clinician or discharging them. The Resentful Stalker rarely gives any advanced warning.

In practice, the first clear indication that you have become the target of an Intimacy Seeker is usually a declaration of love. It is important to immediately make clear you have no interest in a relationship with them – that your only interest is in providing medical treatment and you have no wish to have contact with them outside of the hospital and clinic. Practising in relatively small towns and cities can mean that you have had prior contact with the patient in the community and your social circles may even overlap. In that circumstance you should make clear you wish to avoid any further contact. Brutal frankness is the order of the day which leaves no doubt about your feelings (not that that will always stop the patient reinterpreting your words). Certain all-too-common responses should be avoided at all costs, such as 'I do not have personal relationships with patients' or 'I have a partner'. The first invites the patient to discharge themselves and turn up as 'not your patient anymore' and the second places your partner in the role of potential target.

Having made clear your total lack of any interest in a relationship, it is best to end the interview, saying someone will be in contact with them about their future treatment (irrespective of whether they are an in- or out-patient). After making a full note in the records, a discussion of the events with colleagues is essential. In most instances you should have no future role in managing the patient, though occasionally in those with schizophrenic or manic illnesses there may be a case for continuing on the grounds that recovery from the acute symptoms will resolve the problem.

The best early management does not always prevent the progress of the stalking. When you are being stalked, those with whom you live and work should be told to prevent them either unknowingly aiding the stalker or from ignorance failing to provide protection. The primary aim is to avoid all direct communication, contacts or conflicts with the stalker. Keep a copy or record of all communications (letters, emails, phone calls). Make notes of all attempted contact. Where possible, decline to accept deliveries from the stalker. Intrusive contacts, threats or assaults should precipitate contacting the police if you have not already done so. The copies and records of attempted contacts and communications are important in providing grounds on which the police can act. In most urban areas the police nowadays are reasonably well informed and responsive in cases of stalking.

The Resentful Stalker usually declares themselves by making a malicious complaint. Again, make sure your colleagues are informed and follow the same procedures for unwanted communications and contacts. Contact your protection society or union at the earliest opportunity. It is little use contacting complaints organisations in advance as they will just proceed with their processes regardless.

Forensic professionals should take preventative measures to protect themselves from future harassment. Your phone should be extra-directory. Your home address should not be on the voters' register or any public database. Good home security is worth considering.

Threats to Harm and Kill

Threats to kill need to be taken seriously. But how seriously, given such threats are part of the common currency of everyday speech for a significant number of our fellow citizens? Mental health professionals are reasonably comfortable dealing with a patient's threat to kill themselves but far less comfortable when the threat is to kill other people. We lack the research basis which informs our management of threats of suicide. There are studies of clinical samples of threateners and of those convicted of threats to kill which show a positive association with subsequent violence, including homicide [13, 14], but how representative they are of those we see in forensic practice is uncertain. What we can say is the studies that exist should make us just as cautious about our patient's threats to kill others as we are of their threats to kill themselves.

Threats to kill can be conveyed verbally or in writing. They can be direct or implied. They can be made to the presumed target or to others. Whatever way they are uttered, they express an intention to harm. At its simplest, any action requires an intention and sufficient commitment to carry out that intention – to which can be added the opportunity, ability and method to realise the commitment. The clinical question is usually what was the function of the threat, and what is the degree of commitment to act on the expressed threat. Certain threats create special problems: threats to kill prominent people [4–7], threats to commit a massacre and above all threats related to terrorism. These 'special threats' are considered later but what follows, however, is not entirely irrelevant. It is all too easy to be distracted by the content of the threat and miss the characteristics, mental state and motivations of the person making the threat. There is also an overlap or progression from persistent complainers to threateners [8].

If you will forgive another typology, the following separation of threats to kill is based on their function for the threatener and the level of associated commitment to act on the threat [15].

(1) *Screamers* whose threats are little more than expletives uttered in moments of excitement. They lack any commitment to action being an end in themselves which gives voice (they are almost always verbal) to irritation, frustration, disappointment or a brief moment of anger. The context is important because it can occasionally create concern as in the domestic situation where oft-repeated screams can take on a more sinister aspect.

I was asked to see one of my long-term patients who was facing court, having been arrested the previous day for making threats to kill. He was a huge man who had served a five-year sentence for manslaughter following a drunken bar fight. Anybody would have been intimidated faced with his anger, particularly if they knew of his history, which the target had known. The threat had been made in the context of the next-door neighbour, not for the first time, knocking over his rubbish bin and leaving the mess spread over my patient's driveway. In the years since his release from prison my patient had remained abstinent from drugs and alcohol, had maintained regular employment and had established a long-term relationship. The court accepted that the threat expressed anger and frustration, not an intent to harm. My patient received counselling about the effect he had on others which precluded him indulging in expressing his feelings through outbursts likely to frighten people.

(2) *Shockers* threaten either to cause distress to a target or to create a drama which brings attention to themselves or a current grievance. Both variants are an end in themselves, rarely having any associated commitment to act. There is always an element of calculation in making this type of threat. Unlike screamers, this is not a cathartic discharging of their own current emotions but an attempt to evoke fear in the target. They can be uttered in any modality.

Those who threaten to distress their target are more likely to be encountered not in the clinic but personally or by report, in our everyday. Threats to accuse someone of a non-existent offence, often of a sexual nature, are more common than death threats and far more effective at producing fear. There are exceptions.

One disturbed and substance-abusing man I assessed developed a habit of threatening to commit a terrorist outrage when he wanted to cause fear or distress. The police and members of his family were frequent targets. These threats occurred so often and were so implausible that they were ignored or treated with contempt for a long time. This provoked him to try and make his threats more plausible and frightening. Unfortunately, in the present climate it is all too easy to have terrorist threats taken seriously, particularly when you are a Muslim. He talked himself into prison but could not talk himself out.

One young woman had from her early teens repeatedly phoned the police saying she was about to kill herself by jumping off a high building. This ploy began to lose its effectiveness. A tragedy happened involving a psychotic man setting a fire in a homeless shelter in which a man died and several were seriously injured. This provided her with a new script. She now phoned saying she had set a fire in a shelter or hotel to kill the people inside. This was so successful she ended up in court facing a potential prison sentence. She had a horrendous history of abuse and neglect as a child. Although of normal intelligence, she was illiterate and had never had gainful employment. Since absconding from a children's home, she had lived on the streets with occasional brief psychiatric admissions. She had no friends and no contact with family. She claimed her only friends were the police. Various attempts by mental health and social services to engage with her had failed. Making threats were her only way to affect the world and bring her the attention she craved. She had been remanded in custody for the report to be prepared. She had been unable to cope on the remand wing and finished up in the psychiatric unit which she found even more distressing. When seen, one thing she was clear about was that she never wanted to come back to prison. With this in her mind, when she was placed on a community order, she cooperated with the clinical psychologist and social services. Many problems remained, but with occasional reminders of consequences, the threats ceased.

(3) *Shielders* make threats in an attempt at self-protection. In the animal kingdom, threat displays are mostly to ward off attack or avoid conflict. Those of us who grow up in rough neighbourhoods out of self-protection often fostered a threatening aspect and demeaner with the threat to kill as the last strategy before turning tail and running.

A man referred for a court report had been caught on video brandishing a machete at a train station. He was a reclusive individual in his forties who lived on a modest inheritance. His passions were music and his large garden. His only social activity was joining a group of fellow music lovers, every week or so, to go to concerts in the city. Some months previously on the late-night train home he had witnessed a gang of youths seriously assault another passenger in the same carriage. He had subsequently given a statement to the police. He was too fearful to join the group on their next few outings but was persuaded by phone calls from fellow members to recommence attending. On the next return journey, he thought he glimpsed one of the attackers in the next carriage. He was left in a state of terror until he reached home. He decided that rather than stop the outings he would place in his briefcase a Gurkha knife which had hung for years on a wall at home. With this reassurance he continued his outings as, he said, he thought this would scare them off should they come for him. The talisman worked for some weeks until one night as he left the train he thought he saw the gang from the attack gathered at the other end of the platform. When they seemed to be moving towards him, he pulled out the blade and began brandishing it while threatening to kill. Management included insisting he took a taxi home from the city which, though expensive, he could well afford, and that he forgo threatening people with weapons of any sort.

The commitment of the shielder is to avoiding the harm threatened by the other. These are threats uttered from fear. If they fail to deter, and escape is not an option, that very fear may, on rare occasion, lead to responding with greater violence than the original aggressor. Assessing those who have killed in fights in bars or the street, not infrequently the victim was the one with the greater reputation and history of violence, and the killer just the more fearful.

(4) *Schemers* utter threats to influence others to act in the manner the threatener desires. Their threats take the general form of 'I will do x if you don't do y.' Their commitment is to gaining advantage from the threat rather than directly injuring the target. If their manipulations fail, they may progress to more sinister strategies.

(5) *Warnings* are threats to which some degree of commitment attaches to the utterance. Warnings are promises. Some promises are kept, some are not. With threats to kill, a tiny fraction will be followed by homicide; some will be followed by a non-lethal attack, though most will not be acted upon. The first problem is separating a warning from other types of threat. Humans, like most animals, are quite good at recognising which threats need to be taken seriously; after all, over past generations our survival has been at stake. The combination of context and not finding the threat frightening usually helps exclude most threats. Sensitivity to a threat, however, depends in no small part on the target's prior experience of the threatener and their prior experiences of victimisation. Those threatened by an ex-partner often underestimate the risk, whereas threats from strangers, for understandable reasons, tend to be overestimated.

Assessing and Managing the Threatener

When we are faced with assessing someone who has made a threat to kill, a process of selection has usually occurred which excludes most of those who present a low risk of launching an attack. Typically, the target of the threat (or those monitoring the threatener's communications) has been sufficiently alarmed to report the threat to the police or other authorities (including health services), who in turn take the threat seriously enough to set in motion further enquiries by the courts, security services, hospital managers and so on, who then have been sufficiently concerned to make the referral. As noted earlier, this does not exclude all those at little risk of acting on the threat but does ensure all need careful assessment.

The research base is scanty but suggests, unsurprisingly, that the chances of an attack following a threat to kill are higher in those with a history of prior violence, who are substance abusers, are the target's ex-partner or have previously received a diagnosis of schizophrenia. Some general idea of the level of probable commitment can be gathered from the following variables.

The level of preoccupation with the victim and with doing them harm should be established. Those caught up in insistent and persistent fantasies of inflicting violence are obviously at greater risk of acting on their threats given the opportunity and means. Those for whom it is an occasional passing thought raise far less concern.

The plausibility of their acting on the threat needs to be considered. I was once asked for an emergency assessment on an in-patient making threats to kill his ex-partner's new lover. He was described as a one-time member of the army special forces with a history of violence in civilian life. In the event, he was a severely depressed man confined to a wheelchair. He had lost both legs and one arm when, a couple of months earlier, he had attempted suicide by throwing himself in front of a train. I was impressed by the patient's force of personality which was able to produce such anxiety in the team caring for him.

Evidence of planning, particularly in association with preparations, is a red light. I was once asked to assess a university student who had written an essay in which he described his desire to commit a campus massacre. In interview he revealed having legally acquired both a rifle and a handgun to put his well-developed plan into action. The essay was a last-ditch attempt to have someone stop him. As he said, at least it showed his tutor sometimes read his essays, and sometimes took him seriously. A potential killer giving the play of chance a last opportunity to stop them has occurred in a number of my cases. The police removed the guns and his licence. The patient was seen long term in the clinic.

Loss–gain calculations should be explored. Although occasionally we are asked to assess those who uttered a verbal threat in the heat of the moment, for the most part we see threateners who have published or spoken in a more considered manner. If the impulsive threat is followed by violence, it usually happens at the time. In assessing the more cold-blooded threat, it helps to explore the patient's view of what they will lose if they act on the threat as compared with what they may gain. Of particular concern are those who believe they have nothing to lose, such as the depressed and those overwhelmed by a life crisis. Equally concerning are those who believe that to act on the threat would be justified and would bring meaning to either their lives or their deaths. Threats to kill which have been repeated again and again still need to be taken seriously and assessed on their merits at the time, just as with recurrent threats of suicide.

The final consideration in those you judge to be issuing a warning is: why make a threat? We face the same question with threats of suicide. One answer is that the threatener hopes to evoke some intervention to stop, or make unnecessary, the violence. A far less comforting answer is that the threat is a kind of rehearsal which makes real for them the possibility that they will act on the threat. The most troubling answer is that the uttering of the threat can be for the threatener a way of binding themselves to commit the act. The problem we all face in assessing a threat is obtaining sufficient information from the patient or from available sources. The error is not to access and consider what is available.

One patient had killed a lawyer. He had been treated over several years for a delusional disorder centring on a conspiracy by a large section of the legal profession. Over the years he had occasionally threatened to kill lawyers – any lawyers. In the weeks prior to the killing, he had once more been talking about killing a lawyer. He was being managed in the community with weekly sessions with a counsellor, regular visits from a community nurse and six-weekly visits to a psychiatrist. The final psychiatric assessment a week prior to the killing noted he was his usual bland self, full of reassurances about how well he was progressing. Tucked away in the records were the recent counsellor's notes which gave details of intrusive fantasies of acting and of tentative plans about how and when. The nurse's notes filed separately expressed concerns about his recently cutting off all social contacts and seeming more agitated and preoccupied than usual about his delusions. The pressure on public mental health services is such that reading all the recent notes, let alone communicating with all involved professionals prior to a routine assessment, has become a counsel of perfection. Perhaps one day bean counters will realise that the cost of coronial inquests, trials, imprisonment and compensation payments, let alone government enquiries, could buy a lot of good-quality mental healthcare.

A threat to kill to which a degree of commitment to act attaches does not occur in a vacuum. Whatever the stated provocation which motivates the threat, behind this is a person with an often troubled personal history who has current social and psychological problems. In many, their psychiatric state is playing a part. Most such threateners who reach our clinic are despairing if not clinically depressed; they are often socially isolated and in some form of crisis; alcohol and drug abuse are common, some are psychotic; all could benefit from mental health support and treatment.

A threat to kill oneself judged to be a warning which might be enacted would almost always result in the provision of mental healthcare, often as an in-patient or sometimes in the community. The patient's refusal of such care would trigger consideration of compulsory treatment. In these circumstances a bias towards involuntary treatment would be usual. There is no reason why when assessing someone who has made a threat to kill, acting on which is considered a real possibility, a similar process should not be followed. There is an implicit assumption that suicide is the result of mental disorders, many of which would have been treatable. The same assumption is not made about homicide, though mental disorders are common in such offenders and those who kill after making threats have high rates of depression and psychotic disorders. These people are our core business. Just as with the risk of suicide, management is about attempting to improve their psychiatric, psychological and social functioning while in many cases addressing their substance abuse problems.

When a Credible Threat Is Communicated to You

When a credible threat is communicated to a health professional, there is in some US states a legal obligation to warn the potential victim and/or the police. No such laws exist in most jurisdictions in the English-speaking world. No common law obligation to rescue exists. This places the professional responsibility on how to respond on the clinician. In forensic practice we often see those referred because of threats. In this situation the courts, police or other referring agency are aware of the threat. The problems begin when a patient being seen for other reasons communicates a credible threat to kill someone.

It is important to tell the patient you take the threat seriously. An attempt should be made to explore with the patient:

- The reasons for the intention to kill and why it has surfaced now.
- How they plan to carry out the killing.
- Have they made any preparations?
- Whether they have guns and/or a current gun licence.
- Fantasies about the killing – for how long and how often have they been entertained.
- The likely effect on their life should they act on the threat, including any thoughts of proceeding to suicide.

Their current mental state, particularly depressive and psychotic symptoms, needs to be explored for any possible justification for immediate compulsory admission. An offer of voluntary admission can be made. If accepted, it needs to be organised immediately. I know of cases where the patient was allowed home to collect a few things and used the chance to kill the target of their threat. In one, the social worker was waiting by the front door while the patient killed his partner in the kitchen.

The patient should be told you intend to do everything you can to stop them ruining their lives in this way. Now is the time to manipulate any positive feelings (transference) which may exist. If you are not inclined to immediate admission, the patient should be told you will be discussing the situation with colleagues to decide how best to help them. Should the patient ask if you are going to inform the potential victim, I would be inclined to say yes on the grounds that the question was an invitation to step in to prevent the tragedy. In case you are wrong, the victim and/or the police need to be informed before the patient has a chance to act. The patient should ideally be kept in the clinic long enough to warn the victim.

In the early days of attempting to run a threatener's clinic, the police's cooperation was reluctant at best. This changed when an experienced clinical psychologist reported to the police that a patient on a court order was making what she considered a credible threat to kill. She let the police know the likely victim and that the man might have a gun. The police had not acted on this information when 12 hours later there was a siege at a petrol station involving the man holding the named victim hostage. The police, to their credit, brought the psychologist to the scene where she brokered a peaceful resolution. We subsequently received full police cooperation, possibly in part because no mention was ever made of the earlier request for intervention.

When You Are Threatened by a Patient

When you are threatened, always respond by saying you take the threat seriously and are frightened, irrespective of your actual thoughts or feelings. To do otherwise amounts to a challenge to prove they are serious. The worst response is to ignore the threat or say something silly like 'You didn't mean that.' If a patient takes the trouble to threaten you, the least you can do is show them some respect as an individual with desires and the agency to act. Once the threat is acknowledged, a decision needs to be made whether to continue or terminate the interview. This decision is a test of clinical acumen, not of personal courage. Should you continue, why the patient felt the need to threaten you requires exploration in detail. Do not be put off by claims of not really meaning it or not wanting to talk about it. Be prepared to acknowledge responsibility and apologise if they identify any inopportune words or actions by you or a colleague. If they raise an unjustified grievance, where possible also apologise on the grounds of failing to communicate adequately. In the acute situation, the aim is to restore as much calm and rapport as possible. Whether the interview continued or was suspended, there will need to be discussions with colleagues about how to proceed. Document the discussions in your notes.

References

1. Mullen PE, Pathe M, Purcell R. *Stalkers and Their Victims*, 2nd ed. Cambridge, Cambridge University Press, 2009.

2. Mullen PE, Pathé M. Stalking and the pathologies of love. *Australian & New Zealand Journal of Psychiatry* 1994; 28 (3): 469–77. doi: 10.3109/00048679409075876.

3. Pathé M, Mullen PE. The impact of stalkers on their victims. *British Journal of Psychiatry* 1997; 170 (1): 12–17. doi: 10.11 92/bjp.170.1.12.

4. James DV, Farnham FR, Allen P et al. Threats to public figures and association with approach, as a proxy for violence: the importance of grievance. *Frontiers in Psychology* 2022; 13: 998155.

5. James DV, Mullen PE, Meloy JR et al. The role of mental disorder in attacks on European politicians 1990–2004. *Acta Psychiatrica Scandinavica* 2007; 116, 334–44. doi: 10.1111/j.1600-0447.2007.01077.x.

6. Dietz PE, Martell DA. Mentally Disordered Offenders in Pursuit of Celebrities and Politicians. Washington, DC, National Institute of Justice, 1989.

7. James DV, Mullen PE, Pathé MT et al. Attacks on the British royal family: the role of psychotic illness. *Journal of the American Academy of Psychiatry and the Law* 2008; 36: 59–67.

8. Mullen PE, Lester G. Vexatious litigants and unusually persistent complainants and petitioners: from querulous paranoia to querulous behaviour. *Behavioral Sciences & the Law* 2006; 24: 333–49. https://doi.org/ 10.1002/bsl.671.

9. MacKenzie RD, James DV. Management and treatment of stalkers: problems, options, and solutions. *Behavioral Sciences & the Law* 2011. doi: 10.1002/bsl.980.

10. Eastwood C, Barton D. *Play Misty for Me.* Motion picture, USA, 1971.

11. McEwan I. *Enduring Love*. London, Cape, 1997.

12. Scheler M. *Ressentiment* (trans. W. W. Holdheim). New York, Free Press, 1961 [1910].

13. Macdonald JM. The threat to kill. *American Journal of Psychiatry* 1963; 120: 125–30.

14. Warren LJ, Mullen PE, Thomas SDM et al. Threats to kill: a follow up study. *Psychological Medicine* 2008; 38: 599–605.

15. Warren LJ, Mullen PE, Ogloff JRP. A clinical study of those who utter threats to kill. *Behavioural Sciences and the Law* 2011; 29: 141–54.

Sexual Offending

Danny H. Sullivan

Introduction

Sexual offending is astonishingly prevalent and is associated with significant mental health and psychosocial consequences for victims. It is also the basis of a range of severe criminal justice sanctions, which in various jurisdictions can include indeterminate sentences as well as post-sentence restrictions. Of all forms of offending, it is sexual offending which is most stigmatised and despised, and this may lead to vigilantism and persecution of offenders or those perceived to be offenders [1].

However, it is an area of forensic psychiatry which may be neglected in training and in which empirical evidence can easily give way to prejudice and supposition. The stigma of sexual offenders may also be projected onto those psychiatrists who deal with them, who in turn may be presupposed to condone or excuse offending.

Forensic psychiatrists assessing and treating sexual offenders must be conscious of their own attitudes, transference and counter-transference; and in some cases they may need to rely on reflective practice and other protective measures to maintain the empathic – yet boundaried and objective – stance which is necessary to work effectively with sexual offenders.

Much of the field of sexual offending involves other disciplines, particularly forensic psychology. However, there are specific roles for forensic psychiatry, including the assessment and management of problematic sexualised behaviours across the lifespan, determination of its association with mental disorder, the provision of expert evidence – including risk assessment – often in ethically complex situations and the management of high-risk sexual offenders, on occasion using medication.

As will be seen, the skills of forensic psychiatrists are of particular use in assessing complex aberrant human behaviour and drawing on multiple frameworks to provide plausible and cogent formulations for cases of sexual offending. These tasks require the capacity to engage effectively with offenders or those at risk of offending, to manage ethical conflicts that may arise, and to translate their opinions effectively for clinical, legal and public audiences.

Normative Human Sexuality

A comprehensive theoretical understanding of human sexuality remains elusive. A range of biological, cognitive, psychodynamic and cultural theories – and blends of these – fail to capture the complexity of human sexual arousal and drives. In addition, the boundary between normative and deviant sexuality is not clearly defined, and varies over time and culture. Nor is individual sexuality static or easily catalogued, or even straightforward to describe and define [2].

Nevertheless, sexual offending is more straightforwardly defined when the expression of sexual desire involves lack of consent, violence and/or vulnerable victims. Specific victims do not need to be apparent, as in offences associated with viewing images of unknown children who have been exploited for sexual purposes. Some offences will be defined by their seeming motivation in preparation for sexual offending, such as interactions with vulnerable people geared to sexual purposes; others are indicative of concerning deviant arousal – perhaps as 'pre-crime'.

In numerous international jurisdictions, various sexual practices and orientations may be criminalised and subject to public censure and sanction, at times justified by the spurious conflation of sexual orientation or practice, with religious sin or antisocial behaviour.

Theories of Sexual Offending

It cannot be claimed that any one theory of sexual offending provides a satisfactory and comprehensive explanatory framework, but elements of several theories underpin treatment programmes. Some common elements of theoretical frameworks can be identified and may provide some understanding of the motivations or factors underlying individual offending.

Common elements in sexual offending involve poor self-regulation, deviant arousal and antisocial attitudes, although different theoretical models may use different nomenclature to describe these factors. Not all elements need be apparent in an individual offender, but one or more will help in better understanding features of the offending and also facilitate treatment planning [3].

Self-regulation relies on the capacity to inhibit sexual desires, and may be impaired through executive dysfunction, cognitive impairment, personality vulnerabilities or acute intoxication. Deviant arousal includes abnormal focus of sexual interest, cognitive distortions about sexual activity and the behaviour of victims, or extreme preoccupation and hypersexuality. Antisocial attitudes reflect the cognitive distortions prevalent in sexual offenders, empathy deficits and a willingness or predisposition to exploit others for one's own gratification.

Theories of sexual offending may also draw on the effects of adverse childhood experience on offenders – including themselves being a victim of sexual abuse – on attachment, emotional insight and self-regulation. Developmental and learnt factors, as well as cultural, familial and social influences, may be associated with disrupted psychosexual development, development of problematic sexual scripts and other factors associated with increased offending risk.

In addition to explanatory theories grounded in individual factors, situational and contextual factors are important to understanding sexual offending. These may reflect dynamic risk factors overlapping with those for other forms of offending, as well as the opportunity for offending. In many cases, the function of the offending is of relevance not only to understanding but also to treatment and to reducing reoffending risk.

Sexual Deviance

There are diagnostic criteria for paraphilias in both the *International Classification of Diseases 11th Revision* (ICD-11) [4] and the *Diagnostic and Statistical Manual of Mental*

Disorders – 5th Edition (DSM-5) [5]. These align poorly with other mental disorders, particularly because many with paraphilic sexual interests are not distressed or impaired by them, until the criminal justice system intervenes. The introduction of the DSM-5 was preceded by years of debate in academic journals over the framing of criteria, reflecting that paraphilias are not like other forms of 'mental disorder' [6]. The end result was that *paraphilias* were separated from *paraphilic disorders*, with the former simply indicating an 'intense and persistent sexual interest other than sexually interest in genital stimulation or preparatory fondling with phenotypically normal, physically mature, consenting human partners' and the latter involving, in addition, 'distress or impairment to the individual . . . [or] personal harm, or risk of harm, to others' [5].

The natural history of deviant sexual interests is poorly understood, based on self-report of selected samples such as those assessed for courts, or catalogued by self-report questionnaires. In particular, the genesis, trajectory and persistence of deviant sexual interest is not clear. It is likely that many experience deviant arousal but do not act on it in ways which transgress the law. Nevertheless, deviant sexual arousal is, in the main, considered a strong and persistent risk factor for sexual offending and reoffending, and when encountered may be striking in its qualitative and quantitative difference from normative human sexuality [7].

Paraphilias are divided into so-called courtship disorders, disorders involving anomalous sexual targets and sadomasochistic categories. Courtship disorders, in which approaches to potential sexual partners are distorted, include voyeurism, exhibitionism and frotteurism. Where there is no contact, these are complex to prosecute and may involve alternative charges of stalking, trespass or acquisitive offences rather than sexual acts. Forensic psychiatrists become adept at exploring seemingly innocuous behaviours or minor public order offences which demonstrate offence-paralleling behaviour.

Anomalous sexual targets may include fetishes, involving sexual arousal significantly directed at specific body parts or sexual activities, to the exclusion of the person, as well as preoccupations with items of clothing or fabrics, including wearing clothing of another gender, or non-human items. This is also taken to include sexual attraction to children, although determining the age limits or characteristics of these categories for legal purposes is complex. As a result, many jurisdictions distinguish criminal charges when victims are younger children, and youths who are sexually mature but legally defined as below the age of consent.

Deviant arousal to the infliction or reception of pain may also be contentious, where the sexual assault of another may be taken for some legal purposes to constitute a paraphilia and considered indicative of a predisposition to rape [6]. The notion of a rape paraphilia differs from sexual sadism but may be grounds for preventative detention, although much adult rape is not clearly preceded by sexual fantasies or preoccupation of the sort defined as paraphilia. Indeed, studies of those convicted of rape demonstrate more in common with violent offenders and criminal histories similar to general offenders rather than sexual offenders [8].

When deviant sexual arousal is present and associated with offending or distress, it often warrants intensive psychological treatment. If associated with marked risk of future offending, treatment may also include anti-libidinal medication.

Sexual Offending and Mental Disorder

There are associations with a range of mental disorders which may be of relevance in the assessment and treatment of sexual offending. Psychodynamic explanations initially dominated the field, but in more recent years commentators have remarked on the features of sexual offenders which are similar to impulse control disorders and obsessive-compulsive disorders, and sought evidence of biological markers or correlates with offending.

Cognitive impairment is relevant to sexual offending, whether through disinhibition, reduced controls over underlying deviant arousal or direct effects on sexual appetite. Specific conditions including Klüver-Bucy syndrome and Huntington's disease may be associated with sexual offending through limbic system impairments. Dementia, in particular behavioural variant frontotemporal dementia, may be associated with sexually disinhibited behaviour and assaults and is particularly problematic when a person with dementia is placed in a setting with others vulnerable to assault [9].

People with intellectual disability may have an increased rate of sexual offending, but for a range of reasons. These may relate to limited sexual knowledge or opportunity, or identification with children, as well as social skills deficits and impairments in social cognition and emotional regulation associated with disability. Some with autism spectrum disorder may demonstrate unusual sexual preferences which meet criteria for a paraphilia diagnosis but reflect rigid and stereotyped interests, as well as impaired capacity for empathy [10].

There is a limited association with psychotic illness, most apparent when delusions have a strong sexual content and motivate action; however, sexual offending in psychotic illness tends to be more disorganised rather than being driven by sexualised delusions. Despite elevated sexual drive being evident in manic illness, this is infrequently associated with sexual offending and tends to be more impulsive.

The most prominent associations with sexual offending are with personality disorder or personality difficulty. Traits of dissociality and borderline pattern are particularly prominent. However, negative affectivity and anankastia may also be apparent, particularly in courtship disorders, as well as problematic pornography use; and disinhibition and detachment may also be present and relevant in the formulation of offending behaviour. Furthermore, negative emotional states are often associated with sexual offending as a contextual factor, a setting factor for opportunistic offending.

Special Groups

Children and Adolescents

The boundary between sexual experimentation and sexually abusive behaviour may be hard to determine in children. Coercion and behaviour directed at much younger children may be associated with the protagonist having themselves been victimised, concerning exposure to pornography, as well as developmental disabilities. A small number may also reflect developing paraphilia or ongoing risk of reoffending. Treatment programmes directed at children and adolescents differ from those for adults, and may incorporate a greater strengths-based focus. Optimism about the benefits of intervention is necessary, but a small number of adolescent or childhood offenders may require ongoing intervention due to ongoing offending risk [11].

Adolescent sexual offenders are likely to have different risk factors to adults, including being themselves subject to childhood sexual abuse, and early and significant exposure to pornography. It is commonly held that sexual deviance is less likely to be evident, although efforts to assault stranger adult females may raise concerns about aggressive sexual fantasies.

Furthermore, interventions for children and adolescents may be effective in developing appropriate templates for sexuality before these become more entrenched, and also in addressing psychosocial adversity which may underpin sexually abusive behaviours by minors.

Female Offenders

The prevalence of sexual offending among women is likely underestimated. There is limited research and a dearth of validated assessment tools or treatment interventions for female offenders, the number of which is much lower than for men. Although some will meet paraphilia diagnoses and have sadistic features, most have vulnerabilities related to their own childhood sexual abuse or personality structure [12].

Elderly Offenders

Some elderly offenders are simply those who have offended in the past or long held deviant arousal, and in older life have renewed opportunity through contact with grandchildren or other roles. It is noted that the sexual offenders are over-represented among elderly prisoners [31], reflecting less on persistence of offending and more on increasingly lengthy sentences and willingness to prosecute historical sexual offences.

Particular challenges are posed by elderly men with cognitive impairment in residential settings who engage in sexually aggressive behaviours towards other residents. Treatment options may be limited by capacity to consent, physical health comorbidities and capacity to participate in or retain information from treatment. Such behaviours are likely to result in marked difficulty in finding residential placements.

Learning Disability

Risk factors for offending in populations with learning disability (LD) are likely to differ from sexual offenders without LD. In particular, a lack of opportunity for healthy sexual expression and deficits in sexual knowledge or social cognition may be associated with offending. The assessment and treatment of behaviours of concern in LD is a specialised field and includes some specific risk assessment tools, as well as treatment programmes modified for cognitive impairment. In those who are poorly motivated or seem not to benefit from treatment interventions, the use of anti-libidinal medications may be of use but is associated with significant concerns about capacity to consent and the vulnerability of LD populations. However, this is a population who without effective intervention are often subject to protracted and excessive restriction of liberty.

Child Exploitation Material and Viewing Child Pornography

The internet has facilitated the viewing of pornographic material featuring children, and also assisted adults to make contact with minors for sexual purposes. A significant minority of those who view pornography featuring minors will also engage in contact offending [13]. Many who have deviant sexual arousal to minors will view pornography but make no effort to engage in contact offending. However, the use of pornography can escalate, bring offenders into contact with others who normalise the sexual abuse of children or promote the trading or creation of images [14]. The discourse around viewing child pornography has increasingly focussed on participation in an international market which harms children, particularly those from developing countries.

Assessment

Medical and psychiatric training does not necessarily encompass how to approach an in-depth psychosexual history. Sexual offenders are likely to be sensitive to critical or embar-rassed approaches; an objective, dispassionate approach in the interviewer will yield the most information. Eliciting an account of behaviours and cognitions before testing incon-sistencies through Socratic questioning may provide insights into cognitive distortions, contextual factors and mental state abnormalities associated with offending behaviours. Unless specific questions are asked of those being evaluated, spontaneous disclosure of more unusual deviant ideation is unlikely. A range of other techniques may be used according to the individual case [15].

Self-report questionnaires tend to be of little utility except as a structured checklist of associations with deviant arousal and behaviour. Under-reporting of deviance is the norm in forensic settings. Physiological assessments including penile plethysmography have been used but remain accessible only in specialised settings and are of limited validity in correlation with behaviour. Advocates of polygraphy attest to benefit in monitoring com-pliance with court orders for those conditionally released into the community, but admissi-bility and fairness remain problematic, as does the reliability of responses and the rate of false-positive and -negative responses. Other assessment techniques which rely on salience have some validity but may be limited in availability outside specialised services [15].

There is limited utility of biological or neuropsychological investigations in assessing sexual offenders. Neuroimaging and electrophysiological measures may show abnormalities but these are not diagnostic or correlated with disorders or behaviour. Testosterone levels may be elevated in sexual offenders compared to non-sexual offenders, and in cohorts, higher levels may correlate with increased violence in offending compared to those in lower ranks, but levels do not correlate with offending. The exception is with serial monitoring of testosterone levels in those treated with anti-libidinal medications, which demonstrates compliance and correlates with suppression of sexual drive and reduced offending risk [16].

Risk assessment in sexual offending involves actuarial scales, structured professional judgement tools and a plethora of specialised instruments for specific types of offending. These have validity for triaging offenders to various levels of intensity of treatment inter-vention, but in this highly polarised and publicly scrutinised arena may be subject to lay commentary. In preventative detention or indeterminate sentencing situations, forensic psychiatrists can expect sophisticated and challenging cross-examination focussed not only on the threshold decision but also on the reliability and validity of tools, their sensitivity and specificity, and the ethics of the legislation underpinning such decisions. There is no doubt that this is a fraught area and one in which experts should tread warily.

Treatment

In recent years, increasingly punitive attitudes to sexual offending have become prominent. This is reflected in lengthy sentences, indeterminate sentences or post-sentence orders, sex offender registers and associated constraints, civil commitment, and electronic monitoring. The consequences of sex offender status may also include exile from communities, media furore and extra-judicial vigilantism. In many jurisdictions, there are limited opportunities for those with proclivities to sexual offending to receive treatment without mandatory notification or marked stigma. Consequently, treatment of sexual offending is almost always under legal mandate. Treatment may be 'voluntary' but with legal consequences for non-compliance or refusal to participate [17]. This is relevant to engagement and motivation.

Motivation for treatment may be initially external, but one major goal is to engender internal motivation so that after treatment is completed, those who have sexually offended will continue to use strategies to avoid further offending. Consequently, the initial phase of intervention is often geared to treatment readiness.

The treatment of sexual offending involves, variously, combinations of social and environmental restrictions, psychological intervention through group and individual modalities, and in cases marked by recidivism and significant risk, the use of specific medications. Risk factors for reoffending from large meta-analytic cohorts provide guidance for treatment targets [18]. Offence-paralleling behaviours [19] may also be targets, and a strengths-based theoretical focus may also underpin programmes [20].

The evidence for effectiveness of treatment remains somewhat equivocal. There is some evidence that offenders assessed at low risk of reoffending may have worse outcomes if they undergo psychological treatment, but a small but significant reduction in reoffending from those assessed at moderate to high risk of reoffending [21, 22].

However, following a 2017 review of the effectiveness of English specialist sex offender treatment programmes by the National Offender Management Service [23], treatment programmes were suspended before eventual reinstatement. Currently the evidence for therapeutic programme effectiveness is guardedly optimistic: it appears that factors supporting effectiveness relate to programme fidelity to core evidence-based treatment targets, and the skills of clinicians. It is also likely that the heterogeneity of offender groups impacts upon effectiveness, and tailoring programmes and selecting offenders may enhance the effectiveness of intervention [24, 25].

'Psychologically Informed' Treatments

Behavioural interventions remain salient for offenders with strong deviant arousal. These generally include techniques which seek to pair deviant sexual arousal with aversive responses, including: masturbatory reconditioning; imaginal desensitisation; the use of smelling salts, pain or flash cards with unpleasant content; and covert sensitisation [26]. These all require motivation for an offender to use the techniques prior to or during situations of increased risk due to arousal.

A relapse prevention approach may also frame intervention, translated from substance use treatment. This relies on identifying and anticipating high-risk situations or risk factors for offending, and may include cognitive behavioural interventions, stress management and relaxation, as well as significant lifestyle modification.

Psychologically informed treatment programmes are generally correctional, although some may take place through non-government organisations, privately or in forensic mental health settings. These are structured, group-based programmes, sometimes delivered individually when necessary due to specific service, offender or offence characteristics. The targets are criminogenic needs and may include modules geared at, for instance, fantasy control, cognitive distortions or schemas, and emotional regulation [27].

Other interventions include Circles of Support and Accountability, in which volunteers and professionals support offenders to reintegrate into society while holding the offender accountable for their behaviour and continued focus on not reoffending [28]. Individually tailored treatment will also take into account other treatment needs, particularly mental disorder, substance use and personality vulnerabilities.

Specific challenges exist when an offender maintains that they did not commit an offence. Denial or clinically significant minimisation was, in the past, grounds for denying treatment and parole but increasingly is seen as a specific challenge for treatment programmes. This has resulted in programmes developing methods of engaging in treatment those who persistently deny their offending [29]. Other cognitive distortions include blaming the victim (externalising), denying personal responsibility (internalising denials) and rationalisation (denying the wrongness of behaviour such as paedophilia) [30].

Medication

The use of medication has followed surgical castration, which was a drastic but likely effective and symbolic treatment in the mid-twentieth century. Some jurisdictions still pursue surgical castration, likely in part due to its punitive connotations. However, in recent years there has been increasing evidence for medications, particularly for those with high-risk behaviours or entrenched offending underpinned by deviant sexual arousal. This has been set out in a well-regarded consensus statement [16].

The use of medication requires informed consent in those with capacity, or in some jurisdictions may be authorised by a legal decision-maker informed by medical evidence, especially when decision-making capacity is impaired. This is a contentious area because of the vulnerability of offenders, particularly those with cognitive impairment or disability.

Initially these included oestrogens and typical anti-psychotics, despite limited evidence of effectiveness and significant adverse effects. In more recent years there has been a developing evidence base for selective serotonin reuptake inhibitor (SSRI) medications, which have been hypothesised to reduce reoffending through reduction of impulsive or compulsive behaviour, or through improvement in negative emotional states which may be associated with or predispose to sexual or violent offending. These are obviously palatable due to their relatively limited adverse effect profile and ubiquity [16].

Medroxyprogesterone acetate was used for some time, once more because it was ubiquitous but also because its long-acting injectable nature was relevant to compliance. However, significant adverse effects – metabolic, thrombotic and an association with meningioma – have reduced the use of medroxyprogesterone acetate [16].

Cyproterone acetate is a testosterone agonist which markedly reduces testosterone levels and has a clear evidence base as a first-line agent for reduction of deviant sexual arousal. In some jurisdictions it is available in injected formulation [16]. Unfortunately, tolerance often develops.

Increasingly, and particularly for higher-risk patients, gonadotrophin hormone-releasing hormone (GnRH) analogues or agonists have become the predominant agents used. The side-effect profile is predominantly associated with its effect on sex hormones; as an injected medication, compliance is assured. Initial testosterone flare can be managed through concurrent prescription of cyproterone and environmental management. Suppression of testosterone to castration levels is in most cases reversible, and reduction of offending is supported by good-quality empirical evidence [16].

Conclusions

The management of sexual offending is a specialised component of forensic mental health which specifically involves psychiatrists. The development and maintenance of expertise and adherence to expert guidelines requires collaboration and networking, as well as effective working with other disciplines. However, good practice in the management of sexual offending benefits the community through reduction of risk and offenders through the provision of high-quality care, which might afford the opportunity to return to the community with offending risk managed effectively.

References

1. Thomas T. *Sex Crime: Sex Offending and Society*. London, Routledge, 2015.

2. Bancroft J. *Human Sexuality and Its Problems*. New York, Elsevier Health Sciences, 2008.

3. Ward T, Polaschek D, Beech AR. *Theories of Sexual Offending*. New York, John Wiley & Sons, 2006.

4. https://icd.who.int/browse11/l-m/en#/http%3a%2f%2fid.who.int%2ficd%2fentity%2f334423054.

5. American Psychiatric Association. *Diagnostic and Statistical Manual of Mental Disorders: DSM-5*. Washington, DC, American Psychiatric Association, 2013.

6. Beech AR, Miner MH, Thornton D. Paraphilias in the DSM-5. *Annual Review of Clinical Psychology* 2016; 12: 383–406.

7. Laws DR, O'Donohue WT (eds) *Sexual Deviance: Theory, Assessment, and Treatment*. New York, Guilford Press, 2008.

8. Prentky RA, Burgess AW. *Forensic Management of Sexual Offenders*. New York, Springer Science & Business Media, 2000.

9. Saleh FM, Grudzinskas Jr AJ, Bradford JM, Brodsky DJ. Sex *Offender: Identification, Risk Assessment, Treatment and Legal Issues*. Oxford, Oxford University Press, 2009.

10. Craig LA, Lindsay WR, Browne KD (eds) *Assessment and Treatment of Sexual Offenders with Intellectual Disabilities: A Handbook*. New York, John Wiley & Sons, 2010.

11. Barbaree HE, Marshall WL (eds) *The Juvenile Sex Offender*. New York, Guilford Press, 2008.

12. Gannon TA, Cortoni F (eds) *Female Sexual Offenders: Theory, Assessment and Treatment*. New York, John Wiley & Sons, 2010.

13. Seto MC, Eke AW. Correlates of admitted sexual interest in children among individuals convicted of child pornography offenses. *Law and Human Behavior* 2017; 41 (3): 305.

14. Quayle E, Taylor M. *Child Pornography: An Internet Crime*. London, Routledge, 2004.

15. Russell K, Darjee R. Practical assessment and management of risk in sexual offenders. *Advances in Psychiatric Treatment* 2013; 19 (1): 56–66.

16. Thibaut F, Cosyns P, Fedoroff JP, et al. The World Federation of Societies of Biological Psychiatry Task Force on Paraphilias: 2020 guidelines for the pharmacological treatment of paraphilic disorders. *The World Journal of Biological Psychiatry* 2020; 21 (6): 412–90.

17. McSherry B, Keyzer P. *Sex Offenders and Preventive Detention: Politics, Policy and Practice*. Alexandria, NSW, Federation Press, 2009.

18. Hanson RK, Morton-Bourgon KE. The characteristics of persistent sexual offenders: a meta-analysis of recidivism studies. *Journal of Consulting and Clinical Psychology* 2005; 73 (6): 1154.

19. Daffern M, Jones L, Shine J (eds) *Offence Paralleling Behaviour: A Case Formulation Approach to Offender Assessment and*

Intervention. New York, John Wiley & Sons, 2010.

20. Andrews DA, Bonta J, Wormith JS. The risk-need-responsivity (RNR) model: does adding the good lives model contribute to effective crime prevention? *Criminal Justice and Behavior* 2011; 38 (7): 735–55.

21. Hanson RK, Thornton D. *Static 99: Improving Actuarial Risk Assessments for Sex Offenders*. Ottawa, ON, Solicitor General Canada, 1999.

22. Schmucker M, Lösel F. The effects of sexual offender treatment on recidivism: an international meta-analysis of sound quality evaluations. *Journal of Experimental Criminology* 2015; 11 (4): 597–630.

23. Mews A, Di Bella L, Purver M. *Impact Evaluation of the Prison-Based Core Sex Offender Treatment Programme*. London, Ministry of Justice, 2017.

24. Gannon TA, Olver ME, Mallion JS, James M. Does specialized psychological treatment for offending reduce recidivism? A meta-analysis examining staff and program variables as predictors of treatment effectiveness. *Clinical Psychology Review* 2019; 73: 101752.

25. Tyler N, Gannon TA, Olver ME. Does treatment for sexual offending work?

Current Psychiatry Reports 2021; 23 (8): 1–8.

26. Saleh FM, Grudzinskas Jr AJ, Bradford JM, Brodsky DJ. *Sex Offenders Identification, Risk Assessment, Treatment and Legal Issues*. Oxford, Oxford University Press, 2009.

27. Craig LA, Gannon TA, Dixon L (eds) *What Works in Offender Rehabilitation: An Evidence-Based Approach to Assessment and Treatment*. New York, John Wiley & Sons, 2013.

28. Clarke M, Brown S, Völlm B. Circles of Support and Accountability for sex offenders: a systematic review of outcomes. *Sexual Abuse* 2017; 29 (5): 446–78.

29. Marshall LE, Marshall WL. Motivating sex offenders to enter and effectively engage in treatment. In Wilcox D, Donathy M, Gray R, Baim C (eds) *Working with Sex Offenders: A Guide for Practitioners*. London, Taylor & Francis, 2017.

30. Kennedy HG, Grubin DH. Patterns of denial in sexual offenders. *Psychological Medicine* 1992; 22: 191–6.

31. Davoren M, Fitzpatrick M, Caddow F et al. Older men and older women remand prisoners: mental illness, physical illness, offending patterns and needs. *International Psychogeriatrics* 2014; 27: 1–9. doi: 10.1017/S1041610214002348.

Chapter 14

Terrorism-Related Assessments

Paul Gill and Frank Farnham

Introduction

This chapter is about forensic psychiatric assessment of terrorism cases. As will become clear, this may not be a straightforward exercise in that it can be difficult to decide whether the case actually involves terrorism, let alone what contribution mental disorder may or may not make. Nonetheless, psychiatric assessment is often requested and assessment of the terrorism offender relies on the same basic principles of good-quality assessment, utilising a multi-agency approach, that is applicable when assessing any complex criminal, or potentially criminal, behaviour involving mental disorder.

What Is Terrorism?

If 'terrorism studies conference bingo' existed, you would be delighted to see 'audience question on defining terrorism' on your card. The debate appears endless. Terrorism is an emotive term ripe for politicisation. It comes with notions and normative assumptions of whose violence is (il-)legitimate. It opens accusations of double standards when applied selectively. It often overlooks the violence of the state. It can be difficult to distinguish from other forms of non-state political violence. It is not that terrorism is difficult to define. There are, after all, over 250 definitions of it at the last count [1]. The problem, for many, is the lack of consensus definition. Some of the non-consensus stems from terrorism studies' multi-disciplinary history. Historians, political scientists, psychologists and criminologists focus on and prioritise different definitional facets. Terrorism has been depicted as a problem of historical activities, a problem that war can overcome, a problem for the criminal justice system to sort and increasingly a problem that those in mental healthcare can prevent [2]. Schmid outlines many different attributes of terrorism definitions, including terrorism's

> often symbolic character, its often indiscriminate nature, its typical focus on civilian and non-combatant targets of violence, its sometimes retributive aims, the disruption of public order and the putting in danger of public security, the creation of a climate of fear to influence audiences wider than the direct victims, its disregard for the rules of war and the rules of punishment, and its asymmetric character (armed versus unarmed; weak versus strong) . . . usually an instrument for the attempted realization of a political or religious project that perpetrators lacking mass support are seeking, that it generally involves a series of punctuated acts of demonstrative public violence, followed by threats of more in order to impress, intimidate and/or coerce target audiences. [1] (p. 39)

Schmid sought to create a 'good enough' definition through three rounds of large-scale expert surveys [1] (pp. 86–7). The consensus definition has 12 components:

1. Terrorism refers, on the one hand, to a doctrine about the presumed effectiveness of a special form or tactic of fear-generating, coercive political violence and, on the other hand, to a conspiratorial practice of calculated, demonstrative, direct violent action without legal or moral restraints, targeting mainly civilians and non-combatants, performed for its propagandistic and psychological effects on various audiences and conflict parties.

2. Terrorism as a tactic is employed in *three main contexts*: (i) illegal state repression, (ii) propagandistic agitation by non-state actors in times of peace or outside zones of conflict and (iii) as an illicit tactic of irregular warfare employed by state- and non-state actors.

3. The physical *violence* or threat thereof employed by terrorist actors involves single-phase acts of lethal violence (such as bombings and armed assaults), dual-phased life-threatening incidents (like kidnapping, hijacking and other forms of hostage-taking for coercive bargaining) as well as multi-phased sequences of actions (such as in 'disappearances' involving kidnapping, secret detention, torture and murder).

4. The public(-ised) terrorist victimisation initiates threat-based communication processes whereby, on the one hand, conditional demands are made to individuals, groups, governments, societies or sections thereof, and, on the other hand, the support of specific constituencies (based on ties of ethnicity, religion, political affiliation and the like) is sought by the terrorist perpetrators.

5. At the origin of terrorism stands *terror* – instilled fear, dread, panic or mere anxiety – spread among those identifying, or sharing similarities, with the direct victims, generated by some of the modalities of the terrorist act – its shocking brutality, lack of discrimination, dramatic or symbolic quality and disregard of the rules of warfare and the rules of punishment.

6. The main direct *victims* of terrorist attacks are in general not any armed forces but are *usually civilians, non-combatants or other innocent and defenceless persons* who bear no direct responsibility for the conflict that gave rise to acts of terrorism.

7. The *direct victims are not the ultimate target* (as in a classical assassination where victim and target coincide) but serve as message generators, more or less unwittingly helped by the news values of the mass media, to reach various audiences and conflict parties that identify either with the victims' plight or the terrorists' professed cause.

8. Sources of terrorist violence can be individual *perpetrators*, small groups and diffuse transnational networks, as well as state actors or state-sponsored clandestine agents (such as death squads and hit teams).

9. While showing similarities with methods employed by organised crime as well as those found in war crimes, terrorist violence is *predominantly political* – usually in its motivation but nearly always in its societal repercussions.

10. The immediate *intent* of acts of terrorism is to terrorise, intimidate, antagonise, disorientate, destabilise, coerce, compel, demoralise or provoke a target population or conflict party in the hope of achieving from the resulting insecurity a favourable power outcome, such as obtaining publicity, extorting ransom money, submission to terrorist demands and/or mobilising or immobilising sectors of the public.

11. The *motivations* to engage in terrorism cover a broad range, including redress for alleged grievances, personal or vicarious revenge, collective punishment, revolution,

national liberation and the promotion of diverse ideological, political, social, national or religious causes and objectives.

12. Acts of terrorism rarely stand alone but form part of a *campaign* of violence which alone can, due to the serial character of acts of violence and threats of more to come, create a pervasive climate of fear that enables the terrorists to manipulate the political process.

While this looks great for more standardised approaches in the scientific study of terrorism, there remain major gaps in legal definitions of terrorism across state boundaries. Some countries have 'rational codes', devised at a time of no national security panic, which seek to be all-encompassing and well thought through. Others have a series of panic legislations responding to 'the politics of the last atrocity'.

What constitutes a criminal offence differs across national counter-terrorism legislations. The line in the sand in the conflict between public safety and individual rights to liberty, privacy and free expression dramatically differs cross-nationally. This has major knock-on effects for the practice of risk assessment and management. For example, the UK has an expansive set of legislation that criminalises a wide range of precursor and terrorism-related behaviours. These laws reach far higher 'upstream' than many other national contexts and include (a) membership of proscribed organisations, (b) exclusion orders barring travel into the UK, (c) contributing, receiving or soliciting financial support for terrorism, (d) collecting or possessing information of a kind likely to be useful to a person committing or preparing an act of terrorism, (e) the publication of statements likely to be understood by their audience as a direct or indirect encouragement to the commission or preparation of terrorist offences, (f) dissemination of terrorist publications and (g) attendance at a place used for terrorism training.

In recent years there has been renewed interest in involving a range of agencies in formulating a response to terrorism. The overt focus on mental health and complex needs necessitates a look at what the evidence base says about their relationship to terrorist engagement.

The Evidence for Mental Disorder, Complex Needs and Terrorist Engagement

Debates surrounding the presence and relevance of mental disorders and terrorist engagement date back to the origins of terrorism studies in the late 1960s [3–4]. For the most part, however, while debates raged, empiricism lagged. The past decade, though, witnessed a renaissance in data from a plurality of sources. Sources include openly available data compiled systematically, closed-source data such as police and intelligence files, first-hand interviews and general population surveys. The field is now in a better place to make finer-grained assertions thanks to these efforts. The discourse has changed from 'it's all about mental disorders' to 'it has nothing to do with mental disorder' to a greater consideration of the role mental disorders and associated complex needs can play, in what circumstances and for whom.

Recently, Gill et al. conducted a systematic review of the evidence base of the relationship between mental disorders and terrorist engagement [5]. We can draw six main conclusions from their synthesis.

First, it is a myth to suggest there is no presence of mental disorders within terrorist samples. This myth largely sprung from misunderstandings and previous literature reviews from the turn of the century which highlighted the severe lack of supporting data *at that time* [4]. The data renaissance is a very recent phenomenon. Of the 28 samples identified by Gill et al. [5], 24 were published in papers since 2013. Pooling the results of 19 samples that both measured confirmed (rather than suggested) diagnoses and clearly articulated the sample size (n = 1705) demonstrates a rate of 14.4% with a confirmed diagnosis. However, these samples were underpinned by different data collection methods. In those studies involving clinical examinations (n = 236 subjects), the prevalence rate jumps to 33.4%.

Second, Gill et al. [5] demonstrate that the types of mental disorders found in terrorist samples vary hugely. There is no common diagnosis. Diversity reigns. Different studies found examples of depression, Asperger syndrome, schizophrenia, attention-deficit hyperactivity disorder, psychotic disorder, borderline personality disorder, post-traumatic stress, primary dissocial problems, narcissistic disorder, schizoaffective disorder, delusional disorder, bipolar disorder, anxiety disorder, obsessive-compulsive disorder, sleep disorder, unspecified personality disorders, mood disorders, and intellectual disabilities [6–12]. To understand pathways into terrorism necessitates understanding equifinality [13]. People with different initial states can end at the same outcome (in this case terrorist engagement) after traversing different routes to get there.

Third, there is also no one common outcome of terrorist engagement. Some become lone actors, some co-offend in larger groups, some act locally, some travel to foreign battlefields, some purposely die in their actions, some live to fight another day and others prefer facilitating from the shadows. Within this diversity of outcomes, we might find a greater propensity for certain types of people more likely ending in one outcome than others. For example, there appears to be an inverse relationship between co-offending and the presence of mental disorders. The more embedded the co-offending, the fewer mental disorders are present (11, 14–16). Lone actors also appear to more often have diagnoses of schizophrenia, autism and delusional disorder than the general population [16]. Clinical interviews and personality tests suggest (failed) suicide bombers appear different than other terrorist roles [17]. Suicide bombers more likely present diagnoses of avoidant-dependent personality disorders, depressive symptoms and more readily displayed suicidal tendencies.

Fourth, mental disorders, when present, may play a different role in an individual's terrorist engagement. Gill et al.'s review shows examples of mental disorders (a) being the biggest influence directly driving the behaviour, (b) being a more subtle cause of a cause that exacerbated other stressors, (c) being the result of, rather than the reason for, terrorist engagement and (d) being present but seemingly playing no role. The synthesis also notes that factors that might explain sympathy for a cause may not neatly map onto the factors that explain mobilising to violence on behalf of that cause [5].

Finally, it is insufficient to only examine mental health disorders. Other adverse life experiences and complex needs tend to co-occur. Evidence is abundant here. Formulations of risk could additionally consider issues related to self-harm [18], suicidal ideation [19–22], poor interpersonal and family relationships [23–28], bereavement [7, 29–31], discrimination and victimisation [19, 32–40], economic pressures and unemployment [6, 23, 41–54], homelessness [41, 55], experiences of neglect, physical, sexual and/or psychological trauma [18, 22–23, 41, 56–61], and substance misuse and addiction [18, 20, 24, 41, 62–63].

Risk Assessment and Management

Collectively, the evidence base demonstrates that the types of risk factors commonly included across general and interpersonal violence risk assessment instruments are also present for terrorist samples. Terrorist risk assessment and management can learn a lot from the much more established field of general violence risk assessment. One immediate area for learning is to disregard the tendency for policy to treat 'extremism' as the main problem. For the individual, extremism is often the solution to other problems ongoing in their life. It is these problems, we suggest, which require addressing first before any work can be done on extremist tendencies.

The risk assessment and ongoing management of individuals deemed to be a risk to national security are core components of the policing and intelligence agencies worldwide. The number of individuals 'on the radar' far outnumber those who can be actively managed at any one time. The scrutiny of the effectiveness and quality of an individual's risk assessment, and the subsequent management of that risk, come to the fore when terrorist attacks occur. This was the case in the UK following the 2017 terrorist attacks in Westminster, Manchester, London Bridge, Finsbury Park and Parsons Green. As noted publicly, among the perpetrators were those known to authorities, an active subject of interest, a closed subject of interest and individuals referred to the upstream prevention services.

The scale and number of attacks in 2017, plus the fact that some perpetrators were on MI5's or counter-terrorism policing's (CTP's) 'radar', prompted a series of detailed internal and external reviews of MI5 and CTP counter-terrorism processes. Two official reports were released in the public domain. First, Lord Anderson QC independently assessed nine classified internal reviews conducted by MI5 and CTP. Second, Parliament's Intelligence and Security Committee examined 'what needs to change' in the wake of the 2017 attacks.

Lord Anderson's review, published in December 2017, provided an independent assessment and assurance of the MI5 and police internal reviews following the London and Manchester attacks. One pivotal internal review, examined by Lord Anderson, was the Operational Improvement Review (OIR) which considered:

- whether there are any further improvements that can be made in how leads, prioritisation and triage processes operate;
- the process by which individuals are categorised as a closed subject of interest, and how cases are then reviewed and escalated where indicators of potential re-engagement in terrorist-related activity are identified;
- what data sources, tools and approaches, both tactical and strategic, can best support this work;
- which partners can contribute, and how we can further strengthen joint working in managing this risk;
- how data is shared and links are made with other organisations/interventions (such as PREVENT or community policing), where appropriate;
- any policy, legal or ethical questions associated with this issue that require consideration;
- the overall level of assurance it is possible to provide in this area, and the resource and prioritisation challenges associated with managing this risk.

Most, if not all, of these considerations bear directly on the issue of the effective risk assessment and subsequent management of individuals of concern. This covers a range of potential assessment points, including those who are in the pre-offence space, those who are within the prison system, closed cases and those released from prison. There are a range of commercial risk assessment products available and presumably a number of non-published 'in-house' risk assessment instruments. Undoubtedly, structured professional judgement (SPJ) approaches are currently in vogue and widely seen as best practice among those who have responsibility for risk assessment in a variety of clinical, forensic and custodial settings.

Most terrorism risk assessment tools follow suit and either explicitly or implicitly; for example, identifying vulnerable people (IVP) identifies itself as a SPJ approach. However, the grounds by which they self-identify as SPJ differ. The likes of IVP, extremist media index (EMI), online violent extremist screening tool (OVEST) and violent extremist risk assessment (VERA) encourage the first two steps of SPJ (e.g. gather information and resources; determine the relevance of factors to individual risk) but do not provide advice on formulation, scenario planning and management strategies. The extremism risk guidelines (ERG22+) go a step further than IVP and use formulation but not scenario planning. The terrorist radicalisation assessment protocol (TRAP-18) and multi-level guidelines (MLG) are the closest match to typical SPJ development guidelines. This is particularly so with the MLG whose developers were also heavily involved with Historical Clinical Risk – 20 (HCR-20), the Guidelines for Stalking Assessment and Management (SAM) and other highly rated risk assessment tools for other types of violence.

Overall, there is no specific psychiatry of terrorism. Rather, given the range of social and personal factors, as well as the possible variations in psychological make-up and mental state, emphasis in the UK has been on systems for assessing risk and individual need through forms of case identification and multi-disciplinary assessment, including psychiatric input. Alongside the various criminal justice routes are a range of early prevention initiatives within the UK. For example, the Channel programme seeks to identify referred individuals vulnerable to becoming involved in (violent) extremism [64]. Practitioners conduct risk assessments in order to inform decisions regarding whether and how to intervene with such individuals to prevent them from becoming radicalised and progressing further towards harmful behaviour.

One of the key areas of concern emanating from the government reports mentioned earlier was the need for development and piloting new models for managing risks posed by 'closed and closing subjects of interest involving greater multi-agency working at a local level' [64] (p. 26). One such process is the national multi-agency centres (NMAC) which were unveiled in the updated CONTEST strategy in June 2018. The NMAC works in partnership to better understand the national security risk posed by individuals who are or have been subject to national security investigations, in recognition that some of these people may continue to pose a risk.

These centres, initially based in London, the West Midlands and Greater Manchester, were designed to enable greater information sharing between MI5/CTP and partners including government departments, devolved administrations and local authorities. With greater information sharing, the intent is to improve risk assessment abilities and enrich the number of local interventions available for the purpose of safeguarding and/or disengagement from extremism. As stated in its launch document, the NMAC pilots will contain 'a spirit of experimentation and rigorous evaluation, designed to drive an innovative approach that addresses the challenges' currently faced [64] (p. 42).

Other tailored approaches, such as the newly formed Counter-Terrorism Vulnerability Hubs (CTVH), have also recently been established, which draw on previous models of multi-agency liaison and diversion [65]. They consist of a joint National Health Service (NHS) and CTP team of consultant forensic psychiatrists, consultant forensic and clinical psychologists, and forensic nurse specialists who work alongside detectives. There are three 'hubs' in total, offering coverage over a large part of England and Wales.

Where a case is identified through the UK's PREVENT arrangements as having a defined counter-terrorism risk and there is concern about potential underlying mental disorder, the hubs liaise with the individual's healthcare provider in order to share appropriate information and make a fully informed risk assessment. The hubs also attempt to divert subjects into appropriate healthcare services where appropriate and provide counter-terrorism police colleagues with advice and guidance about mental illness and mental disorder.

The hubs offer a support service only and do not take on a case management role. The hubs are not agents of the security service and do not make covert enquiries or any enquiries with the NHS for investigative purposes. Maintaining health confidentiality boundaries is important, as is avoiding further stigmatisation of the mentally ill.

Ultimately, psychiatric assessment, including risk assessment and management, depends upon careful clinical interview and evaluation of all relevant sources of information. In this regard, forensic psychiatric assessment of terrorism is no different to forensic psychiatric assessment of any other complex multifactorial behaviour.

References

1. Schmid AP (ed.). *The Routledge Handbook of Terrorism Research*. London, Taylor & Francis, 2011.

2. Augestad Knudsen R. Between vulnerability and risk? Mental health in UK counter-terrorism. *Behavioral Sciences of Terrorism and Political Aggression* 2021; 13 (1): 43–61.

3. Corner E, Gill P, Schouten R, Farnham F. Mental disorders, personality traits, and grievance-fueled targeted violence: the evidence base and implications for research and practice. *Journal of Personality Assessment* 2018; 100 (5): 459–70.

4. Gill P, Corner E. There and back again: the study of mental disorder and terrorist involvement. *American Psychologist* 2017; 72 (3): 231.

5. Gill P, Clemmow C, Hetzel F et al. Systematic review of mental health problems and violent extremism. *The Journal of Forensic Psychiatry & Psychology* 2021; 32 (1): 51–78.

6. Bakker E. *Jihadi Terrorists in Europe*. The Hague, Cliengendael, 2006.

7. Knight S, Woodward K, Lancaster GL. Violent versus nonviolent actors: an empirical study of different types of extremism. *Journal of Threat Assessment and Management* 2017; 4 (4): 230.

8. Leygraf N. Zur Phänomenologie islamistisch-terroristischer Straftäter. *Forensische Psychiatrie, Psychologie, Kriminologie* 2014; 4 (8): 237–45.

9. Van Leyenhorst M, Andreas A. Dutch suspects of terrorist activity: a study of their biographical backgrounds based on primary sources. *Journal for Deradicalization* 2017; 12: 309–44.

10. Weenink AW. Behavioral problems and disorders among radicals in police files. *Perspectives on Terrorism* 2015; 9 (2): 17–33.

11. Corner E, Gill P, Mason O. Mental health disorders and the terrorist: a research note probing selection effects and disorder prevalence. *Studies in Conflict & Terrorism* 2016; 39 (6): 560–8.

12. Gill P, Corner E, McKee A, Hitchen P, Betley P. What do closed source data tell us

about lone actor terrorist behavior? A research note. *Terrorism and Political Violence* 2022; 34 (1): 113–30.

13. Borum R. Radicalization into violent extremism II: a review of conceptual models and empirical research. *Journal of Strategic Security* 2011; 4 (4): 37–62.

14. Gruenewald J, Chermak S, Freilich JD. Distinguishing 'loner' attacks from other domestic extremist violence: a comparison of far-right homicide incident and offender characteristics. *Criminology & Public Policy* 2013; 12 (1): 65–91.

15. Hewitt C. *Understanding Terrorism in America: From the Klan to al Qaeda.* London, Psychology Press, 2003.

16. Corner E, Gill P. A false dichotomy? Mental illness and lone-actor terrorism. *Law and Human Behavior* 2015; 39 (1): 23.

17. Merari A. *Driven to Death: Psychological and Social Aspects of Suicide Terrorism.* New York, Oxford University Press, 2010.

18. Oppetit A, Campelo N, Bouzar L et al. Do radicalized minors have different social and psychological profiles from radicalized adults? *Frontiers in Psychiatry* 2019; 10: 644.

19. Bouzar D, Martin M. What motives bring youth to engage in the Jihad? *Neuropsychiatr Enf Adolesc* 2016; 64 (6): 353–59.

20. Ilardi GJ. Interviews with Canadian radicals. *Studies in Conflict & Terrorism* 2013; 36 (9): 713–38.

21. Corner E, Gill P. Psychological distress, terrorist involvement and disengagement from terrorism: a sequence analysis approach. *Journal of Quantitative Criminology* 2020; 36: 499–526.

22. Simi P, Sporer K, Bubolz BF. Narratives of childhood adversity and adolescent misconduct as precursors to violent extremism: a life-course criminological approach. *Journal of Research in Crime and Delinquency* 2016; 53 (4): 536–63.

23. Jasko K, LaFree G, Kruglanski A. Quest for significance and violent extremism: the case of domestic radicalization. *Political Psychology* 2017; 38 (5): 815–31.

24. Aly A, Striegher JL. Examining the role of religion in radicalization to violent Islamist extremism. *Studies in Conflict & Terrorism* 2012; 35 (12): 849–62.

25. Bazex H, Mensat JY. Qui sont les djihadistes français? Analyse de 12 cas pour contribuer à l'élaboration de profils et à l'évaluation du risque de passage à l'acte. *Annales Médico-psychologiques, revue psychiatrique* 2016; 174 (4): 257–65.

26. Bazex H, Bénézech M, Mensat JY. 'Le miroir de la haine'. La prise en charge pénitentiaire de la radicalisation: analyse clinique et criminologique de 112 personnes placées sous main de justice. *Annales Médico-psychologiques, revue psychiatrique* 2017; 175 (3): 276–82.

27. Sieckelinck S, Sikkens E, Van San M, Kotnis S, De Winter M. Transitional journeys into and out of extremism: a biographical approach. *Studies in Conflict & Terrorism* 2019; 42 (7): 662–82.

28. Rink A, Sharma K. The determinants of religious radicalization: evidence from Kenya. *Journal of Conflict Resolution* 2018; 62 (6): 1229–61.

29. Böckler N, Leuschner V, Zick A, Scheithauer H. Same but different? Developmental pathways to demonstrative targeted attacks – qualitative case analyses of adolescent and young adult perpetrators of targeted school attacks and jihadi terrorist attacks in Germany. *International Journal of Developmental Science* 2018; 12 (1–2): 5–24.

30. Beardsley NL, Beech AR. Applying the violent extremist risk assessment (VERA) to a sample of terrorist case studies. *Journal of Aggression, Conflict and Peace Research* 2013; 5 (1): 4–15.

31. Botha A. Political socialization and terrorist radicalization among individuals who joined al-Shabaab in Kenya. *Studies in Conflict & Terrorism* 2014; 37 (11): 895–919.

32. Ali RB, Moss SA, Barrelle K, Lentini P. Does the pursuit of meaning explain the initiation, escalation, and disengagement of violent extremists? *Aggression and Violent Behavior.* 2017; 34: 185–92.

33. Ferguson N, Burgess M, Hollywood I. Crossing the Rubicon: deciding to become a paramilitary in Northern Ireland. *International Journal of Conflict and Violence (IJCV)* 2008; 2 (1): 130–7.

34. Florez-Morris M. Joining guerrilla groups in Colombia: individual motivations and processes for entering a violent organization. *Studies in Conflict & Terrorism* 2007; 30 (7): 615–34.

35. Denov M, Gervais C. Negotiating (in)security: agency, resistance, and resourcefulness among girls formerly associated with Sierra Leone's Revolutionary United Front. *Signs: Journal of Women in Culture and Society* 2007; 32 (4): 885–910.

36. Glaser J, Dixit J, Green DP. Studying hate crime with the internet: what makes racists advocate racial violence? *Journal of Social Issues* 2002; 58 (1): 177–93.

37. Schafer JA, Mullins CW, Box S. Awakenings: the emergence of white supremacist ideologies. *Deviant Behavior* 2014; 35 (3): 173–96.

38. De Waele M, Pauwels LJ. Why do Flemish youth participate in right-wing disruptive groups? *Gang Transitions and Transformations in an International Context.* New York, Springer, 2016, pp. 173–200.

39. Victoroff J, Adelman JR, Matthews M. Psychological factors associated with support for suicide bombing in the Muslim diaspora. *Political Psychology* 2012; 33 (6): 791–809.

40. Doosje B, Loseman A, Van Den Bos K. Determinants of radicalization of Islamic youth in the Netherlands: personal uncertainty, perceived injustice, and perceived group threat. *Journal of Social Issues* 2013; 69 (3): 586–604.

41. Baron SW. Canadian male street skinheads: street gang or street terrorists? *Canadian Review of Sociology* 1997; 34 (2): 125–54.

42. De Bie JL, De Poot CJ. Studying police files with grounded theory methods to understand Jihadist networks. *Studies in*

Conflict & Terrorism 2016; 39 (7–8): 580–601.

43. Fair CC. The educated militants of Pakistan: implications for Pakistan's domestic security. *Contemporary South Asia* 2008; 16 (1): 93–106.

44. Dean G. Criminal profiling in a terrorism context. *Criminal Profiling: International Theory, Research, and Practice.* Clifton, NJ, Humana Press, 2007, pp. 169–88.

45. Gill P, Corner E, Conway M et al. Terrorist use of the Internet by the numbers: quantifying behaviors, patterns, and processes. *Criminology & Public Policy* 2017; 16 (1): 99–117.

46. Gill P, Horgan J, Deckert P. Bombing alone: tracing the motivations and antecedent behaviors of lone-actor terrorists. *Journal of Forensic Sciences* 2014; 59 (2): 425–35.

47. Horgan J, Morrison JF. Here to stay? The rising threat of violent dissident Republicanism in Northern Ireland. *Terrorism and Political Violence* 2011; 23 (4): 642–69.

48. Horgan J, Shortland N, Abbasciano S, Walsh S. Actions speak louder than words: a behavioral analysis of 183 individuals convicted for terrorist offenses in the United States from 1995 to 2012. *Journal of Forensic Sciences* 2016; 61 (5): 1228–37.

49. Ducol B. Devenir jihadiste à l'ère numérique: une approche processuelle et situationnelle de l'engagement jihadiste au regard du Web (doctoral dissertation, Université Laval).

50. Jacques K, Taylor PJ. Myths and realities of female-perpetrated terrorism. *Law and Human Behavior* 2013; 37 (1): 35.

51. Meloy JR, Roshdi K, Glaz-Ocik J, Hoffmann J. Investigating the individual terrorist in Europe. *Journal of Threat Assessment and Management* 2015; 2 (3–4): 140.

52. Reynolds SC, Hafez MM. Social network analysis of German foreign fighters in Syria and Iraq. *Terrorism and Political Violence* 2019; 31 (4): 661–86.

53. Altunbas Y, Thornton J. Are homegrown Islamic terrorists different? Some UK evidence. *Southern Economic Journal* 2011; 78 (2): 262–72.

54. Bhui K, Silva MJ, Topciu RA, Jones E. Pathways to sympathies for violent protest and terrorism. *The British Journal of Psychiatry* 2016; 209 (6): 483–90.

55. Weenink AW. Adversity, criminality, and mental health problems in jihadis in Dutch police files. *Perspectives on Terrorism* 2019; 13 (5): 130–42.

56. Post JM. Terrorist on trial: the context of political crime. *The Journal of the American Academy of Psychiatry and the Law* 2000; 28 (2): 171–8.

57. Stern JE. X: A case study of a Swedish neo-Nazi and his reintegration into Swedish society. *Behavioral Sciences & the Law* 2014; 32 (3): 440–53.

58. Klausen J, Campion S, Needle N, Nguyen G, Libretti R. Toward a behavioral model of 'homegrown' radicalization trajectories. *Studies in Conflict & Terrorism* 2016; 39 (1): 67–83.

59. Speckhard A, Ahkmedova K. The making of a martyr: Chechen suicide terrorism. *Studies in Conflict & Terrorism* 2006; 29 (5): 429–92.

60. Bubolz BF, Simi P. The problem of overgeneralization: the case of mental health problems and US violent white supremacists. *American Behavioral Scientist* 2019. https://doi.org/10.1177/0002764219831746.

61. Dhumad S, Candilis PJ, Cleary SD, Dyer AR, Khalifa N. Risk factors for terrorism: a comparison of family, childhood, and personality risk factors among Iraqi terrorists, murderers, and controls. *Behavioral Sciences of Terrorism and Political Aggression* 2020; 12 (1): 72–88.

62. Stys Y, Gobeil R, Harris AJR, Michel S. Violent extremists in federal institutions: estimating radicalization and susceptibility to radicalization in the federal offender population. Ottawa, Correctional Service Canada, 2014.

63. Denov M, Gervais C. Negotiating (in)security: agency, resistance, and resourcefulness among girls formerly associated with Sierra Leone's Revolutionary United Front. *Signs: Journal of Women in Culture and Society* 2007; 32 (4): 885–910.

64. https://assets.publishing.service.gov.uk/government/uploads/system/uploads/attachment_data/file/716907/140618_CCS207_CCS0218929798-1_CONTEST_3.0_WEB.pdf.

65. James DV, Kerrigan TR, Forfar R, Farnham FR, Preston LF. The Fixated Threat Assessment Centre: preventing harm and facilitating care. *The Journal of Forensic Psychiatry & Psychology* 2010; 21 (4): 521–36.

Forensic Psychotherapy
and Psychological Therapies
in Forensic Mental Health Settings

Gwen Adshead and John Marshall

Forensic Psychotherapy
Gwen Adshead

'Forensic psychotherapy' is a shorthand term for the treatment of offenders with psycho-dynamic psychotherapy. Over the last decade, a range of psychological therapies for offenders have been developed, often based on improved therapies for personality disorder. In this section, I discuss what distinguishes forensic psychotherapy from other psychological therapies offered to offenders, and which offenders might benefit most from psycho-dynamically focussed therapy.

It may be easier to begin by describing the *similarities* between forensic psychotherapy and other interventions offered to offenders. Like these other therapies, the outcomes of forensic psychotherapy are improved mental health and reduced risk of further offending. Like other therapies, forensic psychotherapy assumes that the offence has meaning for the offender and thus may fulfil some positive psychological function. Finally, just as with other therapies, forensic psychotherapy is most effective when there is a therapeutic alliance with the patient, and a sense of trust which allows for curiosity and reflection.

People who have had a good experience of forensic psychotherapy say that they have learned more about their own minds and the minds of others, and understand more about how they came to offend. They describe being better able to reflect on their mental function and that of others; that is, they are better able to *mentalise* their feelings and thoughts, and experience a greater sense of agency over their minds and choices, which aids in desistance from future offending [1].

Theoretical Base

Forensic psychotherapy draws on psychodynamic accounts of mental function and is based on three key assumptions. First, forensic psychotherapy assumes that early childhood experience has an influence on the development of the antisocial state of mind. An early empirical contribution by Bowlby [2] observed that young people who stole repeatedly often had histories of childhood neglect and deprivation. Bowlby hypothesised that the stealing behaviour represented an unconscious solution to unresolved distress and anger; that is, the stealing had a psychological soothing function, both consciously and unconsciously. He argued that therapy which addressed both the unconscious distress and the conscious motives for stealing could provide a 'secure base' from which to support psychological change [3].

Later research by Bowlby in collaboration with ethologists and child development specialists showed how exposure to childhood trauma and adversity at the hands of parents could lead to the development of an 'insecure' state of mind, which in turn is associated with poor mental health. Attachment insecurity is common in offenders and a risk factor for criminal rule-breaking, especially violence [4]. Exposure to childhood trauma increases the risk of chronic severe violence [5, 6], which is likely to be mediated by an insecure attachment system. Attachment insecurity in offenders may also explain why victims of violence are commonly partners and family members.

Forensic psychotherapy's second assumption is that humans develop organised and persisting patterns of cognitions and feelings which help them manage high levels of interpersonal distress (both conscious or unconscious). These patterns are usually termed 'defences' because they protect the individual from feeling overwhelmed with distress. First described by Freud, defences have been subsequently studied in terms of their relevance to lifespan stress management [7], psychological change in response to therapy [8] and personality maturation [9]. Exposure to overwhelming distress in childhood causes a child to develop a range of defences that help ward off pain and distress and make the child feel safe and strong.

However, childhood defences can become dysfunctional if they persist into adulthood. They may not be able to manage adult distress, and this also causes problems because the adult now acts like a child when under stress, which makes them unpopular with others and can lead to rule-breaking. Further, an individual with dysfunctional defences is at risk of externalising or 'acting out' their distress rather than symbolising it using language and then mentalising the distress [10]. An act of violence is prima facie evidence that a person's defences were overwhelmed, which is also more likely to happen in a person with an insecure attachment system. Studies of psychological defences in forensic patients have found high levels of immature defences [11, 12].

Finally, forensic psychotherapy assumes that human beings are narrators who seek to make meaning of interpersonal experience, and who may use complex communications in their relationships with others. In this context, acts of violence can be understood as highly individual and complex communications to the victim. This assumption implies that violence is heterogeneous, idiosyncratic and relational; so any actuarial data about violence must be appraised and integrated with the offender's narrative of themselves and others. This assumption about the complexity of human minds also implies that we should not take everything the offender patient says at face value. What they say may represent a kind of 'truthiness' about their world, but their narrative needs to be triangulated with views from third parties and the wider society to which the offender patient belongs. Forensic psychotherapists practise holding these kinds of uncertainties and tensions about 'truth' as part of the work.

Critics of forensic psychotherapy sometimes suggest that it pays too much attention to unconscious processes and not enough to conscious experience. But most contemporary psychological theorists accept that we have good evidence that a significant amount of psychological function operates out of consciousness; therefore, what people consciously say or assert may not reflect *all* that they believe or feel. For example, a patient may insist that they are well, and do not need to be in hospital, but comply with all treatment and never apply for a tribunal or seek to go on leave, saying that they are waiting for a sign from God that they are ready. No amount of medication shifts this view. The forensic psychotherapist will suggest that this patient unconsciously knows that all is not well, and that under the surface denial, the patient 'knows' they need help and fears being discharged and feeling uncared for.

Forensic Psychotherapeutic Treatment: Implications for Services

Before treatment starts, the forensic psychotherapist will carry out an extended assessment which covers the patient's developmental history, their relationships and how they think about them, and their narrative of the index offence. This assessment allows for the development of a formulation that offers a hypothesis about why this offence happened at this time, and what needs to change for the offender to be able to manage their risk more safely. The forensic psychotherapist will want to help the offender understand the meaning of the violence to them, and then include that understanding in a plan for managing risk in future.

All patients and diagnoses may benefit from forensic psychotherapy, except for those patients who struggle to engage with any therapy, such as those who are very paranoid or dismissing of need. Timing is an issue; forensic psychotherapy is not indicated for people in crisis and may often be most effective after a period of therapy that helps people regulate their moods and understand basic cognitive processes (such as cognitive behavioural therapy (CBT) and dialectical behaviour therapy (DBT)). Non-verbal patients (or where the therapist and patient do not share a language) may still be able to benefit from creative therapies that are also based on psychodynamic theories of the importance of symbolic thought.

In terms of individual technique, forensic psychotherapy is especially useful for helping patients think about their index offence, its meaning and its impact. Therapy focusses on exploring the patient's narrative of their offence and the defences involved, and gently allowing them to build new defences that are less risky. In general populations, the evidence base suggests that 18 months of individual psychodynamic therapy can be effective as other therapies, especially for complex cases [13], and the process of change is evident at the neurobiological level [14]. There is no obvious reason why this would not be true in forensic services, and case reports suggest that forensic patients find relief in talking about their offences, especially when these have been traumatic for them.

Forensic psychotherapy's reliance on attachment theory connects 'security of mind' with forensic mental health services' duty to provide secure care, whether physical, procedural or relational. Attachment insecurity is associated with poor mentalising skills, which are common in offenders [15], and therapy which improves mentalising (mentalisation-based therapy (MBT)) has been shown to be effective in a range of disorders [16], especially personality disorders. The Offenders with Personality Disorder (OPD) programme in prisons and probation is based on MBT [17] and is now the subject of a national treatment trial with offenders with antisocial personality disorder in the community. MBT is an essential intervention in forensic services because of the evidence of its efficacy in personality disorder which is so prevalent in forensic populations.

MBT has a group component, which is likely to be one of the factors relevant to its efficacy. Group therapy was first recommended for antisocial people in the 1960s because participation in a therapy group is a pro-social act in itself. Participation in groups allows group facilitators to observe offenders' relationships with others and their capacity for mentalising and perspective-taking. Group therapy also allows participants to practise being pro-social and thinking about other people's perspectives; it can also reduce shame and hopelessness to be in a group with people with similar offending histories [18]. No forensic service can afford to be without a group work programme and forensic psycho-therapy should be one of the disciplines involved in this.

Forensic psychotherapy is also useful to support thinking about group/institutional dynamics in forensic services. Relational security entails thinking about relationships in services, and this includes relationships between staff and patients and staff and staff. Early work by Menzies Lyth [19] indicated that organisations can be anxious if they have a difficult primary task to complete; and when organisations are anxious, they can do odd things and act unprofessionally. Given the well-publicised and sadly frequent concerns about failed care and abusive staff in different kinds of hospital and care home, managing organisational anxiety should be an important issue for all forensic services. The Royal College of Psychiatrists Quality Guidelines for secure units recommend that a forensic psychotherapist is employed to provide reflective practice spaces for all staff: from ward based to senior management.

Forensic Psychotherapy and Risk Assessment

Forensic psychotherapy is not only a treatment intervention; it can be especially useful in relation to good-quality risk assessment. When humans assess chance or risk, they tend to first use a basic mode of thought (system 1) based on the last conscious emotion or cognitive appraisal they made, and then engage a deeper more reflective mode of thought (system 2), which is more reality based [20]. Risk assessments made in system 1 mode only tend to be unreliable and irrational but those made using system 2 are more coherent. Psychodynamic models of thinking prioritise system 2 modes, which make risk assessment better for patients and professionals alike.

Further, the psychodynamic model assumes that each act of violence requires a complex analysis of individual risk factors. Violence risk assessment is always multi-factorial, but the last factor that triggers the violence may be a memory, a relationship, a smile or a sudden panic, often associated with unresolved fear from the past [10]. The psychodynamic model offers a relational perspective on complex violence which com-plements the actuarial.

Finally, the psychodynamic model of trauma argues that unresolved distress can lead to unconscious repetition of interactions with others, in a search for relief. This process has been described as 'repetition compulsion' or 're-enactment' of toxic attachment patterns; and in cases of relational violence, the forensic psychotherapist anticipates repetition of offence-related thoughts and feelings in relationships with staff and others. These concepts mirror that described as 'offence paralleling' [21]; another example of the overlap between forensic psycho-therapy and clinical/forensic psychology.

Conclusion

Forensic psychiatry is a branch of healthcare, where patients present with complex needs in tragic and distressing circumstances, in some ways similar to spinal rehabilitation units or palliative care. In such services, it makes sense for patients to be able to access a range of therapists who can address different aspects of their needs using different kinds of interven-tion. As a member of a team of therapists, the forensic psychotherapist offers efficient and effective therapy to help make the offender patient's mind more intelligible, coherent and safe.

Psychological Treatments in Forensic Mental Health Settings

John Marshall

Psychological Treatment of Violence, Sexual Harm and Other Offending

The interplay between early childhood experiences including adversity, temperament, neurodevelopment and resultant emotion or information processing difficulties are core psychological drivers for violence, sexual harm and other forms of offending [22]. Information processing refers to the automatic cognitive processes that occur during all forms of aggression. Emotional dysregulation also commonly underpins violence. Theoretical and scientifically informed psychological formulations are a critical component to reducing violence or sexual harm, as they attempt to unpick an individual's complex information processing signature. The way someone thinks and feels, as well as what they do, are key maintaining factors for violence. Formulations form the bedrock of psychological intervention or treatment planning.

Formulations also focus on helping professionals and their patients to understand the motivations underlying violence, and consequently their function. For example, a person who is violent after experiencing high levels of stress in the context of an intimate partner relationship may be trying to (maladaptively) exert control over their environment and communicate to the victim. They may possess insufficient coping skills to manage this scenario adaptively. They may possess attitudes that promote the use of violence and lack of concern for the victim by minimising the impact of their actions. Psychological assessment often identifies this confluence of chronic difficulties with emotional regulation skills stemming from temperamental and/or adverse childhood experiences. There are multiple targets in this example for psychological intervention, but a good formulation helps determine relevance, priorities and the sequence of psychological treatments.

Before tackling the critical drivers for violence, psychological therapists should build trust, raise hope, shift the barriers to change and locate that change to within the individual and away from the violent person's perception of being buffeted by externalised events, as is often the case. Managing emotional states, developing empathy and becoming aware of thinking states so that the patient can be changed are key. Being aware of complex trauma is important in understanding how violence and sexual harm emerged. From developmental perspectives, trauma may also be a core need for intervention because of the adverse impact on learning and maladaptive coping [23]. Appropriately accredited clinical or forensic psychologists, as well as appropriately trained and supervised psychological practitioners, have a lead role to play in advancing relevant formulation and treatment plans for violent individuals.

Psychological Treatment of Violence

The Risk Need Responsivity (RNR) model traditionally underpins psychological treatment for violence [1]. RNR is a set of principles of effective intervention where a wide variety of therapeutic interventions can be applied depending on risks and underlying needs. RNR recognises that violence or violent offending is complex and multifactorial. This means in practice that specialist high-intensity psychological treatment should be earmarked for people engaged in higher-risk offending, using structured clinical judgement methods to assess the risk.

Needs Principle

With regards to need, RNR principles draw upon well-established empirical literature about factors associated with offending. These factors include antisocial behaviour, antisocial personality, impulsivity, bold or daring temperament, pleasure-seeking, aggressive behaviours, and a callous disregard for others. Associated risks consist of poor emotional self-control, anger-management difficulties and problem-solving deficits. Commonly the targets of treatment, therefore, are to enhance these latter skills. Antisocial cognitions, including attitudes, values, beliefs and a personal identity favourable to crime, are also key areas of change. Antisocial associates, isolation from pro-social individuals or improvement in the quality of relationships are vital. Problematic domestic, social and workplace relationships are also intervention targets. Finally, substance abuse problems also need to be targeted in order to produce a positive direction of change.

The RNR model considers personal, interpersonal and social factors as being involved in the development and maintenance of criminal behaviours, such as violent offending [24]. In the case of mental disorders, where symptom issues can understandably dominate the thinking of clinicians, it is critical that criminogenic needs should also be the focus of treatment [25]. Where violent people are patients detained due to mental disorders such as psychosis as part of a schizophrenia spectrum disorder, the importance of RNR-based or criminogenic need interventions still holds. Witt et al. examined 110 eligible studies reporting on 45,533 individuals, 8,439 (18.5%) of whom were violent. A total of 39,995 (87.8%) were diagnosed with a schizophrenia spectrum disorder. These researchers found that the impact of psychotic symptoms on violence was modest compared to antisocial and aggressive traits, low empathy and pro-violent attitudes [26]. It is not an either/or but a both/and in terms of prioritisation of mental health and criminogenic needs. A good psychological formulation threads examples of these concepts together, attempting to explain the trajectory of the individual engaging in violence and identifying targets for change. It is imperative that psychiatrists and psychologists ensure that psychological factors associated with violence are tackled beyond clinical symptoms.

Responsivity Principle

Non-criminogenic factors such as personal distress have previously been viewed as tertiary, not the focus of treatment, except that such issues are relevant to the third principle of effective intervention; that is, the responsivity principle. The responsivity principle consists of two components: general and specific responsivity. The general responsivity principle states that effective interventions tend to be based on cognitive, behavioural and social learning theories. The specific responsivity principle suggests that the treatment offered is to be matched not only to criminogenic need but also to those attributes and circumstances of individuals that render them likely to benefit from that treatment [27]. However, there are also models of intervention, particularly for mentally disordered offenders which integrate responsivity and criminogenic issues through a clinical formulation. A person who engages in violent offences and, for example, meets the criteria for post-traumatic stress disorder (PTSD being viewed as a responsivity issue) may have angry outbursts and substance abuse problems (a criminogenic treatment target) because of their intrusive (PTSD) recollections or hypervigilance. In other words, PTSD symptoms, anger and substance abuse problems may act as direct drivers for violence. A clinical formulation might lead to targeting PTSD symptoms to impact on criminogenic needs and risk first, in parallel with or after CBT anger and substance abuse programmes (notwithstanding the fact that depending on the severity of difficulties, all three approaches might be required).

Although this chapter focusses on group and individual psychological treatment in order to ensure parity of service delivery, building psychological principles into daily care and treatment of violent offenders and patients using professional and scientific evidence is an important strategy. Research has consistently shown the importance of psychological aspects of care to improve health outcomes. Psychologically informed care can help people who offend using violence to reduce their distress and cope better. This is particularly true for detained patients. Infusing psychologically informed principles into nursing care may make patient hospital stays shorter and reduce their risk of reoffending. Psychological interventions described here tend to be more effective when implemented within a 'whole-systems' approach.

Matched Stepped Care

In Scotland, the Scottish Parliament and Government have promoted the creation of a number of national frameworks to allow for evidence-based care and psychological treatment to be promulgated, as well as psychological therapy protocols devised to meet the needs of specific forensic populations and allow for national treatment pathways to be delivered [28]. This Forensic Matrix prescribes a number of psychological therapies placed on a matched stepped care delivery continuum [29]. Stepped care is a system of delivering and monitoring treatments so that the most effective and least resource-intensive psychological treatment is delivered to patients first, then only 'stepping up' to intensive/specialist services as clinically required. Matched stepped care and an appropriate governance framework ensure services deliver evidence-based practices, targeting 'underlying needs', and ensure that clear treatment pathways exist, low to high-intensity interventions are provided with good fidelity, and the right people skills are in place to deliver these interventions.

The requirement to step up in intensity and expertise level of treatment is based on a clinical formulation and risk. Having the right service in the right place, at the right time delivered by the right professional, is critical to reducing risk among people who are violent. NHS Education for Scotland and the Forensic Network via the School of Forensic Mental Health (SoFMH) have also developed low-intensity psychological training for staff in forensic services to increase access to psychological therapy in forensic settings. This example of a national forensic framework ensures that psychological treatments are high up the policy and service delivery agenda.

Psychological Therapies in Intimate Partner Violence (IPV)

By way of contrast with general violence, violence against an intimate partner often reoccurs within relationships and can continue for years, with high recidivism rates and risk of lethal outcomes [30]. Typically, women who physically survive IPV are left with resultant chronic psychological difficulties [31].

CBT interventions are designed for perpetrators of IPV following the assumption that intimate partner violence is a problem located within the male perpetrator. While males do perpetrate IPV more often, one complication is that there are estimates of two-way violence in up to 50% of couples reporting IPV, albeit male violence is more serious and can be lethal [31]. Traditionally, this 'power and control' approach, where IPV was assumed to be about men maintaining power over women, took the stance of 're-educating' males [32]. CBT is still the most used and evaluated approach to IPV focussed on intra-male/perpetrator issues. However, there have been mixed outcomes for CBT to address IPV. A recent systematic review concluded that there is insufficient randomised controlled trial evidence to confirm that cognitive behavioural group therapy for perpetrators of IPV has a positive effect [33]. CBT is often delivered to groups of men. These typically men-only group CBT formats have high dropout rates and can even increase risk among men who have lower risk levels prior to commencing treatment [34]. Importantly, the design of interventions does not sufficiently take account of LGBTQIA+ relationships.

Nevertheless, there are promising psychological therapies focussing on the maladaptive communication between (heterosexual) couples. Treatment with couples may be more suited to tackling cognitive distortions fuelling violence, addressing victim-blaming and empathy. Expert psychological risk assessment and formulation is critical to ensuring the safety of victims among couples, and careful advice is needed as to whether couples therapy is indicated. With these caveats in mind, there are promising outcomes reported by helping couples solve problems together and communicate more effectively following couple-based CBT with a substantial conflict management focus [35].

Systemic couples therapy tackles relationship patterns where there is often a myriad of dysfunctional qualities. The focus of this therapy is on communication difficulties, conflict management issues, sexual problems and any other diverse concerns that might be viewed as driving violence within a psychological formulation. The key point is that the formulations need to include the couple and wider family system. A critical limitation of psychological therapies for IPV is that the interventions described in the literature concern mild to moderate situational couple violence. Situational couple violence refers to mild mutual levels of violence among partners connected to specific stressors or life events where violence is a medium maladaptively used to 'resolve' conflict. This sharply contrasts with 'intimate partner terrorism', characterised by severe physical abuse and systematic partner domination, coercion and exploitation of the woman in the relationship. Psychological approaches involving couple therapy in high-risk scenarios like these are ethically and practically questionable, and there are risks of violence during therapy where one or both partners have unreasonable expectations [36]. The focus instead should be on risk and safety planning for the likely victim where chronic abuse occurs.

Psychological Therapies for Forensic Patients

One of the challenges of treatment of forensic patients with high levels of complex difficulties is matching the available or emerging evidence base to the individual. The majority of forensic patients with psychosis, for example, also present with personality disorder, comorbid with the mental illness, substance misuse disorders and/or cognitive deficits. Such extremely complex and enduring problems demand highly specialist, individually tailored psychological interventions delivered by psychological practitioners with the highest levels of training. However, forensic patients may also have simpler underlying or associated difficulties which may respond to less intensive interventions. A model of matched stepped care can, therefore, be applied in the absence of evidence, or where evidence is emerging.

Where no standardised or single treatment is available or suitable, the appropriate approach will be to seek to understand and treat the underlying problems. In these cases, highly specialist psychological practitioners are required to use the available evidence to select, modify, adapt and evaluate psychological treatments to match the patient's risks and needs and be responsive to their particular learning styles and any cognitive deficits. Although this could be perceived as 'off-road', a number of factors are taken into account to ensure the safe and effective delivery of psychological therapies in forensic mental health services. The Forensic Mental Health Matrix is a guide in Scotland to help providers of NHS mental health services deliver evidence-based psychological therapy for patients who pose a risk of harm to others. It is intended to apply to both community and in-patient services. It is written as an addition to the general services' 'Guide to Delivering Evidence-Based Psychological Therapies in Scotland' – known as the 'Matrix'. The principles contained in that document are endorsed, and a model of matched stepped care for forensic patients is included.

The 'Forensic Mental Health Matrix' was commissioned in recognition of the specific needs of patients in forensic mental health services. These patients present with a range of clinical problems in common with other users of mental health services and in the absence of specific outcome research with samples of forensic patients, the evidence tables contained in the Matrix can be used as guides in treatment planning.

A number of key themes are set out with regards to the psychological treatment of the forensic patient:

(1) Formulation of psychological needs and delivery of psychological therapy must be carried out as part of a risk assessment and management process.

(2) Review patients' progress in psychological therapy in terms of the impact on risk.

(3) Although personality disorder is rarely the reason someone presents to mental health practitioners, understanding the effects of personality disorder plays a crucial role in addressing offending behaviour. Psychological interventions for those with personality disorders should aim to (1) help staff formulate, interact with and manage the patient, (2) improve personality functioning through specific therapies and (3) reduce the risk of reoffending through appropriately responsive offending behaviour programmes.

(4) All forensic patients in Scotland are or were subject to the Care Programming Approach (CPA). This ensures adherence to an appropriate risk assessment and management process and provides a mechanism for reviewing risk management plans, including those addressing psychological needs.

(5) Motivation to engage in treatment, known as 'readiness to change', seems to influence a person's response to psychological work. While motivational strategies with individual patients may help, a positive therapeutic ethos is also essential for readiness. Effective multidisciplinary working, robust supervision and reflective practice systems, a psychologically minded workforce, and paying close attention to the organisational, physical, social and psychological environment are important factors in this.

(6) Strengths-based approaches, such as the 'Good Lives' model, show promise. Interventions should be designed to enable individuals to make positive choices and

changes in their lives and to capitalise on natural opportunities to develop non-offending and mentally healthy lifestyles.

(7) The rights of the patient must be carefully balanced against the rights of the public to be protected from harm.

(8) Mental health services have a duty to cooperate with other agencies. This may require information sharing about patients' psychological needs or progress in therapy which is relevant to their risk management.

(9) Low-intensity interventions are brief interventions aimed at current distress or transient or mild mental health problems but may have a limited effect on overall functioning or risk of reoffending.

(10) High intensity denotes a standardised psychological therapy delivered to a formal protocol or model for mental health problems with a significant effect on functioning and where there is a significant effect on the risk of reoffending and future risk of harm.

(11) Specialist interventions are standardised high-intensity psychological therapies developed and modified for specific patient groups. These are aimed at moderate and severe mental health problems with a significant effect on functioning. The interventions themselves are generally targeted at patients with more complex risk and needs and are directly related to offending behaviour and its causes.

(12) Highly specialist interventions are psychological therapies or interventions based on case formulations that may be drawn from a range of psychological models and are individually tailored to the patient's mental health problems and where risk assessment and management are key drivers in the execution of the therapy.

In practice, a range of approaches from structuring clinical care through to high-intensity interventions are applied to forensic patients in Scotland. Training approaches from the Matrix include themes of increasing 'psychological-mindedness' (thinking about psychological issues and applying key principles related to these in day-to-day practice); 'psychological literacy' (having a good understanding of theories and models underpinning psychological practice) and how psychological theory and practice is used to help forensic patients to change.

According to the Forensic Matrix stepped care approach, different levels of intensity of interventions can be used to address forensic patients' needs. For example, a forensic patient may require psychological work aimed at improving their management of basic emotions first (low intensity) before the patient will be able to cope with the demands of treatment for sex offending or violence (specialist/highly specialist). Several psychological interventions which address different but common underlying needs of forensic patients have now been developed as part of the Forensic Matrix suite of interventions. However, there is now a critical need to evaluate the effectiveness of these therapies. Forensic patients may also require psychological interventions to address clinical symptoms that may be relevant to triggering or maintaining violence, such as Cognitive Behavioural Therapy for Psychosis (CBT-P), before addressing offending needs.

Examples of low-intensity interventions are On the Road to Recovery (OTRTR), which is a brief, group psychological intervention delivered across the Scottish Forensic Mental Health Managed Care Network ('Forensic Network'). The OTRTR protocol was written in 2011 by a working group of clinical and forensic psychologists within the Forensic Network. The programme is based on the principles of cognitive behaviour therapy with a focus on compassionate mind training [6]. The core purpose of OTRTR is to engage then open a negotiation about recovery and inculcate in patients hope that recovery is possible. It is intended to be one of the first psychological treatments offered to patients on their journey to recovery from mental health difficulties, prior to engaging in more demanding and longer-term therapies. Patients may complete OTRTR prior to high-intensity interventions for violence such as Life Minus Violence (LMV). LMV consists of a minimum of 125 treatment sessions (approximately 300 hours of therapy) of group work as well as individual cognitive rehearsal sessions to enhance learning. There is limited but emerging evidence on reduced violence, impulsivity and anger control issues post-LMV for detained patients with a mental disorder.

Psychological Therapies for People Who Sexually Harm

Balancing public fear and anxiety about people who sexually harm versus the need to ensure our communities remain safe is a challenging line to walk for professionals engaged in treatment. The role of psychological treatments in addressing the needs of people who sexually harm is critical to reducing risk. Psychological treatment for people who sexually harm has been historically dominated by CBT. It is critical to know the magnitude of the effects of these interventions and how they can be delivered with optimum impact. Meta-analysis is where researchers systematically combine and pool the findings from multiple studies to draw overall conclusions. The RNR model [25] has also been the prominent approach to the treatment of people who sexually harm others. Treatment approaches consistent with the RNR principles have been demonstrated to lead to reductions in sexual offence recidivism [37]. By contrast, criticisms levelled at RNR are that RNR-based programmes are over-focussed on criminogenic needs and risk. Criminogenic needs are general factors, such as impulsivity, that are specifically linked to offending. Proponents of a different approach known as the Good Lives Model (GLM) argue that RNR does not take account of personal and holistic needs along with practical everyday decisions people make in their lives which might promote desistence from offending [38]. Although the GLM was for a time seen as a potential replacement for RNR-based models of treatment, a consensus is emerging that there is considerable overlap between CBT and GLM models despite the difference in language. Moreover, there is a mature literature about the impact of RNR-based interventions, for example using CBT offence-focussed interventions [39]. Moving beyond the type of intervention, the role of clinical psychologists in delivery and expert supervision of treatment for people who sexually harm has become increasingly critical.

An important meta-analytic study attempted to answer the question about whether psychological treatment of people who sexually harm or offend was effective [21]. This work was imperative because a Home Office study in the English prison service showed that treatment was associated with increased recidivism. More treated sex offenders committed at least one sexual reoffence (excluding breach) during the follow-up period when compared with matched comparison offenders (10.0% compared with 8.0%) [40]. Meta-analysis also tells us which treatment strategies are most effective in reducing recidivism among people who sexually harm.

Kim et al. considered (1) effect sizes across the meta-analytic literature (i.e. a review of meta-analysis). These researchers examined effect sizes across different target populations (e.g. adolescents vs. adults) in order to examine how sex offender treatments have performed across populations, and (2) effect sizes across different types of sex offender treatments. Every meta-analysis found significant effects of treatment, and the mean effect size was d = −0.36 (range −0.15 to −0.80). These mean effect sizes suggest that the sex offender treatments produced an overall 22% reduction in recidivism [21]. However, effect sizes in treatment for adolescents compared to adults are 3.8 times greater [41]. Sex offender treatments occurring in the community produced about an overall 17% reduction in recidivism, while the grand mean effect size of institutional treatments was smaller, d = −0.20, suggesting about a 10% reduction in recidivism. In other words, psychological treatments for people who sexually offend are considered as to be 'proven or at least promising' [21, 42]. The important caveat is that the effectiveness of interventions reduces in prison [43]. There is also a lack of high-quality evidence for patients in secure hospital services, though there are examples of promising interventions [44]. The general totality of research outcomes is positive despite the historical over-focus on the ineffective prison interventions, most likely due to poor programme integrity and monitoring.

Previous treatment interventions took the form of manualised programmes. Such programmes require a psychological therapist to follow a highly detailed treatment manual. Programmes like these, if presented in a psychoeducational or didactic style, may not sufficiently take account of individualised need. People who sexually harm have substantial heterogeneity of psychological and mental health needs. It may be inappropriate to require all those who sexually harm to follow the same treatment programme rigidly. In delivering psychological treatments for sexual harm, the approach should be matched to the individual's abilities and learning styles. The general psychotherapy literature is relevant in that it identifies the need for flexibility in applying psychological treatment.

With regards to CBT interventions, although denial and minimisation do not predict future risk, it is the role of therapists to reduce denial and minimisations in order to make interventions personally relevant. People who sexually harm others should, with support, attempt to overcome denial (claiming they did not commit an offence) and minimisation (it was not their fault, or it was 'consenting' sex, or they did no harm, for example). People engaging in any harm aim to develop an internal locus of control; in other words, take some responsibility for their lives and going forward to implement new coping. Psychological therapists infuse motivational approaches throughout therapies as well as displaying warmth, empathy and support, to assist in reducing the defences of those engaging in sexual harm while at the same time being able to provide a counterpoint to developing a new approach to life.

In all psychological interventions, therapists must establish and maintain mutual trust. Building attachments, particularly for all patients in secure forensic in-patient settings, provides people with a safe base to develop trust and explore new possibilities for coping in life, including taking responsibility for problems in the past and future. People who sexually harm others, particularly those with other co-occurring mental disorders, experience profound loneliness in their lives, deficits in intimacy and attachment difficulties, and may experience high levels of shame. Even in cases of severe mental illness such as psychosis as a key offence driver, developing an internal locus of control and taking responsibility for past maladaptive coping (e.g. substance abuse, avoidance) is critical to recovery journeys. Good-quality patient–therapist relationships result from various features of the therapist's behaviour and characteristics.

People who sexually harm often have problems with emotional self-regulation. The general psychological research evidence shows that management of emotions is essential to the development of effective emotional self-regulation. Poor emotional management leading to anger, mood instability, over-excitement or low mood diverts patients from considering the long-term impacts of their behaviour to narrowing attention towards immediate satisfaction. Instant gratification or speedy satisfaction can lead to a perception of having control over a stressful environment. In other words, being emotionally dysregulated, for example, can 'work' in the short term by pushing people away. Underlying motivations like this must be considered in the formulation of sexual harm. A corollary of this for those with sexual harm interests may be the speedy satisfaction or pursuit of (deviant) sexual gratification. Managing and shifting sexual deviation is another treatment goal. These targets of interventions again are driven by a detailed individual psychological formulation.

Common chains of distorted thoughts, feelings, and behaviours link up and may lead to a sexually harmful act. Bringing these chains to the patient's awareness assists in the reduction of further risk. Learning to reduce avoidance and dealing with goals that engage with others is more likely to aid motivation and build skills for a better life.

Patients with mental disorder and/or who sexually harm others have often experienced high levels of childhood adversity, such as physical, sexual and emotional abuse or neglect in their childhoods. Ensuring that patients develop secure attachments to pro-social relatives, friends, volunteers and professional staff is a steppingstone to delivering the nuts and bolts of evidence-based interventions. This content of interventions is as important as how the interventions are delivered. Process should not usurp content and vice versa.

Psychological Therapies for People with Intellectual Disabilities

One of the most common reasons that people with intellectual disabilities (ID) come to the attention of mental health services is due to anger problems. Anger feelings strongly predict aggression and violence. Aggressive behaviour impacts on work, leisure, education and relationships generally. In secure forensic settings, problems with aggression set back recovery from other mental health problems as well as hindering progress towards lower levels of security and ultimately community placements. Where anger and violence are concerned, a risk assessment that is attuned for a person with ID leads to a formulation targeting factors which are amenable to change. Key dynamic factors in violence which are potentially changeable are feelings of anger, substance abuse, impulsiveness, antagonistic attitudes and deficits in coping skills. The mainstay of interventions for violence among people with ID is CBT; however, the challenge is to ensure responsivity in that CBT interventions are adapted for ID. The focus of CBT where anger is a driver is to normalise it, then use skills to improve emotional self-regulation such as self-monitoring, learning relaxation, changing thinking and problem-solving. Stress inoculation is critical because as a behavioural component of CBT, the person is introduced gradually to more provoking or challenging situations to apply new skills.

There is a positive evidence base for CBT approaches in ID such as randomised control studies on people with mild to moderate ID with, for example, key workers reporting their patients more able to cope with provoking situations [45]. Some studies have even tried to separate out the key treatment components of CBT for people in forensic ID settings. Relaxation training, for example, has been identified as a critical component for efficacious treatment [46]. In addition, stress inoculation techniques which involve the application of new coping skills to challenging situations are critical. Stress inoculation also includes rehearsal of skills for provoking social situations then using pro-social strategies in these situations instead of aggression.

When adapting CBT for people with ID, a number of strategies are required. These include Socratic dialogue, behavioural practice in the form of judicious use of role-playing, simple communication using short sentences and words with few syllables, checking understanding and working closely with relatives [47]. Information needs to be carefully chunked in CBT interventions for people with ID. Memory aids, the use of clear brief structure and visual supports and prompts are critical. Growing interest is also emerging in the use of mindfulness techniques and how these are integrated with CBT.

Therapeutic Safety and Security

Frontline staff who have frequent face-to-face contact with people with ID in forensic secure settings can have severe challenges to manage. These challenges can involve threats to working in a safe environment due to violence and aggression and the need to balance safety, security and opportunities for growth, along with the use of restrictive measures to prevent violence that may be counterproductive. Restrictive approaches can increase the anger, frustration and stress of patients with ID in forensic secure services [48].

Ward Atmosphere and Structured Clinical Care

In forensic secure settings, ward, climate or atmosphere can lend itself to improving the therapeutic milieu which supports individual or group treatment or conversely reinforces difficulties. Structured clinical care, which can shift ward climate, can be a psychological intervention in its own right. A high-quality social and physical environment can promote pro-social behaviour and problem-solving. However, there is limited research on the effectiveness of group climate impacts within forensic secure settings and patients with ID.

Positive Behavioural Support

A promising therapeutic milieu or staff training intervention is positive behavioural support (PBS). PBS includes a detailed functional analysis of problematic behaviours, de-escalation techniques, staff engaging in positive shaping and reinforcement of coping and pro-social skills. Patients are closely involved in their PBS plans. Evaluation of PBS in medium-secure settings demonstrates increased staff confidence in working with patients with ID in forensic contexts [49]. Increasing self-confidence and understating of contextual drivers of aggression rather than locating the problem inside the patient might help reduce the risk of occupational stress and burnout for staff. Staff training such as PBS does impact on how staff interact and provide feedback to patients with ID. However, the impact of staff training to change staff behaviour and the ecology of a forensic ward setting has been shown not to reduce challenging behaviour among ID patients [50]. This meta-analysis by Knotter and colleagues brought together different training programmes focussed on disparate challenging behaviour such as self-harm and violence, which may have affected the findings. Many training models do not aim to reduce the frequency or severity of aggressive behaviour in the first place but focus on daily structure. The future focus may be on staff training programmes that marry changes in ward or unit ecology with understanding the individualised function of aggressive behaviour for each patient.

Psychological Therapies for Violent Extremism

Radicalisation is currently the key concept underpinning risk for violent extremism. Psychological treatment for radicalisation is a controversial area with extreme limitations around definitions, the complexity of potential links between radicalisation and violence, such as terrorism, and whether interventions are or can be effective, particularly in secure or prison contexts. Radicalisation has been functionally defined as enhanced planning and groundwork for intergroup conflict and a heightened engagement to it. Radicalisation refers to a change in beliefs, feelings and behaviours that justify intergroup violence and the demand for sacrifice in defending their ingroup [51].

There are many strategies and prevention approaches at a societal and political level for deradicalisation, but the focus here is on the psychological. Some authors posit that there are many mechanisms involved in radicalisation such as cognitive openings [52], perceived injustices, ingroup–outgroup views, developing new radicalised identity to reduce uncertainty, increase pro-violence attitudes, peer group radicalisation processes, extreme religious beliefs (religiosity) or political beliefs and highly focussed goals reducing ambiguity about one's own life. Complex social psychological processes such as cohesive group identity decrease fear of death and increase the valence of self-sacrifice ideas.

For psychiatrists or psychologists, taking a categorical approach, assessing for mental disorder or illness such as psychosis, it is generally agreed that those with an extremist or radicalised proclivity are generally unlikely to be mentally ill or disordered. However, when clinicians take a dimensional approach to mental health, then problematic personality traits are more often found, as well as subclinical symptoms [53, 54]. Identification of symptoms or traits may be as relevant to a radicalisation formulation and treatment as a full diagnosis. Formulations are needed to consider the personal significance of radicalised belief systems or ideology.

Deradicalisation means rejecting an explicit commitment to violence to achieve one's means. In the UK, the PREVENT programme has been the flagship approach. PREVENT is part of the government counter-terrorism strategy CONTEST2 and aims to reduce the threat to the UK from terrorism by stopping people from becoming terrorists or supporting terrorism. PREVENT focuses on all forms of terrorism and functions in a 'pre-criminal' space'. The PREVENT strategy is focussed on providing support and re-direction to individuals at risk of or in the process of being groomed and radicalised into terrorist activity before any crime is committed. It is recommended that a thorough mental health assessment and formulation for radicalised people is important to identify mental health precursors to radicalisation and the interplay of diagnoses, psychosocial impairments, trauma, personal factors, social dynamics and environmental stressors. Treatment of these problems may be critical, and although they may be linked to radicalisation or extremism, individual, social, political and operational factors may also need to be carefully considered.

Psychological Treatment of Other Offending (Stalking, Fire-Setting)

Fire-Setting

Fire-setting refers to the intentional setting of fire that targets property or person, ignited without supervision or permission from authority. The term is common in the adolescent-based literature. Based on the Multi-Trajectory Theory of Adult Firesetting (M-TTAF), psychological interventions for adult forensic patients include the following treatment targets: (1) inappropriate fire interest and scripts, (2) offence-supportive cognitions, (3) Self-regulation and emotional regulation issues and (4) communication problems [55]. Moreover, general antisocial cognitions, scripts and values along with specific pro-fire-setting cognitions must be shifted in interventions. Interest or fascinations with fire to reduce arousal or gain pleasure may also be a key change treatment goal. Randomised control trial evidence reports efficacy of psychological interventions among adult prisoners for CBT-based group work interventions to reduce fire-setting risks [56].

Stalking

There is no one type of person who stalks. Stalking is a complex, heterogeneous problem. In the rare cases where stalking is fuelled by delusions or other symptoms of psychosis, psychiatric assessment and multidisciplinary treatment is warranted. Violence risk and threats of violence in stalking should be regarded seriously using validated structured risk assessment systems and priority given to victim self-protection measures. People who stalk share some common attitudinal states and skills deficits. Frameworks for readiness to change are important in preparation for psychological treatment. For most engaged in persistent stalking, serious and pervasive psychological problems are present [57]. Promising outcomes over 12 months have been shown for recidivistic stalking using DBT, though a more recent study indicated positive outcomes for intensive CBT for anger and DBT, suggesting high-intensity psychological support focussed on emotional regulation and positive self-management yielded benefits in different treatment modalities [58]. For the majority of stalkers, the behaviour is underpinned by more serious and pervasive problems and treatment can be a difficult and challenging endeavour.

Conclusions

Psychological treatments can be effective in reducing risk for violence and aggression, such as sexual harm in community contexts and violence among ID forensic patients. In other areas, the evidence for a positive outcome is improving, such as systemic couple approaches to IPV. One clear finding, whether the focus is on sexual harm, violence or domestic violence, is that the hands-on presence of a suitably qualified and registered psychologist, whether via supervision or delivery or both, is associated with lower levels of post-treatment recidivism [59]. Finally, there is a paucity of outcome evidence in stalking and in deradicalisation or extremist-based violence.

Despite the different pace of outcome literature, one theme remains constant, and that is that psychological formulation, taking account of likely causal mechanisms, forms the bedrock of psychological treatment planning. Understanding the multifaceted aetiology of violence among different groups is an important stepping stone towards high-quality formulation and treatment applied to the individual. Although the intensity of a psychological approach, whatever the modality, may be beneficial in some areas, CBT interventions remain the mainstay of current approaches but adapted substantially to the individual, for example CBT for psychosis or CBT adapted for ID patients. In in-patient forensic settings, group or individual therapies must be embedded within an enriching therapeutic milieu, such as delivering structured or psychologically informed care. National policies should reflect the best emerging psychological treatment evidence using stepped care models to deliver the best intervention at the right time by the most competent professional to benefit forensic patients and potential victims. Psychological treatments are a key pillar of a range of interventions for patients who are violent and present with complex forensic needs.

References

1. King S. Transformative agency and desistance from crime. *Criminology & Criminal Justice* 2013; 13 (3): 317–35.

2. Bowlby J. Forty-four juvenile thieves: their characters and home-life. *International Journal of Psycho-Analysis* 1944; 25: 19–53.

3. Bowlby J. *A Secure Base: Parent-Child Attachment and Healthy Human Development*. London, Routledge, 1988 (3rd ed., 2012).

4. Ogilvie CA, Newman E, Todd L, Peck D. Attachment and violent offending: a meta-analysis. *Aggression and Violent Behaviour* 2014; 19 (4): 322–39.

5. Fox BH, Perez N, Cass E, Baglivio MT, Epps N. Trauma changes everything: examining the relationship between adverse childhood experiences and serious, violent and chronic juvenile offenders. *Child Abuse & Neglect* 2015; 46: 163–73.

6. Hughes K, Bellis MA, Hardcastle KA et al. The effect of multiple adverse childhood experiences on health: a systematic review and meta-analysis. *The Lancet Public Health* 2017; 2 (8): e356–66.

7. Vaillant GE. *Ego Mechanisms of Defense: A Guide for Clinicians and Researchers*. Washington, DC, American Psychiatric Press, 1992.

8. Perry JC, Bond M. Change in defense mechanisms during long-term dynamic psychotherapy and five-year outcome. *American Journal of Psychiatry* 2012; 169 (9): 916–25.

9. Cramer P. Psychological maturity and change in adult defense mechanisms. *Journal of Research in Personality* 2012; 46 (3): 306–16.

10. Yakeley J, Adshead G. Locks, keys, and security of mind: psychodynamic approaches to forensic psychiatry.

11. Huband N, Duggan C, McCarthy L, Mason L, Rathbone G. Defence styles in a sample of forensic patients with personality disorder. *Personality and Mental Health* 2014; 8 (3): 238–49.

12. Tapp J, Cottle L, Christmas M et al. A psychometric evaluation of the Defence Style Questionnaire-40 in a UK forensic patient population. *The Journal of Forensic Psychiatry & Psychology* 2018; 29 (2): 288–307.

13. Steinert C, Munder T, Rabung S, Hoyer J, Leichsenring F. Psychodynamic therapy: as efficacious as other empirically supported treatments? A meta-analysis testing equivalence of outcomes. *American Journal of Psychiatry* 2017; 174 (10): 943–53.

14. Buchheim A, Viviani R, Kessler H et al. Changes in prefrontal-limbic function in major depression after 15 months of long-term psychotherapy. *PloS One* 2012; 7 (3): e33745.

15. Fonagy P, Levinson A. Offending and attachment: the relationship between interpersonal awareness and offending in a prison population with psychiatric disorder. *Canadian Journal of Psychoanalysis* 2004; 12 (2): 225–51.

16. Bateman AW, Fonagy PE. *Handbook of Mentalizing in Mental Health Practice*. Washington, DC, American Psychiatric Publishing, Inc., 2012.

17. Benefield N, Joseph N, Skett S et al. The offender personality disorder strategy jointly delivered by NOMS and NHS England. *Prison Service Journal* 2015; 218: 4–9.

18. Marshall WL, Burton DL. The importance of group processes in offender treatment. *Aggression and Violent Behavior* 2010; 15 (2): 141–9.

The *Journal of the American Academy of Psychiatry and the Law* 2013 41 (1): 38–45.

19. Lyth, IM. *Containing Anxiety in Institutions: Selected Essays, Vol. 1.* London, Free Association Books, 1988.

20. Kahneman, D. *Thinking, Fast and Slow.* London, Macmillan, 2011.

21. Daffern M, Jones L, Shine J (eds) *Offence Paralleling Behaviour: A Case Formulation Approach to Offender Assessment and Intervention* (Vol. 48). Chichester, John Wiley & Sons, 2010.

22. Ireland J, Ireland C. Therapeutic treatment approaches for violence: some essential components. In JL Ireland, CA Ireland, P Birch (eds) *Violent and Sexual Offenders: Assessment, Treatment and Management* (2nd ed.). New York, Routledge, 2019, pp. 319–41.

23. Hacker H. Trauma and its treatment in forensic settings. In JL Ireland, P Birch, CA Ireland (eds) *Routledge International Handbook on Aggression.* London, Taylor and Francis, 2017.

24. Ogloff JTP, Davis MR. Advances in offender assessment and rehabilitation: contributions of the risk-need-responsivity approach. *Psychology Crime & Law* 2004; 10: 229–42.

25. Andrews DA, Bonta J. *The Psychology of Criminal Conduct* (5th ed.). New Providence, NJ, LexisNexis Matthew Bender, 2010.

26. Witt K, van Dorn R, Fazel S. Risk factors for violence in psychosis: systematic review and meta-regression analysis of 110 studies. *PloS One* 2013; 8 (2).

27. Andrews D, Bonta J, Hoge R. Classification for effective rehabilitation. *Criminal Justice and Behaviour* 1990; 17: 19–52.

28. *Mental Health in Scotland: A Guide to Delivering Evidence-Based Psychological Therapies in Scotland – The Matrix, 2011* (NHS Education for Scotland and The Scottish Government, 2011 and 2015).

29. *The Matrix, A Guide to Delivering Evidence-Based Psychological Therapies in Scotland,* 2015.

30. Vatnar SKV, Bjørkly S. Lethal intimate partner violence: an interactional perspective on women's perceptions of lethal incidents. *Violence and Victims* 2013; 28 (5): 772–89.

31. Hurless N, Cottone RR. Considerations of conjoint couples therapy in cases of intimate partner violence. *The Family Journal;* 2018, 26 (3): 324–9.

32. Armenti NA, Babcock JC. Conjoint treatment for intimate partner violence: a systematic review and implications. *Couple and Family Psychology: Research and Practice* 2016; 5 (2): 109–23.

33. Nesset MB, Lara-Cabrera ML, Dalsbø TK et al. Cognitive behavioural group therapy for male perpetrators of intimate partner violence: a systematic review. *BMC Psychiatry* 2019; 19 (1): 11.

34. Babcock J, LaTaillade J. Evaluating interventions for men who batter. In Vincent J, Jouriles E (eds) *Domestic Violence: Guidelines for Research-Informed Practice.* Philadelphia, PA, Jessica Kingsley Publishers, 2000, pp. 37–77.

35. Karakurt G, Whiting K, van Esch C et al. Couples therapy for intimate partner violence: a systematic review and meta-analysis. *Journal of Marital Family Therapy* 2016; 42 (4): 567–83.

36. Zahl-Olsen R, Gausel N, Zahl-Olsen A et al. Physical couple and family violence among clients seeking therapy: identifiers and predictors. *Frontiers in Psychology* 2019; 10: 2847.

37. Hanson RK, Bourgon G, Helmus G et al. The principles of effective correctional treatment also apply to sexual offenders: a meta-analysis. *Criminal Justice and Behavior* 2009; 36: 865–91.

38. Laws DR, Ward T. *Desistance from Sex Offending: Alternatives to Throwing Away the Key.* New York, The Guilford Press, 2011.

39. Looman J, Abracen J. The risk need responsivity model of offender rehabilitation: is there really a need for a paradigm shift? *International Journal of Behavioural Consultation and Therapy* 2013; 8 (3–4): 30–6.

40. Mews A, Di Bella L, Purver M. *Impact Evaluation of the Prison-Based Core Sex Offender Treatment Programme* (Ministry

of Justice Analytical Series). London, Ministry of Justice, 2017.

41. Walker SC, Bishop AS. Length of stay, therapeutic change, and recidivism for incarcerated juvenile offenders. *Journal of Offender Rehabilitation* 2016; 55 (6): 355–76.

42. Nagayama Hall GC. Sexual offender recidivism revisited: a meta-analysis of recent treatment studies. In Database of Abstracts of Reviews of Effects (DARE): Quality-Assessed Reviews. York, Centre for Reviews and Dissemination (UK), 1995.

43. Lösel F, Link E, Schmucker M et al. On the effectiveness of sexual offender treatment in prisons: a comparison of two different evaluation designs in routine practice. *Sex Abuse* 2020; 32(4): 452–75.

44. Clarke C, Tapp J, Lord A, Moore E. Group-work for offender patients on sex offending in a high security hospital: investigating aspects of impact via qualitative analysis. *Journal of Sexual Aggression* 2013; 19 (1): 50–65.

45. Willner P, Rose J, Jahoda A et al. Group-based cognitive-behavioural anger management for people with mild to moderate intellectual disabilities: cluster randomised controlled trial. *The British Journal of Psychiatry* 2013; 203: 288–96.

46. Bellemans T, Didden R, Van Busschbach J et al. Psychomotor therapy targeting anger and aggressive behavior in individuals with mild or borderline intellectual disabilities: a systematic review. *Journal of Intellectual and Developmental Disabilities* 2019; 44: 121–30.

47. Lindsay W. Adaptations and developments in treatment programmes for offenders with developmental disabilities. *Psychiatry, Psychology and Law* 2009; 16: S18–S35.

48. Hawkins S, Allen D, Jenkins R. The use of physical interventions with people with intellectual disabilities and challenging behaviour: the experiences of service users and staff members. *Journal of Applied Research in Intellectual Disabilities* 2005; 18: 19–34.

49. Davies B, Griffiths J, Liddiard K et al. Changes in staff confidence and attributions for challenging behaviours after training in positive behavioural support within a forensic medium secure service. *The Journal of Forensic Psychiatry & Psychology* 2015; 26: 847–61.

50. Knotter M, Spruit A, De Swart J et al. Training direct care staff working with persons with intellectual disabilities and challenging behaviour: a meta-analytic review study. *Aggression and Violent Behaviour* 2018; 40: 60–72.

51. Trip S, Bora CH, Marian M et al. Psychological mechanisms involved in radicalization and extremism: a rational emotive behavioral conceptualization. *Frontiers in Psychology.* 2019; 10: 437.

52. Wiktorowicz Q. *Radical Islam Rising: Muslim Extremism in the West.* Lanham, MD, Rowman and Littlefield Publishers, 2005.

53. Gøtzsche-Astrup O, Lindekilde L. Either or? Reconciling findings on mental health and extremism using a dimensional rather than categorical paradigm. *Journal of Forensic Science* 2019; 64: 982–8.

54. Bhui K, Otis M, Silva MJ, Halvorsrud K, Freestone M, Jones E. Extremism and common mental illness: cross-sectional community survey of White British and Pakistani men and women living in England. *Br J Psychiatry.* 2019: 1–8.

55. Gannon TA, Ciardha CÓ, Doley RM, Alleyne E. The Multi-Trajectory Theory of Adult Firesetting (M-TTAF). *Aggression and Violent Behaviour* 2012; 17 (2): 107–21.

56. Gannon TA, Alleyne E, Butler H et al. Specialist group therapy for psychological factors associated with fire setting: evidence of a treatment effect from a non-randomized trial with male prisoners. *Behaviour Research and Therapy* 2015; 73: 42–51.

57. MacKenzie RD, James DV. Management and treatment of stalkers: problems, options, and solutions. *Behavior Science & Law* 2011; 29: 220–39.

58. Rosenfeld B, Galietta M, Foellmi M et al. Dialectical behavior therapy (DBT) for the treatment of stalking offenders: a randomized controlled study. *Law and Human Behavior* 2019; 43 (4): 319–28.

59. Gannon TA, Olver ME, Mallion JS, James M. Does specialized psychological treatment for offending reduce recidivism? A meta-analysis examining staff and program variables as predictors of treatment effectiveness. *Clinical Psychology Review* 2019; 73: 101752.

Forensic Aspects of Medical Negligence

Damian J. Mohan

Introduction

Patients who have suffered a personal injury as a result of clinical negligence should be compensated appropriately and as quickly as the circumstances in their cases allow. Historically, the clash between the plaintiff's right not to be harmed and the defendant's right to retain a good reputation has led to the evolution of an adversarial court system as a means of resolving the litigation. Future direction will involve the development of alternative systems and case management process to deal with clinical negligence claims. The alternative systems proposed will be discussed later in this chapter. Meanwhile, for the practising forensic psychiatrist, there are two aspects of interest – how to avoid being found negligent and how to give expert evidence in relation to clinical negligence. The focus of this chapter is on the latter rather than the former.

Many patients who are the victims of medical negligence, such as failed surgery or misdiagnosis, go on to develop psychiatric complications, such as a depressive disorder or an adjustment disorder, associated with the disability arising out of the said negligence. In these cases, a psychiatric expert is instructed to undertake a psychiatric evaluation and provide an expert report on 'condition and prognosis'. This chapter seeks to provide an overview of the legal and medical principles that underpin medical negligence litigation, including the definition of medical negligence, what constitutes a psychiatric injury, the psychiatric evaluation and practical issues which commonly arise when undertaking a psychiatric assessment in the context of clinical negligence litigation. A more in-depth discussion of the subject can be found in two excellent textbooks, *Psychiatry and the Law* [1] and *Clinical Practice and the Law* [2].

Less frequently, a psychiatric expert will be instructed to provide an expert report on the standard of psychiatric care provided, usually following a death or misadventure, such as a suicide. In such cases, the psychiatric expert will be required to undertake a 'psychiatric autopsy', which will involve a forensic examination of the clinical records and hospital policies and an expert opinion on whether the standard of care provided met the threshold of care that 'an ordinary, prudent professional with the same training and experience in good standing in a same or similar community would practice under the same or similar circumstances'.[1] This type of system analysis is outside the scope of this chapter.

Tort of Negligence

A tort is an act or omission that gives rise to injury or harm to another and amounts to a civil wrong for which courts impose liability. Negligence 'is the omission to do something which

---

[1] *Vaughan v Menlove* [1837] 3 Bing NC 468, 132 ER 490 (CP).

a reasonable person, guided upon those considerations which ordinarily regulate the conduct of human affairs, would do or doing something which a prudent and reasonable person would not do'.[2]

The tort of negligence will arise when three criteria are met:

- The defendant owes the plaintiff a duty of care.
- There is a breach of the expected duty.
- As a result of that breach, the plaintiff is injured.

Criminal Negligence

Most legal actions that relate to clinical practice are civil actions for medical negligence. In a small number of cases, gross medical negligence can lead to criminal liability. If a doctor's actions are so negligent as to cause the death of a patient, then they may be charged with manslaughter, which is known as 'gross negligence manslaughter'.[3] There have been several such cases in the UK.[4]

In 2015, a doctor was found guilty of 'manslaughter by gross negligence' in Nottingham Crown Court before a jury. The judge sentenced her to a two-year jail term suspended for two years. She appealed twice to the Court of Appeal and lost both times. In April 2019, the trainee paediatrician was allowed to return to practice under close supervision after a medical practitioners' tribunal deemed her to be a low risk to patients. The tribunal found 'extensive and substantial' mitigating factors in her case, including remorse, insight and remediation, as well as the support of her employers and her Deanery. It imposed a range of conditions on her practice for a period of two years, beginning in July 2019, when her current suspension ended.

Medical Negligence

There are three main elements to clinical negligence: (a) duty of care, (b) breach of duty and (c) causation.

Duty of Care

In medical negligence claims, the existence of the duty is usually clear. The class of persons to whom the duty is owed, generally patients, is usually readily identifiable.[5]

Some exceptions can be identified where a doctor is engaged to assess a person who is not ordinarily a patient of the clinician in question. Examples include: (i) patients who are referred for a pre-employment medical examination; (ii) a doctor who is called to a police station to examine a patient; (iii) examination on behalf of an insurance company; and (iv) an examination by a public health doctor for child welfare or other reasons.

In some common law jurisdictions, there is an emerging body of law which suggests that, in some circumstances, the mere fact that a doctor is retained to examine a person on behalf of a third party does not exempt the doctor from owing a duty to that patient. Following a UK Supreme Court decision in *Jones v Kaney*,[6] expert witnesses are now exposed to the

---

[2] *Blyth v Birmingham Waterworks Co.* [1956] 11 Ex Ch 781 at 784.
[3] *The People (AG) v Dunleavey* [1948] IR 95.
[4] *R v Adomako* [1995] 1 AC 1; *R v Misra* [2004] EWCA Crm 2375.
[5] See *Barnett v Chelsea & Kensington Hospital Management Committee* [1969] ALL RE 1068.
[6] *Jones v Kaney* [2011] UKSC 13.

risk of being sued in respect of evidence given in court. In Ireland, a High Court Judge, after hearing an expert who omitted details of relevant past medical history, formed the view that the expert's 'failure to do so was reprehensible', and directed that his judgment be forwarded to the Irish Medical Council.[7]

Vicarious (Institutional) Liability

Vicarious liability is a form of secondary liability whereby an employer may be liable for acts of its employees committed in the course or scope of their employment. This is an important concept when assessing liability. In general, 'The hospital system within which medical people operate is required to be such that it supports the competence and level of professional expertise that attends a busy maternity unit. Those professionals attending women in childbirth are entitled to the support which proper hospital administration provides to professionals working within that system.'[8]

Standard of Care and Breach of Duty

Addressing the question of standard of care will be a matter for the instructing lawyer. The principles applicable in cases of medical negligence are relatively clear from *Bolam v Friern Hospital Management Committee*[9] and more latterly in *Bolitho v City and Hackney Authority*.[10]

A modern view of the principles which underpin the assessment of a medical negligence claim can be found in the 'Dunne Principles'. The guidelines which govern the assessment of expected standards of care for medical practitioners are clearly set out in *Dunne (a Minor) v National Maternity Hospital & Anor* [1989][11] and are summarised in Box 16.1.

Box 16.1 Dunne Principles.

1 The true test for establishing negligence in diagnosis on the part of the medical practitioner is whether he has been proved to be guilty of such failure as no medical practitioner of equal specialist or general status and skill would be guilty of, if acting with ordinary care.

2 If the allegation of negligence against the medical practitioner is based on proof that he deviated from a general and approved practice that will not establish negligence unless it is also proved that the course he did take was one which no medical practitioner of like specialisation and skill would have followed, had he been taking the ordinary care required from a person of his qualifications.

3 It is quite in order for an honest difference of opinion to arise between two doctors as to which is the better of two ways of treating a patient and the following of one course rather than the other does not imply negligence.

4 It is not up to the judge to decide which of two alternative courses is in his opinion preferable, but his function is merely to decide whether the course of treatment followed complied with the careful conduct of a medical practitioner of like specialisation and skill to that professed by the doctor in question.

---

[7] *Waliszewski v McArthur & Co.* (steel and metal) Ltd [2015] Barton Justice.
[8] *HM v HSE* [2011] IEHC. [9] [1957] 2 All RR 118. [10] [1997] 4 All ER 771. [11] [1989] IR 91.

It will be noted that the principles are applied expressly to matters of diagnosis and treatment. The standard applicable to alleged non-disclosure of operative risks remained unclear for a considerable time until a decision of the Irish High Court in *Geoghegan v Harris*.[12] The decision of the United Kingdom Supreme Court in *Montgomery v Lanarkshire Health Board*[13] eventually brought English (and Scottish) law into line with the rest of the common law world.

Causation

(i) Definition of causation: 'Causation' means the issue of whether the act of the defendant caused the plaintiff the damage complained of. It is the plaintiff, as the person alleging negligence, who must introduce expert medical evidence. There is an obligation on any party intending to sue another, alleging professional negligence, to obtain a supportive expert opinion first before embarking on this course.[14] Supreme Court Denham J. stated: 'It is important in professional negligence cases to act reasonably. Proceedings must have an appropriate basis; Counsel has a duty of care.'[15]

(ii) Causation – informed consent and foreseeability: It will be a matter for the instructing solicitor to be satisfied about the prospects of success on the issue of breach of duty and /or causation. Often proving causation in medical negligence cases is difficult as the client may have elected for treatment, even if warned of the risk. The guiding principles relating to informed consent are set out in *Montgomery v Lanarkshire Health Board*[16] as follows:

> The doctor is under a duty to take reasonable care to ensure that the patient is aware of any material risks involved in any recommended treatment and of any reasonable alternative or variant treatment. The test of materiality is whether in the circumstances of the particular case, a reasonable person in the patient's position would be likely to attach significance to the risk or the doctor is or should be reasonably aware that the particular patient would be likely to attach significance to it.

Hence, before commencing any procedure or treatment, consent must be tailored to the individual and provided in a form of language easily understood by the patient. The treating doctor should know and understand the patient's views and values. In undertaking a medical negligence evaluation, where the issue of consent is retrospectively called in to question, the psychiatric expert may be asked to retrospectively assess the patient's capacity to provide informed consent at the time of the alleged medical negligence. A detailed examination of medical records should take place to see whether the patient's version of events is supported by the medical records.

(iii) Causation – the 'but for' test: Causation is often more hotly contested in medical negligence than in other forms of negligence. Sometimes it happens because the case is so complex that liability or causation have been difficult to determine or are in dispute. An obvious reason for this might be a medical negligence claim, whereby the plaintiff is usually someone with a pre-existing illness or someone undergoing

---

[12] [2000] 3 IR 536. [13] [2015] UKSC 11, [2015] 2ALL ER 1031, [2015] 2 WLR 768.
[14] *Reidy v National Maternity Hospital* [1997] IEHC 143 HC. [15] *Connolly v Casey* [1998] IEHC 90.
[16] *Montgomery v Lanarkshire Health Board* [2015] UKSC 11.

a procedure that, even if competently performed, could have significant risks. As a result, it is often more difficult to prove that negligent treatment, rather than the original illness, or the procedure or treatment being provided, was the cause of the ultimate damage. Put simply, the 'but for' test asks whether the plaintiff would have been unscathed 'but for' the negligent act.

The classical illustration of this principle is found in the case of *Barnett v Chelsea and Kensington Hospital Management Committee*.[17] In this case, a number of night watchmen presented at the accident and emergency department of the defendant hospital complaining of stomach pains, having accidentally consumed arsenic. The defendant doctor refused to see them, thus breaching his duty of care. However, the medical evidence before the court demonstrated that even if the men had been treated when they arrived at the hospital and had been afforded with the best available treatment, the poisoning was sufficiently serious that they would have died anyway. It was the arsenic, and not the negligent failure to treat, that killed the men.

(iv) Causation – 'material contribution': The obligation is on the plaintiff to show that their case on causation is the more likely than not. In doing so, the expert should differentiate between the effects of poor treatment and the underlying pathology. The expert should always consider the 'but for' test and form an opinion on whether the treatment complained of may have 'materially contributed' to the patient's injury.

(v) Causation – 'loss of chance': Loss of chance arises where the plaintiff suffers no direct harm as a result of the negligence; instead, the acts or omissions of a defendant cause the patient to lose a chance of recovery that they might otherwise have had. Loss of chance claims often arise in delay in diagnosis of cancer cases.

(vi) Causation – the doctrine of *res ipsa loquitur* in clinical negligence cases: The onus of proof always rests with the plaintiff. The plaintiff must prove on the balance of probabilities that the alleged act or omission caused the alleged damage as well as proving that the act itself was negligent. Sometimes, the patient will not have to prove that a specific act caused the damage. For example, if a healthy person is subject to an anaesthetic and there is a failure to return the patient to consciousness, this scenario is called *res ipsa loquitur* or 'the facts speak for themselves'. In such cases, the court may be permitted to draw an inference of negligence from the facts that have been proved. Where a claim of *res ipsa loquitur* is made, the onus is on the defendant to explain the plaintiff's injury and to show that it did not result from any negligence on the part of the defendant.

(vii) Causation – psychiatric specifics and clinical negligence cases: In providing care for psychiatric patients, there is an obligation to act to vindicate the right to life and prevent suicide. In *Savage*[18] the claimant said that the defendant hospital had been negligent in failing to prevent her daughter escaping from the mental hospital at which she was detained and committing suicide. The Trust failed in their appeal against a refusal to strike out the claim that they had been negligent in having inadequate security. This is consistent with Article 2 of the European Convention on Human Rights (ECHR) in which the authorities are under a duty to protect persons in custody or in a vulnerable position.[19]

---

[17] *Barnett v Chelsea and Kensington Hospital Management Committee* [1969] 1 QB 428.
[18] Savage v South Essex Partnership NHS Foundation Trust and Another CA 21-Dec-2007.
[19] *Keenan v. the United Kingdom – 27229/95* [2001] ECHR 242 (3 April 2001).

Negligence Claims: Statute of Limitations and Date of Knowledge

There is a limited time within which patients can make a medical negligence claim against a doctor. The reason for having a statute of limitations is to ensure that the defendant is not unfairly prejudiced by the passage of time. The term 'statute of limitations' refers to the length of time within which a person must make a personal injury claim following an injury. The general rule for adults in the UK who are considering making a claim for personal injury compensation is three years from the date of the injury in which to bring a claim. There are many variants on this internationally. In the Republic of Ireland, the rules surrounding this time limit are set out in the Statute of Limitations Act 1957. A person has two years, less one day, from the 'date of knowledge' to bring a claim forward. It is not uncommon for the plaintiff's solicitor to issue proceedings without an expert report to prevent a claim becoming 'statute barred'.

The cause of action in most medical negligence cases will be the date of the actual injury from a particular operation, procedure or treatment. In cases where the plaintiff does not realise that they had a cause for action or has developed a medical problem from a particular operation or procedure after the limitation period has expired, the 'date of knowledge' is examined.

The 'date of knowledge' of an injured patient is the date on which they first knew that they had been injured and that the injury was significant and attributable to the wrongful act of another identified person or persons. The 'date of knowledge' test provides that the three-year period (two years in Ireland) within which the plaintiff who is claiming to have suffered medical negligence will not begin until the date upon which the plaintiff becomes aware of all the following pieces of information:

- That the plaintiff has suffered an injury.
- That the injury suffered is significant.
- That the injury was caused by the fault of someone else.
- The identity of the person who caused the injury.
- If the fault for the injury lies with someone other than the person who is liable to compensate the plaintiff, the identity of the person who actually caused the injury and the legal basis as to why this person is liable.

When undertaking a psychiatric assessment for the purpose of preparing an expert report in a medical negligent action, inquiries should be made to determine the 'date of knowledge'.

The 'date of knowledge' test can prevent injustice from occurring in many scenarios. Take, for example, a situation where a doctor prescribes a patient with inappropriate medication over a period which has the effect of causing them serious organ damage. While the injury may be very serious in nature, it might well not manifest itself for several years. If the patient does not begin to experience serious symptoms until three years after the medication has been taken, an absolute application of the three-year (two in Ireland) rule would mean that any claim against the doctor would be barred by the 'statute of limitations', notwithstanding the fact that the patient could not possibly have known that they were the victim of medical negligence at any time in that period. However, the application of the 'date of knowledge' test in such a case would mean that the three- (or two-)year period would only start to run from the date that the patient found out that they had suffered a serious injury (organ damage) and that this injury was caused by someone's negligence (the doctor's prescription of inappropriate medication).

Allowances are made for minors (i.e. children under 18 years). An injured minor has a three-year period (two years in Ireland) from the date of their 18th birthday in which to initiate legal proceedings. A minor can, however, pursue a claim before their 18th birthday provided a parent or guardian acts as their 'next friend'; that is, as an individual who acts on behalf of another individual but does not have the legal capacity to act on their own behalf.

Plaintiffs who are mentally disabled have a period of three years (two years in Ireland) from the date on which they cease to be under the disability or the date of their death. This allows a permanently mentally disabled person to take legal action through their 'next friend' in relation to any alleged medical negligence at any time.

Expert advice and its effect on statutory limitation periods was considered by the Supreme Court in *Green v Hardiman*.[20] The decision of Charleston J considered that in circumstances where expert advice is required to establish undiscovered injuries caused by negligence, incorrect expert advice about the injury could have the effect of stopping the clock for the purposes of the statutory limitation.

Psychiatric Injury

After the shock, trauma and pain of physical injury or disease as a result of clinical negligence, it is not uncommon for patients to develop psychiatric injuries, such as depression, anxiety or post-traumatic stress disorder (PTSD). Such conditions can often be debilitating. The effects can be life-changing and the severity of psychiatric injuries should not be underestimated. The courts have recognised that psychiatric illness or injury, including 'nervous shock', can constitute harm.[21]

If a person who has suffered a physical injury has also suffered a psychiatric injury, appropriate compensation can be sought to compensate them for their pain and suffering and, perhaps more importantly, to ensure that any future necessary treatment is provided for.

In many cases, victims of clinical negligence do not necessarily realise that they have suffered a psychiatric injury. The plaintiff's solicitor will be aware of the possibility of psychiatric injury and, in cases where it may be relevant, will refer the plaintiff for evaluation and preparation of an expert medicolegal report.

'Nervous Shock' and 'Recognised Psychiatric Illness'

Claimants must prove that their psychiatric damage amounts to 'a recognised psychiatric illness'. 'Nervous shock' is the legal term for psychiatric or psychological injury. Psychiatric Injuries include depression, PTSD and anxiety or panic attacks. Mental distress and mild anxiety falling short of psychiatric or psychological injury do not give rise to liability. There is no recovery for mere distress, emotional upset or 'shock' in the ordinary everyday sense. Hence, the primary function of the psychiatric expert is to carry out a detailed assessment and to form an opinion as to whether the injured person is suffering from a 'recognised psychiatric disorder'.

---

[20] *Green v Hardiman* [2019] IESC 51. [21] *R v Morris* [1998] 1 Cr App R 368.

Eggshell Rule

In taking a careful history, inquiries should be made about the presence or otherwise of a pre-existing psychiatric disorder. Lawyers refer to the term 'eggshell rule'. The so-called eggshell rule requires the defendant to take the claimant as they find them. In other words, if the injured party has a pre-condition which left them more vulnerable, so that an injury would have a far more significant impact on that party, then the defendant cannot raise this as a defence and must compensate accordingly.

Psychiatric Diagnosis

In setting out the psychiatric diagnosis, if any, a paragraph on each diagnosis will suffice. It is usual to use *International Classification of Diseases* (ICD)-10 or the *Diagnostic and Statistical Manual of Mental Disorders* (5th ed.) (DSM-5) diagnoses and to use code numbers. The doctor should determine the existence of any psychiatric disorder and its relationship to the medical negligence.

In his book *Expert Psychiatric Evidence* [3] (p. 127), Rix makes the following recommendations when formulating an opinion on psychiatric injury:

- 'Justify the diagnosis by reference to symptoms and signs. Indicate the extent to which the evidence from the medical records supports the diagnosis. Indicate to what extent there is other corroborative evidence. Make clear if the diagnosis is based entirely on self-report.'
- 'If diagnoses have been suggested by other experts and these are not supported, indicate this and say why.'
- 'Commonly there may be a range of reasonable opinion as to diagnosis. State what other diagnoses may reasonably be made and indicate why your diagnosis is to be preferred.'

Mental Injury and the Law: Hillsborough Disaster – Primary and Secondary Victims

The Hillsborough Disaster refers to the events of 15 April 1989 when a human crush occurred in the Leppings Lane stand of Hillsborough Stadium in Sheffield during an FA Cup semi-final, with 96 fatalities and over 760 injuries. Hillsborough is remembered primarily for the physical injuries. The disaster also inflicted psychological damage on family members who were seated in different sections of the stadium to their loved ones and watched helplessly as the crush developed. Live broadcast on television and radio meant that the trauma was transmitted directly to thousands who had family at the game. Many witnesses went on to develop PTSD.

Hillsborough was to become a key event in determining legal precedent and the resultant case law would determine how law would deal with psychiatric injury. In the years immediately following the tragedy, controversial judicial decisions in cases such as *Alcock*[22] developed the English common law in relation to the rules on 'primary victims' and 'secondary victims' of negligently inflicted psychiatric injury. A claimant can only claim for psychiatric harm if they suffer or have suffered from a recognised medical condition, such as PTSD. *Alcock* added that the condition must be induced by shock. Damages cannot

---

[22] *Alcock v Chief Constable of South Yorkshire* [1991] UKHL.

be awarded for the ordinary grief or sorrow caused by a person's death. In the *Alcock* case, it was Lord Oliver's judgment which created a formal distinction between 'primary' and 'secondary' victims, namely those in the area of danger or at risk of danger (primary) and those who witnessed the events (secondary).

The rules for primary victims are relatively straightforward. The claimant must have suffered a recognised psychiatric disorder, and there must be reasonable foreseeability of the risk of physical injury following the defendant's negligence, even if the psychiatric harm itself was not reasonably foreseeable. In contrast, for claims brought by secondary victims, although the requirement to have suffered a recognised condition remains, there are additional criteria that claimants must satisfy. In the 1991 case of *Alcock*, 10 claimants sought damages for the mental injuries they incurred following Hillsborough. They made their claim as secondary victims. None had been present in the stands where the crush occurred. The relation to the event was not primary, in that they were not the ones in imminent danger of being crushed. Instead, they were indirect victims. Their injury was as the result of processing the harm that had been inflicted on their loved ones. The claims of all 10 were dismissed. In his judgment, Lord Oliver outlined four cumulative criteria that set an extremely high benchmark for any claim to succeed. These are termed the 'Alcock Principles'. To qualify for damages, a victim of mental injury sustained after witnessing harm brought upon a loved one through the negligence of a third party must:

1. Have a relationship of love and affection with the primary victim. This was presumed to exist only between parent and child and spouses. Claimants who lost siblings, grandchildren or others were therefore excluded.

2. Have a direct perception of the event with unaided senses. This clause disqualified the witnessing of the events via television or radio.

3. Have proximity to the event or its immediate aftermath. Proximity was whether one's injury occurred close enough in time to the event, which was determined by the judges. The period of eight hours that expired before the mother identified her son's remains in the mortuary was deemed excessive.

4. Experience psychological injury from a single nervous shock. By this the judges argued that an event could only refer to a single incident that occurred in a single moment in time and not a series of interconnected developments that spanned many hours.

Other jurisdictions have other interpretations. The Irish courts remain reluctant to adopt the categorisation of nervous shock victims as 'primary' or 'secondary' victims. In Ireland, the starting point for determining liability in negligently inflicted psychiatric injury of persons in a close relationship with the primary victim are the principles set out in *Kelly v Hennessy*.[23] This case sets out the tests required for 'proximity of the relationship, spatial proximity and temporal proximity'. The recent High Court case of *Lisa Sheehan v Bus Éireann/Irish Bus and Vincent Dower*[24] presents a useful summary of the law on negligently inflicted psychiatric injuries.

---

[23] *Kelly v Hennessy* [S.C. No. 159 of 1993].
[24] *Lisa Sheehan v Bus Éireann/Irish Bus and Vincent Dower* [2020] IEHC 160.

Loss of Consortium

Being the victim of medical negligence can have a devastating effect not only on the patient but also on their family. As outlined in the previous subsection, in the UK the law does allow for psychiatric injury claims to be made by 'secondary victims'; that is, those that may have suffered a loss as a result of the medical negligence involving a loved one (primary victim) but have not themselves suffered physical harm. For example, where a person is significantly injured by medical negligence, the partner of that person may have a claim for 'loss of consortium'. For a spouse to succeed in such a claim, it must be proved that they have suffered the total loss of the ordinary incidents of an ongoing marital relationship and that, as a matter of probability, the legal and factual cause of such loss was an injury to their spouse that resulted from negligence or breach of duty on the part of the defendant.[25]

Accepting Instructions

What Is an Expert?

The reader is referred to the textbook *A Guide to Expert Witness Evidence* [4]. The expert must be qualified in the field in which expertise is claimed. The function of expert witnesses is to assist the court in evaluating the facts proven in evidence. An expert should not go beyond their field and should not give opinion on the final issue [5, 6]. The independent role and function of an expert in court is clearly outlined in the *Ikarian Reefer* judgment[26] and updated in the *Anglo Group plc* judgment.[27] Box 16.2 displays the duties of an expert witness as set out in the *Ikarian Reefer* judgment.

Discovery

If you are satisfied that you have the requisite expertise and are not conflicted, the next step is to seek a formal letter of instruction outlining the background to the case and the issues to be addressed. It is important to have a copy of the book of pleadings, which include the Personal Injuries Summons and Replies to Particulars.

Medical reports and medical records should also be made available to the expert in advance of meeting the plaintiff. Often the plaintiff may have attended several hospitals. It is essential that notes are taken up from all the hospitals in which the patient was treated, and not just from the hospital which is the subject of the complaint. Primary care physician records are essential. Often there is a telling note or letter in the non-offending hospitals records or the primary care physician notes that may be crucial to the matter under litigation. If you are the expert engaged by the plaintiff's solicitor, the instructing solicitor should be the person who coordinates the taking up of the medical records. If you are engaged by the defendant's solicitor, a court order may be required for discovery of medical records in cases where disclosure is not forthcoming.

---

25 *Andaloc v Irarnrod Eireann and others* [2014] 3 IR 516.
26 *National Justice Compania Naviera S.A. v. Prudential Assurance Co. Ltd* [1993].
27 *Anglo Group Plc v Winther Brown & Co Limited and BML (Office Computers) Limited [2000] 72 Con LR 118 (TCC). 343. ITCLR 559.*

> **Box 16.2 Ikarian Reefer: duties of an expert [7, 8].**
>
> 1 Expert evidence should be the independent product of the expert uninfluenced by the exigencies of the litigation.
> 2 An expert should give objective unbiased opinion in relation to matters within his expertise.
> 3 An expert should state the facts and assumptions upon which his opinion is based and not omit to consider material facts which could detract from his concluded opinion.
> 4 An expert should make it clear when a particular issue falls outside his expertise.
> 5 An expert should indicate if insufficient data is available in which case his opinion is provisional.

The Psychiatric Interview

This will involve the patient meeting with a consultant psychiatrist in a professional setting, where a full assessment can take place. From personal experience, patients referred for assessment in the context of medical negligence cases are fearful, sometimes angry and nearly always distrustful of the medical profession. These emotions are entirely understandable. The expert should be well prepared in advance to ensure that the patient is met with sensitivity and professionalism. The interviewing psychiatrist should allocate extra time when undertaking an evaluation of a patient who is the victim of medical negligence. The consultation will not go well if the already injured patient feels that they are being rushed.

Consent to Proceed with Psychiatric Evaluation

As with all medical interventions, consent should be sought in advance of the assessment. Patients should be informed about the nature of the interview and who will have access to the clinical information obtained during the psychiatric evaluation.

The General Medical Council (GMC) provides guidance on the exchange of information between a patient and a third party who is requesting an expert report, such as a medical indemnity provider.[28] These principles also apply to the psychiatric expert undertaking an evaluation in the context of a medical negligence claim. The GMC guidance seeks to balance the duty of care the expert has to the patient with the expert's obligation to the third party, such as the insurance provider. The GMC provides advice on what information to disclose and how, as well as guidance on seeking the patient's consent to disclose.

Given the potential level of distrust that exists between the plaintiff who is complaining of medical negligence and the medical profession, the need for the expert to adhere to a formal process in seeking consent to proceed with the psychiatric evaluation is even more relevant. The issues that should be explored when obtaining consent to proceed with a psychiatric evaluation are outlined in Appendix 16.1.

Preparation of the Expert Report

The psychiatrist's primary duty is expressing an opinion and giving evidence to the court. If the psychiatrist is called to give evidence to the court, the doctor will be cross-examined on the content of the report. It is important that the psychiatrist is satisfied that they can stand over the content of the report in court. The Medical Protection Society provide a very

---

[28] www.gmc-uk.org/-/media/documents/gmc-guidance-for-doctors–confidentiality–disclosing-infor mation-for-employment–insuran-70064157.pdf.

> **Box 16.3** Learning points.
>
> 1 A third-party examination does not exempt the doctor from owing a duty to that patient.
> 2 The plaintiff's solicitor may issue proceedings without an expert report to prevent a claim becoming 'statute barred'.
> 3 Inquiries should be made to determine the 'date of knowledge'.
> 4 The primary function of the psychiatric expert is to form an opinion as to whether the injured person is suffering from a 'recognised psychiatric disorder'.
> 5 It is essential that notes are taken up from all the hospitals and primary care physician clinics in which the patient was treated, and not just from the hospital which is the subject of the complaint.
> 6 The expert should adhere to a formal process in seeking consent to proceed with the psychiatric evaluation.
> 7 The expert should allocate extra time when undertaking evaluations in medical negligence cases.

helpful guide on the layout and structure of an expert medical report, laid out in Appendix 16.2.[29] See also Appendix 16.3.

In most countries, the rules of the court require that the report includes a statement by the psychiatrist acknowledging that one's duty as an expert is to assist the court as to matters within one's area of expertise and that this duty overrides any obligation to any party paying the psychiatrist's fees. The court also requires that the clinician preparing the report disclose any financial or economic interest to the author of the report or any person connected to the author in any business or economic activity of the party retaining the expert to include a sponsorship or contribution to any research being carried out by the expert or any university or institution, or any other body to which the expert is connected (see Appendix 16.4). See Box 16.3 for a summary of the learning points from this chapter.

Future Directions and Improving Systems for the Management of Clinical Negligence Claims

At present, clinical negligence litigation in common law jurisdictions is mostly dealt with in an adversarial system which results in pitting doctors against patients. This only adds further anxiety to an already stressful situation for both sides.

Managing clinical negligence claims, such as a catastrophic birth injury, is much more complex than managing many other types of personal injury claims, such as a claim arising out of a road traffic accident. Liability or causation may have been difficult to determine or in dispute. Clinical negligence claims will involve the plaintiffs and their families, who in many cases, have suffered enormous trauma and pain. Modern jurisdictions are looking to introduce practices and procedures to reflect this complexity, in a move away from the traditional adversarial court system, while maintaining fairness to ensure that no one is undercompensated and no one is overcompensated [9]. Best practice in dealing with clinical negligence claims should include the following procedures.

---

[29] www.medicalprotection.org/uk/articles/eng-guide-to-writing-expert-reports.

Pre-Action Protocol

A pre-action protocol explains the conduct and sets out the steps a court would normally expect parties to take before commencing proceedings. In the UK the obligation to have a pre-action protocol came into force in July 2000 for professional negligence cases.

Case Management

Procedures for allowing for case management of clinical negligence are being implemented in many jurisdictions. The benefits of active case management can be summarised as follows:

(i) Identification of what the issue is going to be.

(ii) Having an active case management system directs the expert to identify what is agreed and what is not agreed.

(iii) Witness statements are accepted and therefore victims do not have to go into the witness box and deal with the distress associated with this. Many people express concern that in some cases, parents of children who have been catastrophically injured as a result of clinical negligence have to undergo the additional trauma of giving evidence in the court and being cross-examined on their evidence.

(iv) Active case management leads to early engagement between the parties and facilitates meetings between lawyers in a meaningful way at an early stage.

(v) Settlement can be achieved by case management which may not be easily achieved by having a meeting of lawyers without there being active case management. Case management can act as a catalyst to settle a claim.

Dedicated Clinical Negligence Court

In some jurisdictions it is proposed that there should be a dedicated list in the High Court to deal with the management and hearing of clinical negligence claims. This would improve efficiency and help avoid unreasonable delays.

No-Fault Compensation

In recent years many governments around the world have been troubled by the financial and socioeconomic cost of clinical negligence. In 2016 the Scottish Government consulted on a 'no blame redress scheme' for adverse incidents arising out of clinical treatment. In 2017, the Law Reform Commission of South Africa included a no-fault compensation scheme in its research into potential solutions to address the rising cost of clinical negligence. In 2018, a no-fault compensation scheme was included in the scope of an expert review commissioned by the Irish Government into how civil justice could be reformed and made more affordable. This expert review group ultimately rejected the introduction of a no-fault compensation scheme on constitutional grounds. In the UK a report was commissioned by Dickinson et al. which looked at no-fault compensation. New Zealand introduced a no-fault compensation scheme in 2005. Claimants in New Zealand are unable to go to court without first going through the no-fault system.

In general, family advocates do not favour the introduction of a no-fault system as advocacy improves the delivery of safer healthcare by identifying systemic problems.

A useful international comparison of the advantages and disadvantages of no-fault compensation schemes can be found in *No Fault Compensation: Advantages and Disadvantages* [10].

Vaccination and Condition-Specific Compensation Schemes

The establishment of a compensation scheme to deal with certain vaccine damages was discussed prior to the onset of COVID-19. There is a strong moral argument that those who encourage vaccines could support a compensation scheme. The difference of opinion usually lies in the level of the award. There is concern that any compensation awarded may not be in line with that what the court might award. Other condition-specific compensation schemes have been set up in countries where there are many claims arising out of systemic negligence, such as Hepatitis C claims caused by infected blood transfusions or the underperformance of cervical screening programmes. The establishment of such case-specific compensation schemes lends itself to a speedy and effective determination of claims. These hearings are usually held in private.

In summary, active case management is desirable and assists with identification of contentious issues followed by a pragmatic and effective way to separate out complex cases from mainstream court cases. The development of improved procedures is likely to reduce the delay in defendants coming to the table and lead to a more effective and speedy determination of cases relying on inquisitorial rather than adversarial skills.

Conclusion

Medical negligence claims are a complex area of the law, and the process of handling a claim can be long and expensive, with numerous developments along the way, including fraudulent behaviours, that only become apparent following full discovery of medical records. The medical expert witness should have the relevant expertise and a good working knowledge of the Legal process. This chapter has sought to introduce some of the basic principles of law that a psychiatric expert engaged in clinical negligence litigation should be familiar with.

As with all areas of medicine, the expert must comply with the ethical, professional and legal obligations of doctors. Patient privacy and confidentiality of personal health information must be protected. Most, if not all, patients referred by their solicitors, or by the defendant medical indemnity body, will already feel betrayed and let down by the medical profession. They will be fearful and distrustful. On the other side, there is a clinician who fears reputational damage.

Appendix 16.1 Template for Consent to Proceed with Psychiatric Evaluation

'Ms X signed a declaration confirming that she was informed that the examination was being conducted at the request of the solicitors acting on behalf of the Defendant. I was satisfied that she understood the limits of confidentiality and that she was consenting to proceed with the evaluation.'

Appendix 16.2   Medical Protection Society Guide to Writing an Expert Medical Report

<u>Title Page</u>
  1 Date of report.
  2 Date of any examinations.
  3 The identity of the parties to the action.
  4 Full name (and date of birth) of the Plaintiff.
  5 The party providing the instructions.
  6 The nature of the report.

Numbered pages, short, numbered paragraphs, and appropriate subheadings.

Personal details of the expert – name, current post, and summary of previous experience.

A Statement of the Opinion the expert has been asked to provide and details of relevant knowledge/experience enabling him/her to comment on the issues.

<u>Chronology and Summary of the Relevant Evidence</u>
  7 Giving exact dates wherever possible.
  8 When referring to important parts of the records, quoting relevant entries verbatim, identifying it as a direct quote – e.g. by the use of italics.
  9 Identifying disputed facts and stating the sources of the information set out, e.g. 'history given on admission to hospital on 4.01.2020'.
 10 Explaining relevant technical terms and abbreviations.
 11 Reviewing the evidence for a sufficient period of time before and after the incident – to put the events in context and highlight other relevant features of the history.

<u>The Opinion</u>
  (a) Should comment on each of the Plaintiff's injuries separately quoting the allegation whenever possible.
  (b) Where the allegation appears to repeat or overlap with another, or seems misdirected, explaining why and referring to other relevant paragraphs.
  (c) The opinion should justify the conclusions reached by reference to the evidence in the case and his/her specialist knowledge:
   • Where dealing with an issue on which there is a range of opinion, providing reasons for the view expressed.
   • Where the expert takes sides in the area of factual dispute, giving an explanation of why s/he favours one version over another.
   • Where there is evidence undermining the expert's opinion, outlining that evidence, and explaining why it is not persuasive.

<u>The Concluding Paragraph</u>
  (a) This should return to the issues the expert has been asked to consider and/or the statements of the case, to make sure that an Opinion has been given on all relevant matters with proper attention to the legal tests to be applied.

(b) Finally, the report should be free standing. The reader should be able to glean the key issues in the case, understand the evidence available and reach a clear understanding of the range of expert opinion, without needing to look at any other document.

Appendix 16.3 Template for Medical Negligence Expert Opinion

(a) Whether the plaintiff suffered any injury as a result of the alleged medical negligence, and if so, the extent of same.
(b) Whether the plaintiff's psychiatric injury was caused wholly/partly by their underlying condition and whether the plaintiff's pre-existing psychiatric condition was exacerbated by the outcome of their treatment.
(c) Current condition: whether Ms X has recovered from the alleged injuries and, if not, whether such ongoing symptoms can be attributed to their underlying psychiatric condition.
(d) The plaintiff's prognosis for the future.
(e) Conclusion.

Appendix 16.4 Declaration of Compliance with Duties of Expert

(a) I am Mr/Mrs/Dr/Professor.
(b) I understand that my primary duty is to assist the court with matters within my field of expertise and that this duty overrides any obligation to the party by whom I am engaged or the person who has paid or is liable to pay me.
(c) I understand that in preparing reports and/or giving evidence, I must maintain professional objectivity and impartiality at all times.
(d) I have attempted to the best of my ability, in preparing this report, to be accurate and complete. I have mentioned all matters and facts which I regard as relevant to the opinions I have expressed and any details of any literature or other material which have been relied on in making the report are contained within the report.
(e) I have no conflict of interest of any kind, other than any conflict disclosed in this report. If a conflict has been disclosed, I do not consider that any interest disclosed affects my suitability as an expert witness on any issue on which I have given evidence or intend to give evidence. I hereby give an undertaking to advise the instructing party if, between the date of the expert's report and the final hearing, there is any change in circumstances which affects my ability to give independent unconflicted evidence.
(f) Wherever I have no personal knowledge, I have indicated the source of factual information.
(g) I have not included anything in this report which has been suggested to me by anyone, including those instructing me, without forming my own independent view of the matter.
(h) I confirm that I am not appointed or instructed under any contingency fee arrangement or that I have entered into any agreement whereby the payment of my fees is in any way dependent of the outcome of the case.

References

1. Casey P, Brady P, Craven, C et al. *Psychiatry and the Law* (2nd ed.). Dublin, Blackhall Publishing, 2010).

2. Mills S. *Clinical Practice and the Law*. Oxford, Butterworths, 2002.

3. Rix KJB. *Expert Psychiatric Evidence*. London, The Royal College of Psychiatrists, 2011.

4. Tottenham M, Prendergast EJ, Joyce C, Madden H. *A Guide to Expert Witness Evidence*. London, Bloomsbury, 2019.

5. Kennedy HG. Limits of psychiatric evidence in civil cases: science and sensibility. *Medico-Legal Journal of Ireland* 2004; 10: 1–16.

6. Kennedy HG. Limits of psychiatric evidence in criminal cases: morals and madness. *Medico-Legal Journal of Ireland* 2005; 11: 1–17.

7. Kenny A. The psychiatric expert in court. *Psychological Medicine* 1984; 14 (2): 291–302.

8. Grounds A. On describing mental states. *British Journal of Medical Psychology* 1987; 60 (Pt 4): 305–11.

9. Meenan C. *Justice Expert Group Report to Review the Law of Torts and the Current Systems for the Management of Clinical Negligence Claims* (January 2020). www.gov.ie/en/publication/ffb23-expert-group-report-to-review-the-law-of-torts-and-the-current-systems-for-the-management-of-clinical-negligence-claims.

10. Rowles M. *No Fault Compensation: Advantages and Disadvantages*. www.imo.ie/news-media/events/2019/medical-negligence-the-ca/Melanie-Rowles-No-Faults-Claims-Systems.pdf.

Child and Adolescent Forensic Mental Health Services

Saima Ali, Enys Delmage, Heidi Hales and Alexis Theodorou

Introduction

This chapter covers the differences between adolescent and adult forensic mental health. These differences include consideration of:

- a developmental perspective when considering adolescents
- different systems around a child and their evolution through adolescence
- diagnostic presentations including neurodevelopmental needs, developing personality disorders, conduct disorder and first-presentation psychosis
- the minimum age of criminal responsibility
- adolescent-focussed risk assessment
- the complexity of adolescent forensic services in the community and secure establishments.

The following vignettes provide a walk-through process for some of the above areas.

YP1 – First Presentation

John is a 15-year-old boy charged with murder. He is alleged to have stabbed a 14-year-old boy at a local park. During a police interview without an appropriate adult he admitted to the offence, stating that he had committed it for 'the clout'. Since being in custody he has tied a ligature around his neck necessitating emergency medical intervention and has presented as aggressive and tearful.

YP2 – First Presentation

Charlie is a 14-year-old, brought to the emergency department by ambulance following a car crash in which he was driving – his girlfriend was also in the vehicle and sustained severe injuries. He stated that he was speeding because he was being followed, and admitted to cannabis and alcohol use at the time. Police attended the crash scene and found a kitchen knife on his person and a nail-studded baseball bat in the car boot.

YP3 – First Presentation

Joe is a 16-year-old boy who is well known to the local Youth Offending Service with a long history of offending starting when he was 14, first with theft and then including drug possession, drug dealing and violent offences. Joe has become threatening and aggressive at home and his parents are concerned about his risk to his siblings.

Development through Adolescence

Adolescence is a time of transition between childhood and adulthood. It represents a period of significant change, encompassing puberty, separation from caregivers and identity acquisition. Every child's journey to cognitive, emotional and biological maturity is unique, and development in each domain is independent and occurs in its own time [1]. Adverse experiences during childhood and adolescence negatively impact development and influence life-long outcomes, including development of mental illness [2, 3].

The activation of the hypothalamic-pituitary-gonadal axis marks the onset of puberty and sexual development [1]. Dynamic brain development occurs throughout adolescence and neuronal maturation continues until the mid-20s [1, 4, 5]. White matter appears to mature hierarchically, with integration of executive and emotion systems occurring last [1, 6].

Erikson suggested that the primary psychosocial task of adolescence was identity formation [7]. This involves gaining social and emotional independence from parents or caregivers, subsequently developing capacity for intimacy. This does not negate the need for guidance and support. Removal from this trajectory can be deeply damaging for adolescents as crucial developmental tasks are missed [8].

During adolescence, peers take on a more central role [9]. Although this is a key aspect of maturation, some peers may be a negative influence. This is especially pertinent when considering adolescent offending. Children show a heightened susceptibility to peer influence during adolescence, resulting in a reward-sensitive motivational state that may increase risky behaviour [10]. Adolescents are more likely to commit delinquent acts in groups, whereas adults are more likely to offend alone [11]. Those with neurodevelopmental or attachment and emotional regulation difficulties may be particularly vulnerable to gang culture, increasing their offending risk alongside that of violent victimisation [12, 13].

Society and culture have a significant influence on adolescent development. Societal expectations have varied across history and continue to differ globally. There is often a mismatch between a young person's cognitive or emotional capacity and the societal expectations placed upon them, perhaps best illustrated by global variations in the age of criminal responsibility (Figure 17.1).

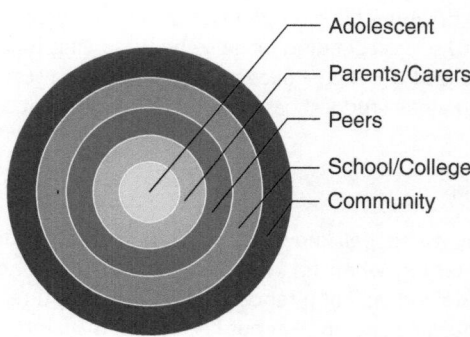

Figure 17.1 Systems around a child.

A systemic approach and transparent communication are key to effective intervention when treating adolescents with any difficulties. Each system plays a critical role in the young person's world. Creating an open dialogue between different systems and the young person is crucial. One example of systemic working within the family itself is family therapy, which is an evidence-based treatment widely used in Child and Adolescent Mental Health Services (CAMHS) to help resolve conflicts; multi-systemic therapy has demonstrated efficacy in the United States but not the United Kingdom. Multi-agency networks around a young person at risk support the development of a co-created, integrated care plan [14].

YP1 – Systems

John is an only child. His parents had a volatile relationship and were both under the care of community mental health teams. Between the ages of one and seven, he lived between his parental home and both grandmothers due to frequent police involvement for suspected domestic violence and alcohol misuse. When he was 13 years old, he was excluded from school, began to smoke cannabis with older boys in his housing estate and started expressing a fascination with knives and drill music. A referral was made to social services, but the family engaged minimally and eventually the case was closed.

Systems needs considered – Difficulties at home and school led to a social care referral but poor family engagement led to case closure, despite the apparent parental neglect. Furthermore, a need for contextual safeguarding is noted, with him at risk of being criminally exploited as a child and groomed into local gang activity as a replacement care system.

YP2 – Systems

Charlie left school at 16 and worked in a supermarket, but has missed a number of shifts over the past three months. His father was contacted via telephone and reported that Charlie sometimes goes missing and has been away from home, and of unknown address, for one month.

Systems needs considered – Charlie has a supportive family around him who should be informed of his assessment in the emergency department. He has been missing from home for a month, indicating vulnerability to child criminal exploitation and subsequent grooming by local gangs.

YP3 – Systems

Joe lives with his parents and two younger siblings. His mother has repeatedly asked for support from local services and was offered parenting groups, which they attended. They have struggled to get him to appointments, and he never engaged in assessments. They have felt judged by professionals and are now struggling to trust those working with them. Social care have been involved for the past two years, supporting the family with him being a child in need. They have recently re-referred him to CAMHS and he is awaiting assessment.

Systems needs considered – Joe's family have tried hard to meet his needs, asked for help and engaged with all the support given. However, Joe has been a 'difficult-to-parent' child and their situation has escalated to the extent that they are ready for him to be taken into the care of the local authority because of his risk to his siblings. The opportunity for early assessment and treatment was missed due to his behaviour being labelled as 'naughty' rather than in need of assessment.

Diagnoses in Adolescent Forensic Psychiatry

Young people presenting to adolescent forensic services have a variety of diagnoses and needs which overlap with those seen in adults, including substance misuse, psychosis, affective and neurodevelopmental disorders, emotional dysregulation, and antisocial behaviour. However, their presentations may differ from those in adult services because it is their first presentation to services. As with adult clients using forensic services, there is much comorbidity. Levels of mental health needs in young people placed in secure services in England were described in 2016 [15] and in youth custody internationally [16].

Oppositional Defiant Disorder and Conduct Disorder

These are the most common diagnoses in childhood [14]. Oppositional defiant disorder describes defiant and disobedient younger children who may later develop conduct disorder. Those with conduct disorder get involved in fights, damage property, set fires, steal, lie, break rules, disrespect and disobey authority. The context of such behaviour is important, whether alone (unsocialised conduct disorder), in the home or with others (socialised conduct disorder).

There are several seminal longitudinal studies investigating the risk factors, development and outcome of childhood delinquency including studies in: Camberwell, South London in the UK, starting in 1953 [17]; Dunedin, New Zealand, starting in 1972 [18]; the Great Smokey Mountains, North Carolina in the US, starting in 1992 [19]; and Avon, UK, starting in 1991/1992 [20]. These studies have shown that most delinquency develops in early adolescence (late onset) and ends by the end of adolescence and early 20s (adolescent limited). However, some show signs of oppositional defiant disorder as young as three years (early onset) and some, often those with early onset but including some with late onset, continue criminal behaviour through their adult life (life-course persistent). The majority of those with criminal behaviour in adult life have had conduct disorder in childhood but the majority with conduct disorder in childhood do not have a persistent pattern of offending.

Causes of conduct disorder are multifactorial. Twin studies have shown that there is a 50% heritable component [21] along with significant gene environment interaction with childhood antisocial behaviour restricting opportunities, and environmental risks and childhood adverse experiences affecting the young person's experience of and interaction with the world [22]. Investigators have studied the development of psychopathic personality traits [23] and fracture points in childhood which may offer opportunities for intervention [24].

Emotional Dysregulation

Many young people presenting to adolescent forensic services show signs of emotional dysregulation. Many have suffered adverse childhood experiences and neglect, leading to poorly developed strategies to manage their emotions. Risk assessments, as with adult services, often focus on risk to others; risk to self must also be considered.

Neurodevelopmental Disorders

There is growing concern that a disproportionate proportion of young people involved with youth justice services have neurodevelopmental disorders, including attention deficit hyperactive disorder (ADHD), autistic spectrum condition (ASC) and learning disability (LD)

[15, 16, 25, 26]. Having a mild neurodevelopmental disability appears to make young people vulnerable to being recruited into gang activity because they are keen to belong to a peer group. Comorbidity is common [15].

YP1 – Diagnosis

John's family described him as a 'loner' child who enjoyed his own company, being particularly interested in his collection of toy dinosaurs. He struggled in school, especially on transfer to secondary school, being unable to form lasting friendship groups. He was frequently excluded for disruptive behaviour before eventually being expelled at the age of 13.

Differential diagnoses – Social communication difficulties with increasing difficulties at secondary school transfer raise the possibility of ASC. He is likely to have comorbid emotional dysregulation following the traumas of witnessing domestic violence at home and changes of caregivers between his parents and grandmothers.

Treatment needs – He requires further assessment for ASC, attachment patterns, trauma symptoms and emotional difficulties. Management plans need to be holistic and ASC informed, considering all of his complex needs. It is likely he would benefit from a comprehensive care plan including social skills training, emotional literacy and review of family relationships/family therapy.

YP2 – Diagnosis

Charlie stated that his friends had been telling him he was in trouble with the government and had also been hearing his name mentioned on the radio. He stated that the crash was unintentional and seemed unconcerned about the damage to himself and his girlfriend (he sustained minor lacerations – she was admitted to the intensive care unit) and the potential for death through his actions. Charlie had no suicidal ideation. He made allusions about harming others and is increasingly wary of people who are bald, which he says is a sign of a government agent. His main priority was to get out of hospital as soon as possible to record this latest development in his diary, as he was building a case to take to the police. He does not want to stay in hospital because he does not consider himself to be unwell.

Differential diagnoses – It appears that Charlie may be suffering from a first episode psychosis which has been precipitated and worsened by cannabis use [45].

Treatment needs – Charlie will need admission to hospital, likely under the Mental Health Act. His risk to others needs to be considered when thinking about the level of security of the adolescent ward. The mainstay of treatment will be anti-psychotic treatment, but he will also benefit from substance misuse work and psychoeducation to support compliance with medication.

YP3 – Diagnosis

Joe is described as impulsive. His mother said that he was always on the go. Although he managed primary school, he was frequently in trouble for being in fights and disrupting the class. He suffered bullying from his peer group. In secondary school his difficulties in the classroom became increasingly apparent. He struggled with the curriculum and could not sit still in the classroom. He frequently left the class and walked out of school. He was excluded when aged 14 and placed in the local alternative school provision. He has extremely poor attendance and tends to go in at the beginning of school but then leave to meet his friends who are also avoiding school. He smokes cannabis daily.

Differential diagnoses – Joe presents with symptoms of ADHD and difficulty with learning. It is not clear whether his difficulty with learning is related to impulsivity and inattention, substance misuse or specific or global LD. His behaviour now fulfils the criteria for conduct disorder likely developed secondary to ADHD.

Treatment needs – Joe and his family need outreach work from the professional network to build up trusting relationships. He needs further assessment of ADHD (collateral history, observations and Conners) and LD (cognitive assessment and functional needs assessment). He needs a co-created integrated multi-agency care plan including support for his parents and individual work with him. In view of his difficulty in engaging, a mentor may be best placed for initial engagement. If he has ongoing symptoms of ADHD, medication will be useful to reduce impulsivity. However, young people often dislike the side effects of lack of appetite and feeling 'dampened'.

The Minimum Age of Criminal Responsibility (MACR)

The MACR can reasonably be defined as the age below which children are presumed to be unable to have the capacity to commit an offence. In most jurisdictions internationally, this can be described as a conclusive presumption – which means that it cannot be rebutted by evidence. Children below this age fall outside of the jurisdiction of the youth criminal justice systems. Where they have committed illegal acts, such children are managed by civil law interventions including placement in secure children's homes, hospital settings, residential educational settings or highly supported placements under the auspice of social services.

When compared to adult criminal justice proceedings, youth offending and the detention of children has a broader set of safeguards in place. These are drawn from the Convention on the Rights of the Child (1989) which states that 'the arrest, detention or imprisonment of a child ... shall be used only as a measure of last resort'. The aim set out is to ensure the child remains within the broader familial network, with greater employment of non-custodial alternatives [27].

In 2007, the United Nations released the first advisory recommending that the MACR should be no less than 12 years old [28]. Subsequent neurodevelopmental research has demonstrated that adolescent brains undergo extensive pruning and neuronal remodelling. This raises significant doubts about a child's capacity to have *mens rea* if they lack the ability to understand the impact of their actions, or indeed the ability to follow court proceedings. As such, this recommendation has been revised to the age of 14 [29].

Despite this, global prevalence estimates of children (those under the age of 18) held on remand and in prison range between 160,000 and 250,000 [30]. A contributing factor to this is likely to be the wide international differences in relation to where the MACR is set. For instance, 66 countries are currently operating *doli incapax* (a defence for children in circumstances where they did not know that their behaviour was seriously wrong), 25 vary the MACR according to seriousness of offence, 10 have different MACRs for boys versus girls, 5 have Sharia law in operation alongside state-mandated or federal law, 13 have no MACR, at least 1 has multiple established legal processes (Gaza – where tribal adjudication, military law, precedent and common law all interface) and 5 have a position yet to be established. Within the UK, the MACR is 10 years in England, Wales and Northern Ireland, whereas in 2019 Scotland increased their MACR to 12 from a previous age of 8 years. In the Republic of Ireland it is 10 years, and 12 for less serious offences.

YP1

Legal needs highlighted – In England and Wales all children must have an appropriate adult (their mother or someone appointed by social care) with them when they are interviewed. There are also protocols to reduce the length of time any child is in police custody because it is not age appropriate. However, in the rush to move children on from custody, interviews may inadvertently be held without an appropriate adult. For serious crimes, such as alleged murder, the child is likely to be remanded into custody, though occasionally they can be remanded in local authority care. Placements need to be found quickly.

Assessment and diversion from police custody – Children may find custody even more distressing than their adult counterparts. Their safety is paramount. In England and Wales there are Youth Justice Liaison and Diversion workers who can assess young people in custody during working hours. If the child is very unsettled and a risk to themselves, they may need assessment in hospital.

YP2

Balancing legal and health needs highlighted – While Charlie is alleged to have committed several offences (dangerous driving and possession of a weapon), the primary consideration on presentation to the emergency department is his physical and mental health needs. Police may attend the emergency department and wait for the outcome of assessment to know if he is to be admitted or discharged into their care.

Risk review in the emergency department – The health professionals assessing in the emergency department need to consider his acute risk to himself and others, considering the weapons he was carrying and manner of car crash. Security from the hospital may be needed to ensure that everyone remains safe.

Risk Assessments in Young People

Many young people will engage in delinquent activity during adolescence but only a small minority engage in serious or persistent violent crime. The purpose of risk assessment has traditionally been to understand who will desist and who will persist. Structured protocols can help to formally highlight areas of concern within a young person's life and identify areas for multi-agency intervention. Rather than focussing on a particular offence, robust assessments consider a young person's risk from holistic developmental, systems-based and trauma-informed perspectives [31]. Tools used in adolescence differ from adults because of their focus upon encouraging a strengths-based approach to risk reduction.

Adolescence is a time of significant change and regular re-evaluation of risk is strongly advised. Furthermore, considering the importance of the different systems and people around adolescents, it is important to highlight risk scenarios rather than giving one overall rating. This, again, will enable integrated care plans to consider the safest placement where risk management plans can be implemented.

Young people who are engaged in lone-actor terrorism/mass-shooting behaviour should not be assessed using standard risk assessment tools alone – in these circumstances practitioners would be advised to consult with colleagues in adult forensic services for advice, or locate their nearest Fixated Threat Assessment Centre for guidance (see Table 17.1).

Table 17.1 Risk assessment tools in adolescent forensic psychiatry

Risk Assessment Tool	Risk Assessed	Composition and Application
SAVRY Structured Assessment of Violence Risk in Youth	• Violence	• Contains 24 items in 3 risk domains: historical, social/contextual and individual/clinical. • Includes protective factors: prosocial involvement, strong social support, strong attachments, positive attitude towards intervention and authority, strong commitment to school, and resilient personality traits [32].
START-AV Short Term Assessment of Risk and Treatability: Adolescent Version	• Violence • General offending • Harm to self • Victimisation	• Developmentally informed adaptation of START tool used with adults. • 25 dynamic factors assessed according to strengths and vulnerabilities. Reported to be able to assess change in risk because of the use of dynamic factors. • Factors are divided into 3 domains: individual adolescent, relationships and environment, and responses to interventions [33].
YLS/CMI 2.0 Youth level of service/case management inventory	• General offending • Recidivism	• Uses an adjusted actuarial model. • Contains 42 items relating to risk and need in seven domains: Education/Employment, Attitudes/Orientation, Peer Relations, Leisure Activities, Substance Abuse Treatment, Personality/Behaviour and Family Circumstances/Parenting [34].
SAPROF-YV Structured assessment of protective factors of violence risk: youth version	• Protective factors against violence	• Intended to be used in conjunction with other risks assessment tools, e.g. SAVRY. • Comprising 16 dynamic protective factors assessed in 4 domains (resilience, motivational, relational and external). • The assessor is asked to name 'key factors' – factors crucial in preventing violence, and 'goal factors' – factors holding promise for the future [34].
AIM 3 Assessment, intervention, Moving On	• Harmful sexual behaviour	• Used with young males in the assessment of harmful sexual behaviour. 25 items are assessed in five holistic domains (sexual, non-sexual, developmental, environmental, self-regulation) to help consider relevant targets for intervention. • Difficult to complete if there are no convictions for sexually harmful behaviour and young person denies all allegations. • Where AIM 2 gave the need for overall risk monitoring, updated AIM 3 gives a holistic formulation of need [36].

PROFESOR

Protective + Risk Observations For Eliminating Sexual Offense Recidivism

- Sexual offence risk assessment tool

  - Structured checklist.
  - Describes protective and risk factors for individuals who have committed sexual offences.
  - Age range is 12–25.
  - NOT designed to predict future risk of offending – but assists with planning interventions to reduce sexual offending.

PCL-YV

Hare Psychopathy Checklist: Youth ersion

- Psychopathic traits

  - Although not strictly a risk assessment tool, this does inform risk: youth with higher PCL-YV scores tend to be recidivists, both in general and violent offending [37].
  - Used to assess psychopathic traits and behaviours.
  - Comprises 20 items that assess psychological and behavioural traits.

YP1 – Risk History

Information from the local Youth Offending Service shows that John has a long history of offending since exclusion from school.

Risk assessment – John presents with risk to self and to others. A SAVRY risk assessment would be useful as he has a long history of offending. This will identify areas in his life which increase his risk, including the difficulties at home and in the community and his social communication difficulties and impulsivity from emotional dysregulation.

YP2

Risk assessment – It may be useful to complete a SAVRY with Charlie, though if he does not have a long history of offending and the current violent thoughts are new, related to this first psychotic episode, this may not be useful.

Adolescent Forensic Services

Adolescent forensic mental health services include community and secure in-patient services. Community services in England and Wales have recently expanded to include a national framework of community forensic CAMHS [38] and Youth Justice Liaison and Diversion services to screen all young people who have contact with local police services. The aims of such services are to support local children's agencies, including youth justice, CAMHS and social care, in understanding the needs of young people showing risk behaviour and developing a co-created integrated care plan.

In each jurisdiction, detention of young people in secure settings can be under mental health, secure welfare and youth justice legal frameworks. However, the weighting of these settings varies globally [39, 40] and across time [41]. Secure services in England were described in 2016 [42] (see Figure 17.2).

Of note, services continue to evolve with regards to the establishment and closure of units. There is discussion in England about the development of secure schools in the youth justice estate [43]. Also of note, medium-secure psychiatric units are being developed in Scotland and the Republic of Ireland.

While all forensic settings need to ensure that they work towards least restrictive principles, this is especially important when considering detaining children, as they are still developing. While detention in a secure setting may sometimes be necessary, care needs to be taken that detention is underpinned by a philosophy of rehabilitation, to avoid it being experienced as an adverse childhood experience, causing further trauma to young people.

Future Directions

Adolescent forensic mental health is a continually developing field with ongoing research [44] and service evolution.

Current developments include:

- greater links between academic research about development and those developing preventative community services
- greater understanding of frontal lobe development, enabling consideration of specific needs of young people and young adults

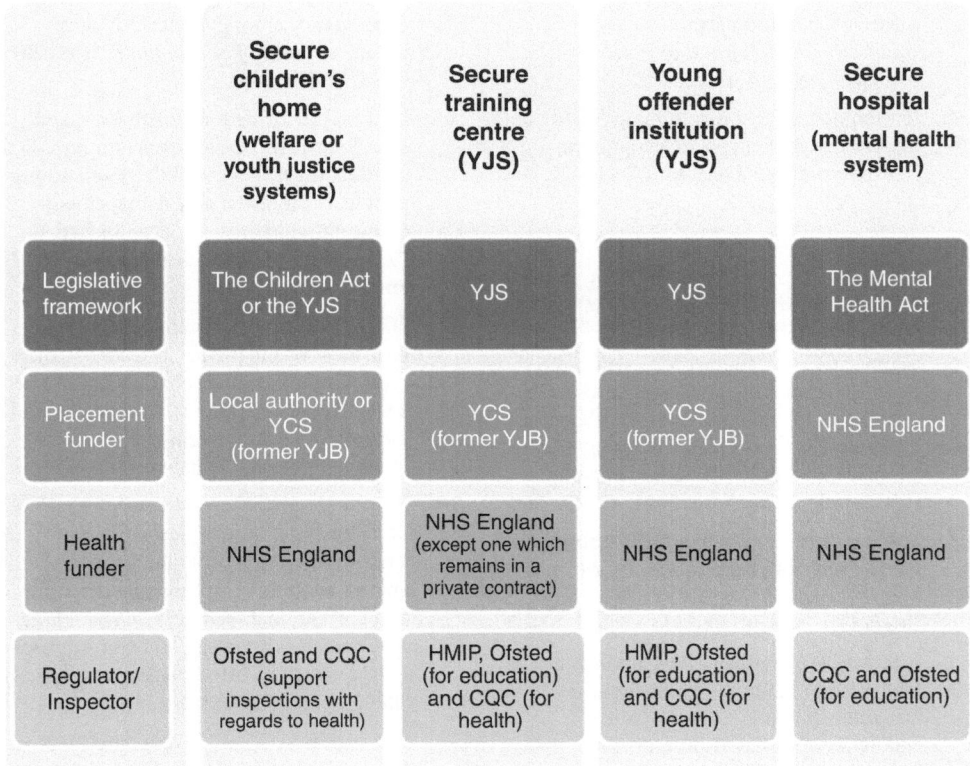

Figure 17.2 The secure estate for young people in England in 2016 [14].

- greater understanding of effects of neurodevelopmental comorbidity; what this means as a diagnosis, where care is best offered and what works for whom
- collaboration and agreement between clinicians in discussion about 'emerging personality disorder'; where care is best offered and what works for whom
- development of community forensic CAMHS services
- reduction in number of detained young people internationally
- ongoing discussion about what services are needed and where
- development of medium-secure units, including in the Republic of Ireland and Scotland
- increasing international collaboration to learn what works and for whom.

References

1. Sawyer, SM, Azzopardi, PS, Wickremarathne, D, Patton, GC – The age of adolescence. *Lancet Child Adolesc. Health* (2018); 2(3): 223–228.

2. Chapman, DP, Whitfield, CL, Felitti, VJ, Dube, SR, Edwards, VJ, Anda, RF – Adverse childhood experiences and the risk of depressive disorders in adulthood. *J. Affect. Disorders* (2004); 217–225.

3. Felitti VJ, Anda RF, Nordenberg D et al. Relationship of childhood abuse and household dysfunction to many of the

leading causes of death in adults: the Adverse Childhood Experiences (ACE) study. *American Journal of Preventive Medicine* 1998; 14(4): 245–58.

4. Huttenlocher PR. Morphometric study of human cerebral cortex development. *Neuropsychologia* 1990; 28 (6): 517–27.

5. Pfefferbaum A, Mathalon DH, Sullivan EV et al. A quantitative magnetic resonance imaging study of changes in brain morphology from infancy to late adulthood. *Archives of Neurology* 1994; 51 (9): 874–887.

6. Simmonds DJ, Hallquist MN, Asato M, Luna B. Developmental stages and sex differences of white matter and behavioral development through adolescence: a longitudinal diffusion tensor imaging (DTI) study. *Neuroimage* 2014; 92: 356–368.

7. Sokol JT. Identify development throughout the lifetime: an examination of Eriksonian theory. *Graduate Journal of Counseling Psychology* 2009; 1 (2): 1–11.

8. Petersen AC, Nancy L, Barbara G et al. Promoting mental health during the transition into adolescence. In Schulenberg J, Maggs JL, Hurrelmann K (eds) *Health Risks and Developmental Transitions during Adolescence.* Cambridge, Cambridge University Press, 1997, pp. 471–97.

9. Welborn BL, Lieberman MD, Goldenberg D et al. Neural mechanisms of social influence in adolescence. *Social Cognitive and Affective Neuroscience* 2016; 11 (1): 100–9.

10. Albert D, Chein J, Steinberg L. The teenage brain: peer influences on adolescent decision making. *Current Directions in Psychological Science* 2013; 22 (2): 114–20.

11. Zimring F. *American Youth Violence: Studies in Crime and Public Policy.* New York, Oxford University Press, 1998.

12. Taylor TJ, Peterson D, Esbensen FA, Freng A. Gang membership as a risk factor for adolescent violent victimisation. *Journal of Research in Crime and Delinquency* 2007; 44 (4): 351–80.

13. Nydegger LA, Quinn K, Walsh JL, Pacella-LaBarbara ML, Dickson-Gomez J.

Polytraumatization, mental health and delinquency among adolescent gang members. *Journal of Traumatic Stress* 2019; 32 (6): 890–8.

14. National Institute for Health Care and Excellence. Antisocial behaviour and conduct disorders in children and young people: recognition and management. Clinical Guideline CG158 published 27 March 2013. www.nice.org.uk/guidance/cg158.

15. Hales H, Warner L, Smith J, Bartlett A. Census of young people in secure settings on 14 September 2016: characteristics, needs and pathways of care. 2018. www.england.nhs.uk/publication/secure-settings-for-young-people-a-national-scoping-exercise.

16. Beaudry G, Yu R, Langstrom N, Fazel S. An updated systematic review and meta-regression analysis: mental disorders among adolescents in juvenile detention and correctional facilities. *Journal of the American Academy of Child and Adolescent Psychiatry* 2020. https://jaacap.org/article/S0890-8567(20)30061-7/pdf.

17. Farrington DP, Coid JW, Harnett L et al. Criminal careers and life success: new findings from the Cambridge Study in Delinquent Development. Home Office Briefing, 2006. www.crim.cam.ac.uk/people/academic_research/david_farrington/hofind281.pdf.

18. Broidy LM, Nagin DS, Tremblay RE et al. Developmental trajectories of childhood disruptive behaviour disorders and adolescent delinquency: a cross-national replication. Developmental Psychology 2003; 39 (39): 222–45.

19. Rowe R, Maughan B, Pickles A, Costello EJ, Angold A. The relationship between DSM-IV oppositional defiant disorder and conduct disorder: findings from the Great Smoky Mountains Study. *Journal of Child Psychology and Psychiatry* 2002; 43 (3): 365–73.

20. Barker ED, Maughan B. Differentiating early-onset persistent versus childhood-limited conduct problem youth. *American Journal of Psychiatry* 2009; 166 (8): 900–8.

21. Polderman TJ, Benyamin B, de Leeuw CA et al. Meta-analysis of the heritability of human traits based on fifty years of twin studies. *Nature Genetics* 2015; 47 (7): 702–9.

22. Lahey BB, Rathouz PJ, Applegate B, Tackett JL, Waldman ID. A developmental propensity model of the origins of conduct problems during childhood and adolescence. In Lahey BB, Moffitt TE, Caspi A (eds) *Causes of Conduct Disorder and Juvenile Delinquency*. New York, The Guilford Press, 2003, pp. 76–117.

23. Viding E, McCrory EJ. Understanding the development of psychopathy: progress and challenges. *Psychological Medicine* 2018; 48 (4): 566.

24. McCrory EJ, Gerin MI, Viding E. Annual research review: childhood maltreatment, latent vulnerability and the shift to preventative psychiatry – the contribution of functional brain imaging. *Journal of Child Psychology and Psychiatry* 2017; 58 (4): 338–57. doi: 10.1111/jcpp.12713.

25. Hughes N, Williams H, Chitsabesan P, Davies R, Mounce L. Nobody made the connection: the prevalence of neurodisability in young people who offend. Office of the Children's Commissioner, 2012. www.childrenscom missioner.gov.uk/wp-content/uploads/201 7/07/Nobody-made-the-connection.pdf.

26. Office of the Children's Commissioner. 'I think I must have been born bad'; Emotional wellbeing and mental health of children and young people in the youth justice system. 2011. www.childrenscom missioner.gov.uk/wp-content/uploads/201 7/07/I_think_I_must_have_been_born_ba d_-_full_report.pdf.

27. United Nations. Convention on the Rights of the Child. General assembly resolution 44/45, New York, United Nations, 2 September 1990. www.ohchr.org/en/inst ruments-mechanisms/instruments/conven tion-rights-child.

28. United Nations Committee on the Rights of the Child. General comment No. 10 (2007).

29. United Nations Committee on the Rights of the Child. General comment No. 24 (2019).

30. United Nations global study on children deprived of liberty (A/74/136, 11 July 2019).

31. Viljoen JL, Jonnson MR, Sheperd SM. Assessing risk for violent, general and sexual offending in adolescents: recent advances and future directions. In Wormith JS, Craig LA, Hogue TE (eds) *The Wiley Handbook of What Works in Violence Risk Management: Theory, Research, and Practice Part II – What Works in Violence Risk Assessment*. Hoboken, NJ, Wiley, 2020, pp. 223–51.

32. Borum R, Bartel P, Forth A. *Manual for the Structured Assessment for Violence Risk in Youth (SAVRY)*. Odessa, FL, Psychological Assessment Resources, 2020.

33. Nicholls TL, Viljoen JL, Cruise KR, Desmarais SL, Webster CD. *Short-Term Assessment of Risk and Treatability: Adolescent Version (START: AV) (Abbreviated Manual)*. Coquitlam, Canada, BC Mental Health and Addiction Services, 2005.

34. Hoge RD, Andrews DA. *Youth Level of Service/Case Management Inventory 2.0 (YLS/CMI 2.0): User's Manual*. Toronto, Multi-Health Systems, 2011.

35. De Vries R, Geers M, Stapel M et al. *SAPROF Youth Version: Guidelines for the Assessment of Protective Factors for Violence Risk in Juveniles (English Version)*. Utrecht, Forum Educatief, 2015.

36. Marcella L, Hackett S. *The AIM 3 Assessment Model: Assessment of Adolescents and Harmful Sexual Behaviour*. AIM Project, UK, 2019. https://aimproject .org.uk/aim3-assessment-model-assess ment-of-adolescents-and-harmful-sexual- behaviour-leonard-hackett-2019.

37. Forth AE, Kosson DS, Hare RD. *The Hare Psychopathy Checklist: Youth Version*. Toronto, Multi-Health Systems, 2003.

38. *National Evaluation of Community Forensic Child and Adolescent Mental Health Services* (Community F:CAMHS). London, Anna Freud Centre, 2021. https:// d1uw1dikibnh8j.cloudfront.net/media/166 52/community-fcamhs-final-report.pdf.

39. Fleur SA, Dekkers TJ, Bulanovaite E et al. Overview of European forensic youth care:

towards an integrative mission for intervention and prevention strategies for juvenile offenders. *Child and Adolescent Psychiatry and Mental Health* 2019; 13(6). https://capmh.biomedcentral.com/articles/10.1186/s13034-019-0265-4.

40. Hart D. Correction or care? The use of custody for children in trouble. Prison Reform Trust. Winston Churchill Memorial Trust, 2015. www.wcmt.org.uk/sites/defaul t/files/report-documents/Hart%20Diane%2 0Report%202015%20Final_0.pdf.

41. Case S. *Youth Justice: A Critical Introduction*. London, Routledge, 2018.

42. Warner L, Hales H, Smith J, Bartlett A. Secure settings for young people: a national scoping exercise. NHS England, 2018. www .england.nhs.uk/publication/secure-set tings-for-young-people-a-national-scop ing-exercise.

43. Taylor C. Review of the Youth Justice System: An interim report of emerging findings. Ministry of Justice, 2016. https://assets.pub lishing.service.gov.uk/government/uploads/ system/uploads/attachment_data/file/577105 /youth-justice-review-final-report-print.pdf.

44. Hales H, Holt C, Delmage E, Lengua C. What next for adolescent forensic mental health research? *Criminal Behaviour and Mental Health* 2019; 29: 196–206. DOI: 10.1002/cbm.2124.

45. Flynn D, Smith D, Quirke L, Monks S, Kennedy HG. Ultra high risk of psychosis on committal to a young offender prison: an unrecognised opportunity for early intervention. *BMC Psychiatry* 2012; 12: 100.

Women's Services in Forensic Psychiatry

Vivienne de Vogel

Introduction

In the last two decades, attention has grown for the unique needs of female offenders and more research has been published on the assessment, management and treatment of women in forensic services [1]. Although girls and women represent a minority of the forensic mental health and prison populations, studies worldwide suggest that there has been an increase in the number of females being convicted for committing offences, especially violent offences [2, 3]. Still, most of the tools and treatment programmes currently being used in forensic services have mainly been developed and validated in male samples. More understanding of specific risks and mental health needs of women in forensic services is crucial to be able to provide the most adequate treatment.

This is also important with respect to preventing the intergenerational transmission of violence and crime. Research has yielded evidence that children of antisocial or violent mothers have increased risks of developing multiple mental health problems, including substance abuse and antisocial, violence or other risky behaviours [4, 5]. Furthermore, more attention for female offenders is important for the acknowledgement of their victims. For instance, it still seems to be a taboo – especially for males – to reveal having been sexually or physically abused by a female. The denial of these offences can have major consequences, both for the victim and for the perpetrator.

Gender Differences in Criminological Characteristics

Empirical studies have found substantial gender differences in pathways to offending and nature of offending. First, several studies and theoretical models have stated that girls compared to boys usually have a delayed onset of offending behaviour [6, 7]. However, others have found that girls' criminality and externalizing problems can also peak earlier than in boys, possibly due to early maturation [8]. In a review of 46 studies that examined developmental trajectories of antisocial behaviour in females, Fontaine et al. [9] concluded that there is evidence for different trajectories (e.g. early onset/life-course persistent, childhood limited, adolescence limited, adulthood onset). Mental illness, trauma history, substance abuse and family dysfunction have been identified as gender-specific explanatory factors for offending [10]. Obviously, these factors can also be important explanatory factors for offending in males, but the impact of these factors, especially mental health problems and the often-related history of trauma, is suggested to be stronger for females [3, 10].

Second, it has repeatedly been found that there are gender differences in the nature of offending. In general, women are less often convicted for sexual and violent offences and disproportionately more often for property offences, embezzlement and prostitution.

In forensic services, women are more often convicted for arson compared to men and less often for sexual offences [11, 12]. Furthermore, women are generally found to have different motivations for offending compared to men. For example, women seem more often driven by jealousy, relational frustration and self-defence, whereas motivations for males are more often seen as antisocial, ego driven or resulting from peer pressure [12]. With respect to violent offending, the nature, severity, frequency and victims of violent offences committed by females are significantly different from those committed by males. Overall, violence by girls or women compared to boys or men is more indirect, more reactive and within social relationships and less instrumental or sexual. Victims of female offenders are more often in their direct surroundings, like their children, partner, family or friends. Some types of violence are as common in women as in men, more specifically intimate partner violence, child abuse and in-patient violence by psychiatric patients [1].

Gender Differences in Psychiatric Characteristics

Both men and women who enter forensic services have complex histories with high rates of victimisation and multiple mental health problems. However, some distinct gender differences have been found. Women in forensic services differ from their male counterparts in several aspects, most importantly: (1) more severe trauma history; (2) more comorbidity and internalising disorders; and (3) higher prevalence of self-harming behaviour.

First, the prevalence rate of victimisation, particularly sexual victimisation, has been found to be substantially higher in female offenders than in male offenders and seems to be of particular importance for future risk prediction and prevention [10, 13–14]. To illustrate, in a Dutch multicentre study in forensic psychiatry, it was found that women compared to their male counterparts more often were exposed to a combination of emotional, physical and sexual abuse during childhood and that they more often experienced enduring patterns of victimisation both in childhood and in adulthood [13]. It should be noted, though, that prevalence rates of physical and emotional abuse during childhood were equal and that the prevalence rate of sexual abuse was still alarmingly high in males (26%). However, in females, it was twice as high (52%). Furthermore, in this study, a relation was found between physical abuse and antisocial personality disorder (APD) in men and sexual abuse and borderline personality disorder (BPD) in women. Next to the higher prevalence of (sexual) trauma, gender differences have been found in the nature of trauma and in reactions to traumatic events. Women have experienced more direct trauma (instead of witnessing violence), starting from an earlier age on and more often concerning 'betrayal trauma'; that is, committed by someone they trust, like a family member [15]. Women report more intense feelings of threat and loss associated with trauma and are found to be more susceptible to developing post-traumatic stress disorder (PTSD) following trauma compared to men [15, 16].

Second, notable gender differences have been found in the type of mental health diagnoses with offenders. Women in forensic services compared to men are less often diagnosed with APD or narcissistic personality disorder and more often with internalising disorders and BPD [11–12, 17]. It should be noted here that there might be gender biases in forensic diagnostic processes. For example, impulsivity is often interpreted as a borderline trait in women, while for men it is usually labelled as an antisocial trait. Furthermore, high rates of comorbidity have been found in female offenders, especially with substance abuse and depressive disorders. Women often start using substances as claimed self-medication to sedate feelings of pain and intrusion [18].

Third, female offenders have been found to be more often involved in (non-suicidal) self-harming behaviour compared to their male counterparts [19]. A possible explanation for this higher prevalence is that self-harm is more common in disorders with high prevalence in women like depression and BPD. Self-harming behaviours during stay in forensic services or in prison are also highly prevalent in female offenders, with reported rates varying between 23% and 88% [12, 20]. This self-harming behaviour not only seriously impacts on the woman herself but also on fellow patients who witness this behaviour and (medical) staff who have to respond to it. Moreover, self-harming behaviours are found to constitute a strong predictor for violent incidents towards others during forensic treatment [20–21].

Gender-Sensitive Risk Assessment

Adequate risk assessment and management is of the utmost importance in forensic services to prevent relapse. Despite the major advances in risk assessment over the past decades, few tools have been developed specifically for the assessment of (violence) risk in females. Moreover, research into the psychometric properties of risk assessment tools has been carried out predominantly in male populations. Research results on the predictive accuracy of widely used tools, like the *Historical Clinical Risk Management-20* (HCR-20), versions 2 and 3 [22], have yielded ambiguous results and more recently several gender-sensitive risk assessment guidelines have become available. For example, for adult female forensic psychiatric patients the *Female Additional Manual* (FAM) [23] was developed as an addition to the HCR-20 (version 3). The aim of the FAM is to provide practitioners with a comprehensive violence risk assessment that offers additional guidelines for risk management in women. The FAM contains some additional guidelines to historical items of the HCR-20 (version 3) and eight new items with specific relevance to women, for example prostitution, parenting difficulties and low self-esteem. Furthermore, three extra risk ratings can be coded: the risk of self-destructive behaviour, victimisation and non-violent criminal behaviour. It should be noted that empirical evidence for the gender-specific risk factors is still limited and that recent research found that – although the predictive accuracy of the FAM was significant – the FAM did not yield added value to the HCR-20 (version 3) in predicting violent recidivism [24]. Still, the clinical value of using the FAM for more gender-sensitive risk management strategies has been acknowledged by practitioners.

Gender-Responsive Treatment

Women in forensic services usually have different mental health needs than men and there are indications that many current practices are not sufficiently gender-informed or gender-responsive. The often highly secured and structured environment with a focus on safety and control may not be the most optimal place to treat patients with mental health issues like BPD and internalising disorders considering the possible iatrogenic effects [25]. Moreover, there are additional stress sources within the environment of correctional or forensic services that may lead to depressive feelings or intensify them, like worries about their children, limited resources, overcrowding and possible aggression by other inmates or patients. Long, Fulton and Hollin [26] described the development of a best practice service for women in medium-security psychiatric setting in the UK focussing on trauma treatment and treatment integrity. One of the most important pieces of advice they provide for practitioners working with women is to invest more in emotional relationships instead of physical security.

De Vogel and Nicholls [1] summarised the literature on gender-responsive treatment and stated that treatment for female offenders should: (1) address criminogenic needs; (2) be trauma-informed; and (3) include gender-responsive programmes. First, addressing criminogenic needs is in line with the principles of the risk-need-responsivity (RNR) model which is assumed to be gender-neutral. However, it has been demonstrated that treatment effects are more robust when gender-specific factors are conceptualised as responsivity factors [27]. Second, it is important that practitioners are trauma-informed and that the setting is trauma-responsive; that is, with an emphasis on safety and trust-worthiness, opportunity for choice, collaboration and connection, and that it is strengths-based and skill-building [28]. Third, gender-responsive programmes are needed in which mental health problems, trauma history and the role of social relations are specifically addressed. A number of specific treatment models have been developed for use with female offenders, for instance Beyond Trauma and Beyond Violence [28] and Seeking Safety [29]. These programmes usually focus on recovery from trauma and enlarging coping skills to prevent re-victimisation. Research so far has yielded good results for gender-responsive programmes as compared to gender-neutral programmes [30–31]. More empirical but also qualitative studies are needed concerning treatment of mental health needs of women in forensic services and effects of gender-responsive programmes.

It should be noted here that trauma-informed and trauma-responsive care is also crucial for men in forensic services, but possibly in a distinctive way and with other aims. It has been suggested that traumatised men would benefit most from emotion and behaviour regulation training and social skills development [32], whereas treatment in traumatised women should focus predominantly on enhancing self-esteem, self-efficacy, interpersonal relationships and improving emotional regulation [33].

Recommendations for Working with Women in Forensic Services

Based on the issues discussed so far, several recommendations can be provided for practitioners working with women in forensic services. Generally, it is important for practitioners, but also for managers and policymakers, to be aware of and acknowledge gender differences in offending and (mental health) needs and to further develop and implement treatment programmes that are more responsive to the issues of women. Hence, investing more in monetary and technical support for the implementation of gender-sensitive assessment and gender-responsive programming is recommended.

More specifically, practitioners who are working with women in forensic services should be mindful of the often different nature and motivations for (violent) offending committed by women, be aware of the fact that most current risk assessment instruments are developed for men and keep up with the literature on female violence and offending [34]. It is important to be cognisant of possible gender biases in personality assessments and to test more for internalising problems and effects of trauma, for instance PTSD. Results of widely used tools, like risk assessment tools or tools, to assess psychopathy should be interpreted cautiously as they are mostly validated in males. Further development and validation of gender-sensitive risk assessment tools for adult women are needed, but also for adolescent girls, as there is currently a lack of validated gender-sensitive risk assessment tools for adolescent girls. For both gender-sensitive assessment and gender-responsive treatment it is a prerequisite to have skilled and well-educated staff. Educating staff about differences between male and female patients and training staff in, for instance, coping with severe self-harm of patients in forensic services is important, as well as frequent team interactions/intervisions, coaching, and support from managers.

Finally, it is important to acknowledge potential difficulties in working with women in forensic services. It has been suggested that working with women is more difficult than working with males because it is more time-consuming and emotionally draining as they are sometimes experienced as more manipulative and demanding than men. Particularly the high prevalence of women with BPD in forensic services may affect staff members. In an Italian study in non-forensic patients in out-patient treatment, it was found that paranoid personality disorder and APD were associated with feelings of being criticised/mistreated, and BPD was related to inadequate, overwhelmed and overinvolved countertransference [35]. In a Dutch forensic psychiatric hospital, a pilot study was conducted in which staff members were questioned about their feelings towards their most complex female and male patients [36]. Overall, it was found that staff members felt more helpful, accepting, strong, relaxed, affectionate, sympathetic and receptive towards their most complex female forensic patient and more anxious, threatened and overwhelmed by their most complex male forensic patient. Differences were found between more experienced and less experienced staff members as well as between female and male staff members. For instance, staff members working over five years in this hospital experienced much fewer differences in feelings towards female and male patients.

Concluding, several important gender differences should be acknowledged within forensic services to be able to provide the most optimal treatment for both men and women, with the overall goal to prevent relapse and break the cycle of intergenerational violence.

References

1. de Vogel V, Nicholls TL. Gender matters: an introduction to the special issue on women and girls. *International Journal of Forensic Mental Health* 2016; 15: 1–25. doi: 10.1080/14999013.2016.1141439.

2. Heilbrun K, DeMatteo D, Fretz R et al. How 'specific' are gender-specific rehabilitation needs? An empirical analysis. *Criminal Justice and Behavior* 2008; 35: 1382–97. doi: 10.1177/0093854808323678.

3. Odgers CL, Moretti MM, Reppucci ND. Examining the science and practice of violence risk assessment with female adolescents. *Law and Human Behavior* 2005; 29: 7–27. doi: 10.1007/s10979-005-1397-z.

4. Kim HK, Capaldi DM, Pears KC et al. Intergenerational transmission of internalising and externalising behaviours across three generations: gender-specific pathways. *Criminal Behaviour and Mental Health* 2009; 19: 125–41. doi: 10.1002/cbm.708.

5. Moretti M, Bartolo T, Craig S et al. Gender and the transmission of risk: a prospective study of adolescent girls exposed to maternal versus paternal interparental violence. *Journal of Research on Adolescence* 2014; 24: 80–92. doi: 10.1111/jora.12065.

6. Moffit TE, Caspi A, Rutter M, Silva PA. *Sex Differences in Antisocial Behaviour: Conduct Disorder, Delinquency, and Violence in the Dunedin Longitudinal Study.* Cambridge, Cambridge University Press, 2001.

7. Javdani S, Sadeh N, Verona E. Expanding our lens: female pathways to antisocial behavior in adolescence and adulthood. *Clinical Psychology Review* 2011; 31: 1324–48. doi: 10.1016/j.cpr.2011.09.002.

8. Graber JA, Lewinsohn PM, Seeley JR et al. Is psychopathology associated with the timing of pubertal development? *Journal of the American Academy of Child and Adolescent Psychiatry* 1997; 36: 1768–76. doi: 10.1097/00004583-199712000-00026.

9. Fontaine N, Carbonneau R, Vitaro F et al. Research review: a critical review of studies on the developmental trajectories of antisocial behavior in females. *Journal of Child Psychology and Psychiatry* 2009; 50: 363–85. doi: 10.1111/j.1469-7610.2008.01949.x.

10. Brennan PA, Mednick SA, Hodgins S. Major mental disorders and criminal violence in a Danish birth cohort. *Archives of General Psychiatry* 2000; 57: 494–500. doi: 10.1001/archpsyc.57.5.494.

11. Coid J, Kahtan N, Gault S et al. Women admitted to secure forensic psychiatry services: I. Comparison of women and men. *Journal of Forensic Psychiatry* 2000; 11: 275–95. doi: 10.1080/09585180050142525.

12. de Vogel V, Stam J, Bouman Y et al. Violent women: a multicentre study into gender differences in forensic psychiatric patients. *The Journal of Forensic Psychiatry & Psychology* 2016; 27: 145–68. doi: 10.1080/14789949.2015.1102312C.

13. Bohle A, de Vogel V. Gender differences in victimization and the relation to personality disorders in forensic psychiatry. *Journal of Aggression, Maltreatment & Trauma* 2017; 26: 411–29. doi: 10.1080/10926771.2017.1284170.

14. Green BL, Miranda J, Daroowalla A, Siddique J. Trauma exposure, mental health functioning and program needs for women in jail. *Crime & Delinquency* 2005; 51: 133–51. doi: 10.1177/0011128704267477.

15. Komarovskaya IA, Booker Loper A, Warren JI et al. Exploring gender differences in trauma exposure and the emergence of symptoms of PTSD among incarcerated men and women. *Journal of Forensic Psychiatry &*

Psychology 2011; 22: 395–410. doi: 10.1080/14789949.2011.572989.

16. Valdez CE, Lilly MM. Biological sex, gender role, and Criterion A2: Rethinking the 'gender' gap in PTSD. *Psychological Trauma: Theory, Research, Practice, and Policy* 2014; 6: 34. doi: 10.1037/a0031466.

17. Zlotnick C, Clarke JG, Friedmann PD et al. Gender differences in comorbid disorders among offenders in prison substance abuse treatment programs. *Behavioral Sciences & the Law* 2008; 26: 403–12. doi: 10.1002/bsl.831.

18. Sonne SC, Back SE, Zuniga CD et al. Gender differences in individuals with comorbid alcohol dependence and posttraumatic stress disorder. *The American Journal on Addictions* 2003; 12: 412–23. doi: 10.1111/j.1521-0391.2003.tb00484.x.

19. Völlm BA, Dolan MC. Self-harm among UK prisoners: a cross-sectional study. *The Journal of Forensic Psychiatry & Psychology* 2009; 20: 741–51. doi: 10.1080/14789940903174030.

20. Selenius H, Leppänen Östman S, Strand S. Self-harm as a risk factor for inpatient aggression among women admitted to forensic psychiatric care. *Nordic Journal of Psychiatry* 2016; 70: 554–60.

21. Verstegen N, de Vogel V, Huitema A, Didden R, Nijman H. Physical violence during mandatory psychiatric treatment: prevalence and patient characteristics. *Criminal Justice and Behavior* 2020; 47 (7): 771–89.

22. Douglas KS, Hart SD, Webster CD et al. *HCR-20^{V3}: Assessing Risk of Violence – User Guide*. Burnaby, Mental Health, Law, and Policy Institute, Simon Fraser University, 2013.

23. de Vogel V, de Vries Robbé M, van Kalmthout W, Place C. *Female Additional Manual (FAM): Additional Guidelines to the HCR-20^{V3} for Assessing Risk for Violence in Women, English Version*. Utrecht, Van der Hoeven Kliniek, 2014.

24. de Vogel V, Bruggeman M, Lancel M. Gender-sensitive violence risk assessment: predictive validity of six tools in female forensic psychiatric patients. *Criminal*

Justice and Behavior 2019; 46: 528–549. doi: 10.1177/0093854818824135.

25. Logan C, Blackburn R. Mental disorder in violent women in secure settings: potential relevance to risk for future violence. *International Journal of Law and Psychiatry* 2009; 32: 31–8. doi: 10.1016/j.ijlp.2008.11.010.

26. Long CG, Fulton B, Hollin CR. The development of a 'best practice' service for women in a medium-secure psychiatric setting: treatment components and evaluation. *Clinical Psychology & Psychotherapy* 2008; 15: 304–19. doi: 10.1002/cpp.591.

27. Ashley OS, Marsden ME, Brady TM. Effectiveness of substance abuse treatment programming for women: a review. *The American Journal of Drug and Alcohol Abuse* 2003; 29: 19–53. doi: 10.1081/ADA-120018838.

28. Covington SS. *Beyond Violence: A Prevention Program for Women.* Hoboken, NJ, Wiley, 2013.

29. Najavits LM. *Seeking Safety: A Manual for PTSD and Substance Abuse.* New York, Guilford Press, 2002.

30. Kissin WB, Tang Z, Campbell KM et al. Gender-sensitive substance abuse treatment and arrest outcomes for women. *Journal of Substance Abuse Treatment* 2014; 46: 332–9. doi: 10.1016/j.jsat.2013.09.005.

31. Bartlett A, Jhanjib E, Whitec S et al. Interventions with women offenders: a systematic review and meta-analysis of mental health gain. *The Journal of Forensic Psychiatry & Psychology* 2014; 26: 133–65. doi: 10.1080/14789949.2014.981563.

32. Topitzes J, Mersky JP, Reynolds AJ. From child maltreatment to violent offending: an examination of mixed-gender and gender-specific models. *Journal of Interpersonal Violence* 2012; 27: 2322–47.

33. Salisbury EJ, van Voorhis P, Spiropoulos GV. The predictive validity of a gender-responsive needs assessment. *Crime & Delinquency* 2009; 55: 550–85. doi: 10.1177/0011128707308102.

34. Wright EM, van Voorhis P, Salisbury EJ, Bauman A. Gender-responsive lessons learned and policy implications for women in prison: a review. *Criminal Justice and Behavior* 2012; 39: 1612–32. doi: 10.1177/0093854812451088.

35. Colli A, Tanzilli A, Dimaggio G et al. Patient personality and therapist response: an empirical investigation. *The American Journal of Psychiatry* 2014; 171: 102–8. doi: 10.1176/appi.ajp.2013.13020224.

36. de Vogel V, Louppen M. Measuring feelings of staff members towards their most complex female and male forensic psychiatric patients: a pilot study into gender differences. *International Journal of Forensic Mental Health* 2016; 15: 174–85. doi: 10.1080/14999013.2016.1170741.

Forensic Psychiatry and Intellectual Disability

Harm Boer

A small number of people with intellectual disability (ID) (or learning disability; previously mental retardation) offend or are suspected of having offended. Below average intellectual ability appears to be predictive of future offending behaviour [1] but it is not clear whether those who have a significant ID are over-represented in the criminal justice system (CJS) [2]. Recognising and diagnosing ID in the CJS is notoriously difficult despite screening tools having been developed, such as the Learning Disability Screening Questionnaire (LDSQ) [3]. As people with ID are inherently more vulnerable than the general population, and alternative provision may be available (for instance, through the use of a Mental Health Act), it is important that people with ID in the CJS are recognised, assessed and where appropriate referred for treatment.

Prevalence

The *Diagnostic and Statistical Manual of Mental Disorders*, 5th ed. (DSM-5) and the recent Text Revision (DSM-5-TR) [4, 5] (2013) and International Classification of Diseases (ICD)-10 and 11 definitions [6, 7] of ID are generally accepted and include significant below average intellectual functioning (i.e. with an IQ two standard deviations below average, or on or below 69), deficits in adaptive behaviour and onset before adulthood. The England and Wales Mental Health Act 1983 (amended 2007) includes a definition of 'learning disability' as meaning a state of arrested or incomplete development of the mind which includes significant impairment of intelligence and social functioning. Courts in the United Kingdom have at times accepted evidence that those with an intellectual ability equivalent to an IQ of up to about 74 (and therefore falling within what has been called 'borderline learning disability', particularly if they suffer from additional disorders such as a genetic syndrome) may be classified as suffering from ID.

There are big differences in reported prevalence rates of offenders in the CJS, possibly due to geographical issues and differences in the definition and diagnosis of ID; however, there is a small but significant group of people with ID who are known to the CJS [8]. People with ID may have increased recorded offending rates due to a lower ability to avoid arrest but it is also possible that actual offending is underestimated because of a higher tolerance of disturbed behaviour by both care staff and the police and prosecution or reluctance to involve the police [9].

Studies of the prevalence of ID in the CJS are inherently difficult to conduct, and McKenzie et al. [3] noted that not all studies used all three criteria of ID, for instance not providing information on adaptive functioning. Fazel et al. [10] found substantial heterogeneity, but their results suggested that typically 0.5–1.5% of prisoners were diagnosed with ID (ranging between 0% and 2.8%). A review of prevalence studies carried out since 2006 by Søndenaa et al. [11] suggested prevalence rates which range between 7.1% and 20%.

In the UK, up to 11% of prisoners on remand and 5–7% of sentenced prisoners have been reported to have ID, although there appears to be a problem reliably identifying this group because of insufficient screening [12]. It is therefore likely that people with ID are at risk of receiving insufficient support and treatment despite this population being known to present with multiple comorbid problems (including mental illness, physical problems, autism, attention deficit hyperactivity disorder (ADHD) and substance misuse) more often than the general population.

Offending

People with moderate to profound ID may not have the necessary intent (*mens rea*) to commit a crime, and this is a key issue when it comes to legal perception of the difference between challenging behaviour and criminal behaviour [13]. A person with moderate to severe ID is unlikely to be dealt with through the CJS unless the criminal act is very serious. On the other hand, people with a mild ID may well be charged and convicted.

There have been conflicting arguments as to whether people with mild ID should always be prosecuted. One view is that this may be viewed as oppressive, whereas others may propose that a successful prosecution may prevent more serious offending and make the provision of assessment, treatment and prevention of further offending more likely. Members of staff working with those with ID may be reluctant to report incidents to the police [14]. However, if challenging behaviour remains unchallenged, this may lead to individuals believing that such behaviour is acceptable, leading to further and potentially more serious acts ('learned impunity'), which then in turn may lead to more serious consequences both for society and the perpetrator [13].

There is relatively little research into the behaviours leading to a referral into forensic services. Lindsay et al. [15] looked at people who had committed offences or displayed offending behaviour who had been referred to community and secure in-patient services for people with ID, and found that physical and verbal aggression and contact or non-contact sexual offences were common index behaviours. They found relatively low levels of referrals for fire-setting and theft. However, Lindsay et al. [15] noted that 40% of those referred to secure forensic services had previous offending type behaviours relating to contact sexual offences, and fire-setting was recorded in more than 30%. Perhaps not surprisingly, very few were charged with road traffic offences.

Many people with ID, particularly those who come into contact with the CJS, have additional mental health problems including pervasive developmental disorders, mental illness or substance misuse disorders [16]. Lindsay et al. [17], when comparing a group of people with learning disability who were accepted into forensic services with those who were not accepted into forensic services, found that those who were accepted had significantly higher rates of schizophrenia and ADHD. When a person in police custody appears to be suffering from a mental disorder including ID or appears as if they may need clinical attention, then appropriate help must be sought as soon as possible.

Criminal Justice System

People with ID who come into contact with the CJS may have limited ability to understand the consequences of their actions and may be easily manipulated. They often make no attempt to disguise what they have done, or even 'confess' what they have not done [13, 18].

The screening processes used in police custody may not always detect that a person has an ID [19]. In practice, if those with ID who are in contact with the CJS are assessed, mental health professionals (whether or not ID has been recognised) sometimes express the view that nothing can be done under mental health legislation because the person is not 'mentally ill'. This can happen particularly when the assessing professionals do not have expertise or experience in working with people who have ID. In England and Wales, ID associated with abnormally aggressive or seriously irresponsible behaviour can be seen as a mental disorder which can lead to treatment under the Mental Health Act, even if the person does not have an additional mental illness [13].

In order to assist a vulnerable defendant to understand and participate in court proceedings, all possible steps should be taken to help vulnerable defendants to understand and to participate in court proceedings and the court process should be adapted where necessary. Such adaptations include the defendant having a chance to visit the court out of hours to familiarise themself with the environment, having the proceedings and possible outcomes explained in advance in understandable language, being free to sit with family or a supporting adult during the proceedings, having frequent breaks to aid concentration and having the trial (including cross-examination) conducted in simple, clear and unambivalent language.

The Bradley Report [20] recognised the difficulties inherent in the diversion schemes and the problems resulting from the non-recognition of ID at the court stage. The Bradley Report recommended that the probation service and the judiciary should receive mental health and ID awareness training. Fortunately, (alleged) offenders with ID are more likely to be diverted from the CJS than those without [21].

Forensic Patients in the Community

There needs to be a balance between appropriately diverting people with significant mental health problems from the CJS and ensuring the public are protected. In order to determine whether a community order (rather than admission to hospital or a prison sentence) is appropriate for an offender with ID, a number of factors should be considered, such as the nature of the offence, history of offending, presence of mental illness, comorbid substance misuse, capacity to consent and the need for public protection, but also issues of vulnerability in prison settings and the availability of adapted treatment programmes. Community forensic teams for people with ID can potentially reduce the number of people who would otherwise have risked being given a prison sentence [22–25].

In-Patient Services

Only a small minority of offenders with ID need additional external precautions or physical limitations [26]. In the UK, forensic ID hospital beds exist in high-, medium- and low-secure units, but also in locked units for offenders with ID with names such as locked rehabilitation units and step-down units that are not formally classified as secure units. In England, whereas patients in low-, medium- and high-secure units are generally funded directly by NHS England, those in locked units are currently funded by local Clinical Commissioning Groups.

There are few services specifically for women offenders with ID. This group of patients have high levels of mental illness, are more likely to have suffered from sexual abuse [27] and a small number of these patients are very difficult to manage, often needing very high levels of staffing to keep them and others safe.

Many of the patients admitted to secure units have high rates of psychiatric and developmental morbidities. Most have past experiences of deprivation and abuse, about half have personality disorders, half have substance misuse, a third have mental illnesses and about a third to a quarter have disorders within the autistic spectrum [16, 28]. As a group they also have extensive histories of offending behaviour with risk profiles that are as serious as those detained in generic forensic units [21, 28].

In England there has been pressure through the Transforming Care programme to reduce the number of people in with ID and/or autism in hospital [29]. It was anticipated that the programme would lead to the closure of a proportion of the secure estate with a reciprocal increase in community-based ID forensic services. However, others [30] have argued that reducing beds before appropriate community provision is available is unwise, as in view of the high levels of abuse, neglect and deprivation experienced by many offenders with ID, they need time to develop insight into their difficulties in relating to others, acquire skills in regulating their emotions and acknowledge their future support needs.

Assessment and Treatment

When preparing to assess a person with learning disability it is useful to be aware that such an assessment may take substantially longer, and that repeated assessments may be required. The interviewer may need to use short sentences and simple words, and have a pen and paper to hand as the use of drawings and pictures may be helpful. The importance of informants and supporting documentation cannot be underestimated. In the history, attention to developmental history and the current social situation is particularly relevant.

The mainstream risk assessment instruments are generally used in services for people with ID. Lindsay et al. [31] found that the Violence Risk Appraisal Guide (VRAG), Historical Clinical and Risk Management-20 (HCR 20), Risk Matrix 2000 C and Short Dynamic Risk Scale (SDRS) in men in high-, medium- and low-secure services had predictive validity for violence in the ID population.

As many offenders with ID have additional psychiatric disorders such as schizophrenia, bipolar disorder or depression specific treatment including psychotropic medication should be considered as appropriate. A significant number of in-patients are assessed to have either a diagnosis or traits of personality disorder, and may benefit from relational and psycho-therapeutic treatment. Many patients present with additional psychosocial disadvantages [32] and need a period of stability in a stable environment, allowing for trusting relationships to develop with members of staff prior to active psychological treatment. Motivational work with patients can be both formal (e.g. psychology-led) or informal (e.g. by qualified and experienced unqualified nursing staff).

Specific treatments are available, including cognitive treatment (thinking skills), and offence specific therapies which may concentrate on specific psychological treatment such as anger [33] and sexual offending [37]. Mainstream treatments have also been successfully adapted for use in the ID population such as dialectical behaviour therapy [34].

The length of treatment both in in-patient and out-patient settings may be important. Day [35] found that in-patient offenders with ID with more than two years' in-patient care had a better longer-term outcome than those with less than two years. Sex offenders treated in the community on probation orders for two or more years had better outcomes than those with a one-year order [36].

Conclusion

Although in a minority, people with ID who have offended tend to have a disadvantaged background, poor social skills and impulse control difficulties. They may not be recognised as suffering from ID, may be more difficult to assess and treatment may not always be available. The move to more out-patient services is positive, but in order to ensure future treatment for this vulnerable group of patients, specialised, well-funded and resourced in-patient treatment will also continue to be essential in order to avoid prolonged prison sentences for people with ID.

References

1. West D, Farrington D. *Who Becomes Delinquent?* London, Heinemann Educational, 1973.

2. Holland T, Clare I, Mukhopadhyay T. Prevalence of 'criminal offending' by men and women with intellectual disability and the characteristics of 'offenders': implications for research and service development. *Journal of Intellectual Disability Research* 2002; 46: 6–20.

3. McKenzie K, Michie A, Murray A, Hales C. Screening for offenders with an intellectual disability: the validity of the Learning Disability Screening Questionnaire. *Research in Developmental Disabilities* 2012; 33 (3): 791–5.

4. American Psychiatric Association. *Diagnostic and Statistical Manual of Mental Disorders: DSM-5.* Arlington, VA, American Psychiatric Association, 2013.

5. American Psychiatric Association. *Diagnostic and Statistical Manual of Mental Disorders: DSM-5-TR.* Washington, DC, American Psychiatric Publications Incorporated, 2022.

6. World Health Organization. *International Classification of Diseases. ICD-11 – Mortality and Morbidity Statistics.* Geneva, World Health Organization, 2018.

7. World Health Organization. The ICD-10 classification of mental and behavioural disorders: clinical descriptions and diagnostic guidelines. *Weekly Epidemiological Record* 1992; 67 (30): 227.

8. Talbot J, Riley C. No one knows: offenders with learning difficulties and learning disabilities. *British Journal of Learning Disabilities* 2007; 35:1 54–61.

9. Barron P, Hassiotis A, Banes J. Offenders with intellectual disability: the size of the problem and therapeutic outcomes. *Journal of Intellectual Disability Research* 2002; 46 (6): 454–63.

10. Fazel S, Xenitidis K, Powell J. The prevalence of intellectual disabilities among 12000 prisoners: a systematic review. *International Journal of Law and Psychiatry* 2008; 31 (4): 369–73.

11. Søndenaa E, Rasmussen K, Palmstierna T, Nøttestad J. The prevalence and nature of intellectual disability in Norwegian prisons. *Journal of Intellectual Disability Research* 2008; 52 (12): 1129–37.

12. Singleton N, Gatward R, Meltzer H. *Psychiatric Morbidity among Prisoners in England and Wales.* London, Stationery Office, 1998.

13. Boer H, Alexander RT, Beber E et al. *Forensic Care Pathways for Adults with Intellectual Disability Involved with the Criminal Justice System.* London, Royal

College of Psychiatrists' Faculty of Psychiatry of Intellectual Disability, 2014.

14. McBrien J, Murphy G. Police and carers' views on reporting alleged offences by people with intellectual disabilities. *Psychology, Crime & Law* 2006; 12 (2): 127–44.

15. Lindsay WR, O'Brien G, Carson D et al. Pathways into services for offenders with intellectual disabilities: childhood experiences, diagnostic information, and offense variables. *Criminal Justice and Behavior* 2010; 37 (6): 678–94.

16. Alexander R, Cooray S. Diagnosis of personality disorders in learning disability. *The British Journal of Psychiatry* 2003; 182 (S44): s28–s31.

17. Lindsay WR, Holland T, Wheeler JR et al. Pathways through services for offenders with intellectual disability: a one- and two-year follow-up study. *American Journal on Intellectual and Developmental Disabilities* 2010; 115 (3): 250–62.

18. Finlay WM, Lyons E. Acquiescence in interviews with people who have mental retardation. *Mental Retardation* 2002; 40 (1): 14–29.

19. McKinnon IG, Grubin D. Health screening of people in police custody: evaluation of current police screening procedures in London, UK. *The European Journal of Public Health* 2013; 23 (3): 399–405.

20. Bradley RHL. *Lord Bradley's Review of People with Mental Health Problems or Learning Disabilities in the Criminal Justice System.* London, Crown, 2009, p. 173.

21. Chester V, Völlm B, Tromans S, Kapugama C, Alexander RT. Long-stay patients with and without intellectual disability in forensic psychiatric settings: comparison of characteristics and needs. *BJPsych Open* 2018; 4(4): 226–34.

22. Benton C, Roy A. The first three years of a community forensic service for people with a learning disability. *The British Journal of Forensic Practice* 2008; 10 (2): 4–12.

23. Dinani S, Goodman W, Swift C, Treasure T. Providing forensic community services for people with learning disabilities. *Journal of Learning Disabilities and Offending Behaviour* 2010; 1 (1): 58–63.

24. Devapriam J, Alexander RT. Tiered model of learning disability forensic service provision. *Journal of Learning Disabilities and Offending Behaviour* 2012; 3 (4): 175–85.

25. de Villiers J, Doyle M. Making a difference? Ten years of managing people with intellectual disability and forensic needs in the community. *Journal of Intellectual Disabilities and Offending Behaviour* 2015; 6 (3/4): 165–74.

26. Johnston S. Forensic psychiatry and learning disability. In Fraser W and Kerr M (eds) *Seminars in the Psychiatry of Learning Disabilities.* London, Royal College of Psychiatrists Publications, 2nd ed. (2003), pp. 287–303.

27. Berber E, Boer H. Development of a specialised forensic service for women with learning disability: the first three years. *The British Journal of Forensic Practice* 2004; 6 (4): 10–20.

28. Hogue T, Steptoe L, Taylor JL et al. A comparison of offenders with intellectual disability across three levels of security. *Criminal Behaviour and Mental Health* 2006; 16 (1): 13–28.

29. NHS England. *Transforming Care for People with Learning Disabilities: Next Steps.* London, NHS England, 2015.

30. Taylor JL, McKinnon I, Thorpe I, Gillmer BT. The impact of transforming care on the care and safety of patients with intellectual disabilities and forensic needs. *BJPsych Bulletin* 2017; 41 (4): 205–8.

31. Lindsay WR, Hogue TE, Taylor JL et al. Risk assessment in offenders with intellectual disability: a comparison across three levels of security. *International Journal of Offender Therapy and Comparative Criminology* 2008; 52 (1): 90–111.

32. Holland AJ. Criminal behaviour and developmental disability: an epidemiological perspective. In Lindsay W, Taylor J, Sturmey P (eds) *Offenders with*

Developmental Disabilities. Chichester, Wiley, 2004, pp. 23–34.

33. Taylor JL, Novaco RW, Gillmer BT, Robertson A, Thorne I. Individual cognitive-behavioural anger treatment for people with mild-borderline intellectual disabilities and histories of aggression: a controlled trial. *British Journal of Clinical Psychology* 2005; 44 (3): 367–82.

34. Morrissey C, Ingamells B. Adapted dialectical behaviour therapy for male offenders with learning disabilities in a high secure environment: six years on. *Journal of Learning Disabilities and Offending Behaviour* 2011; 2 (1): 8–15.

35. Day K. A hospital-based treatment programme for male mentally handicapped offenders. *British Journal of Psychiatry* 1988; 153: 635–44.

36. Lindsay WR, Smith AH. Responses to treatment for sex offenders with intellectual disability: a comparison of men with 1- and 2-year probation sentences. *Journal of Intellectual Disability Research* 1998; 42 (5): 346–53.

37. Lindsay WR, Elliot SF, Astell A. Predictors of sexual offence recidivism in offenders with intellectual disabilities. *Journal of Applied Research in Intellectual Disabilities* 2004; 17: 299–305.

Cultural Service Delivery in Forensic Mental Health Services

Brian McKenna and James Cavney

Introduction

In the emerging world of ethnic conflict . . . Western belief in the universality of Western culture suffers three problems; it is false; it is immoral; and it is dangerous. [33]

As contentious as the writings of Samual Huntingdon might be, the quote that opens this chapter epitomises the challenges faced in developing twenty-first-century forensic mental health services (FMHS) to be culturally responsive. Indigenous peoples and other ethnic minorities are increasingly recognised as being disproportionately represented in criminal justice, mental health and FMHS settings. The inadequacy of Western paradigms and systems to meet their needs is evident. In Canada, for example, the Supreme Court recently ruled that the Correctional Service breached its statutory duty to an Indigenous prisoner in assessing his risk of recidivism using actuarial risk assessment tools not validated with Indigenous peoples [2].

The intent of this chapter is to highlight the adverse impact of colonisation and acculturation on Indigenous peoples and ethnic minorities, and to consider the implications for FMHS. It discusses the challenges that arise in developing systemic solutions to address cultural inequity, taking the positive example of the evolution of FMHS in Aotearoa-New Zealand, over the past 30 years, in particular the Auckland Regional Forensic Psychiatry Services (ARFPS).

Culture, Colonisation and Acculturation

Human beings are defined by the cultural groups of which they are a part. The rich tapestry of cultural diversity across time and place reflects diverse habitats and the collaborative response of the group to procure resources for mutual survival [3]. The emergent culture encompasses a shared language, worldview and values, which in turn determine emotional and behavioural responses to the surrounding world. These cultural components are transmitted from one generation to the next, in order to maintain group cohesion and survival [4].

However, as human societies expanded, increased contact between cultures and contestability for resources frequently resulted in cultural dominance, assimilation or attempted annihilation of one group by another. In modern history, this process continued with European colonisation of so-called technologically less advanced Indigenous peoples of the 'New World', through violence and warfare. Conquest typically led to an inherent ethnocentric belief that the dominant culture's way of life was natural, correct and superior [3].

The outcome of colonisation for the usurped group was typically devastating: the loss of identity, self-esteem and resilience through the erosion of cultural institutions such as language, religion and ancestral connectedness to land and social structures. Furthermore, these negative outcomes were not confined to the temporal point of contact but are part of contemporary reality manifest in the intergenerational transmission of trauma, poor mental health, alcohol and substance abuse, and incarceration [3, 4, 5, 6, 7].

The term 'Indigenous' thus has a broader meaning than simply the original inhabitants of the land. Implicit in its meaning is recognition that these peoples have, to varying degrees, been marginalised or otherwise disenfranchised from socio-political influence (self-determination) within their traditional lands [3]. This is due to the development of colonial social institutions that foster discrimination and inequality in power, resources and assimilation through state-sanctioned policies [4]. Non-Indigenous minority migrant groups can face a similar socio-political disenfranchisement and poor social outcomes, particularly if they have had a traumatic migration history.

Implications of Colonisation for FMHS

The devastation of colonisation is reflected in the incarceration rates of Indigenous peoples and the rates of mental illness in such populations. In Australia, Indigenous peoples (Aboriginal and Torres Strait Islanders) experience a relative risk of imprisonment 15.2 times than that of the non-Indigenous population. They constitute 3% of the population and 27% of the prison population, with a staggering imprisonment rate of 2,434 per 100,000 population versus 160 per 100,000 population for non-Aboriginals [8]. Given the growing rate of incarceration of young Indigenous women, the impact on existing communities and future generations is profound [7]. In a representative sample of Indigenous peoples incarcerated in Queensland in 2008, Heffernan et al. [9] found that the 12-month prevalence of mental disorder was 73% among men and 86% among women.

In Canada, Indigenous peoples (First Nations, Inuit and Métis) account for only 4.3% of the general population but represent approximately 21% of the total federal prison population [10]. They have high rates of serious mental illness (psychotic mental illness and major depression) [11].

Furthermore, non-Indigenous ethnic minority groups experience similar inequitable outcomes. For example, 26% of those incarcerated in England and Wales identified with non-white ethnicity, compared with 13% in the general population [12]. This over-representation is not new, remaining relatively constant since 2005. There is growing concern regarding the unmet mental health needs of this population [13].

Colonisation and FMHS in New Zealand

Māori lived in relative cultural isolation in Aotearoa-New Zealand following migration from the Pacific in about 900 AD. Following the arrival of Captain James Cook in 1769, a British colony was established and grew. Initial cross-cultural tensions were assuaged through a humanistic approach with the signing of Te Tiriti o Waitangi (The Treaty of Waitangi) in 1840 [3].

Māori believed the signing secured rights to partnership, protection and equal citizenship, while retaining self-determination over what they valued and controlled. However, Māori came to experience all the devastating hallmarks of post-colonial contact as the British attempted assimilation through land confiscation and the deliberate erosion of Māori cultural institutions [3].

This is exemplified in Māori incarceration rates. In 2017, Māori experienced 7.5 times the risk of imprisonment when compared to New Zealanders of European heritage, with a rate of 704 per 100,000 population [8]. In prison, Māori have higher rates of psychotic symptoms than those experienced by any other ethnic group [14].

Pacific Island peoples (primarily of Samoan, Tongan, Cook Island, Fijian, Nuien, Tokelaun and Tuvaluan descent) immigrated to fill employment need during the 1950s to 1970s. They constitute 7% of the general population but account for 12% of the prison population [15]. Pacific Island people have the highest prevalence rate by ethnicity of any mental illness among prisoners [14].

These prison statistics are reflected in the ethnicity of service users in FMHS in Aotearoa-New Zealand. In an audit of ethnicity undertaken by the authors at the ARFPS, in 2019, in a secure hospital, 43% of service users were Māori and 20% of Pacific Island descent.

Solutions in FMHS in New Zealand

Notwithstanding the devastating impact of colonisation, Te Tiriti o Waitangi has, since the 1970s, provided a powerful mechanism for Māori to seek legal and political redress for many of the injustices suffered as a result of colonisation [16]. This movement has significantly impacted on the development of FMHS over the past 30 years, with renewed attention to resurrect the concept of Māori self-determination (Tino Rangatiratanga) and viable partnerships with the Crown in moving towards a solutions-focussed response to the issues promulgated by colonisation.

In 1988, the Mason Report [17] (commissioned in response to a double homicide in the community and a cluster of 13 suicide deaths within correctional facilities) created the possibility of transformational change and provided a blueprint for service delivery for FMHS in Aotearoa-New Zealand. It recommended the establishment of five regional medium and minimum secure mental health services that interfaced with the community, prisons and courts; multi-disciplinary decision-making; least restrictive care; safe staffing levels; relational security; continuity of care; gradual transition; and cultural responsivity. It also provided an outline for a culturally informed clinical governance structure that included both clinical and cultural leadership [17].

The ARFPS is the largest of the regional services with a catchment population of 1.5 million people in the northern regions of Aotearoa-New Zealand. It provides integrated mental health and intellectual disability services to a 126-bed secure hospital (109-bed mental health and 17-bed intellectual disability), people transitioning to the community, the regions' courts and six prisons. The service is led by a triumvirate of a kaumatua (cultural leader), a clinical director and an operational manager. The associated clinical governance structure explicitly incorporates the views of Māori at all levels of service design and implementation, in which evidence-based medicine and values-based (cultural) practice co-exist.

Models of Care

A model of care is an overarching framework which defines how healthcare services are delivered [18]. Three aspects are important to contemporary clinical models of care in FMHS. These are the concepts of *therapeutic security*, which focusses on the importance of environmental, relational and procedural security; *rehabilitation*, focussing on restructuring lives seriously impacted on by both mental illness and offending; and *recovery-orientated care*, which is person-centred and emphasises hope, empowerment and working towards the self-determination and self-sufficiency of the service user.

The Mason Report [17] highlights that this clinical approach combining therapeutic security, rehabilitation and recovery needs to stand alongside a cultural model of care, given the obligations implicit in the partnership between a Crown agency (ARFPS) and Māori under Te Tiriti o Waitangi. At the ARFPS, Te Ao Māori (the Māori worldview) is integrated through seven core values, being *wairuatanga* (spiritual health), *tikanga/kawa* (boundaries/rules), *whanaungatanga* (family health), *tinana* (physical health), *hinengaro* (mental health), *tūmanako* (hope for the future) and *whakapaitia* (excellence in service delivery) [19].

Clinical Pathway

At the ARFPS, the clinical pathway aligns the recovery paradigm with movement through three levels of security: medium, minimum and open care. Progress is signalled by the achievement of milestones indicating success of therapeutic interventions to the extent that the service user can demonstrate their ability to manage risks at the next level of security [20].

There are four milestones in the pathway (see Figure 20.1). The first marks the acceptance into the rehabilitation streams. Historically, there were two rehabilitative streams in this pathway – a mixed-gender stream (Figure 20.1, Rehabilitation 2) and a male-only stream for men involved in sex offending and very violent offending (Figure 20.1, Rehabilitation 1). The second milestone sits at the interface between medium and minimum security in the rehabilitation streams. The third demarcates that the service user is ready to commence community reintegration under the Forensic Community Reintegration Service (either in a hostel on site or with an external provider of supported accommodation). Milestone 4 is discharge from the FMHS.

Negotiations to accommodate cultural responsivity in the service's model of care led to the development of a third rehabilitative stream – the Kaupapa Māori (Māori approach) stream (Figure 20.1, KMS Rehabilitation). This stream integrates the previously mentioned core Māori values. Daily life on the medium and minimum units in the Kaupapa Māori stream is decidedly different. The day starts communally with *karakia* (prayer); food is prepared and eaten communally in the minimum-secure setting; there are culturally specific gatherings; and visitors are received through ceremonial welcome. Cultural programmes target the development of knowledge and skills required to optimally function in Te Ao Māori. The Kaupapa Māori stream is not exclusive to Māori, although it requires a commitment to participate in the cultural focus of the unit, which is group-orientated.

To assist the multi-disciplinary decision-making for milestone progression, structured clinical judgement has been introduced using a variety of metrics, foremost the DUNDRUM suite of measurements, especially DUNDRUM-3 (programme completion items) and DUNDRUM-4 (Recovery items) [21]. Although the use of the DUNDRUM toolkit with Māori is supported, recent action research has identified the need for additional components to the measures, which capture the cultural and spiritual aspects of Māori recovery [22].

Interventions

Interventions at the ARFPS are grounded in evidence-based practice and targeted to address rehabilitative needs, focussing on physical health, mental health, drugs and alcohol use, problem behaviours, activities of daily living, vocation (in the broad sense of education,

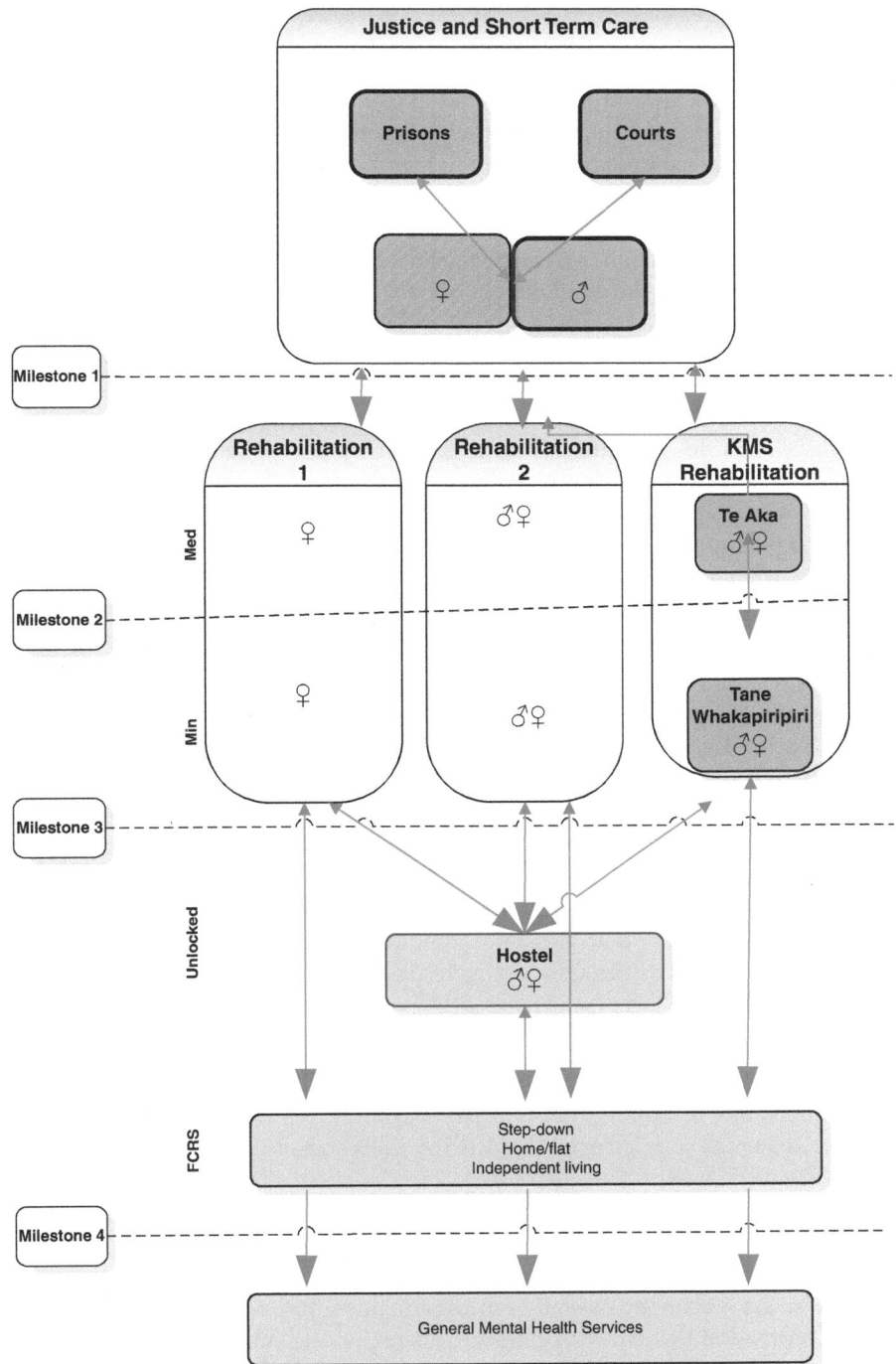

Figure 20.1 The clinical pathway and rehabilitation streams at the ARFPS [20].

occupation and creative expression), and social wellbeing (including family cohesion and intimacy).

There is little evidence as to the effectiveness of many of these programmes in meeting the needs of different ethnic groups. However, the limited studies available comparing the impact of internationally developed, culturally relevant programmes undertaken in correctional settings, compared to standard programmes, have found a positive impact of culturally modified interventions in the reduction of recidivism [23].

To address the needs of Māori in the ARFPS, two broad strategies have thus been undertaken: the modification of existing evidence-based programmes to incorporate a cultural component and the development of specific cultural approaches to meet cultural needs. One example of a culturally modified evidence-based approach is the Tū Tahanga programme, which integrated the Man Alive violence prevention programme with Māori-specific cultural processes [24].

An example of a unique Māori cultural intervention is *hohou i te rongo* (reconciliation). This is practised in de-escalating Māori when aroused and agitated by applying cultural rules to face-to-face engagement undertaken in a culturally safe space (the meeting house), with a focus on restorative obligations [25]. Although research steps have been undertaken to describe both culturally modified evidence-based interventions and culturally specific interventions, a gap remains in determining their efficacy.

Physical Environment

The development of a Kaupapa Māori stream in the ARFPS is also reflected in the physical appearance of the in-patient units. Figure 20.2 shows the carving above the entrance to the Kaupapa Māori medium-secure unit called Te Aka (the vine). Strands representing the vine depict the complexity to be unravelled on entry to the unit (personal communication with Te Rātahi, the carver). It signals the entry to a cultural space, Te Whakamahana, which literally means to bring about warmth. On the walls of this space are cultural depictions of holistic health – physical health, mental health, the health of the family and spiritual wellbeing. This symbolism all taps into deep cultural meaning of wellbeing.

In the minimum-secure unit, there is a traditional meeting house used for ceremonial purposes and cultural activities. The perimeter is a secure fence reminiscent of the traditional fortified hilltop villages (see Figure 20.3).

Workforce

The bicultural nature of the model of care, pathways, interventions and physical space must also be reflected in the competencies (knowledge, skills and attitudes) of the workforce. The workforce in general is expected to have some knowledge and appreciation of Māori culture [17]. However, more important is the alignment of the workforce with the ability to recognise and act on the inequities experienced by Māori through colonisation. This consciousness of critique is referred to as 'cultural safety'.

Cultural safety is achieved by staff of the dominant culture realising and addressing the inequities constructed by their own culture. This requires acknowledgement of the limitations of one's own ethnocentric cultural framework and the associated biases, assumptions and prejudices. It requires a realisation that the correct way forward involves engaging with and empowering those served. It may require accessing the assistance of cultural experts who fully understand the cultural framework under consideration [26].

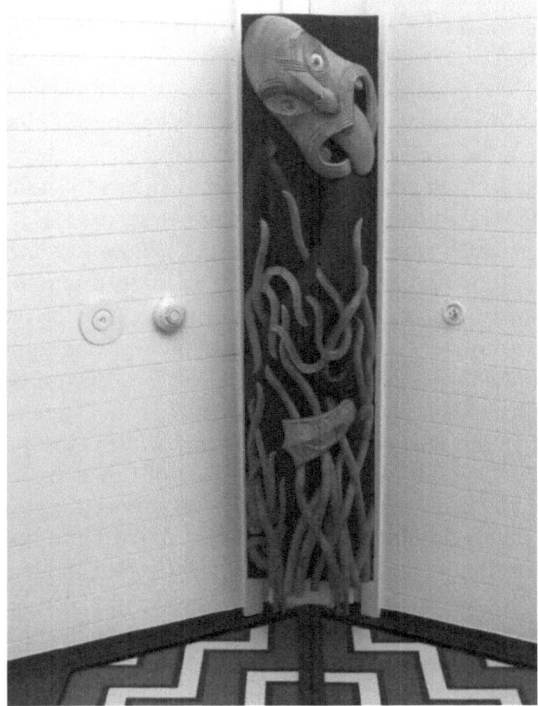

Figure 20.2 Carving in the medium-secure Kaupapa Māori unit (Te Aka).

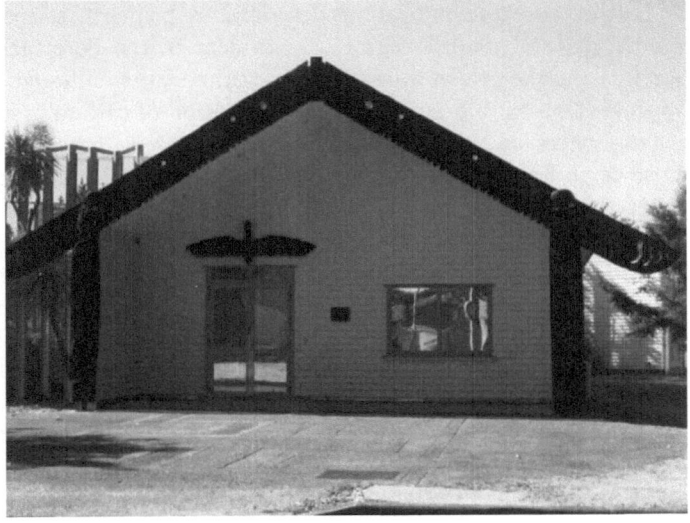

Figure 20.3 The traditional meeting house in the minimum-secure Kaupapa Māori unit (Tāne Whakapiripiri).

This realisation and responsibility to address power differentials arising from colonisation exist at both a personal level and an organisational level. The same processes applied to reflection on individual practice need to be applied at a systems analysis [26]. Leaders of FMHS in Aotearoa-New Zealand are expected to have a knowledge and appreciation of Māori culture [17]. Cultural leadership is expected to sit alongside clinical leadership and be involved in all facets of the decision-making process.

FMHS are also expected to provide Māori health workers in sufficient numbers to meet the needs of the Māori population in each regional service [17]. Presently the health professions do not produce sufficient numbers [27]; however, FMHS in Aotearoa-New Zealand do employ cultural experts (*taura whiri*) as multi-disciplinary team members to assist in the assessment and management of service users; provide training for such teams; assist in developing cultural services; and maintain close working contact with *iwi* (tribes) in the area. Presently in the in-patient units at the ARFPS, every unit has a *taura whiri*.

For some Māori, there is understandable mistrust of the 'system' (state-derived structures and mechanisms). It is the responsibility of *taura whiri* in the hospital to welcome and ease the person into a new setting. An integral part of this is establishing links through *whakapapa* (genealogy). Such links allow core cultural connection through shared ancestry. It is this connection that facilitates the establishment of trust and the ability to engage.

Cultural assessment is a major part of the *taura whiri* role, to identify culturally specific experiences and needs. Assessment is via a holistic model of Māori health, which considers the links between *tinana* (physical health), *hinengaro* (mental health), *whānau* (family and social relationships) and *wairua* (spirituality). This is an understanding that can only be gained by those who live the culture. This perspective is crucial when considering diagnosis, as diagnosis itself is an ethnocentric construct. Diverse lenses are required to determine if experiences are symptomatic of illness or a legitimate cultural reality [3].

Conclusion

What has been described in this chapter as cultural innovation is not without its challenges. As significant as the bicultural progress has been, it has taken over 30 years since the Mason Report in 1988. Furthermore, the innovations described are primarily related to the secure in-patient hospital. Cultural models of care are evident in the Forensic Reintegration Community Services and the prison in-reach teams. In the latter, although cultural input is stretched, improvements have been made in the provision of culturally specific services [28]. Court-related services have yet to articulate a model of care with a cultural component. The ARFPS is also yet to fully address a model of care for the significant minority of Pacific Island service users.

It is also important that cultural responsivity is mirrored in those agencies the FMHS interfaces with (justice, corrections, police and a variety of social care agencies). Failure to do so disrupts the significance of cultural continuity of care. Improvements in the cultural responsivity of aligning agencies are signalled in the recent inquiry into mental health services [29], critique of the criminal justice system [30] and policy shifts in services provided by correctional facilities [31].

It is hoped that the examples presented here provide impetus for cultural transformation in FMHS internationally. Indigenous peoples have a right to culturally safe responses, as embodied in the United Nations Declaration on the Rights of Indigenous People (Article 24) [32]. Such rights need to be extended to ethnic minorities in FMHS. This is not to say that the solutions provided here are appropriate for other services. It is up to each FMHS to negotiate what is appropriate with the culturally diverse people they serve. However, FMHS in Aotearoa-New Zealand have embarked on a culturally responsive journey that has gone too far not to keep going.

References

1. Huntington S. *The Clash of Civilizations and the Remaking of World Order*. New York, Simon, and Schuster, 1996, p. 310.

2. Case in Brief: *Ewert v. Canada (Correctional Service)*. 2018. www.scccsc.ca.

3. Cavney J, Hatters Friedman S. Culture, mental illness and prison: a New Zealand Perspective. In Mills A, Kendall K (eds) *Mental Health in Prisons*. London, Palgrave, 2018. https://doi.org/10.1007/978-3-319-940 90-8_9.

4. Shepherd S, Delgado R, Paradies Y. Inter-relationships, cultural identity, discrimination, distress, agency, and safety among indigenous people in custody, *International Journal of Mental Health* 2018. doi: 10.1080/ 14999013.2018.1431338.

5. Paradies Y. Beyond black and white: essentialism, hybridity and Indigeneity. *Journal of Sociology* 2006; 42: 355–67. doi: 10.1177/1440783306069993.

6. Ogloff J, Pfeifer J, Shepherd S, Ciorciari J. Assessing the mental health, substance abuse, cognitive functioning, and social/emotional well-being needs of Aboriginal prisoners in Australia. *Journal of Correctional Health Care* 2017; 23 (4): 1–14.

7. Sullivan E, Kendall S, Chang S et al. Aboriginal mothers in prison in Australia: a study of social, emotional and physical wellbeing. *Australian and New Zealand Journal of Public Health* 2019; 43: 241–7. doi: 10.1111/1753/1753-6405.12892.

8. Skipworth J. The Australian and New Zealand prison crisis: cultural and clinical issues. *Australian Journal of Psychology* 2018; 53 (5): 1–2. doi: 10.1177/0004867418817375.

9. Heffernan E, Anderson K, Dev A, Kinner S. Prevalence of mental illness among Aboriginal and Torres Strait Islander people in Queensland prisons. *Medical Journal of Australia* 2012; 197: 37–41.

10. Gutierrez L, Helmus R, Hanson R. *What We Know and Don't Know about Risk Assessment with Offenders of Indigenous Heritage*. Research Report: 2017–R009, Ottawa, Public Safety Canada, 2017.

11. Simpson A, McMaster J, Cohen S. Challenges for Canada in meeting the needs of persons with serious mental illness in prison. *Journal of the American Academy of Psychiatry and the Law* 2013; 41: 501–9.

12. Sturge G. *UK Prison Population Statistics Briefing Paper*. Number CBP-04334. 2018. www.parliament.uk/commons-library.

13. Lammy D. *The Lammy Review: An Independent Review into the Treatment of, and Outcomes for, Black, Asian and Minority Ethnic Individuals in the Criminal Justice System*. 2017. www.gov.uk/govern ment/publications/lammy-review-final-report.

14. Indig D, Gear C, Wilhelm K. *Comorbid Substance Use Disorders and Mental Health Disorders among New Zealand Prisoners*. Wellington, Department of Corrections, 2016.

15. Ara Poutama (Department of Corrections). www.corrections.govt.nz/resources/researc h_and_statistics/quarterly_prison_statistics/prison_stats_september_2019#ethnicity.

16. New Zealand Government. Te Kāhui Whakatau (Treaty Settlements). www.govt .nz/browse/history-culture-and-heritage/treaty-of-waitangi-claims/settling-historical-treaty-of-waitangi-claims.

17. Mason K. *Report of the Committee of Inquiry into Procedures Used in Certain Psychiatric Hospitals in Relation to Admission, Discharge or Release on Leave of Certain Classes of Patients* (The Mason

Report). Wellington, Ministry of Health, 1988.

18. Kennedy HG. Models of care in forensic psychiatry. *BJPsych Advances* 2022; 28 (1): 46–59. doi: 10.1192/bja.2021.34.

19. Sweetman L. Ngā waiata o Tāne Whakapiripiri (The music of Tāne Whakapiripiri): cultural expression, transformation, and healing in a Māori forensic psychiatric unit. Doctoral thesis, New York University, 2017. https://pqdtopen.proquest.com/doc/1880347833.html?FMT=ABS.

20. The Mason Clinic. *Te Aranga Hou – Mason Clinic Service User Pathways Future State Map – Milestones Update.* Auckland, Waitematā District Health Board, 2018.

21. Kennedy K, O'Neill C, Flynn G, Gill P, Davoren M. *The DUNDRUM Toolkit: Dangerousness Understanding, Recovery and Urgency Manual* (The DUNDRUM quartet). Dublin, Trinity College Dublin, 2016. www.tara.tcd.ie/handle/2262/39131.

22. Wharewera-Mika J, Cooper E, Wiki N et al. The appropriateness of DUNDRUM-3 and DUNDRUM-4 for Māori in forensic mental health services in New Zealand: participatory action research. *BMC Psychiatry* 2020; 20: 61. https://doi.org/10.1186/s12888-020-2468-x accepted.

23. Gutierrez L, Chadwick N, Wanamaker K. Culturally relevant programming versus the status quo: a meta-analytic review of the effectiveness of treatment of Indigenous offenders. *Canadian Journal of Criminology and Criminal Justice* 2018; 60 (3): 321–53. doi: 10.3138/cjccj.2017-0020.r2.

24. Florencio F. A qualitative descriptive study of Tū Tahanga, a kaupapa Māori adapted violence prevention programme, in a forensic mental health inpatient unit. Master's thesis, Auckland University of Technology, 2020.

25. Wharewera-Mika J, Cooper E, McKenna B et al. Strategies to reduce the use of seclusion with tāngata whai i te ora (Māori mental health service users). *International Journal of Mental Health Nursing* 2016; 25: 258–65.

26. Curtis E, Jones R, Tipene-Leach C. et al. Why cultural safety rather than cultural competency is required to achieve health equity: a literature review and recommended definition. *International Journal for Equity in Health* 2019; 18: 174. https://doi.org/10.1186/s12939-019-1082-3.

27. Te Pou o Te Whakaaro Nui. *Adult Mental Health Forensic Workforce: 2014 Survey of Vote Health Funded Services.* Auckland, Te Pou o Te Whakaaro Nui, 2015.

28. McKenna B, Skipworth J, Tapsell R et al. Impact of an assertive community treatment based model of care on the treatment of prisoners with a serious mental illness. *Australian Psychologist* 2018; 26: 285–9.

29. Paterson R, Durie M, Disley B et al. *He Ara Oranga: Report of the Government Inquiry into Mental Health and Addiction.* Wellington, New Zealand Government, 2018. www.mentalhealth.inquiry.govt.nz/inquiry-report.

30. Burrows C, Gilbert J, Hix Q et al. *He Waka Roimata: Transforming Our Criminal Justice System.* Wellington, New Zealand Government, 2019.

31. Ara Poutama Aotearoa (Department `of Corrections). *Hōkai Rangi. Ara Poutama Aotearoa Strategy 2019–2024.* Wellington, New Zealand Government, 2019.

32. Perdacher E, Kavanagh D, Sheffield J. Wellbeing and mental health interventions for Indigenous people in prison: systematic review *BJPsych Open* 2019; 5 (e95): 1–10. doi: 10.1192/bjo.2019.80.

33. Huntington S. *The Clash of Civilizations and the Remaking of World Order.* New York, Simon and Schuster, 1996, p. 310.

Chapter

2 1

Tackling Ethnic Inequality in Forensic Mental Healthcare

Shubulade Smith and Raj Mohan

Introduction

There are well-known, significant racial disparities in mental healthcare access, experience and outcome. The additional duty of forensic mental health practitioners to be always mindful of public protection means that it is imperative that all steps are taken to reduce the risk that individuals with mental disorder may pose to others, as well as themselves. Forensic mental healthcare focusses on secondary prevention – preventing known patients from relapsing and re-offending – recurrence of violence. The evidence increasingly points to the fact that forensic mental health services are doing this more successfully with some sections of the population we serve than others.

People from all ethnic minority groups (including white minority and people from migrant groups) are more likely to be detained involuntarily than white Indigenous people in white-majority countries [1, 2]. This is particularly the case for those from black African or African-Caribbean backgrounds, who are more likely to be involuntarily detained than any other minoritised group [2]. Furthermore, people of black African and African-Caribbean heritage are 40% more likely than white British people to come into contact with mental health services in crisis and through the criminal justice system, rather than through primary care services such as their family doctor [3, 4, 5]. Once admitted, black people are significantly over-represented in locked wards, psychiatric intensive care and secure care services [6, 7]. This means that forensic mental health practitioners are more likely to have patients from black and other minoritised ethnic backgrounds than expected compared with the number in the general population and compared with other parts of the mental health system. When black people are admitted to hospital, they are more likely to be subjected to restrictive practices such as high-dose anti-psychotic medication, physical restraint and seclusion [6–11].

When black patients leave hospital, they are more likely to be placed under community treatment orders (CTOs), particularly if they are from Caribbean backgrounds (up to 8 × rates of CTOs) and this latter group are significantly more likely to be readmitted involuntarily than any other ethnic group, including people from black African and other black minority groups [2]. Black patients report that their experience of mental healthcare is poor and, unsurprisingly, the evidence indicates that this is likely to interfere with engagement with care and subsequent take-up of services, especially when they are in the community [2]. This increases the chances of relapse and any associated risks to themselves and others [2, 12].

The evidence about access, experience and outcome makes it clear that more could be done. There is little evidence that the current approaches in forensic mental healthcare are really improving outcomes for people from minoritised ethnic communities. Given the higher costs, clinically, societally and financially, of forensic mental healthcare, it is incumbent upon forensic mental health practitioners to be highly competent in caring for patients from minoritised ethnic backgrounds, especially those with the greatest over-representation – black people and people from gypsy, Roma and traveller backgrounds. This means understanding how best to reduce the risk of relapse and associated re-offending in the people from these groups, which requires understanding of how and why black and other minoritised ethnic people are more likely to end up in forensic mental healthcare and how to avoid this happening repeatedly.

The aim of this chapter is to help forensic mental health practitioners understand the nature of racial disparities in mental healthcare and how we might be able to tackle them and in doing so reduce the risk of relapse and recidivism. There will be a focus on the multiple complex factors that are implicated in the increased rates of people from certain minoritised ethnic groups coming into contact with the criminal justice system and forensic mental health services, the greater rate of negative experiences over the life course, social adversity and racism, and the link to worse health outcomes. The chapter will provide practical strategies aimed at reducing racial/ethnic mental health inequality. The wider system approaches as well as strategies for individual clinicians will support services not to perpetuate or exacerbate racial/ethnic disparities and support prevention them in the future in forensic mental healthcare. The chapter will illustrate the problem primarily using the UK context, a multicultural society with evidence of significant disparities in both the criminal justice and mental health system.

Crime and Ethnicity

Most of the crimes in white-majority countries are committed by the majority white population; however, certain ethnic groups are over-represented in the criminal justice system compared with the percentage of people from those groups in the population. For example, in the UK, people from minoritised ethnic groups make up approximately 14% of the general population but 25% of the prison population; in the USA, African-American people make up 12% of the general population but 33% of the prison population, with Hispanic people being 16% of the population but 23% of the prison population; in Australia, Aboriginal and Torres Strait Islanders are 2% of the population but 27% of the prison population; in New Zealand, Māori are 15% of the population but 50% of the prison population; in France, where the majority of Muslims are from the Maghreb, they make up 8% of the general population but an estimated 25–50% of the prison population; and in Ireland, Irish travellers make up 8% of the prison population despite only being 0.7% of the general population [13, 14, 15].

The 2017 Lammy report [13] about the treatment of black, Asian and minority ethnic individuals in the criminal justice system found that people from minoritised ethnic groups are arrested at much higher rates than the white British population, as well as being stopped and searched at far greater rates than white people (53 stop and searches per 1,000 black people, compared with 17.8 per 1,000 for Asian people, 17.5 per 1,000 for mixed-ethnicity people and 7.5 per 1,000 for white people). This disproportionate arrest rate is not matched by the rate of charging decisions, however, with suspects from different ethnic backgrounds being charged at similar rates. From then on, disparities exist within the criminal justice system, with people from minoritised ethnic groups being more likely to be convicted and to receive longer custodial sentences than white people. In 2018, Asian offenders were given longer average custodial sentences for possession of weapons than other ethnic groups, 17.1 months, compared with an overall average of 12.8 months for the same offence.

In the UK, the ethnicity of the prison population varies across the age groups with older prisoners being predominantly white British. However, of concern is that of younger prisoners, 53% of those under 18 are from minoritised ethnic backgrounds. Of these prisoners, two groups stand out: those from black backgrounds and those from gypsy, Roma and traveller (GRT) backgrounds, who are heavily over-represented in the younger prison population. Black people make up 12% of the total adult prison population despite only being 3% of the general population and 20% of children in custody. GRT people are massively over-represented in prison, being less than 0.1% of the general population of England and Wales but 12% of children in custody [13]. Although there are not disproportionate numbers of people from Asian backgrounds in prison, there are marked differences in which Asian ethnic groups dominate in prison, with people from Indian backgrounds being far less likely to come into contact with the criminal justice system, whereas Asian people from Pakistani and Bangladeshi backgrounds are more heavily represented. This likely reflects differences in wealth and deprivation between the groups, as this increases likelihood of contact with the criminal justice system. South Asian people from Indian backgrounds are far less likely to live in deprived areas, compared with people from Bangladeshi and Pakistani backgrounds (only 7% of people from Indian backgrounds live in deprived areas versus 19% of Bangladeshi people and 31% of people from Pakistani backgrounds) [16].

The majority of minoritised ethnic people are not involved in offending behaviour; however, if a person from a minority ethnic background comes into contact with the criminal justice system (particularly if they are black, South Asian or GRT), compared with a white British person they are more likely to be stopped and searched, arrested, convicted and given a longer custodial sentence. Lammy noted that those with the worst outcomes in the criminal justice system have also already suffered marked disadvantage in other institutions that they have come into contact with, such as school, the health system and social care. They have worse scholastic achievement, more school exclusion, greater likelihood of becoming a looked-after child, reduced likelihood of being adopted and worse outcomes with respect to fostering [13].

Patterns of Offending and Ethnicity

In England and Wales, 65% of all crime is carried out by white people; 8.3% by black people; 6.9% by Asian people; 3.2% by those of mixed ethnicity; and 14.8% by those whose ethnicity is unknown. In 2021 in England and Wales, arrests for violent offences accounted for 42% of all arrests for all ethnic groups. However, conviction rates are significantly different from arrest rates and type of conviction varies by ethnicity. For all minoritised ethnic groups, drug offences accounted for by far the largest number of convictions (black people, 40%; Asian, 39%; mixed heritage, 32%; Chinese or other, 31%). For white people, 26% of convictions were for drug offences; violence against the person accounted for 22% of the convictions; theft convictions, 19%; and sexual offences, 3%. For black people, 14% of convictions were for violence against the person; 13% were for theft; and 2% were for sexual offences. Sixteen per cent of convictions against Asian people were for violence; 11% for theft; and 3% for sexual offences. Seventeen per cent of the convictions against people of mixed heritage were for violence; 20% for theft; and 1% for sexual offences [17].

It is of note that most prosecutions and convictions of black people are for drug-related offences and the majority of these were for possession of Class B drugs. When white people committed drug-related offences, they were more likely to be prosecuted and convicted of possession of Class A drugs. Asian people were least likely to be convicted of drug-related offences [18].

Serious violence is overwhelmingly perpetrated by men and there are ethnicity differences in the type of violence perpetrated and the likely victims of that violence. Violent men perpetrate violence in various forms, ranging from punching and kicking to use of weapons, and their victims range from other men to women and children. However, the serious violence perpetrated by black men between the ages of 16 and 24 is likely to involve a knife and their victims are most likely to be other young black men. With serious violence, the perpetrator is likely to be of the same ethnicity as the victim in the majority of cases, although if the perpetrator is of a different ethnicity to the victim, the perpetrator is more likely to be a white man. Substance use is highly correlated with serious violence, with 52% of homicides involving drug users, drug dealers or drugs in some way [19].

The finding that the most prevalent convictions for minoritised ethnic people, particularly black people, are for drug-related offences calls into question what measures are being taken to manage such prolific substance use-related problems/offending. It is known that young people are recruited into drug crime by coercive gang leaders and that gang membership is associated with significant rates of abuse and mental disorder [13, 20]. There is a tendency to view gang membership as simply a risk factor for antisocial behaviour and violence; however, when we encounter people who have been members of gangs, they have likely been exposed to significant trauma and abuse and are thus vulnerable individuals, yet we fail to recognise this. It is of note is that the risk factors for gang membership and entering the forensic mental health system are very similar (see Table 21.1).

The prevalence of drug-related offending is also pertinent to forensic mental health practitioners because substance use is an important mediator of relapse in mental illness and is associated with violence [21]. People from minoritised ethnic backgrounds are less likely to be recorded as having mental health problems, learning disability or having troubled family relationships when they come into contact with the criminal justice system, yet it is clear from their offending patterns that they are a high-risk group for mental disorder. This is particularly so for people from GRT backgrounds [13, 22]. The criminal activity perpetrated by minoritised ethnic groups tends to be related to drugs in a significant proportion of cases and for black people and GRT people, perpetrators are particularly

Table 21.1 Risk factors for gang affiliation [53]

Individual	Relationship	Community/society
• Childhood conduct disorder	• Postnatal depression	• Social disadvantage
• Attachment insecurity	• Child abuse and neglect	• Social inequality
• Learning disabilities	• Domestic violence Non-intact family	• High unemployment
• Low self-esteem	• Poor parental monitoring	• High crime level
• Low academic achievement	• Social exclusion	• Low social capital
• Alcohol and drug use		• Rapid demographic change

likely to be young, between the ages of 16 and 24. This is a key time for the development of mental health problems.

The risk factors for violent offending are very similar to those that increase the risk of developing mental disorder. Thus, people from minoritised ethnic groups who come into contact with the criminal justice system, particularly people from black and GRT backgrounds, are more likely to have suffered adverse childhood experiences (ACEs), are highly likely to have a drug-related issue and are highly likely to have been a victim of violent crime themselves, as well as having witnessed violence against a friend or acquaintance. If they have been involved in gang activity, this puts them at even greater risk of substance use, victimisation, witnessing violence and having some form of mental disorder [20]. All this indicates that there may be significant unmet mental health need in this population and that the root causes and drivers of their issues are not being addressed.

Understanding Ethnic Inequality in Forensic Mental Healthcare

Risk to self or others is the commonest reason for involuntary detention in people with mental illness. Until a few years ago, race was listed as a risk factor for violent behaviour, based on the finding that African-American males were more likely than any other ethnic group to be victims and perpetrators of homicide and that in the USA, violent crime arrest rates were six times higher for black American males than for white American males [23, 24]. There was a tacit assumption that the higher rates seen were related to constitutional characteristics of being black. However, there is minimal evidence that race or ethnicity contribute to the prediction of future violence when deprivation and other socially and structurally determined risk factors for violence are accounted for. The UK Government's Serious Violence Strategy of 2018 [25] outlined a number of risk factors for violent offending. They found no clear evidence of a correlation between ethnicity and serious violence and this was confirmed by a Home Office Report in 2019, a 2019 College of Policing Report and the Haylock systematic review, all of which found no direct association between ethnicity and violent offending. Risk factors associated with serious violence included age (younger), gender (male), ACEs and gang involvement. Being involved with a gang was associated with cannabis use, low scholastic achievement and learning disability, prevalence of use, and availability of cannabis in the neighbourhood [18, 26, 27, 28].

Mental health problems can affect everyone, regardless of socioeconomic background; however, they affect those from impoverished backgrounds disproportionately. Poverty is associated with poorer housing; poorer education; poorer community cohesion; and the resultant social isolation and loneliness. Poverty is a major driver of mental ill-health, with rates of mental disorder being over 2.5 times more likely in those in the lowest two deciles of income compared with those with the highest incomes [29]. In addition, there is a greater risk of being exposed to biological factors that are risk factors for mental disorder or can have a detrimental effect on mental health, such as perinatal complications, lead toxicity, substance use and so on.

It is now well established that social determinants are key to the development of mental disorder in both children and adults. Increased numbers of ACEs are associated with an increased risk of mental disorder [30, 31]. Exposure to trauma experiences and negative life events as an adult is associated with mental disorder. The COVID-19 pandemic highlighted that isolation and loneliness are associated with an increased risk of mental disorder, including suicidal ideation and behaviour [32].

Haylock et al.'s [28] systematic review found that poor mental health and ACEs were associated with an increased risk of youth and gang violence. They noted that socially determined risk factors are responsible for disproportionate rates of violent offending, in particular discrimination and economic inequality. They indicated that interventions to reduce violence risk should focus on reducing social inequality and that research should focus on the link between poor mental health and knife crime and the trajectory into gangs. Young men from deprived backgrounds and minoritised communities are at greater risk of gang involvement and this puts them at higher risk for substance use and mental disorder; thus they should be targeted for more intensive treatment and management [26, 27, 28].

Finally, those who are subjected to greater discrimination are more likely to be poorer, and thus at greater risk of the mental disorder risk factors mediated by poverty, but there is also increasing evidence that discrimination in and of itself is associated with greater risk of mental disorder [33, 34]. There is growing evidence that people from minoritised ethnic groups have greater exposure to the social determinants of mental and physical disorder than people from white-majority backgrounds.

Therefore, people from minoritised ethnic groups may be at higher risk of developing mental disorder and this would be expected for those who are from more deprived backgrounds, which includes South Asian people of Bangladeshi and Pakistani origin, black African and black Caribbean people, and GRT people [16, 22]. It is of note that people from these groups have the worst health outcomes in our society. However, the ongoing poor health outcomes in the more deprived Bangladeshi and Pakistani populations are not seen in the more affluent South Asian people of Indian origin. This demonstrates the importance of disaggregating data and ensuring that as far as possible the different types of people subsumed within each overarching ethnic group are separated out.

The main reason proposed for why black people are more likely to be detained involuntarily is that they are more prone to psychotic illness and people with psychosis are more likely to be subjected to involuntary detention. However, the majority of people with psychosis live in the community; many are cared for by primary care services and have never been hospitalised [35]. Community surveys have found rates of psychosis in black people living in white-majority countries to be up to three times higher than psychosis rates in white people. This is noticeably greater than in black-majority countries where rates of psychosis are similar to or lower than those seen in white-majority countries [36].

The percentage of black people detained in hospital is 9%, but the percentage detained in locked intensive care units is 17% and the percentage detained in forensic secure settings is 12–21% [2]. The detention rate for black people in acute mental healthcare settings is 9%, three times higher than expected for the percentage of black people in the population. The percentage detained in psychiatric intensive care and forensic secure settings ranges from 12% to 21%, up to seven times higher than the percentage of black people in the general population. It remains unclear why there are such disproportionate rates of detention in this group. Despite people from minoritised ethnic populations, particularly those of black African and African-Caribbean heritage, being significantly over-represented in both the criminal justice system and in involuntary detention in mental healthcare, there has been a distinct lack of enquiry into why this is.

Barnett et al. [2] found that almost half of the papers which found higher rates of involuntary detention in minoritised ethnic groups offered no explanation as to why this might be or offered explanations that had no evidential support. The explanations tended to be associated with culture-bound stereotypes of the groups described. The difficulty is that the conclusions reached by these researchers, which had no evidential basis, recurred again and again over a number of years, giving the erroneous impression that these ideas were evidence-based and therefore true. The culture-bound assumptions tended towards immutable characterisations of the group and thus the individuals belonging to that group. If the characteristic behaviour of an individual is immutable, then there is nothing to be done to change that individual's behaviour; the only strategy is to contain it. Barnett et al. suggested that this could explain why after 40–50 years of knowing about these racial disparities, there has been little change; in fact, there has been an increase in disparities over time [2].

Morgan et al. [37] proposed that the excess rates of mental illness such as psychosis that are seen in minoritised ethnic groups, particularly in black people, are more likely to be related to socio-environmental factors than genetic or biological ones. They proposed a socio-developmental model 'that posits greater exposure to systemic social risks over the life course, particularly those involving threat, hostility and violence', and that this might explain the high rates of psychoses in some migrant and minority ethnic groups [37]. This model includes the impact of discrimination, which has been underestimated and needs to be understood in order to better understand not only the disproportionate rates of mental illness and detention but also how to improve the experience for people from minoritised ethnic backgrounds, particularly those who are black. To understand this, one first needs to understand the different forms of discrimination and racism. In her 'gardener's tale', Jones outlines the reasons why discrimination can be harmful for growth and lead to ill-health [38]. When we think of racism, we think of interpersonal discrimination towards another person because of their race or ethnicity, but there are other types of racism that may be impacting our patients – institutional/structural and internalised (see Box 21.1).

Box 21.1 Different types of racism/discrimination, adapted from Jones [38]

Personally Mediated Discrimination/Racism

This is essentially when a person is prejudiced against a group of people based on assumptions about their abilities, motivations and intentions towards others according to their race/sex/gender/sexuality/religion/disability and so on. Discrimination is when there are differential actions against others because of these negative assumptions about their race/sex/gender/sexuality/religion/disability and so on. This can be overt or covert, intentional or unintentional, or acts of omission and commission. It manifests as a lack of respect – such as shopkeepers' vigilance, suspicion around people wearing hijabs, failure to communicate options, poor service, avoidance and so on; devaluation – such as surprise at competence and stifling of aspirations; and dehumanising – such as use of excessive force (police, mental health services) and failure to provide adequate pain relief.

Institutional/Structural Discrimination/Racism

Macpherson described institutional racism as 'the collective failure of an organization to provide an appropriate and professional service to people because of their colour, culture, or ethnic origin' [54]. It manifests as differential access to goods, services and opportunities. It is so commonplace that there are differences in access and outcomes that this is often seen as an 'inherited disadvantage' and is 'codified' into our customs, practice and laws and thus goes unrecognised. For example, in the Victorian era, it was common knowledge that it was detrimental for women to be highly educated because it had been scientifically proven to shrink their ovaries and cause brain dysfunction – education was physically bad for women who would become infertile and decline cognitively, which was clearly bad for society as it would be faced with dwindling fertility and a group of women who would require long-term care. Thus it became customary, 'codified' into our customs, practices and laws, that doctors, lawyers and other professionals were male.

This, however, meant that advances in women's medicine did not progress as quickly as they did for men and to this day women have poorer health outcomes than men. The disadvantages faced by women are not actively enacted by practitioners; in fact, with institutional or structural discrimination, there is often no 'active perpetrator', no deliberate sidelining of a whole group of people, so it may be inadvertent inaction in the face of need. This manifests in differences in access to material conditions such as good-quality education, sound housing, gainful employment, appropriate medical facilities and a clean environment. There are even differences in access to information – including one's own history or that of one's people, differences in access to resources (including wealth and organisational infrastructure) and less of a voice (including voting rights and representation in government). When different institutions combine to uphold existing structures, and more importantly when policies and even infrastructure disadvantage whole groups of people, this is structural discrimination. Examples of deliberate and active structural discrimination include apartheid in South Africa and the white Australia policy.

Internalised Discrimination/Racism

This is when an individual accepts the negative assumptions and stereotypes about the abilities and intrinsic worth of the group they belong to; that is, that they are indeed inherently inferior, leading to low self-esteem and low self-worth by those who are stigmatised. This involves accepting limitations to one's hopes, dreams and aspirations, self-expression, and even autonomy (a sense of less choice). It involves self-devaluation, such as stratification by colour (colourism); using racial slurs as nicknames for oneself or others of the same background; and the belief that the products and services of those from other ethnic backgrounds are 'better'. Importantly, it may result in resignation, such as dropping out of school, failing to vote, engaging in risky health behaviours and feeling less of a citizen. The latter is particularly important for forensic mental health because if a person feels that they are not valued by society and that societal mores and values do not apply to them, then the very incentives that motivate others to conform so that they are accepted are not available to be used as levers for change.

Ethnic Inequality and Unmet Need in Forensic Mental Health

Criminogenic risk factors and the risk factors for mental disorder are very similar (Table 21.1). It is unsurprising then that those who are exposed to greater numbers of these risk factors in their youth are more likely to come into contact with either the criminal justice system and/or the mental health system. The tendency to aggregate people from different ethnic backgrounds together results in masking of the difficulties of particular groups when they are melded with ethnic groups who are doing especially well, such as grouping people from Bangladeshi backgrounds who have high rates of social risk factors and associated very poor health experiences and outcomes with people from Indian backgrounds who have lower rates of social adversity and better health outcomes under the same umbrella term, South Asian. It is likely that a similar thing happens with those from GRT backgrounds, although compounding matters for this group is a lack of recognition of their existence and their different needs at all [22].

When the data is disaggregated, it becomes clear that ethnic minority status in and of itself is associated with worse experience and outcome in various areas of mental healthcare, in particular psychological therapies, even for those ethnic minority people able to access it. Access, experience and outcomes of psychological therapy are especially poor for those from black, Pakistani and Bangladeshi backgrounds [39, 40]. There is a lack of data on those from GRT backgrounds, but it is probable that they are even less able to access psychological therapy.

Black people are significantly more likely to be detained in a forensic setting. This is likely related to an increased number of early life risk factors (ACEs), later life experiences of trauma and some interpersonal racism but also structural discrimination on the grounds of race. The latter is most apparent in the access to the treatments known to help with mental disorder in forensic patients. Apart from medication, black patients are less likely to be offered treatments such as psychological therapy and occupational therapy. Of particular note is that black patients are far less likely to be offered appropriate substance use treatment despite this being a major cause of mental relapse and a mediator of violence in people with mental disorder [21]. The addiction services that are available are often not open to those under forensic mental healthcare and therefore fewer black people who need substance use support will be able to access them because they are more likely to spend their mental health in-patient stay in a secure setting. In addition, addiction services tend to cater for people with opiate use disorders and often having a mental disorder is an exclusion criterion for substance use support [21].

Black patients tend to have issues with Class B drugs, such as harmful use of cannabis and occasionally stimulants such as crack cocaine. This means that the drug and alcohol services as they are currently structured and configured do not and cannot meet their needs. Therefore, the primary risk factor that often brings them into contact with the criminal justice system and forensic mental health services is not and will not be addressed. This is inaction in the face of need and is clearly structurally mediated. This is an example of structural discrimination (see Box 21.1). Understanding the range of unmet need across different ethnic groups will support improvements in care.

Public Health Approach to Reducing Inequality

In 2005, Scotland introduced a public health approach to knife crime and drug use after it was identified as being the most violent nation in the developed world by the United Nations [41]. It developed the Violence Reduction Unit and began to view violence as 'a disease affecting communities ... caused by poverty, inequality and despair' rather than a traditional law and order issue. The Scottish government decided to address the root causes of violence so as to prevent it happening in the first place. As a result, violent crime in Scotland has reduced by nearly a half and crime involving handling a weapon has fallen by 65% [41]. It is the authors' view that a public health approach to addressing the ethnic disparities in forensic mental healthcare is long overdue.

Making Use of Data

Addressing health inequalities relies on awareness and skill to identify them within the healthcare services. Mental health services obtain significant amounts of data, but it is often argued that this data is not optimally used to improve access, experience and outcomes equally for all groups of individuals with protected characteristics. It is essential that any data collected should be meaningful, as well as disaggregated. For instance, data showing that all ethnic minority groups (lumped together) have poorer outcomes is unlikely on its own to lead to solutions. Additionally, the ability to interrogate data in ways that help identify where disparities lie, or what causes them, can lead to potential solutions.

Utilising the Advancing Mental Health Equality System for Change

The National Collaborating Centre for Mental Health (NCCMH) has developed a resource that supports healthcare organisations and commissioners to address health inequalities. They recommend a process consisting of four stages: (1) identify inequalities, (2) design solutions, (3) implement these and (4) evaluate them using Quality Improvement (QI) methodology. It is important that appropriate local data is used to design changes to implement and meaningful measures are used to assess change. The key process that underpins the process is co-production where ideas are created with people who would be affected by the change [42].

The Patient and Carer Race Equality Framework

The NCCMH also supported the development of the Patient and Carer Race Equality Framework (PCREF), an organisational competency framework that uses a maturity matrix approach to improve organisational processes, procedures and policies such that the organisation and the staff working in it better serve the needs of and deliver equitable care to people from minoritised ethnic communities who use the service. QI methodology is used to bring about iterative change. This is currently being piloted in three sites in England, including in forensic settings [43].

Designing and Developing Services That Meet the Needs of Minoritised Ethnic Groups

It is clear that much of the criminality and forensic mental health need in black people is driven by substance use. We need more data to ascertain if this is also the case for those from GRT backgrounds. Admission to forensic healthcare is an opportune time to support people with their substance use issues, even if they themselves fail to recognise the negative impact of the substance on their health and social functioning. Developing services so they can meet the needs of minoritised ethnic people with mental disorder and comorbid substance use is crucial to reducing the likelihood of relapse and associated re-offending. Using approaches such as the Patient and Carer Race Equality Framework (PCREF) to design and develop services co-produced with the people who will be using them will result in services that are more acceptable and more likely to address unmet need for those from minoritised communities.

What Can Individual Clinicians Do to Reduce Inequality?

Individual clinicians often feel powerless when large-scale health disparities are highlighted within their services. It is important to recognise that large statistics are made of individuals, and there are interventions possible that can improve access, experience or outcomes for each individual. This requires a person-centred approach to treatment planning, which takes into account the unique needs of that individual, their psycho-social determinants, and their choices and preferences. National directives recommend person-centred care planning, integrated personalised commissioning, personal health budgets and supporting patient choice [44]. This will involve a culture shift and training and supporting staff to deliver person-centred care consistently.

Cultural Safety and Trauma-Informed Care

Understanding the inequality and inequity in the forensic mental healthcare systems also means that clinicians need to question their standard approaches to the care provided and recognise that no one size fits all. The concept of cultural safety is useful in redesigning services to meet the needs of diverse populations and to provide equitable care. Cultural safety requires care providers to examine the power imbalances in care. Providers must be willing to question their own biases, attitudes, assumptions, stereotypes and prejudices that may be contributing to a lower quality of healthcare for some patients. Cultural safety can prevent 'othering' and takes into account the culture of the clinician and the clinical environment. Cultural safety requires healthcare professionals and their associated healthcare organisations to influence healthcare by reducing bias in the wider system within which they operate, as well as addressing their own biases and thus achieving equity within the workforce and working environment [45]. A trauma-informed approach acknowledging and working with multiple experiences of trauma, disadvantage and deprivation will support the development of a culturally safe environment.

Be Careful about Language

Black men are rated as taller, heavier and stronger than white men [46]. Black people's faces are more likely to be perceived as 'angry' compared with white people [47]. The behaviour of black people is perceived as more violent than that of white people, with 75% rating a 'shove' as violent when the perpetrator was black versus 17% when the perpetrator was white. Forty-two per cent described the same behaviour as 'playing around' when the perpetrator was white [48].

Given the unconscious perceptions of black people as being inherently stronger, angrier and more aggressive, which may not actually match the evidence of the person being assessed or treated, it is important to ensure that the language used is appropriate and evidence-based. Adjectives and adverbs such as 'well-built ... fit-looking ... powerfully ... large ... athletic ... muscular' convey a sense that if the person were to hit someone it would cause significant damage; that the person would be difficult to physically overcome and restrain; and that a higher level of restriction/security would be required to subdue them. If there is evidence that the person does pose a greater risk to others, then this should be documented and evidenced clearly. To reduce the risk of and counter concerns about unconscious bias against a particular group of people, the following is suggested:

What to do?

- Expect everyone to be described in terms of their ethnicity – we need the data to better understand any disparities and unmet need.
- Appearance is important in terms of an indication of mental state and therefore should be recorded for these purposes.
- Physique is important in terms of whether this may be an indication of physical health, such as emaciated, very overweight, jaundiced and so on. A person's physique gives no indication of their capacity for harm and the risk they might pose to others, however.

- See Box 21.2 for a way of critically analysing statements made about risk in an individual's notes and reports and how to approach the statements made in notes/reports to ensure they are more likely to be based on the evidence of the person's behaviour rather than unconsciously driven cultural-bound assumptions.

Box 21.2 Critical analysis of risk statements

1. What was the aggressive behaviour?

- Verbal
- Physical

2. When did it happen?

- Recent historical
- Distant historical

3. What was the context?

- Driven by psychotic process
- Occurred during an act of self-harm?
- In response to provocation
- Excessive response driven by maladaptive coping mechanisms (uses violence as a coping mechanism, disproportionate to provocation)
- Proportionate to provocation
- Self-defence
- In response to being attacked to prevent further harm

4. What helped ameliorate the situation?

- Person calmed themselves down
- Person took themselves away from the situation
- Verbal de-escalation
- Physical intervention
- Time out
- restraint
- Seclusion
- medication

5. What factors about this individual raise concerns about their risk to themselves or others?

- History of violence towards self or others
- Frequency of violence towards self or others
- Severity of violence towards self or others
- Intent to harm self or others

Racial/Ethnic Identity in Forensic Mental Health

Heilbrun et al. [49] stated that race exerts a powerful influence on how people think of themselves and how others respond to them, yet it has received little attention as a formal part of the forensic mental health assessment process. They propose that this should change because a person's experience of racism and their experience of society as a minoritised individual influence their development (psychological and social) in ways that are important to understand when investigating the facts and motivations associated with what might have brought them into contact with the criminal justice system and forensic mental healthcare. It will also have a bearing on their engagement with and response to the treatment offered. The aim of forensic mental healthcare is to rehabilitate people back into the community so that they no longer pose a risk to themselves or others; however, in the case of people from racialised minority groups, we are rehabilitating them back into a community in which they are often feared and reviled. What impact does that societal view have on self-esteem and expectation of others' views, when that expectation is frequently negative and has now been compounded by actions confirming that the person has behaved dangerously?

Heilbrun et al. [49] suggest that racial identity may be relevant to the forensic question and therefore the practitioner must consider how to describe it and how it might affect their management. They suggest questions to appraise racial identity including:

- 'I want to talk a bit about how you see yourself and how you think other people see you, for example when people ask about your race or ethnicity, what do you say?'
- 'How important is that to you?'
- 'Does it make a difference in your life?'
- 'Have you ever been treated differently because of your race? Tell me about that.'
- 'If so, how did you feel about being treated differently? What did you do?'

Heilbrun et al. conclude that forensic mental health assessment (and management) should consistently involve gathering and documenting relevant information about racial identity. When that information is relevant to the outcomes being considered, the relationship between racial identity and those outcomes should be described and explained. For some people, culturally appropriate advocacy may facilitate discussions about and understanding of racial identity and this in turn will support better formulation development.

Use Clinical Formulation to Address Ethnic Disparity

In-depth clinical case formulations can help better understand the complex interplay of psycho-social factors that have impacted on an individual's clinical presentation. The exploration should specifically look at social determinants and experiences of trauma (including racial trauma [50]). It should also involve an exploration of racial/ethnic identity. Developing a deeper understanding of an individual will help engagement and impact on treatment decision-making, and will indicate where there is the need for better use of non-pharmacological interventions along with medications. Improving the provision of appropriate psycho-social interventions which take into account the wider social context of people's lives has the potential to improve outcomes, particularly for people from minoritised ethnic groups.

Conclusion

The consistent finding of higher rates of involuntary detention of people from minoritised ethnic groups, particularly black and GRT people in intensive care and more secure parts of the mental health system, without there being any attempts to address this is a failure to recognise an obvious need, the addressing of which could help reduce relapse and any associated re-offending. The societal influences that increase the likelihood of a person coming into contact with the criminal justice system and forensic mental health services must be recognised and understood in order to develop services which better address the needs of people from minoritised ethnic backgrounds. Nazroo et al. [51] have stated that it is crucial that the public health agenda pays close attention to issues of racism and how they shape the lives of racial/ethnic minority people.

This is not simply a moral or ethical imperative, or to fulfil the legal imperatives; this is also for economic and societal reasons. When forensic patients relapse, both perpetrator and victim are harmed at great personal, social and financial cost. Finally, the severe lack of research into care pathways, experience of and outcomes in secure care for minoritised ethnic patients must be addressed as a matter of urgency. The dearth of research in this area is, in and of itself, an institutional failing.

Arya et al. [52] stress that there is a critical need to better understand why people from minoritised ethnic groups are at increased risk of involuntary psychiatric care and how this is best addressed; the disparities in care and treatment need to be better understood and addressed, including how this might reduce relapse and re-admission and how to introduce more culturally safe service provision. In addition to this, forensic mental health practitioners must add to their armoury the recognition of how racial/ethnic identity may shape an individual's response to services, engagement in treatment and successful rehabilitation into the community.

References

1. Ali S, Dearman SP, McWilliam C. Are Asians at greater risk of compulsory psychiatric admission than Caucasians in the acute general adult setting? *Medicine, Science and the Law* 2007; 47 (4): 311–14.

2. Barnett P, Mackay E, Matthews H et al. Ethnic variations in compulsory detention under the Mental Health Act: a systematic review and meta-analysis of international data. *Lancet Psychiatry* 2019; 6 (4): 305–17.

3. Bhui K, Stansfeld S, Hull S et al. Ethnic variations in pathways to and use of specialist mental health services in the UK. Systematic review. *British Journal of Psychiatry* 2003; 182: 105–16.

4. Archie S, Akhtar-Danesh N, Norman RM et al. Ethnic diversity and pathways to care for a first episode of psychosis in Ontario. *Schizophrenia Bulletin* 2010; 36 (4): 688–70.

5. Halvorsrud K, Nazroo J, Otis M, Brown Hajdukova E, Bhui K. Ethnic inequalities and pathways to care in psychosis in England: a systematic review and meta-analysis. *BMC Medicine* 2018; 16 (1): 223.

6. Modernising the Mental Health Act: Increasing Choice, Reducing Compulsion. London, Department of Health, 2018. www.gov.uk/government/publications/modernising-the-mental-health-act-final-report-from-the-independent-review.

7. NHS Digital. *Mental Health Statistics: Annual Figures, 2018–2019*. NHS Digital, London, 2019.

8. Das-Munshi J, Bhugra D, Crawford MJ. Ethnic minority inequalities in access to treatments for schizophrenia and schizoaffective disorders: findings from

a nationally representative cross-sectional study. *BMC Medicine* 2018; 16 (1): 55.

9. Payne-Gill J, Whitfield C, Beck A. The relationship between ethnic background and the use of restrictive practices to manage incidents of violence or aggression in psychiatric inpatient settings. *International Journal of Mental Health Nursing* 2021; 30 (5): 1221–1233.

10. Bruce M, Smith J. Length of stay among multi-ethnic psychiatric inpatients in the United Kingdom. *Comprehensive Psychiatry* 2020; 102.

11. Kapadia D, Zhang J, Salway S et al. *Ethnic Inequalities in Healthcare: A Rapid Review.* NHS Race & Health Observatory, 2022. www.nhsrho.org/wp-content/uploads/2022/02/RHO-Rapid-Review-Final-Report_v.7.pdf.

12. Bansal N, Bhopal R, Netto G et al. Disparate patterns of hospitalisation reflect unmet needs and persistent ethnic inequalities in mental health care: the Scottish health and ethnicity linkage study. *Ethnicity & Health* 2014; 19 (2): 217–39.

13. The Lammy Review: An Independent Review into the Treatment of, and Outcomes for, Black, Asian and Minority Ethnic Individuals in the Criminal Justice System. 2017. https://assets.publishing.service.gov.uk/government/uploads/system/uploads/attachment_data/file/643001/lammy-review-final-report.pdf.

14. Ministry of Justice. Ethnicity and the Criminal Justice System Statistics 2020. www.gov.uk/government/statistics/ethnicity-and-the-criminal-justice-system-statistics-2020/ethnicity-and-the-criminal-justice-system-2020.

15. Joyce S, O'Reilly O, O'Brien M et al. *Irish Travellers' Access to Justice.* University of Limerick, Report, 2022. https://hdl.handle.net/10344/11203.

16. Raleigh V, Holmes J. *The Health of People from Ethnic Minority Groups in England.* Kings Fund, 2021. www.kingsfund.org.uk/publications/health-people-ethnic-minority-groups-england.

17. UK Government. *Ethnicity Facts and Figures.* Crime, Justice and the Law, 2020.

www.ethnicity-facts-figures.service.gov.uk/crime-justice-and-the-law/courts-sentencing-and-tribunals/prosecutions-and-convictions/latest.

18. Stott C, Radburn M, Kyprianides A et al. *Understanding Ethnic Disparities in Involvement in Crime: A Limited Scope Rapid Evidence Review,* 2021. www.gov.uk/government/publications/the-report-of-the-commission-on-race-and-ethnic-disparities-supporting-research/understanding-ethnic-disparities-in-involvement-in-crime-a-limited-scope-rapid-evidence-review-by-professor-clifford-stott-et-al.

19. Office for National Statistics. *Homicide in England and Wales: Year Ending March 2022.* www.ons.gov.uk/peoplepopulationandcommunity/crimeandjustice/articles/homicideinenglandandwales/yearendingmarch2022.

20. Coid JW, Ullrich S, Keers R et al. Gang membership, violence, and psychiatric morbidity. *American Journal of Psychiatry* 2013; 170 (9): 985–93.

21. Grann M, Fazel S. Substance misuse and violent crime: Swedish population study. *BMJ* 2004; 22(328): 1233–4.

22. House of Commons Women and Equalities Committee. *Tackling Inequalities Faced by Gypsy, Roma and Traveller Communities.* 2019. Seventh Report of Session 2017–19. https://publications.parliament.uk/pa/cm201719/cmselect/cmwomeq/360/full-report.html.

23. Kingery PM, Zimmerman RS, Biafora FA. Risk factors for violent behaviors among ethnically diverse urban adolescents: beyond race/ethnicity. *School Psychology International* 1996; 17 (2): 171–86.

24. Farrington DP, Loeber R, Stouthamer-Loeber M, Van Kammen WB, Schmidt L. Self-reported delinquency and a combined delinquency seriousness scale based on boys, mothers, and teachers: concurrent and predictive validity for African-Americans and Caucasians. *Criminology* 1996; 34: 493–517.

25. HM Government. *Serious Violence Strategy,* 2018. https://assets.publishing.service.gov.uk/government/uploads/system/

uploads/attachment_data/file/698009/ser
ious-violence-strategy.pdf.

26. Smith V, Wynne-McHardy E. An analysis of
indicators of serious violence: findings from
the Millenium Cohort Study and the
Environmental Risk (E-Risk) Longitudinal
Twin Study, 2019. https://assets.publishing
.service.gov.uk/government/uploads/sys
tem/uploads/attachment_data/file/819840/
analysis-of-indicators-of-serious-violence-
horr110.pdf.

27. McNeil A, Wheller L. Knife crime.
Evidence briefing. College of Policing
Report, 2019. https://assets.college.police.
uk/s3fs-public/2022-03/Knife_Crime_Evid
ence_Briefing.pdf.

28. Haylock S, Boshari T, Alexander EC et al.
Risk factors associated with knife-crime in
United Kingdom among young people
aged 10-24 years: a systematic review. *BMC
Public Health* 2020; 20 (1): 1451.

29. UK Government. *Mental Health
Environmental Factors*, 2019. www.gov.uk/
government/publications/better-mental-h
ealth-jsna-toolkit/2-understanding-place.

30. Felitti VJ, Anda RF, Nordenberg D et al.
Relationship of childhood abuse and
household dysfunction to many of the
leading causes of death in adults: the
Adverse Childhood Experiences (ACE)
Study. *American Journal of Preventive
Medicine* 1998; 14 (4): 245–58.

31. Gilbert R, Widom CS, Browne K et al.
Burden and consequences of child
maltreatment in high-income countries.
Lancet 2009; 373 (9657): 68–81.

32. McClelland H, Evans JJ, Nowland R et al.
Loneliness as a predictor of suicidal
ideation and behaviour: a systematic
review and meta-analysis of prospective
studies. *Journal of Affective Disorders* 2020;
274: 880–96.

33. Hatch SL, Gazard B, Williams DR et al.
Discrimination and common mental
disorder among migrant and ethnic groups:
findings from a South East London
Community sample. *Social Psychiatry and
Psychiatric Epidemiology* 2016; 51: 689–701.

34. Pearce J, Rafiq S, Simpson J, Varese F.
Perceived discrimination and psychosis:
a systematic review of the literature. *Social
Psychiatry and Psychiatric Epidemiology*
2019; 54 (9): 1023–44.

35. Rethink Mental Illness. *The Abandoned
Illness: A Report by the Schizophrenia
Commission*, 2012. www.rethink.org/medi
a/2629/the-abandonned-illness_tsc_execu
tive_summary_14_nov.pdf.

36. Morgan C, Cohen A, Esponda GM et al.
Epidemiology of untreated psychoses in 3
diverse settings in the global south: the
International Research Program on
Psychotic Disorders in Diverse Settings
(INTREPID II). *JAMA Psychiatry* 2023; 80
(1): 40–8.

37. Morgan C, Knowles G, Hutchinson G.
Migration, ethnicity and psychoses:
evidence, models and future directions.
World Psychiatry 2019; 18 (3): 247–58.

38. Jones CP. Levels of racism: a theoretic
framework and a gardener's tale. *American
Journal of Public Health* 2000; 90 (8):
1212–15.

39. Harwood H, Rhead R, Chui Z et al.
Variations by ethnicity in referral and
treatment pathways for IAPT service users
in South London. *Psychological Medicine*
2023; 53 (3): 1084–95.

40. Improving Access to Psychological
Therapies Team. *Psychological Therapies:
Annual Report on the Use of IAPT Services
2019–20*. NHS Digital, 2020.

41. Evans L. *A Radical Approach to Tackling
Knife Crime in Scotland*. Cabinet Office,
2019. https://quarterly.blog.gov.uk/2019/0
7/04/a-radical-approach-to-tackling-knife-
crime-in-scotland.

42. National Collaborating Centre for Mental
Health. *Advancing Mental Health Equality
Resource*, 2019 www.rcpsych.ac.uk/improv
ing-care/nccmh/service-design-and-devel
opment/advancing-mental-health-
equality.

43. Smith SM, Kheri A, Ariyo K et al. The
Patient and Carer Race Equality
Framework: a model to reduce mental

health inequity in England and Wales. Frontiers in Psychiatry 2023; 14: 1053502. doi: 10.3389/fpsyt.2023.1053502.

44. Santana M, Manalili K, Zelinsky S et al. Improving the quality of person-centred healthcare from the patient perspective: development of person-centred quality indicators. *BMJ Open* 2020; 10: e037323. doi: 10.1136/bmjopen-2020-037323.

45. Curtis E, Jones R, Tipene-Leach D et al. Why cultural safety rather than cultural competency is required to achieve health equity: a literature review and recommended definition. *International Journal for Equity in Health* 2019; 18: 174.

46. Wilson JP, Hugenberg K, Rule NO. Racial bias in judgments of physical size and formidability: from size to threat. *Journal of Personality and Social Psychology*, 2017; 113 (1): 59–80.

47. Hugenberg K, Bodenhausen GV. Ambiguity in social categorization: the role of prejudice and facial affect in race categorization. *Psychological Science* 2004; 15 (5): 342–5.

48. Duncan B. Differential social perception and attribution of intergroup violence: testing the lower limits of stereotyping of blacks. *Journal of Personality and Social Psychology* 1976; 34 (4): 590–8.

49. Heilbrun K, Kavanaugh A, Grisso T et al. The importance of racial identity in forensic mental health assessment. *Journal of the American Academy of Psychiatry and the Law* 2021; 49 (4): 478–87.

50. Carter R. Racism and psychological and emotional injury: recognizing and assessing race-based traumatic stress. *The Counselling Psychologist* 2007; 35 (1): 13–105.

51. Nazroo JY, Bhui KS, Rhodes J. Where next for understanding race/ethnic inequalities in severe mental illness? Structural, interpersonal and institutional racism. *Sociology of Health and Illness* 2020; 42: 262–76.

52. Arya D, Connolly C, Yeoman B. Black and minority ethnic groups and forensic mental health. *BJPsych Open* 2021; 7 (suppl. 1): S123.

53. Thornberry TP, Lizotte AJ, Krohn MD, Smith CA, Porter PK. Causes and consequences of delinquency: findings from the Rochester Youth Development Study. In Thornberry TP and Krohn MD (eds) *Taking Stock of Delinquency: An Overview of Findings from Contemporary Longitudinal Studies.* New York, Kluwer Academic, 2003, pp. 11–46.

54. Home Office, The Stephen Lawrence Inquiry: Report of an Inquiry by Sir William Macpherson of Cluny, Cm 4262-I, February 1999. https://assets.publishing.service.gov.uk/government/uploads/system/uploads/attachment_data/file/277111/4262.pdf.

Chapter 22

Academic Forensic Psychiatry

Pamela J. Taylor

Forensic psychiatry, of all the specialties in medicine, needs its own strong academic core. Forensic psychiatry is practised at the interface of so many disciplines – clinical and non-clinical – each in their own way striving for 'truth' and informed practice. It is, therefore, vital to understand where there is common ground and where there are differences in acquiring, weighing and conveying evidence for what we do. Medicine and the law, for example, would each be regarded as evidence-based disciplines. Scientific and legal truth-seeking overlap, but their evidence-gathering, reporting and decision-making systems differ. Academic forensic psychiatry is founded in scientific research, with its systematic approach to making and recording observations, formulating hypotheses from them, testing those hypotheses with new observations and accumulating the most comprehensive picture possible in a way that is transparent and replicable. An academic approach supports application of scientific principles as strongly in the individual case as in relevant collective knowledge, and is able to make links between them and communicate all this effectively within and outside the specialty. This requires highly developed and defined specialist training. Academic forensic psychiatry in this sense is the business of all forensic psychiatrists.

In order for forensic psychiatry to thrive, however, it is vital that some forensic psychiatrists further specialise in academic work in terms of additional training, time and immersion in skills that support accurate scientific questioning and testing and, ultimately, the capacity to innovate and keep this cycle active. We need a culture in which every clinician subscribes to the principles of evidence-based practice and development. We need to sustain a lively dialogue between those who are primarily academics and those who are primarily clinicians as this will both inform the most useful research and ensure that research findings become embedded in practice. We need to keep recruitment and retention of forensic psychiatrists high and strong clinical–academic bonds help with this. We need training and continuing professional development, so we must have the skills of those academically trained people who can précis the knowledge, communicate both the knowledge and the practical skills entailed, excite us with new developments, and help us safeguard our health and integrity through circumstances which may challenge them as well as through all the good times.

The Academic Base in Forensic Psychiatry

Dedicated clinical academic posts are under threat and not just in forensic psychiatry. Figures from the latest Medical Schools Council staffing survey, covering the UK, show a decline through this century in the proportion of clinical academic consultants overall – from 7.5% in 2004 to 4.2% in 2017 [1]. Perhaps of most concern is that in many specialties, including psychiatry, the decline has most affected leadership feeder posts – clinical senior lecturers and readers. Smaller specialties, like forensic psychiatry, are disproportionately affected. It is already proving hard to replace retiring chairs. If forensic psychiatry is to remain a viable specialty, it is vital that there is a clear career structure for fully trained academics.

Since universities have moved into funding models that emphasise high grant income and high-impact journal publications and often prioritise higher-income students from overseas, the always small university input to funding academic posts in forensic psychiatry has shrunk further. As advocated across specialties by the Academy of Medical Sciences [2], the best approach for assuring continued forensic psychiatry development is fully integrating research teams across academia and the National Health Service (NHS); independent sector healthcare organisations may be engaged too.

How may this work in practice? Some posts must be embedded in a university base to ensure adequate access to academic training, development and relevant resources. Forward-looking healthcare organisations must, collectively or separately, fund sufficient university posts to ensure that their consultants and trainees, other staff and administrators have the guidance they need to innovate, train and develop staff and develop services. Payback is evident in service developments. All major service reviews that have had implications for successful implementation of major change have included senior academics in the review teams, from the 1975 Butler Report in the UK [3], through the 1992 Reed Report for England and Wales [4], to the current replacement of the Central Mental Hospital in Dundrum, Ireland with a state-of-the-art high-security supported by a fully tiered system [5]. Developers and managers – at national government and local levels – as well as more fully clinical service-orientated colleagues and trainees all benefit.

Close integration also means that clinicians who want to pursue some academic work have the necessary support. Much of the primarily clinician input into academic work lies in recruiting and training forensic psychiatrists for the future. Recruitment follows from engaging trainees, including medical students, through offering supervised, interesting experiences within a clinical, academic or conjoined team. Undergraduates need such experience and information, as career pathways are planned at ever earlier stages [6]. Even student observer status may be worthwhile. Those who spend longer, however, whether medical students in student selected modules or doing an intercalated BSc dissertation, or postgraduates in general professional training, may be involved in tasks which are mutually beneficial; they may perhaps help design and conduct an audit, essential to the consultant's continuing professional development, or a small service evaluation. The academic forensic psychiatrist can be on hand to support clinical colleagues where they would like help with, say, project design, literature searching or data analysis. Job satisfaction surveys have long suggested that active clinician involvement in research is an important factor in job satisfaction and, in turn, retention in post [7].

Training and Professional Development

Specialty registration and training in most countries rests with an independent medical body. In the UK this is the General Medical Council (GMC), where all specialty curricula have been under review since 2017. Here, forensic psychiatry is a recognised specialty of medicine. The emphasis is on skills-based training and, increasingly, on shared medical skills and values to enhance capacity for specialty retraining if required. This review process has stimulated new thinking about what characterises forensic psychiatry as a full medical specialty. Many countries do not recognise forensic psychiatry in this way, leaving psychiatrists to find and attend circumscribed courses in relevant topic areas if they work frequently with offenders or courts or prisons. The latter approach perhaps comes with some potential threat to their medical ethic. The American Academy of Psychiatry and the Law went so far as to develop its own ethical code, apparently rating a category of forensic psychiatry *expert*, or 'forensicist', who in our terms might be distinguished from a forensic psychiatry *specialist*, risking compromising the medical ethic of their members (for a fuller discussion, see [8]).

What clinical attributes make us unique? It is perhaps the combination and weighting of skills required rather than any single skill. In the UK and Ireland and, indeed, in most of Europe and many but not all other countries, forensic psychiatrists not only offer expertise to other professions, particularly to the courts, but also work directly with patients and develop and run specialist clinical services. The new UK curriculum will emphasise 9 'high-level outcomes' and 14 'key capability domains'. The high-level outcomes set the scene with a broad sweep of requirements which would almost certainly be recognised worldwide. These are: (i) professional values, (ii) skills, (iii) knowledge, (iv) health promotion and illness/harm prevention, (v) patient safety and quality improvement, (vi) safeguarding of vulnerable groups, (vii) leadership and team work, (viii) education and training, and (ix) research and scholarship.

The capability domains flesh out some of the common ground we would have with other medical specialists – such as professional relationships with patients which are holistic, empathic, compassionate, realistically optimistic, honest and with clear boundaries. They also highlight our more specialist attributes, for example recognising the emotional impact of the work and the public perception of it, coupled with the exceptional importance in this context of reflective practice. It is recognised that we will need knowledge streams outside medicine as well as a broad spectrum within it, as many of our patients are in poor physical health. Criminology and law are among the other fields specified. The curriculum will also emphasise the range of expert communication skills required – given, on the one hand, the extent of psychopathology and sometimes threat from our patients at stages in their career and, on the other, the wide range of clinical disciplines and non-clinical agencies where we must communicate fluently, without misunderstandings. It captures the special difficulty of working with patients who are both victims and perpetrators of harmful behaviours, of respecting the rights and needs of direct victims of our patients and the importance of preventative strategies at both individual and public health levels.

In preparing the new training guides, we must face questions about the extent to which each skill must be acquired and, in turn, how much lived experience should be mandatory. A number of training domains are not easily accessible for all trainees. It is now unusual for training schemes to be anchored in university departments, so rigour in academic training is hard to access. Should placements in a relevant university-linked centre be required? Availability of training in high-security hospitals is another example of how the allocation of scarce resources may impact on future breadth and depth of training experience. There are just three high-security hospitals in England and one in Scotland. They are not easily accessible to most trainees in the UK, and yet even forensic psychiatrists who never work in high-security hospitals will have to decide for whom these hospitals will be helpful, and sometimes refer people to them and receive their 'graduates'. How much time in training in a high-security hospital is essential?

Academics are interested in developing and evaluating the teaching and training that underpin certification of specialist training, although there is little research into optimal training models specific to forensic psychiatry. One of the most interesting questions, given the multi-disciplinary and inter-agency pattern of working, is about the extent to which it is an advantage to train together across clinical groups and agencies and the extent to which separate intra-specialist training is essential. Almost certainly, we need a combination of approaches. The strength of multi-disciplinary work comes in part from each discipline having unique and robust knowledge and skills to bring to the table. Systematic intradisciplinary training according to a curriculum along the lines just outlined is essential to this. It fosters not only appropriate confidence in relevant skills but also recognition of professional limits. Given robust knowledge and skills, moving on to learning with other disciplines and agencies may extend capacities in all sorts of ways. Generally, there is an ad hoc approach to this; in Scotland, for example, a School of Forensic Mental Health (SoFMH) was established in 2007 to promote such training as well as service developments [9].

How might coming together for training benefit knowledge and skills? On the one hand, it enables us to see disciplinary differences and work with them, and on the other helps us to be more aware and critical of our own approaches. In court, for example, lawyers and doctors deal with the same cases in different ways, sometimes even using the same language differently. Aubert's 1963 summary of six major differences is still widely accepted [10]. First, lawyers tend to dichotomise, doctors to envisage on a spectrum; second, the law uses only one or two simple concepts of probability, such as 'beyond reasonable doubt' or 'on the balance of probabilities' (strictly 49%:51%), and comfortably applies these to an individual while doctors acknowledge both the group derivation of most probability estimates and their limitations (although they sometimes need reminding of those, such as after the miscarriage of justice in *Clark*; see Aitken et al. [11]); third, lawyers test the fit between an event and person using a narrowly defined formula, for example the diminished responsibility defence, while doctors take a more holistic perspective; fourth, lawyers rely on evidence of past events to decide on the future while doctors add consideration of aspects of that future, such as availability of treatment; fifth, lawyers will seek to apply precedent from previous individual cases but doctors make their decisions in the context of how group-based research data applies to the individual; finally, lawyers decide what happened in disputed incidents according to legal rules, which cannot be falsified, only overruled, while doctors at their best are concerned only with scientifically demonstrable or falsifiable causes.

Simply attempting to set out what we know and what we do when talking with people who are confident in their own practice, but relatively ignorant of ours, tests not only our communication and teaching skills but also the extent to which we really understand our own field. This applies to international teaching and learning too. The Ghent Group [12] was set up primarily for forensic psychiatrists interested in teaching from across the European Union, although also welcoming Council of Europe members. Both memberships have common ground in the European Convention on Human Rights [13] but different legal and practice structures. The Ghent Group facilitates learning through two main approaches – one by visiting participating countries in turn to experience the services and national context at first hand, the host country also leading a mini-conference, and the other through annual residential seminars on a theme which requires all participants to explain relevant law and practice in their country and how it is applied in individual cases [14].

Research and Overcoming Problems: Some Themes and Interpretations, Limitations and Applications

Forensic psychiatric research is vital as it underpins the prospect of change for the better. Diseases and behaviours for which there is little prospect of improvement tend to carry stigma – for the sufferers and their doctors alike [44]. There are many problems to be overcome, however, in conducting the kind of high-quality research necessary to assure progress – chief among them resources, bureaucracy and sense of direction. For forensic psychiatry there are likely to be legal barriers, so it is essential that all relevant agencies are engaged in calling out gaps in knowledge and understanding research methods [52].

Resource Pressures and Some Strategies for Meeting Them

In a new field, government initially made some attempts to promote research development in forensic psychiatry. The UK Department of Health funded a special (high-security) hospitals' research unit through the 1970s and 1980s, although largely limited to establishing a special hospitals' case register. As management of these hospitals was devolved, so these limited monies were diverted into a National Programme on Forensic Mental Health Research. This was good for diversifying research. It built knowledge and developed young academics across most disciplines relevant to forensic mental health practice, but this real growth was rewarded by removal of this protected streaming in 2007 [15]. Apart from one small pure research charity (Crime in Mind) and a number of relevant topic-driven or lobbying charities that sometimes commission relevant research, forensic psychiatrists must generally rely on open competition with specialties of much longer duration and often 'harder' science. Thus, funding is tough, but possible through persistence and formal collaborations with academics from other relevant disciplines, often between universities and between university and clinically based staff. By bringing in additional expertise, such cooperation both ensures that methodological approaches are sound and that they are seen to be so. Randomised controlled trials of complex interventions in prisons in England and Wales since 2018 were, for example, only possible in this context, all including partnership with university trials units and between universities and health trusts or boards [16, 17, 18].

Bureaucratic Challenges, Legal Constraints and Some Solutions

A particular challenge to research in forensic psychiatry includes the problem of little relevant specialist experience in ethics committees. Another is the fact that we cannot interfere with legal process, although this in itself is of legitimate academic interest.

Legal limits may affect the nature of research that may be conducted, although perhaps not as much as feared. In modest ways, courts have even been persuaded to permit randomised controlled trials (RCTs) of process – for example, Cosden et al. [19] were able to study randomisation of prospective offender-patients to mental health courts or traditional, adversarial courts in the USA. In the UK, as in some other countries, RCTs have been conducted in prisons (e.g. [16, 17, 18]). As long as there is no interference with due process, the main bureaucratic concern about research in such environments is that it will over-stretch an already stressed, often poorly resourced system. Close work with the relevant host agency at the earliest stage usually ensures both smooth progress of necessary permissions and actual feasibility on the ground, although contingency planning is also advisable. Further, the real possibility that, from time to time, we may truly be working with unique cases is no bar to the use of RCT methodology. It can be as well applied in individual cases [20] and, indeed, *Consort* has developed tools to support such n-1 trials [21] alongside guidance on more conventional RCTs. Where cases are merely rare, subscribing to such an approach between centres worldwide will allow cumulative evidence-gathering on the effectiveness or otherwise of particular approaches.

The RCT is always held up as the gold standard in testing the effects of interventions because it instils good research discipline and reduces some biases. It is vital that we adopt such an approach whenever it is possible to do, but also important to recognise that nothing eliminates all bias and even RCTs may introduce some. For my first RCT [22], for example – nothing to do with the criminal justice system – recruitment was difficult because consultants more often than not refused to allow their patients to be invited to participate on grounds roughly evenly divided between confidence that the intervention (electro-convulsive therapy) worked for schizophrenia and confidence that it did not. This has parallels with expressed concerns that depriving prisoners of 'good experiences' with psychological therapies is wrong. When an ethics committee approves an RCT, this generally follows extensive peer-reviewing for the funding body and sometimes again specifically for the ethics committee, approval from the various host bodies and university or NHS sponsorship (insurance), as well as ethics committee approval per se. With all this hard-won approval in place, colleagues from whom we seek to recruit participants should be reassured that a trial is really necessary.

Further biases may enter, however, through excluding a full range of relevant participants for good reasons – for example, safeguarding people deemed too ill to give free and informed consent or excluding those not ill enough to show change. The main concern expressed about RCTs, however, is that they emphasise group or average results when what we need to know is what works best for whom, under what circumstances, when and perhaps even why. Supplementary work alongside a trial, such as process analysis [23], helps, although such approaches primarily ensure the integrity of the trial. The debate between those who consider that methods can be adjusted sufficiently to ensure 'realist outcomes' [24] and those who do not [25] continues. The most important message is that every research method has its limitations and rather than dreaming of 'gold standards', we would be better served by being aware of those limitations. An important academic skill is knowing how to work with them.

The process of obtaining ethics approval for research – or confirmation that this is not necessary because a study qualifies as a service evaluation or audit [26] – may mean not only prolonged labour but also readiness to educate and to contain well-meaning but potentially damaging interventions. Brown [27] highlighted some key ethical problems over and above the sheer weight of paperwork required in the area of fitness to plead. Such research, by definition, is likely to include people with impairments in capacities for decision-making. Other concerns include the possibility that people under some sense of threat or coercion from the criminal justice system cannot give free consent to research participation. Given a healthy refusal rate for most projects with offenders and offender-patients, the latter seems unlikely to be a major problem, and there are well-recognised ways of building in safeguards, with appropriate assurances of optimal treatment regardless of research participation, allowing plenty of time for completing consent and even consultation with legal advisors if wished. It would be much more serious to deny people any opportunity to take part in research only because they are offenders or offender-patients; in particular, it could deny them critical improvements in treatment because approaches could not be adequately researched with anyone else.

Disclosure of information acquired by researchers was a key issue in Brown's struggles [27]. It is perhaps surprising that, with one or two exceptions required in law, there should be any question of disclosure of research information. Material reported to and recorded by researchers should, after all, in legal terms, be regarded as merely hearsay evidence. Crown Prosecution Service advice to me has been that avoidance of inclusion of high-public-interest cases would generally ensure safety in this regard. The only case found that went to court on this issue – *Bell* – was not part of mental health research. After this case – about research interviews with people thought to have information about the Northern Ireland troubles – some tapes were made public, but the judge ruled: 'in the context of a criminal trial they are just not reliable or fairly obtained evidence'. The reality is that there can be no guarantee of confidentiality in our field, and we have a duty to warn accordingly. In practice, however, no-one in the UK has been placed under pressure to disclose mental health *research* data to the courts, and this case may prove an additional safeguard.

Understanding and Interpreting the Research We Have: Some Successes and Directions

Scientific challenges to forensic mental health research lie mainly in the particular complexity of disorders and social context facing the patients. A considerable advance since the 1980s has been the emergence of studies with large, general population cohorts establishing small but significant associations between various disorders of mental health and various forms of antisocial and criminal behaviour (e.g. [28]) and prisoner studies worldwide showing a high prevalence of various disorders of mental health (e.g. [29]). The order of associations – in both streams – has been remarkably consistent over time and it is arguable that, given the dearth of research resources, further expenditure on cross-sectional counting, however elegantly done, is not needed, although there may be pressure to do so. Already there are voices calling for further prisoner surveys. What is needed is much more knowledge about the sequencing of problems, including points for disrupting damaging pathways and optimising good outcomes and whether there are harms in what is done to offenders.

Many prospective longitudinal studies have advanced knowledge of different patterns in the emergence of antisocial and criminal behaviours. Farrington [30] lists all those that have a cohort size of at least several hundred, are representative of the community, have repeated personal interviews over time, use many different variables from different data sources and span at least five years. Their number, geographical spread and spread over time help to respond to an important criticism that just when such cohorts reach the ages for illness and offending onset, they start to reflect a cultural context that is outdated. Just three examples indicate the growing sophistication of this work – from the early West and Farrington British schoolboy cohort, now of just over 400 who entered the project at age 8 and participated in the latest data collection at age 61 [31], through a New Zealand birth cohort of over 1,000 boys and girls with a remarkably high (95%) follow-up rate from 1972 to 1973 to the latest collection at age 45 [32, 33], to a southwest England cohort of over 14,000, identified during the mother's pregnancy and now followed for about 27 years [34], not included in Farrington [30]. An example of the sophistication that can be achieved in these studies is a finding among the sub-cohort of Dunedin birth cohort boys that a functional polymorphism in the gene encoding the neurotransmitter metabolizing enzyme monoamine oxidase A (MAOA) moderates the effect of childhood maltreatment on subsequent antisocial behaviour, at least partly explaining repeated findings that early trauma increases the risk of later antisocial behaviour but does not make it inevitable [35].

It would be helpful to have comparable sophistication in studies of established offenders and offender-patients, not least because these form only a small subgroup in most population-based studies. What does brain structure or function look like more or less contemporaneously with a serious violent incident when a person was psychotic – or indeed when not psychotic? To what extent do functional brain imaging studies show change which corresponds to changes in symptoms, behaviour or both? There are few studies which clearly anchor the psychopathology or behaviours in time, and only one or two longitudinal prospective studies of brain activity during, say, resolving psychosis. Questions have been asked about the role of neuro-imaging data in court but, in relation to offender-patients, while it may add weight to other clinical evidence, it should be treated with caution [36]; in this field still an absence of evidence does not equate with evidence of the absence of a particular problem.

Psycho-social pathways research also needs more development. Understanding that mental state is likely to improve at least during early imprisonment [37] is helpful, but there is now supplementary knowledge that, with lower staffing and deterioration of prison conditions, the experience of imprisonment may be very different from that in times of higher staffing [38]. Should this be taken into account when considering older work? Every research finding must be interpreted in context – 'treatment as usual' may vary considerably over time and between places, and practitioners are not necessarily even aware of this. This may be particularly hard when trying to interpret research findings from overseas, but it may be unsafe to assume that even *within* any one country practice is constant. Cumulative small incremental changes are difficult to detect. An essential element of that context is that both the problems and strengths of the offenders and offender-patients with whom we work are influenced by what happens between people; the impact of disorder on relationships may be more important than the disorder per se. This has conceptual and methodological implications. Future work should not only map neurobiological and psychological dimensions of mental disorders but also link them to social interactions in the patient's life and in treatment.

This leads to how models of treatment and rehabilitation can be evaluated, given their complexity. We have theoretical models – for example, one relating to high-security hospital patients, drawing on the experiences of a wide range of clinical disciplines and other agency staff [39]. 'Pathological dependence' – the core concern according to this model – is at its most extreme in relation to the most serious offender-patients in the most secure conditions, but the principle of working towards a state of healthy independence through the two main identified processes of 'paving the way' with specific treatments and 'testing out' are likely to hold good in transitions between other levels of service too. In wider clinical practice, concepts of pathways or 'the patient's journey' had already been adopted, but momentum grew in forensic psychiatry with two landmark reports of the 2000s [40, 41] and have been adopted as policy in some areas (e.g. [42]). The task now is to develop strategies for evaluation which go beyond piecemeal approaches [43, 44].

Questions arise too about optimising the legal framework for managing offenders with enduring mental disorder. One key area for consideration in legislation for England and Wales is the 'hybrid order' – mental health legislation allowing for a prison sentence but starting in hospital and with the possibility of repeated movement between hospital and prison (section 45a Mental Health Act 1983/2007). This was introduced to mitigate an unrealised fear of floods of dangerous patients being released after a successful challenge in the European Court of Human Rights to the then absence of right of appeal against restrictions on discharge under section 41 of this Act (*X v. UK*). It was thought at the time that a ground for such appeal might be the untreatability of 'psychopathic disorder', but it was little used in the period after it was introduced. Since then, mental health legislative reform opened the possibility of the imposition of hybrid orders for people with any mental disorder leading to growing concerns about the use of the hybrid order. Discussion about its value started in the courts with *Vowles*. This and subsequent appeal court rulings in cases where the hybrid order was used or might have been used (*Fuller*; *Edwards*; *Fisher*; *Cleland*) have followed judicial case evidence-gathering. This in turn raised questions which have not been adequately answered by research. What are the true advantages and disadvantages of primary health service management with Ministry of Justice restrictions on discharge over primary criminal justice service management under long or indefinite prison sentences?

A research theme that has had relatively substantial investment of thought and money is the assessment of risk of harm to others. Superficially, this has been a somewhat disappointing stream of work. Several reviews have suggested that none of the tools developed offer much if the goal is primarily to show that people with ratings indicative of high risk are the ones who go on to do (more) damaging acts [45, 46]. A rounded academic perspective, however, suggests that this is too simplistic an approach for determining true benefit. The main goal of risk assessment is – or should be – to inform risk management. Effective risk management should reduce the chance of the managed risk occurring. So, correctly used, it should be expected that clinical risk assessment tools will not perform well if the measure of success of a violence prediction is solely of later violence. Therefore, risk assessment tools may be better assessed by studying the impact of their use on practice, and of their other potential advantages, including improved transparency of assessment and decision-making. A further key issue here is to avoid conflation of risk assessment with threat assessment. An individual who is making specific threats of harm to another/others – or indeed to self – is in a different position from someone who is ill, generally distressed and aggressive.

A final point in this necessarily selective tour of research developments is that, in risk assessment, we have generally been preoccupied with secondary or tertiary prevention – that is, our work and inquiry has mainly been about preventing further violence or reducing its impact once some violence has already occurred. A US forensic psychiatrist wisely observed: 'A society sincerely concerned about reducing violence will seek broad measures that address both known risks for violence among persons both with and without mental health problems' [47].

UK academic clinicians are beginning to work along these lines and show success. In Scotland, for example, not only has knife-carrying been targeted but also, according to logical argument, the nature of knives. Most lethal harm follows from knives with a sharp point; making round-ended alternatives preferentially available is beginning to have an impact [48].

Conclusions

Academic forensic psychiatry is the business of all psychiatrists, although we need a group of people who will specialise in it to support the teaching and training and research aspirations of everyone who is primarily concerned with direct clinical service delivery, development or management. Being an academic means reflecting constantly on how we practise – according to good evidence, where there is no evidence, or in spite of the evidence? Seminars, clinical peer reviews and conferences are all essential to the cognitive components of this and should keep us on the first path where possible, ensure that we are aware when we are on the second and united in calling for relevant research and stop us from straying onto or staying on the third. It is not all about cognition, however; feelings and transferences need attention too. This is where psychotherapeutic input to forensic mental health services is so crucial. Bad stuff will happen to most of us at some time and, if we are to remain effective, we need help in managing it.

A few things transcend evidence – in my very first psychiatric post ever I was allowed to admit to a hospital bed a distressed street-living man asking for help with his alcohol dependency – *so that I could learn how pointless that would be*. He did well during his detoxification and was apparently happy but then he discharged himself and we never saw him again. Was that pointless? Did I learn? Sometimes it is important to recognise that our skills and services cannot help, and perhaps even that wrongly applied they could do damage, but my choice would be never to learn to ignore requests for help even in apparently hopeless cases. Kindness and concern are important clinical traits too – and perhaps even these values can be evidenced? Ballatt, Campling and colleagues [49, 50] have developed an important construct of 'intelligent kindness' as an antidote to failing institutions and stress among staff. They suggest that kindness directs attentiveness, which enables 'attunement', which builds trust, which generates a therapeutic alliance, which produces better outcomes, and the whole process, in turn, sets the climate of kinship between staff and staff, staff and patients. Engagement and 'cure' will not always happen, but without an enabling clinical climate it will never happen.

Knowledge is vital but, in clinical practice, there are always limits. Population-based findings may mislead in relation to the individual, credible and evidenced associations do not imply cause and effect, and even prospective longitudinal studies can only hint at many of the answers we crave. Large birth cohorts will, if truly representative of the general population, only include very small numbers of the people who are most prevalent in our highly selected clinical practice – people with schizophrenia or similar psychosis. Psychiatric diagnoses still rely heavily if not exclusively on reported symptoms, although they are not necessarily less valid for that if we approach such data collection systematically – enabling free accounts before applying highly structured tools, comparing the respective findings, examining stability of expression over time, collating the observations of others – family and close associates as well as other professionals – and perhaps adding measures based on relevant theoretical paradigms or physical investigation tools such as neuroimaging. This approach incorporates the best of academic inquiry – ask questions, listen to the answers, record the answers, ask more questions and keep the process going.

The power of the individual case is inescapable. Landmark changes in law and practice have probably more often been driven by individual cases than any other evidence, McNaughton being only one of the best known [51]. Individual cases make powerful stories for the national press, and legislators respond. Relatives and survivors often want a life lost to mean something, a current trend being for a law named for the dead victim. The criminal courts, at least in common law jurisdictions, work on legal precedent as well as statute. Indeed, it is in the application of law and precedent to the individual case that, as forensic psychiatrists, we sometimes seem closest in practice to lawyers. And yet we can add population-based and cohort outcome perspectives into the mix which, without us, the courts lack. Dialogue about these issues within and outside the court matters.

Finally, we have to learn the limits of our expertise and to manage uncertainty. Statistical skills are rare among us, notwithstanding interest in risk assessments, and failures of recognition of this on the part of a renowned academic-clinician – and the court – led to a set of serious miscarriages of justice as further cases followed *Clark*. Statisticians responded [11], but each of us must be able to recognise and be candid about the limits of our expertise. The drive towards ever more sophisticated models of risk assessment perhaps shielded us for a while from acknowledging that, but there is often a limit to the trajectory of our 'getting better'. Academic progress is to acknowledge such limitations within and outside the specialty – in court, in public – and still help to steer offender-patients into appropriate and safe placements.

References

1. Medical Schools Council. *Survey of Medical Academic Clinical Staffing Levels*, 2018. www.medschools.ac.uk/media/2491/m sc-clinical-academic-survey-report-2018.pdf.

2. Academy of Medical Sciences. *Transforming Health through Innovation: Integrating the NHS and Academia*, 2020. https://acmedsci.ac.uk/file-download/23932583.

3. Home Office. *Report of the Committee on Mentally Abnormal Offenders* [Butler]. London, Her Majesty's Stationery Office, 1975, Cmnd 6244.

4   Home Office. *Review of Health and Social Services for Mentally Disorder Offenders and Others Requiring Similar Services* [Reed]. London, HMSO, 1992, Cmnd 2008.

5. Kennedy HG, personal communication.

6. Thomas A. What about forensic psychiatry as a career? Undergraduate and early post-graduate medical perspectives. *Criminal Behaviour and Mental Health* 2012; 22: 247–51. DOI: 10.1002/cbm.1838.

7. Rees MR, Bracewell M. Academic factors in medical recruitment: evidence to support improvements in medical recruitment and retention by improving the academic content in medical posts. *Postgraduate Medical Journal* 2019; 95: 323–7. doi: 10.1136/postgradmedj-2019-136501.

8. Grounds A, Gunn J, Myers WC, Rosner R, Busch KG. Contemplating common ground in the professional ethics of forensic psychiatry. *Criminal Behaviour and Mental Health* 2010; 20: 307–22. DOI: 10.1002/cbm.789,

9. Nedopil N, Gunn J, Thomosn LDG. Teaching forensic psychiatry in Europe. *Criminal Behaviour and Mental Health* 2012; 22: 238–46. DOI: 10.1002/cbm.1845.

10. Aubert V. Researches in the sociology of law. *The American Behavioural Scientist* 7 (4): 16–20 https://doi.org/10.1177/000276426300700405.

11. Aitken C, Roberts P, Jackson G. Communicating and interpreting statistical evidence in the administration of criminal justice. 1. Fundamentals of probability and statistical evidence in criminal proceedings. London, Royal Statistical Society, 2010. www.maths.ed.ac.uk/~cgga/Guide-1-WEB.pdf.

12. The Ghent Group. www.ghentgroup.eu.

13. The European Convention on Human Rights. www.echr.coe.int/Documents/Convention_ENG.pdf.

14. Taylor PJ, Woolfenden N, Nedopil N. Forensic psychiatry training in Europe. *Die Psychiatrie* 2013; 10 (3): 181–7. DOI: 10.1055/s-0038-1670882.

15. Soothill K, Harney K, Maggs A, Chilvers C. The NHS forensic mental health R&D programme: developing new talent or maintaining a stage army? *Personality and Mental Health* 2008; 2: 183–91. DOI: 10.1002/pmh.44.

16. Kirkpatrick T, Lennox C, Taylor R et al. Evaluation of a complex intervention (Engager) for prisoners with common mental health problems, near to and after release: study protocol for a randomised controlled trial. *BMJ Open* 2018; 8 (2): e017931.

17. Forsyth K, Webb RT, Power LA et al. The Older Prisoner Health and Social Care Assessment and Plan (OHSCAP) versus treatment as usual: a randomised controlled trial. *Research Square* 2020. https://assets.researchsquare.com/files/rs-75588/v1/f871ec39-49c9-44cf-aa6a-9fff11d56ab9.pdf.

18. Taylor PJ, Robling M, Playle R et al. A randomised controlled trial of a group psychological intervention to increase locus of control for alcohol consumption among alcohol-misusing short-term (male) prisoners (GASP). *Addiction* 2020. doi:10.1111/add.15006.

19. Cosden M, Ellens J, Schnell J, Yamini-Diouf Y. Efficacy of a mental health treatment court with assertive community treatment. *Behavioral Sciences and the Law* 2005; 23: 199–214. DOI: 10.1002/bsl.638.

20. Mirza RD, Punja S, Vohra S, Guyatt G. The history and development of N-of-1 trials. *Journal of the Royal Society of Medicine* 2017; 110 (8): 330–40 DOI: 10.1177/0141076817721131.

21. *Consort Guidance on N=1 Trials.* www.consort-statement.org/extensions?ContentWidgetId=47627.

22. Taylor PJ, Fleminger JJ. ECT for schizophrenia. *Lancet* 1980; 1: 1380–3. doi:10.1016/s0140-6736(80)92653-7.

23. Moore GF, Audrey S, Barker M et al. Process evaluation of complex interventions: Medical Research Council guidance. *BMJ* 2015; 350: h1258. doi:10.1136/bmj.h1258.

24. Bonell C, Fletcher A, Morton M, Lorenc T, Moore L. Realist randomised controlled trials: a new approach to evaluating complex public health interventions. *Social Science & Medicine* 2012; 75 (12): 2299–2306. https://doi.org/10.1016/j.socscimed.2012.08.032.

25. Van Belle S, Wong G, Westhorp G et al. Can 'realist' randomised controlled trials be genuinely realist? *Trials* 2016; 17: 313. https://doi.org/10.1186/s13063-016-1407-0.

26. UK Research and Innovation, Medical Research Council and NHS Health Research Authority. *Is My Study Research?* 2017. www.hra-decisiontools.org.uk/research.

27. Brown P. Ethical challenges to research in the criminal justice system. *Criminal Behaviour and Mental Health* 2018; 28 (1): 5-12. https://doi.org/10.1002/cbm.2061.

28. Fazel S, Gulati G, Linsell L, Geddes JR, Grann M. Schizophrenia and violence: systematic review and meta-analysis. *PLoS Medicine* 2009; 6: e1000120. doi: 10.1371/jounal.pmed.1002120.

29. Fazel S, Seewald K. Severe mental illness in 33588 prisoners worldwide: systematic review and meta-regression analysis. *British Journal of Psychiatry* 2012; 200: 364–73. doi: 10.1192/bjp.bp.111.096370.

30. Farrington DP. The psychosocial milieu of the offender. In Gunn J and Taylor PJ (eds) *Forensic Psychiatry, Clinical, Legal and Ethical Issues*, 2nd edition. Boca Raton, FL, CRC Press, 2014, pp. 170–85.

31. Farrington DP. Childhood risk factors for criminal career duration: comparisons with prevalence, onset, frequency and recidivism. *Criminal Behaviour and Mental Health* 2020; 30 (4): 159–71. https://doi.org/10.1002/cbm.2155.

32. Poulton R, Moffitt TE, Silva PA. The Dunedin Multidisciplinary Health and Development Study: overview of the first 40 years, with an eye to the future. *Social Psychiatry and Psychiatric Epidemiology* 2015; 50: 679–93. doi: 10.1007/s00127-015-1048-8.

33. Caspi A, Houts RM, Ambler A et al. Longitudinal assessment of mental health disorders and comorbidities across 4 decades among participants in the Dunedin birth cohort study. *JAMA Network Open* 2020; 3 (4): e203221. doi: 10.1001/jamanetworkopen.2020.3221.

34. Lawlor DA, Lewcock M, Rena-Jones L et al. The second generation of the Avon Longitudinal Study of Parents and Children (ALSPAC-G2): a cohort profile. *Welcome Open Research* 2019; 4: 36. https://doi.org/10.12688/wellcomeopenres.15087.2.

35. Caspi A, McClay J, Moffitt TE et al. Role of genotype in the cycle of violence in

maltreated children. *Science* 2002; 297: 851–4.

36. Reagu S, Taylor PJ. Practical legal concerns for use of neuroimaging in the court in England and Wales. In Simpson J (ed.) *Neuroimaging in Forensic Psychiatry: From Clinic to Courtroom.* Chichester, Wiley Blackwell, 2012.

37. Walker J, Illingworth C, Canning A et al. Changes in mental state associated with prison environments: a systematic review. *Acta Psychiatrica Scandinavica* 2014; 129: 427–36.

38. O'Connor S, Bezeczky Z, Moriarty Y, Kalebic N, Taylor PJ. Adjustment to short-term imprisonment under low prison staffing. *BJPsych Bulletin* 2020; 44 (4): 139–44. doi: 10.1192/bjb.2020.2.

39. Jamieson L, Taylor PJ, Gibson B. From pathological dependence to healthy independent living: an emergent grounded theory of facilitating independent living. *The Grounded Theory Review* 2006; 6: 79–107. http://groundedtheoryreview.com/2006/11/30/1222.

40. Bradley K. *The Bradley Report: Lord Bradley's Review of People with Mental Health Problems or Learning Disabilities in the Criminal Justice System.* London, Department of Health, 2009. https://webarchive.nationalarchives.gov.uk/20130105193845/http://www.dh.gov.uk/prod_consum_dh/groups/dh_digitalassets/documents/digitalasset/dh_098698.pdf.

41. Corston J. *A Report by Baroness Jean Corston of a Review of Women with Particular Vulnerabilities in the Criminal Justice System.* London, Home Office, 2007. www.newsocialartschool.org/pdf/Corston-pt-1.pdf.

42. National Offender Management Service and NHS England. *The Offender Personality Disorder Pathway Strategy,* 2015. www.england.nhs.uk/commissioning/wp-content/uploads/sites/12/2016/02/opd-strategy-nov-15.pdf.

43. Forrester A, Hopkin G. Mental health in the criminal justice system: a pathways approach to service and research design. *Criminal Behaviour and Mental Health* 2019; 29 (4): 207–17. https://doi.org/10.1002/cbm.2128.

44. Kennedy HG, Simpson A, Haque Q. Perspective on excellence in forensic mental health services: what we can learn from oncology and other medical services. *Frontiers in Psychiatry* 2019; 10: 733. https://doi.org/10.3389/fpsyt.2019.00733.

45. Singh JP, Fazel S, Gueorguieva R, Buchanan A. Rates of violence in patients classified as high risk by structured risk assessment instruments. *British Journal of Psychiatry* 2014; 104: 180–7. doi: 10.1192/bjp.bp.113.131938.

46. Singh JP, Grann M, Fazel S. A comparative study of violence risk assessment tools: a systematic review and metaregression analysis of 68 studies involving 25,980 participants. *Clinical Psychology Review* 2011; 31: 499–513. doi: 10.1016/j.cpr.2010.11.009.

47. Mossman D. The imperfection of protection through detection and intervention: lessons from three decades of research on the psychiatric assessment of violence risk. *Journal of Legal Medicine* 2009; 30: 109–40. DOI: 10.1080/01947640802694635.

48. Crichton JHM. Falls in Scottish homicide: lessons for homicide reduction in mental health patients. *BJPsych Bulletin* 2017; 41: 185–6. doi: 10.1192/pb.bp.116.054924.

49. Ballatt J, Campling P, Maloney C. *Intelligent Kindness: Rehabilitating the Welfare State,* 2nd ed. Cambridge, Royal College of Psychiatrists/Cambridge University Press, 2020.

50. Campling P. Reforming the culture of healthcare: the case for intelligent kindness. *British Journal of Psychiatry Bulletin* 2015; 39: 1–5. doi: 10.1192/pb.bp.114.047449.

51. Schneider RD. *The Lunatic and the Lords.* Toronto, Irwin Law, 2009.

52. Kennedy HG, Mohan D, Davoren M. Forensic psychiatry and Covid-19: accelerating transformation in forensic psychiatry. *Irish Journal of Psychological Medicine* 2020. doi: 10.1017/ipm.2020.58.

Cases

R v Ivor Bell [2019] NICC 20. Ref: OHA11086

R v Clark [2003] RWCA Crim 1020

R v Cleland [2020] EWCA Crim 906

R v Edwards [2018] EWCA Crim 595

R v Fisher [2019] EWCA Crim 1066, 2019 WL 02551700

R v Fuller [2016] EWCA Crim 1867

X v UK 7215/75 [1981] ECHR 6

R v Vowles; R (Vowles) v SSJ [2015] EWCA Crim 45, [2015] EWCA Civ 56 [2015]

The No-Nonsense Guides

Essential Practical Approaches for the Consultant Forensic Psychiatrist

Mary Davoren, Carolyn Stanley, Sajida Nabi, Katherine Warburton, Kevin Murray, Treena Wilkie and Krishna Pillai

Introduction

We designed this chapter to cover the practical on-the-job knowledge that is rarely, in our experience, covered in books. It is the information new consultants crave the day before commencing that first consultant post; the information new clinical directors wish they had been given six months prior to taking on their management position. There are no references in this chapter and it is not based on clinical trials or guidelines; rather, it is based on experience. In short, we wanted it to feel like having a conversation over a cuppa with a colleague and peer who is 10 years into the job you have just taken up and really wants you to succeed.

The New Consultant Experience

Mary Davoren

Consultant Forensic Psychiatrist, Central Mental Hospital, Dublin, Ireland; Clinical Senior Lecturer in Forensic Psychiatry, Trinity College Dublin, Ireland; Visiting Professor of Forensic Psychiatry, University of Bari 'Aldo Moro', Bari, Italy.

They say you will learn more in your first six months as a consultant than in all your junior doctor training years combined. They are right.

Taking on a new consultant role is both rewarding and daunting, for obvious reasons. You have spent 14 or more years since university working towards precisely this goal, and yet may well feel unprepared in many ways to take this on. In my opinion, much of this stems from the fact that those 14 years contained very little by way of training for a leadership position in a large organisation, and yet that is a key role for any consultant.

An old Irish medical proverb says that in your first six months as a consultant you should buy two new suits and never speak at the consultant meetings – best to observe the dynamics first. Well, I don't know who said that, but frankly it's not bad advice. A vital part of the transition from junior doctor to consultant is to develop an understanding that you will no longer be moving on from that post in six months or a year – this one is for good and the colleagues are for keeps. A clinical director once said to me: a new consultant is for life, not just for Christmas.

Prior to starting your first consultant post, it is vital to maximise the time you have as a higher trainee – develop your special interest areas and develop your CV to its maximum potential – remember, there is a difference between getting a consultant post and getting *the* consultant post you actually want, your first choice. Becoming a doctor is not easy; you have dedicated years of your life from secondary or high school level, through to university and internship, and on to junior doctor training. Do not waste your special interest or research time while on specialist or higher training schemes – this is tantamount to falling at the final hurdle. Regardless of how or where you undertake higher training, the time will fly by and within the blink of an eye you will be applying for your first consultant role.

When you take on your first consultant role as a forensic psychiatrist, a tip is to contact the Mental Health Act office (or equivalent in other jurisdictions), ascertain which tribunals or hearings are approaching quickly and request extensions if possible – this may seem forward and you may be worried how that might look to your new clinical director, but honestly it is far better to have a couple of additional weeks to prepare than to arrive unprepared at your first hearing. When you take up your post, be prepared for the emails – I remember my shock in my first consultant role when I felt that every time I left my desk I returned to 10 or 15 new emails. People seem to incessantly copy in the consultant in almost every email. Some are necessary, some not quite so necessary. Deal with the necessary immediately if you can to keep the decks clear, but also be mindful that you are now the team leader and more junior staff may want your reassurance and support, hence the emails. Part of your new role is to provide that support and reassurance, so actually these emails are part of the job.

The consultant sets the tone on the team in many cases. This is vital to remember – honesty, clarity and behavioural predictability are key in qualities that develop trust in team members. Try to stay as positive and calm as you can, remembering that the hospital is a professional setting. Be a good colleague and swap on-call duties for peers when you can – you may well need that favour in return another day. Be mindful of overtly or repeatedly critiquing the health service or hospital you work in – we all have bad days, and we all work in services where something or indeed many things may need improvement. However, clinical audit and quality improvement (QI) projects are the professional way to set about improving things at work. A less than positive approach about your hospital or trust can undermine the confidence of your team in the service being provided, and is not ideal. In short, don't be a Moaning Myrtle. Remember, you chose to work in this hospital or trust; if you want to make changes, I would suggest focussing your energy into QI in a positive way. Get a good mentor, a senior consultant who can support you through any difficult times; being able to discuss challenging situations with a supportive peer is a very helpful strategy for getting through.

Your office is now a room that team members will gravitate towards, and occasionally professional visitors as well, including board members to welcome the new consultant and so on. A clear desk gives you and everyone else a sense that you are on top of your workload and things are calm and organised. I am a firm believer in styling your office with posters, pictures and other accessories to give it a bit of style and comfort (this was something I picked up in Broadmoor Hospital). Clearing your desk each evening before you leave will allow you to return to an organised calm environment each morning (this was something I tried to pick up in Broadmoor Hospital). But seriously, we spend long periods of time at work, so having a comfortable and calm office matters.

It may sound obvious, but being a hospital consultant is hard work. It is a privileged position and consultants take ultimate clinical responsibility for patient care. We also have a duty and responsibility to uphold the integrity of the medical profession. This is not an easy job and it is vital that you set your own expectations accordingly. Having a balanced work plan or job plan is a way of ensuring you stay fresh and interested in your role. Therefore, you may want to include some management, teaching, committee or research work in your portfolio. I would advise that you do not rush into taking on committees – settle into your role first, but be open when something that genuinely interests you comes along. I would suggest giving priority to committees that might be service-wide or trust-wide, or based in another area such as a prison or university. This can give you time in a setting where you meet a wider peer group and that can help to broaden your professional circle, and is often a real highlight in your work schedule. Go to forensic psychiatry conferences, see what is happening in overseas forensic mental health services and develop international networks. This is a really great way of keeping abreast of new changes in the discipline, engaging with peers and bringing new ideas from international centres of excellence home to your own service.

Be mindful of social media – it can be fun and actually very helpful at times, but it can also set unrealistic expectations. Don't put anything in an email or on social media if you would not be comfortable with it being on the front page of a newspaper. Lastly, I will say, you will settle in more quickly than you know, and pretty soon you will be mentoring new consultants yourself. When the going gets a bit tough, remember there was a time when being in your first consultant forensic psychiatrist role was your dream.

Essential Knowledge for a New Consultant in Forensic Psychiatry
Carolyn Stanley
Consultant Forensic Psychiatrist and Clinical Director, North London Forensic Services, Barnet, Enfield and Haringey Mental Health NHS Trust, London, England, UK.

Congratulations, you've made it! You survived the long, hard slog of higher training and are now a new consultant forensic psychiatrist. You are probably in a state of shock and disbelief; after all, you have taken at least 13 years of your life to achieve this career landmark. It is usually around this time that new consultants start to feel a flash of panic ... or even a tsunami panic. Those 'negative automatic thoughts' we learned about in cognitive behavioural therapy training can really start to kick in if left unchecked. You may start to swim in a sea of worry, feeling that you are not ready, or that your inadequacies are so glaringly obvious that it is like someone has tattooed them across your forehead. Conversely, you may be of the other new consultant breed and be strutting around, bursting with confidence, swanky new suit at the ready, oblivious to the massive wall of stress and consultant accountability that you are walking into.

Breathe: It Is All Okay; You Are Going to Be Fine
Firstly, one of the key things you need to recognise is that you are no longer a higher trainee, specialist registrar or fellow. That chapter is closed. If you have not done so already, you need to get that concept straight in your own head quite sharp and change your approach to the job. Try and get some time off between the transitions of roles, whether that is by annual leave, cleverly placed study leave or unpaid leave before your new start date. It will help you to disconnect and allow for much-needed headspace away from the workplace. Recharge your batteries: that anxiety-ridden road of actually getting the job of your dreams is over.

Get the Basics Sorted
It is important to spend a little time here stating the obvious, but getting some, if not all, of this in hand before you arrive is imperative. No-one will really care that it is your first day

and you have not yet been allocated an office, keys, laptop or phone. They will have their important questions and will need answers. For the sake of your own sanity it is worthwhile sending an email a week or so before your arrival to ascertain who your administrative support is. Politely request that they help set everything up so these housekeeping issues do not dominate your first day. Having to go more than one hour without IT, passwords, security access and your car parking permit is quickly going to get very annoying. Likewise for finding out how to submit travel expense forms and leave requests.

Start as you mean to go on – as organised as possible. It can make for a refreshing contrast to what you may be facing in your clinical areas. The stationery cupboard remains sacred ground to this very day; the Aladdin's cave that is the locked stationery cupboard is still only accessible to the chosen few. Put your orders in early so your office will always be equipped with the essentials.

Being a Leader

I can only really compare the first day of being a new consultant to the first day as a junior doctor. The two are strikingly similar in how you are left feeling as though you know absolutely nothing about the job at hand despite having successfully jumped through all the hoops of training. Rest assured you know more than you think and quite frankly you will no longer have time to worry about such things. Remember, your consultant colleagues will gladly help and support you, so never think they won't.

It is important to recognise that you are a leader and others will be looking to you for direction, motivation and reassurance. There is much written on the topic of effective medical and clinical leadership and you will spend the rest of your consultant career fine-tuning these skills. For now, take stock and decide what type of consultant you want to be. You will have worked alongside plenty of consultants and have seen it done, taking mental notes of what did and did not work well.

Ultimately, the responsibility is now yours, and for the time being make it look like you are taking it all in your stride. The barrage of never-ending questions and being pulled in a hundred different directions will start on day one. The temptation to do everything yourself will be immense just so you can tick if off your ever-growing to-do list. You will never get to the bottom of that to-do list, so strike that unobtainable goal off indefinitely. For these reasons it is essential that you appropriately delegate and utilise surrounding abilities.

It goes without saying that you need to get up to speed fast with your clinical caseload because everyone will treat you as if you know all the minutiae, even if the reality is far from this. The amount of information you need to absorb and filter is vast, and it will take a large amount of your time in the beginning. One of the most important roles of the consultant is to have a clear overview of each case so you can identify key issues and direct the team focus. Then of course there are all the 'unsaid' problem behaviours that everyone else seems to know about in great detail, but there is not one single sniff of it in the patient case notes. You will need to extract these gems of information face to face from your multi-disciplinary team, and if previous consultants are to hand, they will sum it up in a nutshell.

Building strong working relationships with colleagues is invaluable given that forensic psychiatry is a complex and often high-stakes field of work. You cannot and should not be planning to do this alone, so the years ahead will be easier if you put the groundwork in from the start. You will need the expertise of others and they will help you enormously when you need it most. Do you really know the structure of your service and how to manoeuvre effectively within it? Quickly get to know who's who and their skills. Be present on your unit, listen to the chat of staff and meet regularly with your managers to understand the lay of the land and the wider issues you are expected to navigate.

The mental health sector is under strain in almost every country, and your co-workers will frequently be tired and overloaded. More often than not you will find yourself in a similar situation. See this workplace climate for what it is. Do not turn a blind eye to the reality of working in highly demanding conditions and make sure you acknowledge the limits of your team and the individuals within it. This dynamic left unchecked can take its toll, with acrimony and hostility spreading and destroying from within. Yes, be resilient, but no, do not ignore escalating levels of pressure. This will inevitably lead to burnout, increased risk of accidents and lower standards of care. Be kind, supportive and explore this within your team. It is your role to bring people together, supervise and encourage the use of the See Think Act model for reflective practice.

As the weeks pass into months, you will be able to see with increasing clarity the areas requiring quality improvement, the gaps begging for a new business model proposal or other areas where you can sprinkle a bit of your own magic. Again, you will do this better by knowing who to bring in to help you, and you may actually stand a chance of finishing it.

There are several areas of care where you simply cannot let the side down such as meeting national targets for forensic services, for example in the UK the CQUIN targets (NHS Commissioning for Quality and Innovation) or other commissioner-based targets and also in maintaining Mental Health Act compliance. It is essential that you keep on top of this, not to mention that inspections from the relevant regulatory body for your service – the Care Quality Commission in the UK, the Mental Health Commission/Coimisiún Meabhar-Shláinte in Ireland, the Mental Health Commission of Canada/Commission de la Santé Mentale du Canada and so on – can strike at any time! Start as you mean to go on and get into the habit of incorporating good practice into your day-to-day work.

Lastly, workplace politics … they are definitely there. Tread carefully. You will have a period of immunity because you are the new kid on the block, but sooner rather than later you will see the layers. The extent to which you get involved is up to you. Remain professional; remember you are a consultant and that others are looking to you to set an example. Entering into conflict with colleagues can be necessary but also uncomfortable and time-consuming. Keep disagreements factual to bolster what you are saying and do not let it get personal.

Appraisal and Annual Reviews of Consultant Practice

Medical appraisal and maintaining a commitment to lifelong learning is a mandatory part of your working life and will pave the way to your medical council annual revalidation; there is no escaping it and those that do soon find themselves in troubled water. In many ways, appraisal in the UK or continuing professional development (CPD) or continuing professional education submissions in other countries seemed to automatically happen as you were in training while under the all-seeing eye of various supervisors, but now it is solely down to you to organise. Try not to see it as a paperwork chore but rather as something that helps shape both you and your medical career development.

It is worth looking at the key areas of your appraisal or annual CPD requirements from the start and mapping out the year ahead; there is a handy checklist on the NHS England website (www.england.nhs.uk/revalidation/wp-content/uploads/sites/10/2016/03/dctorsmedcl-apprs-chcklst.pdf) to help focus the mind. Your hospital group or hospital trust will send details of their online appraisal e-platform or the group or trust appraisal lead, and in some cases allocate you an appraiser. It is easy to get bogged down under never-ending clinical work, but you must carve out time and protect your schedule for wider growth. Find and join a consultant peer group to discuss your personal development plan and CPD opportunities. Help yourself here by ensuring you are signed up to receive relevant e-bulletins from institutions such as The Royal College of Psychiatrists Faculty of Forensic Psychiatry, the International Association of Forensic Mental Health Services, The International Organisation of Forensic Practitioners and so on. The Royal College of Psychiatrists StartWell framework will be useful, especially if you find yourself geographically isolated from your peers. Each mental health trust should have their own StartWell group, but The Royal College of Psychiatrists, and other international colleges, hold regular events and have an array of online support material for new consultants.

Try to access as much free CPD opportunities as possible; opportunities will crop up within your organisation so make sure you are on all the right email distribution lists. Not only will this tick the CPD box, it will also open up opportunities for networking with colleagues and offer space outside of your usual nine to five for using parts of your brain you forgot you had.

It takes a lot of time to put an appraisal portfolio together; do not leave it until the night before. Endeavour to do a bit each yearly quarter so you are not in complete meltdown trying to reach the submission deadline. If all else fails and your good intentions go to pot, at the very least set up a folder on your computer desktop to drop 'evidence' of your developmental effort along the way.

If, for all sorts of reasons, you find you are getting really stuck with your career, considering finding a mentor or starting with a set of coaching sessions. It's not unusual to not have given life beyond becoming a new consultant forensic psychiatrist much thought, but it is wise to start to think about where you want to be in 5, 10 or even 20 years' time. Tailor your personal development plan (PDP) for your direction of travel; whether it's a future in management, leadership, teaching, research or as a clinical expert, make sure you are weaving this into your yearly goals.

Money, Money, Money

This term has in many ways become a taboo topic, particularly so within some services such as the NHS in the UK, although this can vary significantly in different countries. The reality is that we are all paid a wage; we all have financial outgoings; and some of us still even have a huge student loans to pay off. Consultant pay scales are no secret and are readily available for all to see on the British Medical Association (BMA) website (UK) and Health Service Executive (HSE) website (Ireland), and this is also the case for most international settings, as consultant salaries are typically a matter of public record. So too is the guidance on payment for medical court reports.

From your training you will be aware there is scope to undertake private work within the field of forensic psychiatry, and in many ways this is a necessary requirement if you are to keep your medico-legal skills up to scratch. Hospitals can have widely differing policies on how private work can be incorporated into job planning. If you do intend to carry out private work as a new consultant, you will need to find out what is accepted practice within your unit. Remember to declare private practice at your appraisal if that is required in your country of practice, and update your medical indemnity policy accordingly.

As you develop as a new consultant and find your feet within the service, you may find that opportunities arise to add additional programmed activities (PAs) to your job plan that come with additional payments, including research roles, clinical director, medical lead roles, electro-convulsive therapy (ECT) lead roles and so on. Wonderful! You can start to make a bigger dent in that student loan repayment. But be careful what you wish for here. Ask yourself a few things: are you spreading yourself too thin? Are you really interested or is this just a means to get that winter holiday? Are you really the right person for the role? Does it fit with your longer-term career plan? Alert: extra payments can really mess up your tax situation.

The lists of opportunities as to how you can use your role as a consultant forensic psychiatrist are countless. Some of you may be media savvy and have a promising role in TV and radio; others may foresee a lucrative path in developing medical Continuing Professional Development (CPD) courses unfurling before you. It is up to you to make of it what you will. Ensure that you are always checking your moral compass and that private work in whatever form it may be is not impinging on your contractual obligations and duties as a consultant forensic psychiatrist.

Trainees and Staff Grade Doctors

Junior doctors are invaluable; be thoughtful and nice to them. Give them supervision; at the very least this must be the mandatory 1 hour of weekly clinical supervision. Offer more of your time to help shape their forensic training experience. If you invest in them, they will repay this consideration 10-fold with their input to the team by doing well at their delegated tasks and supporting the rest of the multi-disciplinary team. If you're very lucky, they may even share with you their directory of every random service in every local hospital – a collection of carefully curated telephone numbers and email addresses passed down from one junior doctor to the next over the years like a family heirloom.

Depending on where you are working, you may draw the short straw here and end up with no junior medical staff and be the only medic on the team. Most facilities will have staff grades and/or core trainees and higher trainees. Strictly speaking in England, you are not permitted to perform clinical supervision for trainees within the first year of being a consultant. Use this time to ensure that you have completed your clinical supervisor accreditation in the professional development framework and are ready to say 'yes' to the offer of a trainee. It is not always plain sailing; be sure to familiarise yourself with any Trainee in Trouble policy for your college or health service. If there is not one, then The Royal College of Psychiatrists' policy is very helpful; you will need to seek guidance sooner rather than later and seek specialist support from higher up in the deanery to appropriately manage the situation. Be prepared for these junior doctor situations to be time-consuming. Do not sit on the matter hoping it will all blow over; that is not fair for patients, the workplace or the wellbeing of the doctor in question.

Forensic trainees often feed back that they feel superfluous or too bogged down with inane paperwork. It is your job to support and stimulate their clinical curiosity. Give the time to fully explain the structures within forensic psychiatry and where their role in the team can be vital to shaping the patient care pathway. Show a genuine interest in their future career aspirations and help them think about how they can build their portfolio to achieve this while in post. Remember, these junior doctors will be your future consultant colleagues, or possibly your future clinical or managing director.

Look After Yourself

This leads me onto my last and possibly most important point: self-preservation. It may sound selfish, but the most important person in all of this is you. You are one of the most expensive pieces of kit in any forensic psychiatric healthcare environment, but you are no use to anyone if you are burnt out. As a new consultant you will be bent in every way imaginable. If you cannot find the strength to say no, you will start to feel tired and overwhelmed very quickly.

Stop saying yes to everything; it simply is not sustainable and you do not need to impress anyone anymore. If you are actually sick, take the day off; even if you have a head cold, you may be able to re-arrange your day so you can stay in the comfort of your own home, not spreading germs about, remote working on paperwork. Organisation is going to be paramount here. Make sure you have annual leave booked well in advance; that you are stimulating your professional mind with study leave; and that you actually see in person your friends and family and plan some sort of life outside of work. This warning has been drilled into medics since they first crossed the threshold of medical school, and yet more often than not it is the thing we neglect and sacrifice the most – ourselves. We are by nature (hopefully) a caring bunch, and we want the best for our patients; we want to be helpful and available to our co-workers and be the best for our forensic service. The most important thing to remember here is that nothing is ever set in stone and job plans can be re-negotiated. Opportunities arise as services expand and morph into the new.

Finally, I will add that becoming a consultant forensic psychiatrist is a very rewarding career, and with a sensible and realistic approach to risk management, people management and management of paperwork, you can have a very positive work–life balance. All storms pass sooner or later. Focus on the possibilities, not the problems, and what you focus on will expand.

How to Supervise a Junior Doctor in Forensic Psychiatry

Sajida Nabi
Consultant Forensic Psychiatrist and Associate Clinical Director, Broadmoor Hospital, Crowthorne, England, UK; Lead for the National High Secure Consultants Forum, London, England, UK.

The archetype of a doctor in training as an apprentice is as old as medicine itself and written into the very wording of the Hippocratic Oath. Universities have taken over the awarding of undergraduate degrees, but this relationship continues in a modern form between the trainer and trainee. There is a commonality in the challenges that arise in training in any medical speciality. Forensic psychiatry poses some unique ones of its own and these will be the focus here.

Forensic psychiatry can provoke emotions in a trainee that do not feel familiar in a work context, including, fear disgust, judgement and emotional distress. As established forensic psychiatrists, we can be desensitised to these emotions. However, we can probably remember our first day in a secure hospital. These emotions can be at their most intense at the start of a job and it can help to work closely with a consultant in those first few weeks. In time, the trainee will start to feel more comfortable. It is important to reassure trainees that while the overall risk may be higher, the increased measures in place seek to mitigate that risk. A colleague captured this well when he said that secure hospitals should feel like an abnormal environment and issues arise only when this begins to feel like the norm.

The most difficult aspect can be spotting boundary breaches. As doctors, we want to connect with our patients and this can involve giving something of ourselves. At the early stages of their career, trainees may lack the ability to recognise an eroding of boundaries. They may lack the confidence to enforce them or not understand the need to do so. They are not used to some of the extreme forms of personality pathology. This is an issue that needs to be highlighted by the trainer. Difficult emotions have to be discussed and named. Only then will they form an understanding of where they arise from and how they might be managed.

There is some vital learning to be gained in a forensic psychiatry placement. The trainee may end up in any of the psychiatric specialties, or indeed none of them. Certain knowledge will be applicable for their further careers: an understanding of acute and chronic risk and how to manage this; experience of extreme psychopathology; knowledge of medicine within the criminal justice system; awareness of the psychiatric factors that lead to criminal activity; how to manage risk arising from mental disorder; safe medication prescribing for complex disorder; an understanding of the individual within a societal context.

An awareness of where to access support is paramount. Most deaneries have mentoring and trainee support programmes. There is the clinical supervisor who should provide support and monitor progress through regular supervision. The educational supervisor and training programme directors are also on hand. The Balint Group is an important resource and should be given the time and due importance it deserves. Peers are, and always have been, the greatest support. My advice to trainees is to talk to the people who are having the same experiences as you. Talk to the people who were there before you and came through the other side.

Forensic psychiatry remains a fascinating subject despite the difficulties that can arise. It teaches you how to work in a team and utilise the expertise of others. It provides an understanding of the broader legal and societal context within which medicine operates. It will begin by challenging your emotions and sensibilities, but in the end will make you a less judgemental and more resilient doctor. Sharing this knowledge and expertise with others is beyond rewarding.

Things I Wish I Knew Before Becoming a Clinical Director in Forensic Psychiatry

Katherine Warburton

Statewide Medical Director, California Department of State Hospitals, Sacramento, USA; Associate Clinical Professor, University of California–Davis, USA.

A decade ago, I was installed as the medical director for the largest forensic in-patient system in the USA. This system cares for 44% of all forensic in-patients in the USA. We treat over 6,000 forensic patients on any given day. Forensic patients in California consist of multiple commitment types, including not guilty by reason of insanity, incompetent to stand trial and offenders with mental disorders. The common theme characterising forensic patients is involvement with the criminal justice system due to a serious mental disorder.

Here are three things I've learned in the last 10 years:

1. There are no easy answers to treatment questions in this population.

    Individuals admitted to forensic psychiatric hospitals are exceedingly complex. We are not treating categorical diagnoses that will respond to routine treatment. We are treating a unique and individualised constellation of conditions including refractory psychotic brain diseases, cognitive disorders, trauma, criminogenic risk, violence, personality disorders, substance abuse and consequences of years of inadequate utilisation of preventative medical and psychiatric treatment due to homelessness and incarceration. As such, there is a very limited evidence base to rely upon when developing and delivering treatment protocols. Standard treatment planning methodologies don't address the complexities and salient treatment objectives for this population. Psychopharmacology algorithms are generally exhausted by the time our patients come to us.

2. We are therefore obliged to find the answers ourselves using clinical research. Because there are no adequate guidelines or evidence base to rely upon, we must do it ourselves.

    a. The ability to conduct real-time, in vivo clinical research to help guide clinical protocols is imperative, as this population is not just poorly understood but also constantly evolving. We have engaged multiple academic partners, most notably the University of California–Davis, Texas Tech, Stanford University and Stephen Stahl MD PhD, to help us implement research protocols designed to better understand our population. As Dr Stahl informed us when we asked him for guidelines to treat aggression and criminalisation, 'Looks like you're going to have to do it yourselves.' Through our research partnerships, we've learned that in our hospitals frequent aggression is largely driven by cognitive disorders. We've learned that criminogenic risk is more predictive of violence than positive psychotic symptoms. We've learned that impulsive violence is far more common than psychotic violence. We've learned that predatory violence most often leads to injury. We've learned that systematic psychopharmacology consultation reduces violence. We've learned that almost half of the patients we admit are in an unsheltered/untreated condition at the time of their arrest and most have had repeated criminal justice contact. We've learned that many people with serious mental illness are being arrested because they are paranoid and disorganised and therefore unable to respond appropriately during criminal justice contacts. Our research has taught us that people with serious mental illness are being criminalised rather than treated. Our research has led us to implement a psychopharmacology consultation programme, dialectical behaviour therapy, cognitive behavioural therapy for psychosis and cognitive rehabilitation, and the development of a novel programme for the treatment of violent behaviour. Our research and academic partnerships have guided our development of guidelines for the treatment of violence and guidelines for diversion away from the criminal justice system. Our research has informed the development of a large-scale diversion programme for individuals arrested on felony charges due to symptoms of psychosis. Our clinical team has produced multiple textbooks on prescribing, treating violence and decriminalising mental illness to share the knowledge we've gained.

    b. Outreach to other systems is the other key to finding answers. Visiting and contacting other forensic hospitals provides dual benefits: enrichment through identification of best practices and a comforting elimination of the clinical isolation forensic providers face when treating this complex population. I've visited forensic hospitals throughout the USA, as well as the UK, Italy, Australia and New Zealand.

Many of our most successful initiatives have been inspired by work in other systems. We have learned that regardless of programme size or location, those of us treating this population are facing the same problems. The well of inspired innovation among us is vast, and the more we connect, the better we will all be.

3. We must be advocates and educators, as well as treatment providers.
   The ability to improve and optimise care requires money. Money comes from political processes. Our institutionalised patients stand in the crosshairs of diametrically opposed political advocacy. On one hand, their care is extremely expensive which rankles conservative thinkers. It is also conducted in institutions that remove civil liberties, which offends those in more liberal camps. Therefore, the political landscape is hostile to our institutions, making policy change and the subsequent funding difficult to achieve. Despite this bipartisan political distaste for psychiatric institutions, the patients keep coming. The number of forensic patients in US forensic hospitals increased 76% from 1999 to 2014. Most states in the USA are currently keeping long waitlists for forensic patients, who languish in jails waiting to come in for treatment. It is incumbent upon us, as clinical leaders, to use our knowledge and research to educate and advocate on behalf of these criminalised patients through funding and policy changes. It is only through data-based advocacy by our field that societies will commit to long-term, sustained and adequate care of people living with serious mental illness. Such change would interrupt the clinical deterioration of patients living with psychotic disorders and obviate the need for large forensic systems.

Kevin Murray

Kevin Murray, Honorary Consultant Forensic Psychiatrist, Broadmoor Hospital, Crowthorne, England, UK; West London NHS Trust, London, England, UK; Member, Parole Board, London, England, UK.

Here are three things I wish I'd known before becoming a clinical director in forensic psychiatry:

1 Real and enduring change in organisations takes time and is a team effort. This isn't a bad thing: it means that you get the benefit of other colleagues' ideas and experience, and proposals often improve in consultation. Also it gives organisations a certain stability, which is important in forensic services.
2 Spotting and nurturing talent is a rare privilege. Thinking back over the many colleagues I've worked with and thought 'they will go far' – seeing their careers take off is enormously satisfying and repays the support I had as a senior trainee sponsored by my then clinical director.
3 Things will go wrong from time to time: and when they do, acknowledge it, learn from it, talk about it and plan to avoid it happening again. And make sure you support those most affected.

Treena Wilkie

Forensic Psychiatrist; Chief, Forensic Service, Complex Care and Recovery Program, Centre for Addiction and Mental Health; and Associate Professor, University of Toronto, Toronto, Canada.

I stepped away from my desk on the first day of my role as chief of forensic services at the Centre for Addiction and Mental Health and returned minutes later to 29 new emails; a signal of the rush of information to come in the days ahead. Budgets, new money coming in, more beds from corrections, unfinished re-appointment letters, discussions with architects for the new forensic building, office allocations, implementation of new assessment tools and meetings needing to be booked with the Ministry of Health. It was a breadth of tasks, and a call for expertise in many areas, that I was not expecting. I had had various administrative roles in the hospital over the years, including, most recently, associate chief of the department. Why was there so much I didn't know? Now, a few months in, the three things I wish someone would have told me: always keep the conversation going, maintain balance between administrative and clinical duties, and behold the power of optimism.

Communication has been the key task. The onslaught of emails requires responses: quick, decisive, expressing gratitude and often an acknowledgement as much as a response. What may seem like brief or minor conversations at the time do matter. Listening is sometimes more meaningful than speaking. Be present and keep your door open, literally. Town halls and wide communication within the division keep momentum and a shared vision alive. Communication outside of the forensic division is equally important to disseminate key messages about our field and to develop a shared language that is often missing. Issues do not resolve themselves, and identifying which issues will require our sustained attention (complexity, burnout, resources, systemic inequality) inevitably starts with a conversation.

Despite holding many administrative positions over the years, I have always kept a busy and full clinical practice – in-patients, out-patients, court work, risk assessments. In my mind, this had always been a benefit to my leadership positions – to have active and ongoing experience with patients, families, staff and the bureaucracy of work. As I moved into my new position and reflected on the 'right' balance of administrative to clinical work, the conclusion was clear. In the end, clinical responsibilities always dictate workplace priorities. If there is a patient emergency, or a patient requires intervention, that is where one's attention is focussed. It was important to balance my schedule in a way that supported my capacity to do so – so that I had the mental and emotional capacity, and the actual time, to respond to the people around me in a way that supported patient care within the division. As a result, I decided to move away from in-patient care for the first time in 15 years. This marked the end of a rewarding part of my career, but was a necessary move towards balance.

The final reflection is that people told me many things before I assumed the role, mainly of the problems, the anticipated challenges, the unyielding deficits. The perspective of being a chief has provided clarity regarding this view, yes, but it has also provided a view of the crucial roles played by the helpers, the motivators, the disrupters who have goals of bringing about needed changes, the innovators, the big thinkers and the perceptive observers. The privilege of working with staff, physicians, patients and families requires an acceptance of where we are at and a positive vision for change. Optimism is infectious and those who carry forward positive momentum will be the stabilising force over years to come.

Krishna Pillai
Clinical Director and Consultant Forensic Psychiatrist, The Mason Clinic, Auckland, New Zealand.

When I become a clinical director in December 2019 I wish I had known we were on the verge of a global pandemic that would change all our lives forever. Previously I was perplexed by the mandatory infection control training. Why did I need to know in what order to don and doff a mask and gloves? Aerosol generating procedures? This is a forensic *psychiatric* hospital, for goodness' sake – I don't need to know that stuff. I don't think anybody really could have known what was to come in 2020.

But I wish I had known that becoming a clinical director meant becoming a stranger in my own hospital. Then I would have been prepared to exit my peer review group and supervision dyads gracefully. My colleagues are still the same knowledgeable experts as they always were and I value their advice, but now they are my biggest critics as well as my biggest supporters and I am responsible for their performance reviews. It is like I have come out of the closet or lost my spouse to cancer. I have become the one that people point out from a distance with respect and admiration and sometimes pity. Becoming a clinical director means having to find a new set of peers.

Before I became a clinical director, I imagined that a clinical director had the executive authority to make things happen. As a clinical director I now know that even a boss has a boss, and if anything I feel more constrained by circumstances, obligations and history than ever before. As when I first became a doctor, and then first became a psychiatric trainee, I wish I had known that becoming a clinical director means that you still can't change anything.

Before I become a clinical director I wish somebody had told me 'this is a marathon, not a sprint'. I was given that advice *after* I had taken the job. As with a marathon, there is no point in using your energy to get out in front as you will be overtaken by the mob after only a few miles. Instead, scope out the field and find a small group of like-minded runners to keep pace with. Stay on the shoulder of someone slightly fitter and smarter who will push you a bit. Be courteous and careful and don't trip anybody else. Stay hydrated. But keep your eye on the clock; the race is finite and when the end comes, you need to be there. And when you receive the criticisms or the acclamations, be calm, keep your eyes up, breathe easily and be gracious.

Index